D1558927

Essential Dental Handbook
Clinical and Practice Management Advice
From the Experts

Essential Dental Handbook
Clinical and Practice Management Advice From the Experts

Robert R. Edwab, B.S., D.D.S., Editor

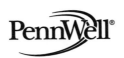

PennWell Corporation

Tulsa, Oklahoma

Copyright © 2003 by
PennWell Corporation
1421 South Sheridan Road
Tulsa, Oklahoma 74112-6600 USA

800.752.9764
+1.918.831.9421
sales@pennwell.com
www.pennwell-store.com
www.pennwell.com

Cover designed by Clark Bell
Book designed by Alana Herron

Library of Congress Cataloging-in-Publication Data
Essential dental handbook : clinical and practice management advice from the experts /
Robert R. Edwab, B.S., D.D.S., editor.
   p. ; cm.
  Includes index.
  ISBN 0-87814-624-5
   1. Dentistry--Handbooks, manuals, etc. 2. Dental care--Handbooks, manuals, etc.
I. Edwab, Robert R., B.S., D.D.S.
  [DNLM: 1. Dental Care--organization & administration. WU 29 E78 2002]
RK56 .E876 2002
617.6--dc21

2002029800

Printed in the United States of America.

1   2   3   4   5   07   06   05   04   03

Contents

Acknowledgements ~~~~~~vii

List of Contributors ~~~~~~~~~~~~~~~~~~~~~~~~~~~~~~~~~~~~~~~viii

List of Figures ~~~~~~xii

List of Tables ~~~~~~xlvi

CHAPTER 1 **Health Status of the Dental Patient** ~~~~~~~~~~~~~~~~1
Robert R. Edwab, B.S., D.D.S.

CHAPTER 2 **Making Dentistry Productive** ~~~~~~~~~~~~~~~~~~~~15
Joseph A. Blaes, D.D.S.

CHAPTER 3 **Children, Parents, Dentists: Dilemmas and Solutions** ~~~~39
Marvin H. Berman, D.D.S.

CHAPTER 4 **Esthetic Posterior Restorations:
A Problem-Solving Guide** ~~~~~~~~~~~~~~~~~~~~~~~105
George Freedman, D.D.S.

CHAPTER 5 **Endodontics** ~~~~~~~~~~~~~~~~~~~~~~~~~~~~~~~~~129
Joe H. Camp, D.D.S., M.S.D.

CHAPTER 6 **Medical Emergencies** ~~~~~~~~~~~~~~~~~~~~~~~~~161
Alan J. Drinnan, M.B, Ch.B., D.D.S.

CHAPTER 7 **Communicating Financially with Your Patients** ~~~~~~~189
Jennifer de St. Georges

CHAPTER 8 **Informed Consent: An Overview** ~~~~~~~~~~~~~~~~~223
Debra S. Reiser, ESQ.

CHAPTER 9 **Temporomandibular Disorders** ~~~~~~~~~~~~~~~~~~251
Henry A. Gremillion, D.D.S., M.A.G.D.

CHAPTER 10 **Oral Surgery** ~~~~~~~~~~~~~~~~~~~~~~~~~~~~~~~~311
Myer Leonard, D.D.S., M.D.

CHAPTER 11 **Crown and Bridge** ~~~~~~~~~~~~~~~~~~~~~~~~~341
Larry Lopez, D.D.S.

CHAPTER 12 **The Impact of Digital Imaging Technology
on the Dental Practice** ~~~~~~~~~~~~~~~~~~~~~~369
Dale A. Miles, B.A., D.D.S., F.R.C.D.

CHAPTER 13 **Orthodontics in the Progressive Dental Practice** ~~~~~~~~387
Elliott M. Moskowitz, D.D.S., M. Sd.

CHAPTER 14 **Removable Prosthodontics** ~~~~~~~~~~~~~~~~~~~~~~~~431
M. Nader Sharifi, D.D.S., M.S.

CHAPTER 15 **Oral Mucosal Disorders Commonly Encountered
in the Practice of Oral Medicine** ~~~~~~~~~~~~~~~~~483
Michael A. Siegel, D.D.S., M.S.

CHAPTER 16 **Periodontics** ~~~~~~~~~~~~~~~~~~~~~~~~~~~~~~~517
Michael Sonick, D.M.D.

Index ~~~~~~715

Acknowledgements

Editing this book was an act of love for a great profession. Dentistry is an important contributing factor to the total health of an individual. As practitioners, we strive for excellence so our patients will be the beneficiaries.

The contributors to this book are all renowned practitioners and educators in the field of dentistry. The information they offer is invaluable. Their dedication to further dental education is what makes them outstanding. My sincere gratitude to them for helping me accomplish this endeavor.

This book is about dentistry. But it would have been impossible without the support of my family—my wife Sherry, my daughter Stacey, and my son Justin. The advice, encouragement, guidance, and patience they offered this past year were extraordinary. I love you all.

Contributors

Chapter 1

Robert R. Edwab, B.S., D.D.S., Brooklyn, New York, is a Diplomate of the American Board of Oral and Maxillofacial Surgeons. He maintains a full time private practice, which ultimately means he performs the same procedures that you do each day. Dr. Edwab has published articles in many of the popular journals and has lectured nationally and internationally at most of the major dental meetings on office oral surgery for the general practitioner. He is appreciated for his knowledge, confidence, and humor as well as his ability to make office oral surgery easy and enjoyable. He is a Fellow of both the American College of Dentists and the International College of Dentists.

Chapter 2

Joseph A. Blaes, D.D.S., Chesterfield, Missouri, has created a unique, innovative, insurance-free, fee-for-service general practice that emphasizes preventive, esthetic, reconstructive, and implant dentistry. Dr. Blaes began writing "Pearls for Your Practice" in *Dental Economics*, and after becoming a trusted resource for new dental material and techniques, he was named editor of *Dental Economics* in 1996. Dr. Blaes is a Fellow of the American College of Dentists, and he currently serves on the Board of the American Academy of Dental Practice Administration.

Chapter 3

Marvin H. Berman, D.D.S., Chicago, Illinois, is a pediatric dentist with over four decades of experience caring for children in a large group practice in Chicago. An Associate Professor at the University of Illinois Dental school, he has lectured world-wide at every major dental meeting in rooms filled to capacity with enthusiastic followers. Thousands of dentists have reaped the benefits of his no-nonsense, drug-free approach to transforming the most reluctant children into happy patients.

Chapter 4

George Freedman, D.D.S., Markham, Ontario, Canada, is a past President of the American Academy of Cosmetic Dentistry and currently is Associate Director of the Esthetic Dental Education Center and scientific chairman of the World Aesthetic Congress (London, UK). A

Diplomate of the American Board of Aesthetic Dentistry, he lectures internationally on dental esthetics, dental technology, and photography. Dr. Freedman maintains a private practice limited to esthetic dentistry in Toronto, Canada.

Chapter 5

Joe H. Camp, D.D.S., M.S.D., private practice of endodontics, Charlotte, North Carolina, attended dental school at University of North Carolina School of Dentistry. He completed graduate training in pediatric dentistry at Indiana University and endodontic training at University of North Carolina. He is an Adjunct Associate Professor at the University of North Carolina School of Dentistry.

Chapter 6

Alan J. Drinnan, M.B., Ch. B., D.D.S., Williamsville, New York, is a Distinguished Service Professor at the State University of New York at Buffalo. He is a graduate in Dentistry (1954) and Medicine (1962) from the University of Bristol (England) and received his D.D.S. from the State University of New York at Buffalo in 1964. He has spent his professional life as a member of the faculty at Buffalo and has a special interest in the medical aspects of dental practice.

Chapter 7

Jennifer de St. Georges, Monte Sereno, California, has been a dental practice educator since 1974. She has spoken at virtually every major meeting in the United States, Canada ,and the United Kingdom, as well as a growing number of leading international conferences. Jenny's common sense and logical approach to management, integrated with her strong emphasis on patient communication, has won her a loyal following in the profession.

Chapter 8

Debra S. Reiser, Esq., New York, New York, admitted to practice in the States of New York and Massachusetts for over 20 years, is a trial attorney concentrating in the areas of medical and dental malpractice. She attended the University of Rochester and received her J.D. from Boston College Law School in 1981. Currently in her own firm in midtown Manhattan, she has previously represented dental malpractice carriers and has litigated numerous dental malpractice cases, on behalf of both patients and dentists.

Chapter 9

Henry A. Gremillion, D.D.S., M.A.G.D., Gainesville, Florida, is a 1977 graduate of Louisiana State University School of Dentistry. He is an Associate Professor in the Department of Orthodontics and holds an affiliate appointment in the Department of Prosthodontics at the University of Florida College of Dentistry. He is Director of the Parker E. Mahan Facial Pain Center, directs a fellowship program in oral facial pain, and is an associate faculty member of the L.D. Pankey Institute for Advanced Dental Education.

Chapter 10

Myer Leonard, D.D.S., M.D., Golden Valley, Minnesota, is Professor Emeritus of Oral and Maxillofacial Surgery at the University of Minnesota. From 1976 to 2001, he was Head of Oral and Maxillofacial Surgery at Hennepin County Medical Center, in addition to being Professor in the Department of Oral and Maxillofacial Surgery. A videotape of the material in this chapter can be obtained from the American Dental Association.

Chapter 11

Larry Lopez, D.D.S., San Antonio, Texas, received his D.D.S. from the University of Texas Health Science Center in Houston and has been in private practice since graduating in 1978. He lectures extensively on crown and bridge dentistry and consults with several companies on new material development.

Chapter 12

Dale A. Miles, B.A., D.D.S., F.R.C.D., Lexington, Kentucky, is a Professor of Oral and Maxillofacial Radiology at the University of Kentucky College of Dentistry in Lexington, Kentucky. He is a Diplomate of both the American Board of Oral and Maxillofacial Radiology and the American Board of Oral Medicine. He also serves as consulting Associate Dean of Clinical Affairs and Faculty Development for the Arizona School of Dentistry & Oral Health. Dr. Miles has a web site for teaching dentists and auxiliaries about digital imaging at www.learndigital.net.

Chapter 13

Elliott M. Moskowitz, D.D.S., M. Sd., New York, New York, is an Associate Clinical Professor in the Department of Orthodontics, at New York University College of Dentistry and Director Emeritus of the Department of Orthodontics and Dentofacial Orthopedics at the Interfaith Medical Center in New York City. He has been in active clinical practice for 30 years and has taught orthodontics on both the predoctoral and postgraduate levels.

Chapter 14

M. Nader Sharifi, D.D.S., M.S., Chicago, Illinois, received his dental education at the University of Illinois and holds a certificate in prosthodontics and Masters Degree in Biomaterials from Northwestern University. A former clinical instructor at Northwestern University, Dr. Sharifi maintains a full time practice of adult general dentistry in downtown Chicago. He has received acclaim for his lectures, nationally and internationally, on the topic of prosthetic dentistry.

Chapter 15

Michael A. Siegel, D.D.S., M.S., Baltimore, Maryland, is an Associate Professor in the Department of Oral Medicine and Diagnostic Sciences at the University of Maryland Dental School. He is an Associate Professor in the Department of Dermatology at the University of Maryland Medical School as well as an Associate Member of the Graduate Faculty at the University of Maryland at Baltimore. Dr. Siegel is a Fellow of both the Academy of General Dentistry and the American College of Dentists, a Diplomate of the American Board of Oral Pathology, and holds a Masters Degree in Oral Pathology.

Chapter 16

Michael Sonick, D.M.D., Fairfield, Connecticut, is a Clinical Assistant Professor of Surgery at Yale School of Medicine, Guest Lecturer, International Program at New York University School of Dentistry, and a member of the editorial board of *Contemporary Esthetics and Restorative Practice*. He is a Diplomate of the American Board of Periodontolgy and currently maintains a private practice devoted to periodontics and the surgical placement of dental implants. He is a frequent lecturer throughout the United States and abroad.

Figures

1-1   Health history questionnaire ~~~~~~~~~~~~~~~~~~~~~~~~~~~~4

1-2   Sample of patient's chart cover ~~~~~~~~~~~~~~~~~~~~~~~~~~13

3-1   Toddler sucking on baby bottle with juice that
        she carries around throughout the day ~~~~~~~~~~~~~~~~~55

3-2   Typical nursing bottle caries pattern in a three-year-old child ~~~~~55

3-3   Rampant neglected carries due to excessive between meal snacking ~~~~56

3-4   Infant food tasting test ~~~~~~~~~~~~~~~~~~~~~~~~~~~~~57

3-5   Recommended tooth brushing position for maximum control and fun ~~~61

3-6   An example of a simple medical history form ~~~~~~~~~~~~~~~~~65

3-7   Chairside communication with mother and children ~~~~~~~~~~~~~~66

3-8   Dental assistant preparing parent for temporary separation from child ~~~~67

3-9   Dental assistant greeting mother and child and explaining the system ~~~69

3-10   Doctor meeting with mother and child in response to her
        refusal to allow her child to enter operatory on her own ~~~~~~~~~~~69

3-11   Baby comfortably nestled in dental assistant embrace ~~~~~~~~~~~~~74

3-12   Dental assistant exhibiting the chairside manner
        essential for establishing rapport with patients ~~~~~~~~~~~~~~~75

3-13a   The art of show-tell-do, acclimating the child to
        the feel of the prophy cup on the fingers first ~~~~~~~~~~~~~~~78

3-13b   Repeating the introduction on the teeth ~~~~~~~~~~~~~~~~~~78

3-14   The "battle station position" with patient more upright, eyes
        open, hands across stomach. Dental assistant right arm resting
        on patient's shoulder next to head. Her left hand resting lightly
        over the patient's hands. Dentist and patient eye to eye. Good
        finger rests. Note the working triangle formed by the dental
        assistant, the dentist, and the patient ~~~~~~~~~~~~~~~~~~~83

3-15   Applying topical anesthetic to injection site ~~~~~~~~~~~~~~~~85

3-16   Administering local anesthesia (infiltration). Note patient's
        eyes open, teeth biting together, soft tissues relaxed ~~~~~~~~~~~85

3-17   Post-operative extraction instructions should be specific and geared
        to your particular practice. Details should be repeated verbally ~~~~86

3-18	Children choosing prizes after dental treatment	89
3-19	Anterior open bite and constricted arches, caused by ongoing thumbsucking and potentiated by the subsequent thrusting of the tongue into the already open space	91
3-20	Toddler enjoying her pacifier and her fragment of blanket	91
3-21	Two year old sucking thumb	91
3-22	Thumbsucking crib in place. Note curved wires that serve as a distraction and not a punishment	92
3-23a	Young boy with cane making his way down the hall accompanied by a dental assistant	94
3-23b	Dental assistant working with special child in his wheel chair	94
3-24	Consultation and case presentation in private office with parent and child. Note up-close and personal approach	97
3-25	Front desk personnel pleasantly attending to business details	97
3-26	Reaping the rewards that are derived from working with children	99
4-1	Composite restoration with inset of previous amalgam filling	105
4-2	The Wand, Milestone Scientific	107
4-3	Fissurotomy bur	107
4-4	Microleakage under an amalgam	111
4-5	Advances in bonding through the generations	113
4-6	Table of adhesive solvents	115
4-7	Conservative cavity preparation	119
4-8	Creating the rounded internal anatomy	119
4-9	Keeping the isthmus narrow	120
4-10a	Matrix in intimate contact with margin (flexiwedge)	121
4-10b	Wooden wedges leave marginal space	121
4-11	Anatomically contoured wedge compared to wooden wedge	121
4-12	Preparation glossy with water after rinse	122
4-13	Preparation glossy with adhesive	122
4-14	Preparation glossy with light-cured adhesive	122
4-15	CCI instrument making tactile interproximal contact	123
4-16	Partial light cure with CCI in composite	123

4-17	Progression of instruments	124
4-18	Duckhead and its adaptation to the occlusal surface	124
4-19	Polishing with paste	126
4-20	Finished restoration	126
5-1 a-b	Referred pain to opposing arch	131
5-2 a-b	Sinus tract traced with gutta-percha point	132
5-3 a-b	Potential misdiagnosis from anatomic structures and patient information	135
5-4 a-c	Deceptive radiographic appearance	135
5-5 a-c	Carbon dioxide ice pencil for vitality testing	137
5-6 a-b	Temporary stopping placed on plastic instrument for heat testing	139
5-7	Infra-orbital injection	141
5-8 a-b	Retreatment of failing root canal	145
5-9 a-c	Coronal calcification of root canal	146
5-10	Torque-controlled electric engine and handpiece	147
5-11 a-d	Severely curved canals	150
5-12 a-c	Lateral condensation filling of rotary nickel-titanium preparations	156
5-13 a-e	Condensation with System B Obturator (analytic technology) of canals prepared with rotary nickel-titanium files	158
5-14 a-b	Bonded restoration sealing coronal orifices	159
7-1	Financial in-office worksheet	207
9-1	Visual analog scale (VAS)	254
9-2	Patient diagrams for self-reporting their pain	254
9-3	Factors that may compromise the adaptive capacity of the masticatory system leading to the development and/or maintenance of temporomandibular disorder	259
9-4	Biomechanics of the temporomandibular joint	268
9-5 a-b	Anteriorly displaced articular disc	273
9-6	Defect in form	275
9-7	Condylar subluxation/dislocation	276
9-8 a-c	Biomechanics of the temporomandibular joint	278
9-9	Mandibular stabilization splint adjusted to suggested criteria	295

11-1   Severe wear resulting from oppositional porcelain restorations   346

11-2   The Alamo crown   346

11-3   Pre-op view   347

11-4   Post-op view of Alamo Crown   347

11-5   Lateral view of tooth to be prepared   347

11-6/11-9 Equal stripping of tooth structure for correct form and material strength   349

11-10   Reduction gauge used to measure occlusal clearance   351

11-11   Diamond bur following gingival margin   351

11-12   Crown with esthetic supragingival margins   351

11-13   Trimmed bite relationship   354

11-14   Artex articulator system   354

11-15   Diagnostic wax-up for lab communication   354

11-16   Photos used for lab communication   356

11-17   Definitive restoration from Figure 11-16   356

11-18   Photo with shade tab in place   356

11-19   Pre-op of broken incisor   357

11-20   Shade map sent to lab   357

11-21   Definitive restoration   357

11-22   Mosaic shade guide for molar shades   359

11-23   Molar restored using mosaic shade guide   359

11-24   Creating the post space length   359

11-25   Creating the post space width   359

11-26   Cleaning and shaping the apical third   359

11-27   The root after preparation   360

11-28   Applying bonding agent   360

11-29   Filling the root with resin sealer   360

11-30   The Fibrefill Obturator/post fully seated   360

11-31   Obturator, post, and core in monobloc   360

11-32   Pre-op PVS impression for a temporary stent   362

11-33   Lab-fabricated temporary restoration   362

11-34   Veneer preparation 363

11-35   Thermal vacuum stent 363

11-36   Application of neck stains 363

11-37   Application of incisal stains 363

11-38   Temporary veneers 364

12-1a,b CEREC 2 CAD-CAM system 371

12-2   PDA screen images 373

12-3a-c Typical digital images 374

12-4   A schematic diagram of the solid-state image capture device 375

12-5   A cross section through several pixels 376

12-6   Diagram of a CMOS-type detector showing amplification
         of the electronic signal at each of three pixels and the
         individualized "read-out" of the charge 377

12-7a   The Gendex DenOptix PSP system 379

12-7b   The Soredex Digora PSP system 379

12-8   Image processing applied to caries detection 381

12-9   "Equalization" procedures applied to a bitewing image 382

12-10a   Various image procedures applied to a maxillary cuspid view 383

12-10b   Digital images taken with two different x-ray machines 384

13-1   Conventional Hawley retainer 389

13-2   A more esthetic removable retainer with a clear
         plastic strip replacing a more visible labial bow 389

13-3   Basic canine to canine Spring Aligner 390

13-4   Additional clasping can be added to the Spring
         Aligner for greater retention 390

13-5   The addition of a posteriorly extended acrylic section adds Spring
         Aligner capabilities to a conventional removable appliance 390

13-6   Severe malocclusion with a significant arch length insufficiency
         resulting in gross crowding and other inter-arch disharmonies 391

13-7   Comprehensive orthodontic treatment with fixed multibonded
         orthodontic appliances. Extractions of first premolars were
         required as part of the overall treatment effort 391

13-8   Inter and intra dental arch disharmonies corrected as a
        result of comprehensive orthodontic treatment ⸺ 391

13-9   An example of localized and relatively mild mandibular incisor
        malpositions. The degree of crowding is less than 3 mm ⸺ 391

13-10   Measuring the available space using brass separating wire
        along the mean arc of the incisal edges ⸺ 392

13-11   Measuring the required space by totaling the mesio-distal
        widths of the mandibular incisors ⸺ 392

13-12   An accurate stone cast from an alginate impression is made ⸺ 394

13-13   A laboratory prescription detailing the type of Spring Aligner,
        the teeth to be reset, and stripping instructions is filled out ⸺ 394

13-14   The mandibular central and lateral incisors
        are removed from the cast with saw cuts ⸺ 396

13-15   The teeth are appropriately reduced in size (simulating
        the stripping that will be performed clinically) and reset ⸺ 396

13-16   The teeth have now been reset to simulate the final desired clinical result ⸺ 396

13-17   A spring wire framework (either .028 or .030 inch diameter
        stainless steel wire) is constructed on the completed set-up cast ⸺ 396

13-18   The acrylic framework portion is fabricated on the
        labial and lingual aspects of the wire framework ⸺ 396

13-19   The cured framework ready to be separated from the cast ⸺ 396

13-20   The completed acrylic framework is trimmed and polished ⸺ 397

13-21   The finished Spring Aligner is placed on the
        cast and is ready to be delivered to the patient ⸺ 397

13-22   At observation visits, the Spring Aligner is adjusted
        with a Howe Plier by gently squeezing the clasps ⸺ 397

13-23   Pre-treatment frontal intraoral view ⸺ 397

13-24   Pre-treatment occlusal view showing the malalignment
        of the mandibular incisors ⸺ 397

13-25   The Spring Aligner in place ⸺ 398

13-26   Additional rotation is needed to correct the mandibular right central incisor ⸺ 398

13-27   After a new in-treatment cast was made and "dimples" were
        placed in the area of needed rotation, the "extra" acrylic in
        this area serves to "supercharge" the rotational movement ⸺ 398

13-28   Pre-treatment occlusal view of patient F.G. 398

13-29   Post-treatment occlusal view of patient F.G. after 10 months of treatment 398

13-30   Frontal intra-oral view of a patient with a severely
         rotated maxillary right central incisor 398

13-31   Occlusal view of the rotated maxillary right central incisor 400

13-32   The Spring Aligner in place 400

13-33   The rotation corrected 400

13-34   A bonded lingual wire was placed to prevent
         relapse of the maxillary right central incisor 400

13-35   Delayed exfoliation of a primary maxillary incisor can cause the
         erupting permanent tooth to assume a lingual crossbite position 400

13-36   Early adverse gingival response of the mandibular
         incisor in a patient with an anterior crossbite 400

13-37   An anterior crossbite of the maxillary right
         central incisor in the mixed dentition 402

13-38   A conventional removable appliance used to correct the crossbite 402

13-39   Auxiliary spring lingual to the maxillary right central
         incisor applies force in a labial direction 402

13-40   The crossbite of the maxillary right central incisor successfully corrected ... 402

13-41   Maxillary removable appliance with occlusal
         coverage used to remove occlusal interferences 402

13-42   The resultant effect of the occlusal coverage in providing
         the necessary "clearance" to resolve the anterior crossbite 402

13-43 a-c Adult patient with a maxillary right lateral incisor in crossbite 403

13-44 a-c A maxillary removable appliance has been constructed with auxiliary
         springs and occlusal acrylic to remove mechanical interferences 403

13-45 a-b The maxillary right lateral incisor crossbite corrected 403

13-46   Dental crossbite - definite occlusal stops and normal bucco-lingual
         inclinations of the opposing molars on the right side. The dental
         midlines coincide, and the left side displays a lingually positioned
         maxillary molar a buccally inclined mandibular molar 405

13-47   "Cross " elastics used to correct dental crossbites 405

13-48   Dental crossbites include buccal crossbites 405

13-49   Functional crossbite—the maxillary and
mandibular dental midlines do not coincide 405

13-50   When the mandible is positioned to its normal transverse
rest position (midlines coinciding), it becomes apparent
that bilateral expansion is required 405

13-51a-c Functional crossbite in the mixed dentition. Note the dental
midline shift towards the side that displays a crossbite relationship
reflecting the mandibular displacement upon closure 406

13-52   A removable expansion device with occlusal acrylic and expansion screw 406

13-53a   Pre-treatment frontal intraoral view illustrating
the initial dental midline relationship 406

13-53b   Post-treatment frontal intraoral view with the midlines coinciding, functional crossbite corrected, and normal transverse mandibular position 406

13-54   Skeletal crossbite with normal bucco-lingual
positions of the maxillary and mandible molars 408

13-55   Clinical photograph of a skeletal crossbite requiring comprehensive orthodontic treatment and orthognathic surgery 408

13-56   Anterior-posterior cephalometric radiograph depicting
the extent of the skeletal transverse disharmony 408

13-57   Maxillary "canine-to-canine" ESSIX retainer 408

13-58   Full arch ESSIX retainer covering all the teeth in the maxillary dental arch 408

13-59   An accurate working cast is fabricated in a "crown and bridge" quality stone 409

13-60   The clear plastic ESSIX retainer is constructed on the working cast 410

13-61   The canine to canine ESSIX mandibular retainer is virtually invisible 410

13-62   Patient requiring implants in need of a transitional
esthetic appliance before the implants are placed 410

13-63   A traditional Hawley type of removable appliance
with pontics replacing the maxillary lateral incisors 411

13-64   Thermoforming process of an ESSIX retainer
with a pontic secured to the working cast 411

13-65   The completed canine to canine ESSIX retainer with pontics in place 411

13-66   Undercut "trenches" have been created on the lingual surfaces of the maxillary lateral incisor pontics to aid retention of the thermoplastic material 411

13-67   The esthetic modified ESSIX retainer serves as an excellent
         transitional appliance until implants and subsequent implant
         supported restorations can be fabricated ～～～～～～～～411

13-68   Full arch Invisalign appliances ～～～～～～～～～～～～～413

13-69   Invisalign appliances on a typodont display their near invisibility quality ～～413

13-70   Adult patient exhibited a significant degree of mandibular incisor crowding ～～414

13-71   The mandibular Invisalign appliance is virtually invisible when worn ～～～414

13-72   Two month progress ～～～～～～～～～～～～～～～～～～415

13-73   Four month progress ～～～～～～～～～～～～～～～～～～415

13-74   Six month progress～～～～～～～～～～～～～～～～～～～415

13-75   The case nearing completion ～～～～～～～～～～～～～～416

13-76   Intraoral center view of the overall occlusion after
         approximately 8 months of orthodontic treatment ～～～～～～416

13-77   A special plier is used to place the elastomeric separator.
         The separator is situated interproximally ～～～～～～～～418

13-78   Dental floss can be used to carry the separator to place in tight
         contacts. The floss is worked from the gingival to occlusal ～～～418

13-79   The elastomeric separator in place ～～～～～～～～～～～418

13-80   A piece of brass separating wire is flattened at one end using a plier ～～418

13-81   The flattened end of the separator is shown ～～～～～～～418

13-82   The flattened end is curved prior to intraoral insertion～～～～～418

13-83   The separating wire is placed between the embrassures.
         The wire is brought to the lingual surface and extended ～～～～420

13-84   Using a Howe plier or hemostat, the wire is twisted upon itself ～～～420

13-85   The wire is then cut with a ligature cutter ～～～～～～～～420

13-86   The excess wire is then pushed interproximally
         so as not to irritate the soft tissues ～～～～～～～～～～420

13-87   Typical band case with numbered sizes of bands. The
         instruments needed from left to right are a band pusher,
         band seating bite stick, and band removing plier ～～～～～～420

13-88   Bands may be "prefitted" on a study cast
         before actually placing them intraorally ～～～～～～～～420

13-89 a-e The fitting, contouring, and cementation steps
in the placement of a mandibular molar band ⸺ 420

13-90 Orthodontic attachments that have been directly bonded
to the facial surfaces of the maxillary mandibular teeth ⸺ 423

13-91 Orthodontic brackets have been directly bonded to an
accurate cast with an intervening bonding material ⸺ 423

13-92 The brackets have been encased in an appropriate template
and transferred to the mouth after preparing the facial surfaces
(similar to the direct technique) ⸺ 423

13-93 Elastomeric modules securing the wire to the orthodontic attachment ⸺ 424

13-94 Elastomeric modules securing the wire to the orthodontic attachment ⸺ 424

13-95 Stainless steel ligature securing the arch wire to the bracket ⸺ 424

13-96 The use of the *In-ovation* bracket (GAC, Corporation) offers a
new dimension in bracket/archwire relationship, which significantly
reduces friction between the arch wire and bracket ⸺ 424

13-97 Multiple missing teeth and resultant tipping
of teeth adjacent to the missing teeth ⸺ 424

13-98 An occlusal view further illustrating a prosthetic dilemma
with respect to the present difficulty in tooth replacement ⸺ 424

13-99 An open coil spring that has been compressed
supplies reciprocal force to reposition the teeth ⸺ 424

13-100 Significant tooth movement has occurred using
the reciprocal force of the open coil spring ⸺ 424

13-101 An occlusal view of the completed tooth movement
and resulting simplified prosthetic clinical situation ⸺ 424

13-102 Pretreatment maxillary midline diastema ⸺ 427

13-103 A sectional appliance with a clear elastomeric thread supplies the force to move
the maxillary incisors along a "track" to effect the desired tooth movement ⸺ 427

13-104 Post-treatment result of the maxillary midline diastema closure ⸺ 427

13-105 The maxillary right second premolar has been fractured below
the alveolar crest, making a predictable restoration difficult ⸺ 427

13-106 A sectional appliance is used with a "box loop" to
forcibly erupt the maxillary right second premolar ⸺ 427

13-107   The maxillary right second premolar and surrounding
          alveolar bone have been repositioned to facilitate the
          fabrication of a full crown on sound tooth structure ⸺⸺427

13-108   The uprighting of tipped posterior teeth to facilitate either
          an implant supported restoration or conventional fixed bridge ⸺⸺427

14-1   An edentulous maxilla with characteristics that will provide
          excellent stability for a complete denture. The ridges are
          high and well rounded, the arch form is U-shaped, there
          are large tuberocities, and the hard palate is of medium depth ⸺⸺434

14-2   An edentulous mandible with characteristics that do not provide
          good stability for a complete denture. The ridges are resorbed to
          basal bone, the arch form is O-shaped, the buccal shelves are
          small, and there does not appear to be a deep lateral throat form ⸺⸺435

14-3   With edentulous areas in the anterior and posterior, the
          path of insertion is best selected from the posterior teeth ⸺⸺439

14-4   The narrow cervical area in the neck of the artificial tooth #7 is due to passing
          through the interproximal contacts to seat with the posterior path of insertion.
          The esthetics are improved here with the use of a subgingival pontic ⸺⸺440

14-5   All occlusal rests should create acute angles ⸺⸺441

14-6   Fracture risk areas are identified. The rest should
          be rounded to all minor connectors and clasp arms ⸺⸺442

14-7   Examples of supra-bulge and infra-bulge clasps ⸺⸺445

14-8   A bilateral distal extension partial denture designed with a
          supra-bulge clasp system and an infra-bulge clasp system ⸺⸺446

14-9   With the tip of the I-Bar distal to the rest seat (B), the clasp arm
          (C) moves downward with the saddle (A) every time a load is applied ⸺⸺448

14-10   An irreversible hydrocolloid impression made by syringing
          blue material into the vestibules and pressing it into the
          occlusal form, then using a green material in the tray ⸺⸺452

14-11   Final impression for complete upper and lower dentures
          made with polysulfide rubber base ⸺⸺453

14-12   Medium-body VPS impression made for an upper complete denture ⸺⸺455

14-13   Four maxillary and five mandibular areas to be border molded ⸺⸺457

14-14   Border molding completed with fast-setting VPS bite registration material ⸺⸺460

14-15   An Alma gauge used to create the starting
         point for size and shape of a wax rim ⸻ 461

14-16   A Fox Plane from Trubyte for creating a
         horizontal plane with an upper wax rim ⸻ 463

14-17   When the lower wax record creates the closest speaking space,
         the incisors are creating the VDO and some of the freeway space ⸻ 464

14-18   A complete denture patient demonstrating the closest speaking space ⸻ 464

14-19   An open bite registration of centric relation obtained with the Coble
         Balancer intra-oral tracing device for a completely edentulous patient ⸻ 466

14-20   Records to be returned to the laboratory for an esthetic wax trial ⸻ 467

14-21   An articulator with a complete denture set up for a wax
         trial. The denture teeth are set in a Class I relationship ⸻ 470

14-22   A set of processed upper and lower dentures
         with undercut areas on the flanges ⸻ 472

14-23   Occlusal indicator wax being used on a denture
         to mark centric occlusion prematurities ⸻ 473

14-24   Pressure-indicating paste brushed onto a complete
         upper denture to identify sore areas ⸻ 476

14-25   The evaluation of the patient's previous and new prosthesis. Areas are
         scrutinized with the patient to educate him/her regarding the benefits
         of a well-extended denture base with ideal occlusal contacts ⸻ 478

15-1   Primary herpetic gingivostomatitis in a 67-year-old grandfather who was
         exposed to HSV by his grandchildren. Note the bleeding and erosion of
         the gingival tissues as well as the involvement of the buccal mucosal ⸻ 485

15-2a   Recurrent herpes labialis: early vesicle ⸻ 488

15-2b   Recurrent herpes labialis: crusted lesions ⸻ 488

15-3   Vesicles on the tip of the nose caused by shedding of recurrent
         HSV along the second division of the trigeminal nerve ⸻ 488

15-4   Localized erosions of the keratinized palatal soft tissues resulting
         from ruptured vesicles of recurrent intraoral herpes following
         extraction of a maxillary premolar tooth ⸻ 490

15-5a   Minor recurrent aphthous ulcerations of the lower lip in a 47-year-old male ⸻ 492

15-5b   Close-up of a single minor recurrent aphthous
         ulceration of the upper lip in the same patient ⸻ 492

15-6a   Major aphthous ulceration of the soft palate in a 66-year-old
male caused by a non-steroidal anti-inflammatory drug ~~~~~~~~~~~~492

15-6b   Major aphthous ulceration of the lower lip in a 27-year-old
male. Note the size and depth of the lesion~~~~~~~~~~~~~~~~~492

15-7a   Asymptomatic reticular lichen planus in a 62-year-old male.
Striae of Wickham of the right buccal mucosa ~~~~~~~~~~~~~~~~~497

15-7b   Asymptomatic reticular lichen planus in a 62-year-old male.
Resolution of the striae following two weeks of topical
steroid therapy employing 0.05% fluocinonide gel ~~~~~~~~~~~~~497

15-8a   Symptomatic reticular lichen planus on the left
lateral tongue border in a 49-year-old male ~~~~~~~~~~~~~~~~~497

15-8b   Low power photomicrograph of saw-tooth rete ridges, and an intense
lymphocytic inflammatory infitrate at the upper level of the connective
tissue in close association with the overlying epithelium ~~~~~~~~~~~497

15-8c   Resolution of the lichen planus following topical steroid therapy ~~~~~~~497

15-9   Atrophic gingival lichen planus in a 40-year-old female
with biopsy-proven cutaneous lichen planus. Note the
intense erythema in the presence of good plaque control ~~~~~~~~~~~499

15-10a   Pseudomembranous candidosis on the tongue
dorsum in a 79-year-old female ~~~~~~~~~~~~~~~~~~~~~~~~502

15-10b   Cytologic preparation of tongue dorsum showing
pseudohyphae of candida albicans ~~~~~~~~~~~~~~~~~~~~~~502

15-10c   Appearance of the tongue following two weeks
of therapy with clotrimazole troches ~~~~~~~~~~~~~~~~~~~~502

15-11a   Erythematous candidosis of the palate in a 44-year-old female under
an ill-fitting maxillary complete denture. Note the pseudomembranous
candidosis along the posterior border of the hard palate ~~~~~~~~~~~503

15-11b   Appearance of the palate following temporary reline of the
denture and two weeks of therapy with nystatin ointment ~~~~~~~~~~503

15-12a   Severe bilateral angular cheilosis in a 71-year-old female patient ~~~~~~505

15-12b   Close-up of the right commissure prior to therapy ~~~~~~~~~~~~~~505

15-12c-d Resolution of the labial commissures following 4 weeks of therapy
using nystatin with triamcinalone acetonide ointment ~~~~~~~~~~~~505

16-1   This patient had resective periodontal surgery 30 years ago. He was
        treated with a full thickness apically repositioned flap. Note the loss
        of interdental papillae. Periodontal pockets have been eliminated,
        however the patient is esthetically compromised ----------------------518

16-2   Teeth and gingiva of a periodontally healthy individual. Gingival color
        is uniform and pale pink. Variation occurs due to differences in
        keratinazation, pigmentation, thickness, and vascularity. The gingival
        margin thins as it moves coronally, and the marginal gingiva is
        scalloped. The embrasure spaces are filled with interdental gingiva ------520

16-3a   Edematous inflamed tissue detaches from the tooth when blown with air
        from a syringe. Sub-gingival calculus is evident in the periodontal pocket ----521

16-3b   Gingival health was attained after patient in Figure 16-3a was treated
        with oral hygiene instructions and scaling and root planning. Tissue is
        firm, pink, fibrotic, and no longer is detachable. Pocket depth is 1 mm ------521

16-4a   Diagram of the biologic width (connective tissue attachment and junctional
        epithelium) with the gingival sulcus. Kois has described the complex
        of biologic width and gingival sulcus as the dentogingival complex ------523

16-4b   Sounding the bone is a technique to determine the position of the
        alveolar bone in relation to the free gingival margin. Under local
        anesthesia, a periodontal probe is placed into the sulcus and pushed
        apically until contact with the bone is made. Thus, the clinician can
        determine the amount of space that exists apical to the potential
        restoration margin so that the biologic width is not invaded -------------523

16-5a   Inflammation around crown with a violated biologic width. The inflamed
        cyanotic reddish margin will remain until the problem is corrected -------524

16-5b   Recession present around teeth # 8, #9, #10, and #11, for the biologic
        width was invaded at the time of cementation. Recession was not present
        at the time of cementation. Note crown recently placed on tooth #7 has
        early recession and inflammation. In time, additional recession will most
        likely occur. When biologic width is violated by the presence of a crown
        margin or restoration, inflammation or recession is usually the result ----524

16-6a   Gingival inflammation is seen in the presence of significant accumulations
        of plaque. Note the rolled reddened marginal gingiva -------------------530

16-6b   Bitewing radiograph of this patient reveals no alveolar bone loss. Patient
        has dental-plaque-induced gingivitis. Progression to periodontitis may
        or may not occur depending upon the patient's resistance to disease ----530

16-7a Gingivitis in a 27-year-old woman before treatment is commenced. Note the reddened edematous tissue and plaque on the teeth. Patient avoids the dentist because "cleanings'" hurt too much ~~~~~~~~531

16-7b The same patient 10 years following root planing and scaling under local anesthesia and instruction in oral hygiene. She has been on a 4-month recall program for 10 years. Periodontal surgery was never needed. Inflammation has been controlled, no attachment loss has occurred and teeth cleanings no longer hurt ~~~~~531

16-8 Pregnancy gingivitis is present in this woman, now in her second trimester of pregnancy. Note the presence of the pyogenic granuloma (pregnancy tumor) associated with the mandibular second bicuspid and an early pyogenic granuloma forming interproximally between the canine and first bicuspid ~~~~532

16-9a Dilantin-induced gingival overgrowth present in a young man. Eating has become difficult due to the significant amount of gingiva present over the teeth. Note the existence of serves outpocketing of gingiva beginning in the papillary areas. The papillae are coalescing and forming "pseudo pockets" ~~~534

16-9b Patient six weeks following periodontal flap surgery to remove hyperplastic gingival tissues. Note the amount of crown that is now visible. Patient is much more comfortable. However, if excellent hygiene is not maintained the hyperplastic will return. Note the immature granulation tissue forming mesial to the mandibular right canine ~~~534

16-10 Herpetic lesions found on the lips of woman one week following periodontal surgery. Oral surgery can trigger the activation of the virus, which lives quiesently in the nerve. Herpes virus usually manifests itself as a cluster of small ulcers ~~~~~~~~~~~~~~~~535

16-11a Gingival sloughing and ulceration seen in a patient with ulcerative lichen planis ~~~~~~~~~~~~~~~~~~~~~~~537

16-11b The patient also demonstrates Wickman's striae on the buccal mucosa, a frequent finding in patients with lichen planis. It presents as a delicate lacy white pattern on the buccal mucosa ~~~~~~~~~~~537

16-12 Gingival redness and desquamation associated with an allergic reaction to chewing gum, contact dermatitis. Note the newly ulcerated marginal gingiva ~~~537

16-13 Gingival sloughing in a patient one week after being instructed in oral hygiene. This self-induced lesion is a result of over-zealous toothbrushing in an attempt to eliminate periodontal disease in one week ~~~~~~~~539

16-14a   Profile of a young female flutist. She has a Class II occlusion and
          anterior flaring of the maxillary anterior teeth. This situation has
          created an open bite in which to place her flute ~~~~~~~~~~~~~539

16-14b   Gingival recession and mucogingival defect are associated with
          mandibular central incisor. The trauma from the flute resting
          against her labial gingiva has resulted in recession ~~~~~~~~~539

16-15   Adult periodontitis present in a patient in her late thirties. Attachment
          loss and alveolar cratering is present throughout her dentition ~~~~~540

16-16a   Localized aggressive periodontitis in a teenage female.
          Note the bony defect distal to the first molar ~~~~~~~~~~~~~542

16-16b   Some bone regeneration was achieved following periodontal
          surgical regenerative (osseous grafting) treatment ~~~~~~~~~542

16-17a   Preoperative radiograph of a teenage patient with localized
          aggressive periodontitis. Angular molar defects are present ~~~~~543

16-17b   Post-surgical radiograph taken eight months following caries
          control and active periodontal treatment, which included
          bone-grafting surgery. The amount of healing is dramatic~~~~~~543

16-18a   Anterior radiographs of a 24-year-old female patient with
          generalized aggressive periodontitis. More than 50% alveolar
          bone loss is present throughout all of her dentition ~~~~~~~544

16-18b   Photograph of same 24-year patient with generalized aggressive perio-
          dontitis. Loss of papillae, recession, and some anterior flaring are evident ~~~~545

16-19   Patient with necrotizing ulcerative periodontitis. Note the inflamed
          gingiva and the blunted papilla. Some of the papilla has already been
          lost. This 19-year-old female is a smoker, was recently hospitalized
          with a life-threatening asthma attack, and had not seen a dentist in
          a few years. Her oral hygiene is fair to poor~~~~~~~~~~~~547

16-20   Same patient as in Figure 16-19 following treatment. Therapy consisted of
          immediate debridement, oral hygiene instructions, and a one-week course
          of penicillin. This was followed up by four visits of root planing and scaling
          under local anesthesia with a reinforcement of oral hygiene instructions.
          Oral hygiene has improved, and tissues are no longer inflamed. However,
          the initial loss of papillae is permanent, and the embrasures are open ~~~~~547

16-21a   Periodontal abscess in an untreated periodontal patient. Note the large
          swelling in the mucobuccal fold over right canine and central incisors.
          The gingival tissues between the central incisors are detachable ~~~~~549

16-21b   Radiograph of abscessed patient reveals alveolar bone loss that approa-
         ches the apical area of the central incisor. Prompt treatment is essential ~~~~549

16-22   Immediate drainage of the periodontal abscess is of paramount
         importance to minimize the amount of bone loss. The abscess
         is curreted, and the patient is place on antibiotics, warm salt-water
         rinses, and chlorhexidine rinses for one week. Initial therapy is
         commenced once the acute abscess is under control ~~~~~~~~~~~~~~~549

16-23a   This 40-year-old patient has seen a dentist only twice in his life.
         The significant amount of calcareous deposits and poor oral
         hygiene bode well for making this a successful case ~~~~~~~~~~~554

16-23b   Lingual view reveals 6 mm ledges of calculus ~~~~~~~~~~~~~~~554

16-23c   The 10-year post-therapeutic result reveals a significant improvement
         with and a return to periodontal health. The patient has undergone
         oral hygiene instructions, scaling and root planing, periodontal surgery,
         minor orthodontics, extraction of his hopeless mandibular incisors, and
         placement of two dental implants. The post-operative result is a testament
         to the benefit of excellent dental care coupled with patient cooperation ~~~554

16-24a   Recession in a 55-year-old patient who received a full mouth
         gingivectomy in the 1960s. This therapy resulted in a loss of attached
         gingiva and the creation of mucogingival defects. All of her affected
         teeth had Class II mobility, and she found it difficult to eat ~~~~~~~555

16-24b   The treatment plan called for mucogingival reconstruction with free
         gingival grafting. Mobility was decreased, attached gingiva and root
         coverage increased, and periodontal health was restored ~~~~~~~~~~555

16-25a   Patient presentation at his initial visit prior to root
         planing and scaling and oral hygiene instructions.
         Oral hygiene is poor, and the gingival tissues are inflamed ~~~~~~556

16-25b   Post-initial therapy the patient is reexamined. Yellow disclosing dye
         reveals much plaque and little if any improvement in oral hygiene.
         This patient is not a good candidate for periodontal surgery and is
         advised to go into a three-month maintenance program ~~~~~~~~~~556

16-26   Complete radiographic examination includes 20 films—4 vertical
         bitewings, 8 anterior periapical, and 8 posterior periapical films ~~~~~~557

16-27a   Panoramic radiographic of the patient is a good screening tool and allows
         one to assess morphologic relationships. However, distortion of up to
         40% can be seen, and fine details are often missed. It is not possible
         to visualize the defect on the distal of the lower left 2nd premolar ~~~~559

16-27b   The periapical radiographic is more accurate and has minimal distortion.
          Vertical defect on the distal of the premolar is seen, as well as root
          resorption at the apical extent of the post ⌐⌐⌐⌐⌐⌐⌐⌐⌐⌐⌐⌐⌐⌐⌐⌐⌐ 559

16-27c   Clinical view of the premolar at the time of surgery. If the only
          pre-surgical radiograph were a panoramic view, this lesion would
          not have been diagnosed, radiographically ⌐⌐⌐⌐⌐⌐⌐⌐⌐⌐⌐⌐⌐⌐⌐⌐ 559

16-28a   Horizontal bitewing radiographs taken during a routine recall visit. They
          are not diagnostic. It is not possible to see the alveolar bone, due to bone
          loss, or to diagnose caries, for the crown margin is not visible in the film ⌐⌐⌐ 560

16-28b   Vertical bitewing radiographs taken the same day as in 16-28a.
          Alveolar bone level can be evaluated and caries diagnosed. It is
          strongly recommended to take vertical bitewing radiographs ⌐⌐⌐⌐⌐⌐ 560

16-29a   Periapical radiograph taken in 1981. Patient felt that x-rays were
          detrimental to her health and refused them for nine years ⌐⌐⌐⌐⌐⌐⌐ 561

16-29b   Periapical radiograph of the area in 29 A taken in 1990. It was the first
          x-ray taken since 1980. Severe bone loss is present in the furcation of the
          first molar, and a perio-endo lesion on the second molar has deemed these
          teeth hopeless. Not taking radiographs turned out to be tooth detrimental ⌐⌐ 561

16-30a   Clinical photograph of a 25-year-old male patient at his initial visit.
          Clinically, severe periodontal disease is suspected. However, the level
          of severity is not truly comprehended until radiographs are taken⌐⌐⌐⌐⌐ 562

16-30b   Radiographs of the patient in 16-30a. The true level of alveolar bone
          loss could not be appreciated until a full mouth radiographic series
          was taken. The patient had 80 to 100 % loss of alveolar bone. His
          teeth were terminal, and they were given a hopeless prognosis ⌐⌐⌐⌐⌐ 562

16-31a   Clinical photograph of a 40-year-old man at his initial periodontal visits.
          However, he has just completed root planing and scaling in the office of
          his restorative dentist. The gingival tissues reveal inflammation and plaque
          is evident at the cervical margins. The patient was advised to redo the initial
          therapy. Little gingival improvement was noted following his second phase
          of initial therapy. This raised suspicion that a systemic problem might exist ⌐⌐ 564

16-31b   Radiographs of the anterior teeth. Radiolucencies are noted at the
          apices of the maxillary lateral incisors and the mandibular incisors.
          This is a reported finding in patients with sarcoidosis ⌐⌐⌐⌐⌐⌐⌐⌐⌐⌐⌐ 564

16-32   Basal cell carcinoma present on the maxillary lip of a 50-year-old female.
          Despite its presence for years, she was never advised to have it removed.
          Undiagnosed lesions should be biopsied or removed en toto ⌐⌐⌐⌐⌐⌐ 566

16-33   Herpetic lesions present on the lip of a patient one week following oral surgery. Trauma is a frequent precipitating factor ~~~~~~~~~~~566

16-34a   Patients wearing complete maxillary dentures will frequently form inflammatory fibrous hyperplasia (epulis fissuratum) in the maxillary anterior region. These folds of excess tissue form in response to ill-fitting dentures and or bone resorption of the alveolar bone that leads to elongated rolls of tissue in the mucobuccal fold area into which the denture flange fits. The tissue is inflamed and serves as a nidus for plaque formation ~~~~~~~567

16-34b   Treatment consisted of removal and grafting with alloderm, an acellular dermal matrix processed from donated human skin ~~~~~~~~~~567

16-34c   Healing at eight weeks was excellent, and a firm keratinized base exists. The patient's denture is relined, and the occlusal is verified ~~~~~567

16-35   Nicotinic stomatitis on the hard palate of a 28-year-old man with a history of smoking two packs of cigarettes a day. Thickening of the epithelium adjacent to the inflamed of the salivary glands is present. The patient is advised to quit smoking ~~~~~~~~~~~~~~~~568

16-36   Blunt trauma present in this 30-year-old homosexual man. He was asymtomatic except for the large ulcer present on his palate. The lesion resolved within two weeks ~~~~~~~~~~~~~~~569

16-37   Initial oral examination tray. It consists of mouth mirror, periodontal probe, furcation (Nabers) probe, single-ended explorer, 2 x 2 piece of gauze, and an 18-inch length of dental floss ~~~~~~~~~~~~570

16-38a   Visual examination of this 24-year-old patient reveals minimal or no periodontal disease ~~~~~~~~~~~~~~~~~~~~~~~~~~~~~~~~572

16-38b   Probing is necessary to reveal 4-mm anterior pocketing and bleeding upon probing. Patient has early gingivitis, which is easily treated at this stage ~~~~572

16-39   Severe periodontitis is easily revealed upon visual examination. Loss of papillae, edema, cyanosis and suppuration, and drifting and shifting of teeth are all evident without probing or radiographs ~~~~~572

16-40   Prior to the initiation of periodontal treatment the papilla is detachable and calculus is present subgingivally. This is the same patient as in Figures 16-3a and 16-3b ~~~~~~~~~~~~~~~~~~~573

16-41a   The periodontal probe is inserted at the line angle parallel to the long axis of the tooth. Pocket depth is minimal ~~~~~~~~~~~~~574

16-41b   The same patient with the probe angled slightly interproximally
          reveals a pocket of 4 mm. It is essential to angle the probe
          interproximally to avoid missing early periodontal disease ~~~~~~~~~574

16-42a   Visual examination of the interproximal gingival tissues
          does not reveal any significant periodontal disease ~~~~~~~~~~~~~~574

16-42b   Reflection of the gingival tissue reveals the extent of the
          disease. It is essential that the probe be angled interproximally
          to diagnose the extent of the bone loss ~~~~~~~~~~~~~~~~~~~~~~~574

16-43   The mesial of the maxillary first bicuspid is predisposed to periodontal
          disease. Anatomically, there are two roots, which may be separate or fused.
          A mesial root groove or furcation is present, depending on whether the
          buccal and palatal roots are bifurcated or fused. Accurate probing of
          this interproximal area should be done on all patients. If the line angle
          is probed, the interproximal bony cratering may be missed ~~~~~~~~~575

16-44   The mesial of the mandibular canine is predisposed to plaque formation.
          The root is broad in a buccal lingual direction. The canine is the
          "cornerstone" of the arch, at the junction between the anterior and
          posterior teeth, and is often missed during oral hygiene. Note the
          absence of bone loss on the premolars and the facial of the canine ~~~~575

16-45   This 78-year-old woman presents with a palatal root groove on only one of
          her maxillary lateral incisors. The left lateral with the root groove probes
          8 mm while the lateral incisor without the root groove probes 3 mm. The
          groove serves as a plaque trap. Treatment should include debridement as
          well as elimination of the groove with a high speed-finishing bur, if possible ~~575

16-46a   Buccal furcations of the molars are easily diagnosed due to their
          accessibility. A furcation (Nabers) probe is used to evaluate the extent~~~~577

16-46b   Flap reflection reveals the horizontal extent of the furcation.
          The vertical extent should also be evaluated ~~~~~~~~~~~~~~~~~~~~~577

16-47a   A curved curate or furcation probe is used to access the
          mesial furcation of the maxillary molar ~~~~~~~~~~~~~~~~~~~~~~~~~578

16-47b   A palatal approach used for the palatal provides better accessibility,
          for they are wider than the buccal embrasures of the maxillary molars ~~~578

16-48   The diameter of most cruets is too wide to enter the furcation
          area, making complete debridement close to impossible ~~~~~~~~~~~579

16-49 a,b Cross sections of the maxillary and mandibular teeth reveal root grooves and concavities present on the furcal aspects of the roots of the maxillary and mandibular molars. Complete root preparation of these areas via instrumentation is not possible ------579

16-50 Class I buccal furcation of a mandibular molar demonstrates early furcal bone loss and a slight enamel projection. Treatment should involve removal of the enamel projection and osseous reshaping to provide easy cleansibility of the furcation ------580

16-51a An early Class II furcation with the Nabers probe showing its extent. It is amenable to guided bone regeneration ------581

16-51b Gore-Tex barrier membranes are placed over the furcations after the roots were debrided with finishing burs, treated with tetracycline for five minutes, and an autogenous bone was placed. The membranes are intimately adapted to prevent the ingrown of gingival connective tissue and epithelium. The buccal gingival flap was then elevated to completely cover the Gore-Tex membrane. The membrane is left for six to eight weeks before removal ------582

16-51c Eight months later, the furcation is closed for bony regeneration has taken place. Probing is not possible ------582

16-52a Root proximity is present between the maxillary first and second molars. Class II furcation involvement exists on the buccal and distal furcation of the maxillary first molar ------583

16-52b Radiograph reveals the extent of the root proximity. The distal buccal root of the first molar is in contact with the mesial buccal root of the second molar. Endodontic therapy was completed in anticipation of the root amputation procedure ------583

16-52c Flap refection reveals the buccal furcation involvement as well as the root proximity. As is, this is a non-maintainable situation ------584

16-52d Post-therapy crowns were placed on the maxillary first and second molars to establish better occlusion. Note the amount of interproximal space that exists between the molars, allowing for cleansibility. Plaque control is excellent (Restoration courtesy of Dr. Peter Ferrara, Westport, CT) ------584

16-53a Class III furcations are present between the first and second mandibular molars. A decision has to be made as to what roots are maintainable from both a periodontal and restorative perspective ------585

16-53b Radiograph of molars showing root proximity, short roots caries, endodontic problems, as well as periodontal disease ------586

16-53c Radiograph of completed case. The mesial root of the mandibular molar was removed, and the remaining three roots treated periodontally and splinted together. It is now possible to clean these teeth easily with a proxybrush ~~~~586

16-53d Photo of the finished case. It lasted 10 years before the margins experienced decay. Periodontally, the case remained stable (Restorative dentistry courtesy of Dr. Keith Rudolph, Westport, CT) ~~~~~~~~~~586

16-54a Gingival flap reflection of trifurcated maxillary molars ~~~~~~~587

16-54b Occlusal view revealing Class III furcation of the maxillary second molar. The third molar is hopeless, and the first molar has a Class II furcation on the distal ~~~~~~~~~~~~~~587

16-54c The distal-buccal root of the first molar was amputated, and the second molar was trisected. It was determined that the palatal and mesial-buccal roots had the best prognosis ~~~~~~~~~~588

16-54d A provisional restoration was fabricated on the altered dentition. The patient is allowed to heal and is instructed in proper home care ~~~~588

16-54e At four months post-surgery, the provisional restoration is removed and patient compliance is assessed. At this stage, a decision is made as to whether the patient can adequately clean the remaining roots. Manual dexterity and patient commitment are essential for long-term stability. This patient demonstrated excellent hygiene, and a decision was made to proceed to the final restoration ~~~~~~589

16-54f Palatal view of final restoration. Patient is adequately maintaining and plaque control is excellent. Monitoring is essential for long-term success (Restorative dentistry courtesy of Dr. Robert Cieri, Wilton, CT) ~~~~~589

16-55a Tunnel preparation was done at the time of surgery. A proxybrush is placed into the tunnel before suturing to maintain the patency of the Class III furcation ~~~~~~~~~590

16-55b Healing is uneventful, and tissue health is excellent. The opening to the Class III furcation is evident ~~~~~~~~~~590

16-55c The patient is maintaining the furcation with a proxybrush dipped in fluoride on a daily basis ~~~~~~~~~~~591

16-55d Radiograph taken 18 months post surgery reveals increasing bone loss and decay of the furcal aspects of the roots. Despite good oral hygiene with fluoride, the roots are still prone to decay. This is not a predictable procedure and is no longer performed by the author ~~~~~591

16-56a   Buccal furcation not amenable to predictable treatment. Restoration is
present in the furcation, making regeneration impossible. With the
exception of extraction, maintenance is the only alternative. The patient
was instructed to irrigate the area on a daily basis with chlorhexidine. This
disturbs the bacteria and may slow down the bone loss in the furcal area.
Maintaining this tooth's furcation does not impact on the adjacent teeth ------592

16-56b   Irrigation device used by patient to deliver subgingival medications
to difficult to maintain areas. Patient was instructed to fill it with
chlorhexidine and irrigate two times a day ------------------------------------592

16-57a   Pretreatment radiograph of a hopeless maxillary
molar with a Class III furcation ---593

16-57b   Post-treatment radiograph of the molar replaced with two implants ------593

16-57c   Post-treatment photographs of mandibular molar restored
with two dental implants. The predictability of this
restoration is in the high 90th percentile ---------------------------------------593

16-58   The blunt end of the explorer and mouth mirror
are used to assess tooth mobility --594

16-59a   Significant generalized occlusal wear in a 40-year-old male bruxer ------597

16-59b   Occlusal view of view through the mandibular incisors. Secondary dentin
is present for the patient has ground his teeth through the enamel, into
the dentin and into the area where the pulp chambers used to be ------597

16-59c   Class II furcations present in mandibular molars. Some clinicians
feel that occlusion "may" be a cofactor in furcal bone loss --------------597

16-60a   Teeth #18 and #19 were lost and never replaced in this patient. The
maxillary molars subsequently drifted into the edentulous space. Implants
were eventually placed. However, there was inadequate interocclusal space ---598

16-60b   Radiographs demonstrate the lack of room to place
an adequate functional restoration --598

16-60c   Final radiograph reveals the multiplicity of treatments that were required
to restore this patient. Maxillary molar crown lengthening, elective molar
endodontics, elective maxillary crown, and a customized UCLA
mandibular prosthesis were all necessary to restore this patient. This
could have been prevented if the space was maintained post-extraction ----599

16-60d   Final photograph of the finished restoration. Plane of occlusion has
been reestablished. The cost was restoration of the maxillary molars
(Restorative dentistry courtesy of Dr. Gary Horblitt, Fairfield, CT) ----599

16-61   Young child beginning tooth brushing. It is never too early
         to begin good oral hygiene habits ～～～～～～～～～～～～～～603

16-62a   This 38-year-old female patient has not seen the dentist in 12 years.
         Significant plaque accumulation with resultant angry red gingivitis is seen ～～～604

16-62b   One week later, after the institution of home care in conjunction with
         oral hygiene instructions, some resolution of inflammation is seen ～～～～～604

16-63   Numerous oral hygiene aids exist to assist the patient in the control
         of dental plaque. They include various types of proxybrushes, dental
         floss, floss threaders, superfloss, stim-u-dents, floss handles, rubber
         tips, disclosing tablets, toothbrushes, etc. ～～～～～～～～～～～～605

16-64   This patient has been flossing. However, the floss has created a gingival cleft,
         for it was not wrapped around the tooth and placed into the sulcus. The floss
         should be placed into the sulcus and wrapped like a C around the tooth ～～～606

16-65   The rubber tip is a useful adjunct in the control of plaque. Patients are
         instructed to begin to gently use the rubber tip one week following
         periodontal surgery. The author finds excellent hygiene, plaque control, and
         minimal pocket depth in the patients that use the rubber tip twice daily ～～～607

16-66   The rubber tip is particularly useful in hard to clean furcations. The
         point of the rubber tip is placed into the furcation, and the patient
         is asked to gently apply pressure. The gingival furcal tissue maintains
         firmness, and oral health is better maintained ～～～～～～～～～～～607

16-67   Proxybrushes are effective at removing interproximal plaque. Embrasure
         space must exist to allow their passage. They are most useful after
         posterior periodontal surgery where there has been attachment loss ～～～608

16-68a   Patient before initial therapy ～～～～～～～～～～～～～～～～～610

16-68b   Patient post initial therapy. Inflammation and pocket depths have
         decreased. However, significant pocketing still remains and pocket
         elimination therapy is indicated ～～～～～～～～～～～～～～～611

16-68c   Pocket elimination surgery has been performed. Gingival tissues are
         healthy, and pocket depth is minimal. However, more of the root has been
         exposed. In an esthetic area, this form of treatment is contraindicated ～～～611

16-69a   This patient has gone through scaling and root planing one
         year ago. The buccal surface of tooth #22 probed 2 mm post
         root planing and scaling. However, she presented with a
         periodontal abscess one year following initial therapy ～～～～～～613

16-69b   Patient probes 6 mm the day of the abscess ～～～～～～～～～～613

16-69c Split thickness flap reflection reveals heavy subgingival calculus. However, the root is calculus free 3 mm apical to the CEJ. The effective area of subgingival instrumentation in this patient was 3 mm ——613

16-69d Thorough root planning was accomplished ——614

16-69e The flap was repositioned with multiple sutures to assure good adaptation, similar to a free gingival graft ——614

16-69f Seven years later, the tissue is firm and the gingival sulcus is non-probable ——614

16-70 Root planing and scaling instrument set up. A variety of curettes are used. Local anesthesia is used 95% of the time to maximize the subgingival depth that can be instrumented ——615

16-71 Ultrasonic instruments are also used for scaling and root planing. In addition, a high-speed prophyjet is used to remove stains. It is more expedient than using a rubber cup and pumice ——615

16-72 High-speed finishing burs are also incorporated in the scaling and root planing armamentarium. The most frequently used burs are 11-fluted finishing burs and the neumeyer bur. They do not cut dentin very well and do not gouge the root surface. Patients experience less hyper-sensitivity than when using ultrasonics or hand instrumentation ——615

16-73 Typical instrument set up for periodontal surgery ——627

16-74a Sulcular incision. The scalpel is placed into the sulcus and directed along the long axis of the tooth in order to preserve all of the attached gingiva ——630

16-74b Care is taken to preserve the entire papilla as well as all of the keratinized gingiva. The scalpel is used to incise as well as to reflect the tissue ——630

16-75a The patient fractured her maxillary lateral incisor subgingivally to the osseous crest. Crown lengthening was indicated in order to avoid invading the biologic width and to expose enough root to achieve crown retention ——632

16-75b Sulcular incisions were made to preserve all of the keratinized tissue as well as the papillae. A palatal approach was used to preserve the entire papilla ——632

16-75c Post-osseous surgery. Note that some bone was removed from the mesial of the central incisor. Some papillary loss will occur ——633

16-75d The flap was sutured to preserve the labial papilla and eliminate pockets from the palatal ——633

16-75e   Final restoration. Esthetics is good with the exception of
           the papilla between the lateral and central, which was lost
           due to the interproximal bone removal. Some recession is
           also seen on the labial of the central incisor ～～～～～～ 634

16-75f   Six years later, the central incisor crown was redone.
           This facilitated the growth of the papilla between the
           central and lateral. Ideal esthetics has now been achieved
           (Restorative dentistry courtesy of Dr. Keith Rudolph, Westport, CT) ～～～ 634

16-76a   Presurgical photograph of a 60-year-old female patient.
           She has only eight teeth remaining. She wears a complete
           maxillary denture. The goal of therapy is to maintain the
           mandibular teeth to support a removable partial denture ～～～～ 635

16-76b   Sulcular incisions are made in order to preserve the attached
           gingiva in anticipation of a bone-grafting procedure ～～～～～～ 636

16-76c   A full thickness flap is elevated exposing the underlying
           alveolar bone. Interproximal defects are evident ～～～～～～～～ 636

16-76d   Autogenous bone is harvested and packed into the interproximal craters once
           they have been debrided and the root meticulously root planed ～～～～ 637

16-76e   The facial and lingual flaps are elevated to achieve primary closure with
           interrupted sutures ～～～～～～～～～～～～～～～～～～～～～～～～～～ 637

16-76f   Lingual view of the sutured flaps ～～～～～～～～～～～～～～～～ 637

16-76g   Surgical view of a probe in place measuring the
           attachment loss of approximately 3.5 mm ～～～～～～～～～～～～～ 638

16-76h   Five-year postoperative result. About 3 mm of attachment
           has been regenerated and the patient is stable. She is
           maintained on a three-month recall program ～～～～～～～～～～ 638

16-77a   Pretreatment photograph of periodontally-involved mandibular
           molar. Probing reveals a circumferential defect ～～～～～～～～ 639

16-77b   Pretreatment radiograph demonstrates vertical
           bone loss and subgingival calculus ～～～～～～～～～～～～～～～ 640

16-77c   Sulcular incisions with a full thickness flap expose the defect.
           Calculus is present on the distal of the mandibular first molar ～～～ 640

16-77d   The root is meticulously debrided with high speed finishing
           burs to reveal a glossy white hard surface, free of endotoxins.
           It will now be treated with tetracycline paste for five minutes,
           prior to application of the bone grafting material ～～～～～～～ 640

16-77e   Autogenous bone graft is placed into the defect ~~~~~~~~~~641

16-77f   A Gore-Tex (ePTFE) membrane is placed over the bone
graft and sutured to place with two circumferential sutures ~~~~~641

16-77g   The flap is coronally repositioned to obtain primary closure. Buccal
periosteal releasing incisions are made to allow tension-free closure ~~~~~641

16-77h   Six year post-treatment radiograph reveals bone fill and crestal cortication ~~642

16-77i   Post treatment, the mandibular molar probes 1 to 2 mm,
a 5 mm gain of probing attachment ~~~~~~~~~~~~~~~~~~~~~~~642

16-78   An inverse bevel is used on the palate where pocket depth is present.
Adequate keratinized tissue is always present on the palate; therefore,
it is impossible to create a mucogingival defect. By design, gingival
tissue is removed, and more of the root will be exposed ~~~~~~~643

16-79a   Dilantin-induced gingival hyperplasia. Excess gingival tissue is present
and is to be removed. An inverse bevel incision is the incision of choice ~~~~644

16-79b   An inverse bevel incision is made in conjunction with a
full thickness mucoperiosteal flap ~~~~~~~~~~~~~~~~~~~~~~~645

16-79c   The flap is apically positioned with a continuous
sling suture. Excess tissue has been removed, root
debridement performed, and the pockets eliminated ~~~~~~~~~~645

16-80   Full thickness flap includes the periosteum and allows
access to underlying alveolar bone. Bone grafting,
osteoplasty, or simple debridement are possible ~~~~~~~~~~~~646

16-81a   Before osseous surgery, significant bony exostosis is seen throughout the
buccal aspect of the maxilla. Patient has veneers on teeth #7, #8, #9, and
#10. She is not satisfied with the cosmetics of the teeth. In addition, the
alveolar bony overgrowth causes her to have a "cheeky" look. The patient
feels that her face appears swollen due to the excess bone ~~~~~~~647

16-81b   Full thickness flap reflection reveals the bony exostosis. The removal
of the excess bone via osteoplasty was the goal of therapy ~~~~~~648

16-81c   Osteoplasty has been completed. In addition, crown lengthening was
performed in order to allow the new veneers to be more harmonious ~~~~648

16-81d   Teeth #6 through #11 have new veneers. Cosmetically they are more
pleasing. Compare to Figure 16-81a. In addition, the excess bony overgrowth
has been removed and the patient is more pleased with her appearance
(Restorative dentistry courtesy of Dr. Mark Samuels, Stratford, CT) ~~~~648

16-82   Diagram of a split (partial) thickness flap. The flap is reflected by sharp dissection, and the periosteum is left attached to the bone ~~~~~~649

16-83   Partial-thickness flap is used to protect the underlying bone from resorption. Note the tooth fenestration on the canine. Once this was observed, partial-thickness dissection was commenced in order to avoid further root exposure. An attempt was made to avoid buccal root recession ~~~~~~~~~650

16-84a   Preoperative view of mandibular canine in need of crown lengthening. Minimal keratinized tissue is present~~~~~~~651

16-84b   A partial-thickness flap was elevated apical to the area of crown lengthening. The attached periosteum was used to apically tack the reflected flap. This technique is used in order to increase the band of keratinized gingiva. The use of a gingival graft is avoided~~~~~~651

16-84c   One-week post crown lengthening surgery, the beginning of a new mucogingival junction is seen. The wound is still healing, but an increased band of keratinized tissue can clearly be seen ~~~~~~651

16-85a   Probing of a patient post initial therapy and pre-periodontal surgery. Patient has generalized severe periodontitis ~~~~~~~~653

16-85b   Radiographs of the maxillary anterior teeth reveal 50 to 80 % bone loss ~~~~653

16-85c   Diagram of the initial incision, an inverse bevel palatal incision ~~~~~653

16-85d   Clinical view of the initial continuous inverse bevel incision. Note the papillae are kept intact~~~~~~~~~~~~~~~~~~~654

16-85e   Diagram of the secondary incision, a continuous sulcular incision ~~~~~654

16-85f   Clinical view of the sulcular incision. The incision begins in the sulcus and connects to adjacent teeth from the palatal line angles of the teeth, so that the papillae are not incised ~~~~~~~~~~~~654

16-85g   Diagram of the two initial palatal incisions ~~~~~~~~~~~~~~~655

16-85h   The third incision connects the inverse bevel and sulcular incisions. An instrument is placed at the base of the sulcular incision and used to elevate the tissue defined by the two incisions off of the bone ~~~~~655

16-85i   The wedge of tissue is removed. It can be used for a connective tissue graft or discarded~~~~~~~~~~~~~~~~655

16-85j   Access is now possible to root plane the palatal and interproximal surfaces. The bone can be treated with osseous surgery, bone grafting, guided tissue regeneration, or simply debrided ~~~~~~~656

16-85k   Buccal view of the suturing technique. Since a buccal
          flap was not elevated, there is no need to suture ~~~~~~~~~~~~~~~~656

16-85l   The palatal tissues are sutured with a continuous sling. In this case,
          a horizontal mattress suture is also incorporated to achieve good
          adaptation of the palatal tissues to the underlying bone ~~~~~~~~~~~~656

16-85m   Labial view of the patient prior to surgery ~~~~~~~~~~~~~~~~~~~~~657

16-85n   Labial view of the patient three months following surgery.
          Pockets have been eliminated, and recession is minimal ~~~~~~~~~~~657

16-86a   Labial view of patient prior to periodontal surgery. Note that the labial
          pocket depth is minimal. Interproximally, the patient probes 7 to 8 mm ~~658

16-86b   Pretreatment radiograph reveals 60 to 80% bone loss ~~~~~~~~~~~~659

16-86c   Five years following periodontal papillary retention flap surgery,
          periodontal probing is 1 to 2 mm. Clinically, the patient is well
          maintained. He is on a three-month recall program ~~~~~~~~~~~~~~~659

16-86d   Radiograph taken five years post periodontal surgery. Note that bone
          level appears to have regenerated. Bone grafting was not performed.
          The author finds that some bone regeneration is possible when
          periodontally involved roots are debrided, excellent oral hygiene is
          maintained, and the patient is on a frequent recall program ~~~~~~~~~659

16-87   No attached gingiva is present on the labial surface of the right
          mandibular central incisor. The tissue is inflamed, and oral hygiene
          is difficult to perform. There is no question that this tooth needs to
          be repaired. Recession has approached the apex of the incisor, and
          the tooth may soon be lost. The prognosis for this tooth is guarded ~~~~~660

16-88a   A 50-year-old woman presents with recession
          of the mandibular anterior teeth ~~~~~~~~~~~~~~~~~~~~~~~~~~~663

16-88b   The recipient site is prepared. The mucoperiosteal bed extends 5 mm
          past the denuded roots apically and one papilla past the roots to be
          covered. This ensures an adequate blood supply to the graft ~~~~~~~~663

16-88c   The graft is harvested from the palate. Note the size of the wound.
          Healing must occur by secondary intention ~~~~~~~~~~~~~~~~~~~663

16-88d   The graft is sutured to place. Initial stabilization occurs by suturing
          to the papillae. Circumferential sutures sync the graft to the root
          surface and the periosteal bed, assuring good blood supply to the
          graft and eliminating a dead space between the graft and the root ~~~~~664

16-88e   One week post-operatively, the graft is edematous and red.
         This is a positive sign of graft vitality 664

16-88f   Five-year post operative result. The graft is healthy, does not probe,
         and 5 mm of root coverage has been achieved 664

16-89a   An incision outlining the free gingival graft is made on the palate 665

16-89b   The graft is harvested, and the wound is dressed with
         a piece of iodoform gauze soaked in cyanoacrylate.
         This serves as an immediate "scab" and helps hemostasis 666

16-89c   A periodontal dressing is applied to the iodoform gauze.
         Once the gauze is soaked in the cyanoacrylate, it hardens,
         thus allowing the periodontal dressing to adhere to it. The
         purpose of the dressing is patient comfort and hemostasis 666

16-90a   Preoperative view of minimal keratinized gingiva 667

16-90b   Bed preparation via split thickness flap. Periosteum is left
         as a base for the free gingival graft 667

16-90c   Free gingival graft sutured to place with simple interrupted
         sutures at the papilla. Additional sutures are not necessary
         when root coverage is not attempted 668

16-90d   Six-month post-operative result. A healthy thickened band of
         keratinized tissue is evident. The graft blends with the papilla,
         for they were de-epithelialized as part of the procedure 668

16-91a   Pre-operative view of recession of teeth #11 and #12. Patient
         complains of sensitivity and is unhappy with the cosmetics 670

16-91b   Preparation of the recipient site. A partial-thickness flap is elevated from the
         line angles of the teeth adjacent to the teeth that are to be grafted. Vertical
         incisions are made at the ends of the flap to assure coverage of the graft ... 670

16-91c   The prepared recipient site is treated with tetracycline paste for
         five minutes. Note the yellowish color of the periosteum. Tetracycline
         treatment is performed in order to disinfect the wound, inhibit tissue
         collagenases, detoxify the root, and open up the dentinal tubules in
         preparation for the connective tissue graft 671

16-91d   The connective tissue graft is transferred to the recipient site and
         sutured with (5-0) gut to the papillae. Additional sutures may be
         placed laterally to stabilize and secure the graft 671

16-91e   The flap is coronally positioned in order to cover the connective
          tissue graft. This serves as an additional blood supply to nourish
          the graft. Vertical and periosteal releasing incisions assure that
          the flap will lie passively over the graft ~~~~~~~~~~~~~~~~~~~~~~~~672

16-91f   At one week post surgery, excellent healing is evident. Hemorrhagic
          edematous tissues at one week are a sign of good healing ~~~~~~~~~~672

16-91g   At two years post surgery, complete root coverage is achieved. It is
          difficult to demarcate the graft from the surrounding tissues. A significant
          benefit of this procedure is the excellent color match of the graft ~~~~~~~672

16-92a   Harvesting of the graft from the palate begins with an incision outline ~~~~673

16-92b   The epithelium is reflected in order to expose the underlying
          connective tissue that will be harvested ~~~~~~~~~~~~~~~~~~~~~~~~~~~~~~673

16-92c   A surgical pick up is used to delineate the connective
          tissue graft from the surrounding palate ~~~~~~~~~~~~~~~~~~~~~~~~~~~~674

16-92d   Connective tissue graft placed on sterile drape ~~~~~~~~~~~~~~~~~~~~~~674

16-92e   The graft site is sutured with circumferential black silk sutures.
          Primary closure is almost achieved ~~~~~~~~~~~~~~~~~~~~~~~~~~~~~~~~675

16-92f   At one week, complete healing is almost achieved. This is an additional
          benefit of this procedure. A free gingival graft creates a much more significant
          wound (see Fig. 16-88c), and healing of the palate takes much longer ~~~~675

16-93a   Pre-operative view of recession on tooth #11. It was recommended
          that this tooth be extracted, for the patient was going through orthodontic
          treatment as well as orthognathic surgery. The patient opted to save
          the tooth, and a subepithelial connective tissue graft was performed ~~~~676

16-93b   One year post operatively and post orthognathic surgery,
          the graft is still stable, and good root coverage maintained ~~~~~~~~~~677

16-93c   Two years later, orthodontics is completed, and the tooth is still stable ~~~~677

16-94a   Anterior view of a 40-year-old man with a six-unit bridge spanning teeth
          #6 through #11. Teeth #7, #8, and #10 were lost in his early 20s due to
          localized aggressive periodontitis (juvenile periodontitis). Significant
          bone loss had occurred, and the alveolar ridge resorbed. Subsequently,
          the pontics replacing these teeth were longer than normal. The result is
          an asymmetrical smile. The central incisors are of different lengths. The
          lateral incisors are also asymmetrical and not in proper proportion to the
          central incisors and canines. Labial concavities are noted over the pontics
          #7, #8, and #10. A shadow is seen that draws the eye to these areas ~~~~~~679

16-94b   Smile view reveals an asymmetrical smile. Esthetic harmony is not
present. Even an untrained eye realizes that something is "just not right" ----- 679

16-94c   Occlusal view with the provisional restoration removed.
Concavities are seen in the areas of the missing teeth.
Note the root prominence of the natural teeth ----- 681

16-94d   A midcrestal incision is made in the pontic area of tooth
#10, and an envelope pouch is made. This is to be the
recipient site of the connective tissue graft ----- 681

16-94e   The connective tissue graft is placed into the recipient site.
A small band of epithelium is kept on the graft, which is
placed occlusally. The prepared pouch is filled with bleeding
connective tissue. Externally, two sutures secure the graft ----- 682

16-94f   The connective tissue graft with a small band of epithelium is being
transferred to the prepared recipient site of the pontic area #7 and #8 ----- 682

16-94g   Occlusal view of the connective tissue graft in place before
external suturing. A resorbable suture is used to tack the graft
in place and prevent it from being dislodged. Note that the
beginning of root prominences is already evident ----- 683

16-94h   The provisional is replaced immediately after surgery.
The provisional had to be altered to accommodate the
connective tissue grafts. Compare to Figure 16-94a ----- 683

16-94i   Two months following surgery, the connective tissue grafts have healed.
Compare this occlusal view to the pre-operative view in Figure 16-94c.
Significant ridge augmentation has been achieved ----- 684

16-94j   Final restoration is in place; a 6-unit fixed bridge, spanning teeth #6
through #11. Harmony has been achieved. Central incisors are of equal
length. Root prominences are seen in the pontic sites #7, #8, and #10.
The gingival height of contour of the canines and central incisors are on
the same plane. The gingival height of contour of the lateral incisors is
approximately 1.5 mm incisal to the centrals and canines. Ten years
post-operatively, the connective grafts remain stable (Restorative
dentistry courtesy of Dr. Keith Rudolph, Westport, CT) ----- 684

16-95a   Intraoral pre-operative view reveals many alterations in ideal dental
and dental gingival relationships. Anterior flaring, diastemata, alterations
in dental gingival heights, and teeth discolorations are evident ----- 685

16-95b   Smile view shows minimal display of teeth due to tooth
wear and decreased vertical dimension ----- 686

16-95c   Postoperative restoration displays re-establishment of proper
dental and gingival relationships. Cosmetic and functional
improvement has been achieved through periodontal
crown lengthening and crowning of maxillary teeth ~~~~~~~~~~~~~686

16-95d   Post-operative smile view reveals improved appearance.
Teeth are in better balance, and more tooth structure is shown ~~~~~686

16-95e   Pre-operative facial appearance prior to beginning dental reconstruction ~~~687

16-95f   Post-operative facial view. Esthetic appearance is greatly improved.
Patient appears happier and more confident (Restorative dentistry
courtesy of Dr. Stephen Rothenberg, Darien, CT) ~~~~~~~~~~~687

16-96a   Initial view of patient's "gummy" smile ~~~~~~~~~~~~~~~~~689

16-96b   Intraoral anterior view reveals slightly altered dental gingival relationships.
The central incisors are short in relationship to the lateral incisors ~~~~~690

16-96c   Extraoral facial view of patient smiling. Excess gingival tissue is evident ~~~~690

16-96d   Provisional restorations were placed in anticipation
of anterior crown lengthening ~~~~~~~~~~~~~~~~~~~~~~~691

16-96e   A diagnostic model was made. Ideal dental gingival
relationships were determined and were used to guide
the surgeon during the crown-lengthening procedure~~~~~~~~~~~~~691

16-96f   Full thickness mucoperiosteal flap was elevated from bicuspid
to bicuspid. Care was taken to preserve the papillae ~~~~~~~~~~~692

16-96g   Ostectomy was begun on teeth #6, #7, and #8.
Compare to the contralateral side ~~~~~~~~~~~~~~~~~~~~~692

16-96h   A periodontal probe measures the distance from crown
margin to bone. This crown had invaded the biologic
width, for it is only 2 mm from the alveolar crest ~~~~~~~~~~~~~693

16-96i   Ostectomy is complete. Bony profiles are symmetrical. Ideal bony relationships are established, for the soft tissue follows the bony architecture ~~~~693

16-96j   The flap is repositioned and sutured to the papilla. No attempt
is made to reposition the gingiva at this time ~~~~~~~~~~~~~694

16-96k   The tissue is allowed to heal unmolested for eight weeks ~~~~~~~~~694

16-96l   Sounding (probing under anesthesia to bone) reveals that 5 mm exist
from the free gingival margin to the alveolar crest. Two millimeters of
gingiva can be removed without violating the biologic width ~~~~~~~~695

16-96m   A caliper is used to measure the length of the central incisor
          on the diagnostic model ⸺⸺⸺⸺⸺⸺⸺⸺⸺⸺⸺⸺ 695

16-96n   The information transferred to the mouth via the caliper ⸺⸺⸺ 696

16-96o   The gingiva is marked with the caliper, and an inverse
          bevel gingivectomy is performed ⸺⸺⸺⸺⸺⸺⸺⸺⸺⸺⸺ 696

16-96p   The collar of tissue is removed, and the distance to bone from
          free gingival margin evaluated. Three millimeters now exist ⸺⸺⸺ 697

16-96q   The gingiva is allowed to heal for two weeks before final
          impressions are taken and the final crowns completed.
          Ideal harmony and esthetics are present in the final restoration ⸺⸺ 697

16-96r   Close up of smile shows ideal amount of teeth. Compare
          to Figure 16-96a. The gummy smile has been eliminated ⸺⸺⸺⸺ 698

16-96s   Full facial view. Patient is much happier with her new smile. A twinkle
          is present in her eyes. Compare to her initial photograph in Figure
          16-96c. (Restoration courtesy of Dr. Fred Kriegle, Hartsdale, NY) ⸺⸺ 698

Tables

5-1   Modified crown-down technique utilizing .04 taper rotary nickel-titanium, by Dr. Ben Johnson ~~~~~~148-149

9-1   Temporomandibular disorder screening questionnaire ~~~~~255

9-2   TMD detailed history—key components ~~~~~256

9-3   Recommended diagnostic classification. Differentiation between arthrogenous and byogenous TMDs, and sub-classifications of each ~~~268

9-4   Acute extracapsular disorders ~~~~~269-270

9-5   Chronic extracapsular disorders ~~~~~271-272

9-6   Intracapsular disorders ~~~~~274-276

9-7   Disc derangement disorders ~~~~~277-279

9-8   Degenerative joint diseases ~~~~~280-281

9-9   Fractures ~~~~~282

9-10   Nonsteroidal anti-inflammatory drugs ~~~~~287

9-11   Steroids ~~~~~287

9-12   Muscle relaxants ~~~~~288

9-13   Antianxiety agents ~~~~~289

9-14   Antidepressant agents ~~~~~291

12-1   Imaging by the "specialties" ~~~~~370

15-1   Medications used to treat herpetic infections ~~~~~487

15-2   Topical medications used to treat recurrent aphthous ulcers ~~~~~494

15-3   Topical medications used to treat lichen planus ~~~~~498

15-4   Topical medications used to treat candidosis ~~~~~506

15-5   Systemic medications used to treat candidosis ~~~~~508

15-6   Medications used to palliate oral mucosal ulcerations ~~~~~510

16-1   Previous classification of periodontal diseases ~~~~~526

16-2   Current classification of periodontal diseases and conditions ~~~~~528

16-3   Initial examination sequence of therapy ~~~~~551

16-4   Extra- and intra-oral examination ~~~~~563

16-5   Examination of the periodontium ~~~~~571

16-6   Furcation classification 576

16-7   Occlusal examination 596

16-8   Menu (treatment options) 601

16-9   Periodontal treatment plan 602

16-10   Initial therapy 602

16-11   Chlorhexidine indications 609

16-12   Surgical flap designs 629

16-13   Mucogingival considerations 661

Chapter 1

Health Status of the Dental Patient

by Robert R. Edwab, B.S., D.D.S.

Dr. Smith has just finished his exam of Mrs. Jones. He has been her dentist for many years. Her signed health history reads "no" for all questions listed. Mrs. Jones requires deep periodontal scaling and preparation of a three-unit bridge. It all can be scheduled for one visit. At the front desk she is given an appointment in four weeks.

Two days later, Mrs. Jones has chest pains and shortness of breath. At the hospital, it is determined she needs a cardiac by-pass procedure and a mitral valve replacement. The procedures are performed, healing is uneventful, and Mrs. Jones is discharged and goes home in one week. During the second week, she is walking around her house, and in week three, she ventures outside. In week four, she attends to some of her easy errands, including her appointment with Dr. Smith.

Upon arrival at the dental office, she is greeted and taken to the operatory, where Dr. Smith gives local anesthesia and completes the proposed scheduled treatments. Everything goes well, and Mrs. Jones is given future appointments to complete the work.

Weeks later, Mrs. Jones develops night sweats, fever, and flu-like symptoms. Diagnosis is endocarditis. Subsequent investigations show that at the dental office, she never received antibiotic prophylaxis for her cardiac situation.

A scenario of what you just read could happen to any dentist. Between visits, patients can develop a myriad of medical conditions and have a plethora of treatments. One simple solution avoids a disaster like the earlier scenario. We must learn to perform a complete medical history and update it every time the patient visits our office. Knowing your patient's health status will help you avoid many acute medical emergencies that might occur in the private office setting.

We live in an extraordinary period of enlightened medical treatments. Many compromised patients who previously would have been confined to their homes, long-term care facilities, or hospitals are now functioning somewhat in society. Many of these patients seek care in our dental offices. All practitioners should develop a scenario so they can identify healthy patients who can receive routine dental treatment regimes and identify those who are medically compromised, requiring their treatments to be modified or delayed.

This chapter will teach the practitioner a six-step sequence, which assists him/her in identifying patients who might prove to be problematic. The sequence can be performed in a short and reasonable amount of time.

The six subject areas are:

- Health history
- Dialog or inquiry history
- Abbreviated vital signs
- Non-invasive physical examination
- American Society of Anesthesiologists physical status classification system
- Treatment modification if required

Health History

The written portion of our patient's health history begins upon his/her arrival in our office. He/she is asked to complete a questionnaire (Fig. 1-1). The health history consists of a series of questions that includes all past and current medical conditions, regardless of whether the patient feels the questions are not related to the current dental visit. Included are current medical care, previous hospital admissions, surgical histories and any related complications, types of anesthesias and their related sequelae, current and past prescribed medications, over-the-counter additives, allergy history (including medications, foods, or environmental conditions), hospital emergency room visits, and any history of smoking (packs per day times how many years) and alcohol (daily quantity times how many years).

There are many variations of commercially-produced medical histories available. The practitioner can combine the attributes of these prepared forms with his/her own criteria and proceed to have the forms duplicated. All questions should have a "yes" or "no" box with a space provided for written answers when required.

Lastly, each medical history form should have a space where the patient places his/her signature and date. Every effort must be made to ensure that the patient completes the form and not his/her escort. The only exception would be a minor who requires a parental signature, someone mentally incapacitated, or someone requiring foreign language translation. In those specific instances, the person completing the form should also sign and state his/her relationship to the patient. A member of your front desk should witness the signing of the form and then sign and date the form in the designated witness area. A sample copy of an office health history follows (Fig. 1-1). It also includes a statement about fees, availability for questions, statement by patient concerning truthfulness, an informed consent statement, and a witness signature area and date. Included is a specialized consent for complications that could arise from local anesthesia and oral surgery.

Patient Information and Health History

Please read this document carefully; be sure to complete fully and sign.

Fees are payable at the time of treatment. If you have any questions concerning this or any other matter, please do not hesitate to discuss them with us.

Please Print

Name _____ Date _____

Address _____

City _____ State _____ Zip _____ Family Dentist _____

Home Tel# _____ Work Tel # _____

Occupation _____ Work Address _____

Date of Birth _____ Soc. Sec. # _____

Purpose of Visit _____

Medical History

Circle Answer

1. Are you in good health?   Yes   No   If the answer to 4 is Yes, please add
2. Are you receiving any medical treatments now?   Yes   No   pertinent information: _____
3. Are you taking any medications now?   Yes   No
   If the answer to 2 or 3 is Yes, please list
   treatments and/or medication(s): _____   5. Are you allergic to any medications?   Yes   No
                                                                                 If Yes, please list: _____

4. Has a physician ever informed you that you had: 6. Have you ever received radiation treatments to the
   a. any heart ailment   Yes   No   head or neck?   Yes   No
   b. high blood pressure   Yes   No   7. Do you take aspirin daily?   Yes   No
   c. diabetes   Yes   No   8. Have you been ill or hospitalized recently?   Yes   No
   d. lung disease or asthma   Yes   No   9. Have you ever had a fractured jaw?   Yes   No
   e. rheumatic fever   Yes   No   10. Are you pregnant or nursing?   Yes   No
   f. any blood disease   Yes   No   11. Please enter your physician's name and address:
   g. hepatitis or liver disease   Yes   No   _____
   h. kidney disease   Yes   No   12. When did you eat last? _____
   i. glaucoma or eye disease   Yes   No   13. Person to contact in an emergency:
   j. any bleeding tendencies   Yes   No   Name: _____
   k. tuberculosis   Yes   No   Telephone # _____
   l. any other medical problems or treatments not listed   Yes   No

My medical history is accurate and complete.

Patient Signature (parent if minor) _____ Date _____

Witness _____ Date _____

We will gladly complete any pertinent insurance forms for you, but inasmuch as there are many differences in the benefits and in the services covered by various plans, office policy is to have any benefit payments sent directly from the insurance company to the patient.

Informed Consent

Occasional complications may arise from oral surgery. These include swelling, discomfort, bleeding, infection, chipped teeth or fillings, bone fracture, jaw joint discomfort, inability to open the mouth fully, and discoloration of the skin.

Some oral surgery procedures including the administration of local anesthesia can cause numbness to the lips, tongue, teeth, gums, or chin. In the vast majority of cases, this numbness is temporary. However, in rare cases, it can be permanent.

My medical history is accurate and complete.

Patient Signature (parent if minor) _____ Date _____

Witness _____ Date _____

Fig. 1-1 Health history questionnaire

Dialog or Inquiry History

Patients don't intentionally lie about their medical history. The problem is that when they get to a question they don't quite understand, it is much easier for them to check "no." One goal is to then query the patient on all questions, especially the ones answered positively and to focus on those aspects of the medical history that might increase our index of suspicion. This helps the patient to recall any pertinent information and also helps him/her rectify any answers incorrectly indicated. A verbal review in question form of the major organ systems follows:

- *Cardiovascular system*—"Ever been told you have high blood pressure, a heart murmur, heart failure, heart disease, angina, rheumatic fever, mitral valve prolapse, or any heart defects? Did you ever have a heart attack, shortness of breath, easily fatigued, chest pains, heart surgery, insertion of a pacemaker or defibrillator, swollen ankles, or palpitations? Is your fatigue, shortness of breath, or chest pain getting worse? Have you ever been told to take antibiotics before dental or medical treatments?"

- *Respiratory system*—"Have you ever had difficulty breathing, sinus problems, or told you have emphysema, asthma, or TB exposure? Do you need more than one pillow to sleep on at night or do you wake up choking or gasping for air?"

- *Allergies*—"Are you allergic to any medicines, codeine, aspirins, local anesthetics in the dental office, or antibiotics? Ever have any past reactions while in the dental office like fainting, palpitations, or rashes, etc.?"

- *G.I and G.U.*—"Ever been told of liver problems, bleeding problems, kidney disease? Ever receive dialysis or told you had hepatitis (A, B, C, etc.) or were jaundiced?"

- *Endocrine and blood systems*—"Have you ever had any history of thyroid problems, diabetes (type 1 or type 2), hemophilia, blood transfusions, bleeding problems, or complications after a previous dental extraction?"

- *Medications*—"Have you in the last few years taken insulin, aspirin, non-prescription over-the-counter drugs, digitalis, antibiotics, blood thinners, antihistamines, high blood pressure or any other heart medicines, birth control pills, or steroids?"
- *Treatments*—"Have you ever received radiation treatments to the head, neck, or any region, cancer chemotherapy, operations, or insertion of something "fake" into your heart, arms, legs, or hips? Ever been treated for fainting spells, blurred vision, stroke, temporomandibular joint (TMJ) problems, endocarditis or an infection of your heart, arthritis, painful swollen joints, high or low blood pressure, or seizures? Are you pregnant, breast feeding, had a large weight loss or weight gain recently?"
- Do you have any conditions that were not mentioned on the health history or that we didn't discuss?

Any positive responses could lead to a discussion and an undisclosed illness. It may also help the patient recall an incident from his/her past medical history that he/she may have forgotten. By mentioning symptoms, the patient might reveal a condition requiring a medical evaluation prior to treatment that could pose a possible problem if we initiated treatment.

Abbreviated Vital Signs

If you do not know the patient's blood pressure when he/she arrives at your office for treatment, you will have difficulty assessing his/her needs if emergency medical treatment is required. For example, if a patient goes into a syncopal (fainting) episode while in your office and you immediately take his/her blood pressure, are you concerned if it is 70 systolic over 50 diastolic? You should not be if he/she has a history of low blood pressure and it is always around 100 systolic over 65 diastolic. But you should be quite concerned if he/she arrives at 210 systolic over 105 diastolic, and after you gave them a local anesthetic injection containing epinephrine he/she passed out and now has a recorded blood pressure of 70 over 50!

Other vital signs such as temperature (infection, etc.), heart rate and rhythm (regular or irregular, etc.), and respirations (number, depth, etc.) are also important, but unless you have specific advanced training, blood pressure should be your most important initial vital sign.

Technology has advanced to a level where you can purchase a reliable automatic blood pressure device for your office at a cost of about $125.00. For accuracy, periodically it can be compared to a manual sphygmomanometer. It is recommended that you place one in your reception area and one in your treatment room.

When a patient arrives for an appointment, your receptionist welcomes and invites him/her into the reception area where, privately, his/her pressure is taken and recorded. As an alternative, the pressure could be taken and recorded upon being seated in the treatment room. This should be done in the dentist's treatment room as well as the hygienist's treatment room.

My personal classification of blood pressures is:

Normal – up to	$\dfrac{139}{89}$
Mild hypertension	$\dfrac{140\text{-}159}{90\text{-}94}$
Moderate hypertension	$\dfrac{160\text{-}199}{95\text{-}99}$

Patients who have blood pressures of 200/100 or greater (either a systolic pressure of 200 or greater, or a 100 diastolic pressure of 100 or greater) have their treatments deferred until we receive a medical consult and clearance. The recordings in each category are relative, since the dental office environment has a tendency to produce an increased blood pressure in many patients. Blood pressures are repeated multiple times in cases where the patient is very nervous and the result is unusually high. But if either the systolic pressure is above 200 or the diastolic pressure is above 100, we defer treatment that day. We will refer to these values again in the "treatment modifications" section.

We also have thermometers in the office when patients have infections and are running temperatures. Odontogenic infections requiring emergency treatments should be referred to the oral surgeon when the temperature is above 101°F.

Non-Invasive Physical Examination

In this section, we use our eyes to carefully observe the patient. Watch the patient walking towards your operatory. Is he/she walking briskly and strong, or does he/she appear weak, walking slowly with assistance? Does he/she need a walker or cane indicating a possible orthopedic, neurological, or circulatory problem? Shake hands and greet your patient. Are his/her hands firm and dry or weak and clammy, indicating a possible syncopal episode brewing? Is he/she out of breath from walking from the waiting room, indicating pulmonary or cardiac problems? If you found the patient already in your chair and ready for treatment, just consider what health problems you can miss.

Now that the patient is in your chair and you are reviewing the signed health history, supplementing it with your dialog/inquiry history and reviewing the patient's abbreviated vital signs, simultaneously look at (examine) him/her carefully from "head to toe." Look for signs of irregular hair loss from radiation treatments or anti-cancer medications. Observe facial asymmetries such as scars, muscle weaknesses, or involuntary movements. Are the pupils of his/her eyes equally round and reactive to the operatory light? Is a ptosis present in the lids? Are the eyes bulging and hands trembling as in hyperthyroid disorders? Are the eyes red, inflamed, and dry from a secretory disturbance? Is the skin pale, indicating anemia, or yellow and jaundiced, indicating hepatitis? Are the neck veins bulging and distended or the face red from hypertension? Is the patient barrel-chested, indicating chronic obstructive pulmonary disease? Are his/her lips and nail beds blue, or is he/she breathing with difficulty, signaling cardiopulmonary dysfunction? Are the fingers deformed from severe arthritis indicating the patient might be on high doses of aspirin and has a potential for a bleeding complication? Are the ankles swollen from heart failure? Do you find bruises indicating the patient is taking blood thinners?

Many medical signs and associated symptoms can be observed if you take the time and effort to look at the patient while he/she is in your operatory chair before commencing treatment. Many of these findings can then be used to expand the discussion in the dialog/inquiry history.

ASA Physical Status Classification System

In 1962, the American Society of Anesthesiologists (ASA) developed a physical classification system to categorize patients scheduled for surgery, according to their medical risk. The system has evolved into a way to classify a patient's risk regardless if he/she is having general anesthesia, IV sedation, or simply local anesthesia. The classifications can be modified and applied in dentistry as follows:

Classification	Description
ASA 1	A normal healthy patient with no positive findings on the health history, dialog/inquiry history, abbreviated vital signs, or chair side physical examination, blood pressure consisting of a systolic up to 139 and a diastolic up to 89
ASA 2	A patient with a mild to moderate systemic disease under control and not life threatening. Examples are mildly elevated blood pressure controlled with medication, 140-159 over 90-94; type 2 diabetes controlled with diet or oral medication; first two trimesters of pregnancy; asthmatic patient who uses an oral spray occasionally; seizure disorder patient under control with medica-

tion; a stable angina patient who has no symptoms unless subjected to a large exertion or emotional situation; extreme anxiety patient who has a history of syncopal episodes in the dental office; patients who have suffered a heart attack more than six months ago but have no symptoms and have returned to normal activity; and, patients over the age of 65.

ASA 3   A patient with a severe systemic condition limiting his/her activity, but is not incapacitating. It could be life threatening if not given special consideration. Examples are type 1 diabetics who are insulin controlled; frequent angina attacks; shortness of breath, chest pain, or fatigue with minimal exertion or stress; blood pressure of 160-194 over 95-99; last trimester of pregnancy where the patient is compromised in certain positions and uncomfortable, hindering venous return; compromised patients with chronic obstructive pulmonary disease including chronic bronchitis or emphysema; swollen ankles; frequent asthmatic attacks or seizures; and patients who have suffered a heart attack more than six months ago, but still have symptoms, *i.e.*, angina, shortness of breath, fatigue, etc.

ASA 4   A patient with a severe systemic disease limiting his/her daily activity and is a constant threat to his/her life. It includes the patient who has chest pains or shortness of breath while sitting in a chair with no activity; the patient who awakes during the night with chest pains or shortness of breath; patients with angina that is getting worse and requires increased doses of medications; patients brought to your office wearing a nose piece and receiving oxygen indicating no cardiac reserve; a patient who has had a heart attack or cerebral vascular accident (stroke) within the last six months, and a blood pressure where the systolic pressure is over 200 or the diastolic pressure is over 100.

Treatment Modifications

After collecting all of the data on your patient, one must decide if the patient is healthy enough to withstand dental treatment. Are there any questions concerning the patient's medical condition that you don't understand? Are you familiar with all of his/her medications and their intended use? Do you need additional information? Will the patient require antibiotic premedication as suggested by the American Heart Association and the American Dental Association recommendations? Calling the patient's physician usually answers most of your questions and also provides suggestions that aid in your treatment. The physician is consulted to aid in determining if a patient can tolerate specific dental procedures, learn any new information about the patient, and assist in determining what treatment modifications are necessary, including pre-medications. The dentist must be able to evaluate all of the available information, as the chance of a medical emergency occurring in the dental office increases as the quantity and severity of the patient's medical conditions increase. All information gleaned from this conversation is then entered on your chart with the physician's name, date, telephone number, and suggestions offered. The end result of this exercise should be to decrease the risk of the patient having an acute episode in the office while under your care.

The ASA categories add additional information to your decisions. ASA 1 patients are healthy and require no modifications to their treatment plan. The ASA 2 patient is under control and if he/she follows a prescribed regimen usually requires no additional modifications. The ASA 3 patient routinely requires consultation, review, and treatment modifications. He/she is moderately medically compromised and cannot withstand many of the dental office stresses.

The ASA 4 patient is so severely medially compromised that he/she should only be treated in a controlled environment of a hospital dental setting. His/her cardiac and systemic reserve is so depleted that you cannot provide dentistry and be prepared for any unusual occurrence that has a good chance of happening. It is not that the quality of dentistry performed in the hospital setting will be improved. This environment ensures that your patient will be adequately attended to if he/she has a medical emergency during dental treatment. An entire department of emergency physicians is available and can provide the immediate assistance needed to treat any unexpected event. Prior consultation and preparation also add solutions to any liability problems should they arise.

Treatment is also deferred for six months following a heart attack or coronary bypass operation. A high percentage of patients who have suffered a heart attack have a second one within six months without even going to the dental office. Coronary bypass patients have occurrences of arrythmias for six months following their surgical procedures that could prove disastrous with the use of local anesthetics and the stress of the dental office.

The American Dental Association in 1997 published new guidelines for the prevention of bacterial endocarditis.[3] After consultation with the patient's physician and determining the cardiac problem, the dentist should be able to dispense oral medications as recommended. Dentists are referred to this important publication to learn the cardiac conditions described and medications and doses recommended. In addition, the American Dental Association in 1997 published guidelines for the antibiotic recommendations for the dental patient with a total joint replacement. Both references are included for additional information.[4]

Some treatment modifications suggested include short appointments, oral sedation, nitrous oxide and oxygen analgesia supplementation, decreased vasoconstrictor in their local anesthetics, early morning appointments before the patient becomes fatigued, premedication with his/her own emergency medications, positioning the patient to avoid syncope, and lastly, most important, profound local anesthesia to ensure that the patient is not stimulated with any painful stimuli.[5] Drugs used by the patient (asthma inhaler, nitroglycerine, etc.) are placed on the bracket table in full view, which tends to offer confidence to the patient worried about a medical emergency being precipitated. This helps to decrease the amount of stress we place on our patients so we can treat them and accomplish our care with minimal risk of a medical emergency.

The amount of written material tends to increase rapidly in a patient's chart. Repeated health forms, procedural documentation, x-rays, pictures, consultations, dental laboratory orders, insurance forms, etc. increase with every visit. Going through all of this material every time the patient seeks treatment can be quite time consuming. Figure 1-2 is an example of a fictitious patient. All of the pertinent medical problems, allergies, premedications, ASA classification, etc., are written on the front of the chart. This serves many purposes. When a patient calls the office for an appointment, your front desk person can identify the special needs of the patient and immediately ask you for special instructions for the patient. When the patient reports for hygiene care, your hygienist can identify and make any appropriate changes to the normal treatment plan. It also allows the practitioner to immediately be aware of the patient's pertinent medical conditions, discuss any changes when he/she arrives in the office, and then make any appropriate changes for treatment. This allows for immediate identification of potential problems and attending to possible solutions to avoid any precipitated emergencies. With the medical information on the front of the chart, the staff must be aware of the confidentiality and sensitivity of the information and the need to ensure that all of the information is protected.

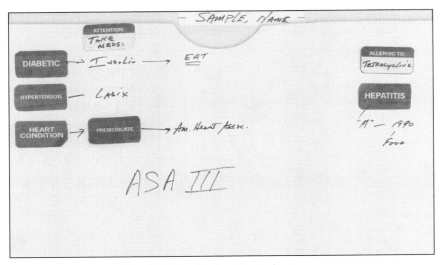

Fig. 1-2 Sample of patient's chart cover

These six steps enable the dental practitioner to decide who to treat, who needs a medical consultation before treatment, who needs a modified appointment, and who should be treated in a controlled hospital environment. More detailed information is available in textbooks and articles, specifically focusing on the treatment of the medically compromised patient.

Notes

[1] Donoff, R.B. *Massachusetts General Hospital Manual of Oral and Maxillofacial Surgery*, 3rd ed., St. Louis: Mosby, 1996

[2] Malamed, S.F., et al. *Medical Emergencies in the Dental Office*, 5th ed., St. Louis: Mosby, 1999

[3] DaJani, A.S., et al. Prevention of Bacterial Endocarditis; Recommendations by the American Heart Association, *JADA* 128(8), 1997, pp. 1,142-1,151

[4] American Dental Association, American Academy of Orthopaedic Surgeons: Advisory Statement; Antibiotic Prophylaxis for Dental Patients with Total Joint Replacement, *JADA* 128(7), 1997, pp. 1,004-1,008

[5] Edwab, R.R. When to Modify Treatment Plans, *Dentistry Today* 17(11), 1998, pp. 106-107

[6] Chestnutt, I.G. and Gibson, J., eds. *Churchill's Pocketbook of Clinical Dentistry*, 1st ed., London: Churchill Livingstone, 1998

Chapter 2

Making Dentistry Productive

By Joseph A. Blaes, D.D.S.

The future of dentistry belongs to those who make the most efficient use of their clinical time. You must organize your practice with highly structured, effective systems that simplify the workplace and consistently produce a quality product at a low level of stress.

The purpose of this chapter is to introduce the reader to five keys that can help organize the clinical portion of the dental practice by introducing systems. Many practices have written policies to help everyone understand the underlying principles of the office. However, if these policies are not backed up with systems, the day-to-day operation of the office suffers.

Systems are the oil that keeps the practice running smoothly day in and day out. Look at it this way, every practice has a financial policy, but few have taken the time to work out the systems needed to implement it. Systems are the written how-to-do-it instructions for the implementation of the policy. It is easy to say that your practice is insurance free, but how does the staff present that to the patients? It had better be in a very consistent manner or you will have a lot of patients leaving the practice. I cannot over-emphasize the power of systems. Within the five keys are a number of systems.

The five keys to a successful practice are:

- Communication skills
- Strong team
- New patient process
- Active hygiene program
- Great scheduling system

Communication Skills

Let's start with what I feel is the keystone of all great practices—communication. Through the years as I built my practice, I was always amazed at how inept I was at talking to the person that we call patient. I have tried every sales trick in the book, thinking that these techniques would help me get my patients to accept more dentistry. But, in the long run, they did not impact my practice as I thought they would.

I am an innovator and picture myself as one who changes quickly when I can see a new path. I must tell you that I did not catch on quickly to the need for being a great communicator. My "ah ha" experience occurred when I met Terry Goss. Terry is a master trainer of Neuro Linguistic Programming or NLP for short. She was able to teach my team this wonderful method of communicating with our patients and all the techniques that went with it. Soon the techniques become second nature, and you use them all the time to quickly get into rapport with your patients. I still use them to this day unconsciously when I meet people.

It is a proven fact that until the person we call patient is in relationship with someone in the office, nothing significant is going to happen. I am firmly convinced that this relationship does not even have to be with me (the dentist). During my years in practice, I have observed the following scenario many times: *The patient needs some dental procedure. I spend some time with the patient explaining what needs to be done and the best way to do it. I show him/her models, x-rays, photos, slides, intra oral photos, and tell them about all the wonderful cutting edge materials I am going to use to fix the problem. I tell the patient how much it will cost and ask if there are any questions or if I can clarify anything that he/she does not understand. I get up to leave and as I am walking out of the door, I hear those familiar words being asked to someone else, "Well, what do you think?"*

How can this be? I have just given the patient my very best and yet he/she asked a clinical assistant or a hygienist whether or not he/she should proceed. Patients do this because they are in relationship with that other person and not in relationship with you. Once a trust relationship has been established, the patient will be comfortable doing important dentistry. The other problem is that we sell "piecework." We sell crowns, fillings, dentures, and root canals instead of the benefits of keeping your own teeth for the rest of your life. We need to get out of this mode and learn to communicate with people.

In order to gain information about our patients, part of our new patient process is an interview. The clinical assistant does the interview and she "seeks first to understand." This is Steven Covey's first principle from his best selling book, *Seven Habits of Highly Effective People*. In other words, she seeks to get the patient's story. That new patient was once a patient in another dental office and left. Now he/she is at your office— why? What dental experiences did he/she have in the previous office? We need some historical information.

The first question that is always asked is "What are your expectations of our office?" If you will ask this question and then just sit back and listen, the patient will tell you. Sit back and *listen*—not so easy is it? Most of us have an extremely difficult time truly listening to someone else. Usually we are trying to think of what we will say when it is our turn to impress you, and we missed everything that you said. We should learn to be a better listener. If we will simply ask more questions, we will receive more information. That is the power of questions. The more you ask, the more you will receive. Listen with an empathic or caring ear. Most people need for you to care about them.

Once you have gathered all the information, it is time to tell your story or as Covey puts it, "seek to be understood." Now is the time to tell the patient about your wonderful dental practice. Now is the time to continue building rapport with the patient. The words you use and how you say them are critically important. I am not a fan of "scripting" because it sometimes causes our conversations to be too rigid rather than spontaneous. Please don't forget the power of how you look when you say things. Body language is extremely important to the way we deliver our message.

Strong Team

Teamwork is the fuel that allows common people to attain uncommon results. Developing a great group of people to work with is a time-consuming process, but well worth it. For years, I have supported the value of all members of the dental staff. It is impossible to practice without them today. All members of the dental team should be considered equal. It is of primary importance that dentists strengthen their relationships with staff and strive for the development of a true team concept in their practices. I have developed the team concept with large and small groups of people in the dental practice. There is no ideal number, but a group of key factors do exist.

There must be a leader who is committed to both the practice and the team. The leader must be the dentist. This responsibility cannot be given to a consultant or an office manager. The year 1999 did not start off well for the St. Louis Rams. In the third preseason game, the exciting new quarterback, Trent Green, went down with a broken leg. The St. Louis fans were crushed because the backup quarterback was an unknown who had come up from the "arena football league." Coach (leader) Dick Vermel has a positive attitude and he is a great motivator. He did not hesitate in naming Kurt Warner to be his new starting quarterback, and he knew the St. Louis Rams would win with Kurt. Kurt Warner stepped up knowing this was his destiny. He became a leader on the field, set several records, and was named the NFL's Most Valuable Player that year—and the Rams won the Super Bowl. As dentists we must look into ourselves and develop that positive attitude of life so we can all be winners in this wonderful profession. In today's world of dentistry, there is not much to feel negative about.

There must be a level of trust among the members of the team. When people don't trust each other, they become suspicious of each other's intentions and will not function well together. They become a group of individuals going their own ways. If someone who is working with you has a problem with being totally honest, talks about others behind their backs, does not follow office policies and systems, or constantly criticizes the leader—it is time to find that person a new home. There must be a mutual trust between all team members, and that includes the dentist/leader.

The team members must have confidence in each other's abilities. Let's go back to the football analogy. For a quarterback to be an outstanding passer, he must have confidence that his offensive line is going to hold back the defenders while he stands in the pocket. It is this confidence that gives a quarterback the edge over other quarterbacks. Watch the great ones play, and you will see this confidence in everything they do. Likewise in the dental office, if you have a staff member who is obviously incompetent and you keep that person around because you don't like firing people, then you are undermining the ability of the other staff members to function as a team. This does not set a good example for the other members of the staff, and they will not come together as a team.

Team members must be educated and trained on a regular basis. Changes occur daily in the concepts, techniques, materials, and equipment of dentistry. Each team member must be updated continually if competence is to be maintained. In-service education and training sessions, on the job education, and off-site education courses must be planned and carried out on a routinely scheduled basis. Staff education takes time and costs money, but it pays great rewards for the team, including higher personal self-esteem, more job efficiency, and better patient care. I am continually amazed by how many dentists take continuing education courses without their team members. It is impossible to take the experience that you had in a course home to your team. There are no second-hand experiences.

In all the independent surveys on job satisfaction, knowing that we make a difference is always either first on the list or at least near the top. How can our team know that what they are doing is correct unless we tell them? Financial rewards are tangible and expected, but praise is the greatest payment of all. Praise motivates and satisfies your team members. Genuine praise for work accomplished well should come not only from the leader, but also from one staff member to another. It is important for the leader to praise each team member six times a day. This will reap benefits in team loyalty that cannot be imagined. Be careful with criticism, it can often be destructive. I do not believe that there is such a thing as "constructive" criticism. Find tactful ways to let team member know that they can improve in certain areas.

You must compensate your team at an acceptable level. Check around your area and find out what people whose education and experience are similar to those of your auxiliaries are earning in other positions. At one point in my career, I found that the checkers in the local supermarket were making more than my team members. I gave immediate raises to my team members. Very few people can continue to do excellent work without some tangible reward in addition to salary. There are a number of ways to give monetary bonuses—just be sure they are fair to everyone involved, including the leader. Other rewards include days off, extra vacation, paid continuing education, recreational gifts, parties, dinners, and staff lunches. One of the most appreciated things that I ever did for our team was a monthly team dinner at an exclusive restaurant that included their significant other. A great book on this subject is *555 Ways to Reward Your Dental Team* by Dr. Nate Booth and myself (PennWell, ISBN 0-96495-002-2).

One of the most difficult tasks for the leader can be true delegation of responsibilities to the team members. I find this very difficult, because I am such a controller. Leaders should delegate, educate their team members about the delegated tasks, and expect results. Most team members will respond with enthusiasm! Just as in my example of the football team, each of our team members has an important role in the success of the practice, and there should not be a hierarchy of importance among team members. Equality for team members should be the goal of the leader, with constant reminders about the importance of each and every person on the team. On busy clinical days, it is easy for one group of staff people to fall behind in their tasks, especially just before the end of the day. In such situations, all team members should help the group that is behind. In this way, everyone is able to leave the office together!

Some final pointers on the team:

- *No secrets*—Everyone knows what is going on at all times with the practice, including long-term plans and performance expectations
- *No whining*—Each team member must accept his/her role in every interaction and participate in solving problems
- *No politics*—Everyone is entitled to the same level of respect and opportunity. The days of playing one group against another are gone
- *No surprises*—Open the books and involve the staff in budgeting, production goals, and cost controls. The results are amazing when a team "buys in"
- *No distractions*—Leave personal problems and issues at the door, and save heart-to-heart discussions until after hours
- *No confusion*—Make sure the whole staff is familiar with equipment operations, financial procedures, and anything else important to the practice. Document internal processes and reinforce training frequently
- *No waste*—Everyone must be careful with the business' resources, including time. Little things add up to big things

The development of a great dental team can result in excellent dental care for the patients, and it can provide the dentist and the staff members with a sense of well-being, support, stability, and satisfaction that is not otherwise obtainable.

New Patient Process

The practice must have a system to introduce the new patient to the practice. This is an extremely important asset and must be nurtured and protected. We discovered that our new patient exam experience was lacking, so we embarked on a year-long quest to change that experience. This is how our new patient process began. We spent many staff meetings brainstorming on how it could be made better for the patient and for us. One of the first things we all agreed upon was that we hated to go to the doctor's office that has a little window in the wall with the sign "Please ring the bell." You ring the bell and then wait until someone slides open the window and says, "What do you want?" When she finds out, she pushes a clipboard to you with some papers attached and says, "Fill these out!" We decided that we would have no windows, no little sliding doors, no clipboards, and no papers to fill out!

Our new patient process begins when the patient calls the office for the first time. Whoever takes that call is trained to follow the process. We thank the person for choosing our office and tell him/her that we look forward to meeting him/her. We ask if he/she is having any type of dental problem that requires immediate treatment and schedule accordingly. Since we pre-block our appointment book, we can always appoint a new patient in a week to 10 days. We ask for the name of the person calling and a phone number where we can reach him/her during the day or night. We ask if he/she has any other questions and then say we are looking forward to meeting him/her at the appointed time. Our main goal is to get the new person into our office to experience our team and the office. We cannot project this over the phone! Get them into the office!

During the morning huddle, we assign a clinical assistant to the new patient. If another patient referred this new person, then we assign that patient's clinical assistant, who will already have something in common with that new person. When the person arrives at the appointed time, they are greeted by name and told that Barb (the assigned clinical assistant) will be with them in just a few minutes. Barb comes into the reception area and introduces herself to the new person and makes reference to the referring patient in that introduction. Her main task is to be friendly and supportive of the new patient so he/she will feel welcome and at home. She escorts the new person to the treatment room (it could be a conference room if you have one) and seats him/her in the chair without a bib. She seats herself comfortably next to the patient and adjusts only the height of the chair to assure that both her eyes and the patient's eyes are on the same level.

Barb now begins the most important part of our new patient process—the new patient interview. The purpose is to gain information AND build rapport! Barb begins by asking the new person why he/she chose our office and what his/her expectations are of us. Now Barb uses her listening skills to gain an insight into why this patient is here. She probes to get the information that she needs. During this interview, Barb will get a dental history, a medical history including allergies, drugs being taken, etc. We find that we get more information by asking the questions than by the patient filling out the typical questionnaire. Barb also uses this interview time to begin to build rapport with this new person. The desired outcome here is to bond with this new person and start building a relationship.

This "relationship" is the most important step in our office. It has been shown by many psychologists that this person we call "patient" must establish a relationship with someone in the office before we try to "sell" him/her anything. I know that many dentists think that the relationship must be with him/her, but in most offices the strong relationship is probably with someone else. Remember the "Well, what do you think?" scenario? Knowing this, we start by consciously trying to build a relationship during the interview session. Barb will then become this patient's clinical assistant. Barb will be with the patient whenever he/she visits the office. This person is not my patient; he/she is Barb's patient.

If this during the interview, the patient expresses concern about a particular dental problem, I want Barb to pick up a mouth mirror and take a look at the area of the mouth. The intention here is not to diagnose, but simply to observe and talk to the patient about possible options. At this time Barb begins to plant "seeds" in the patient's mind about the possibilities of treatment to correct a problem. This is a relaxed time for the patient. Barb is trained in techniques that help the patient realize he/she is in the right place. When Barb feels that the time is right, she will excuse herself by telling the patient that she feels it is time for him/her to meet the dentist.

Barb finds me and I disconnect from whatever I am doing. This is an extremely important time, and I need to be totally focused on the information that Barb is about to pass on to me. In two to three minutes, Barb will summarize all the information that she has received from the new person. I will interrupt only for clarification. With that completed, we return to the patient and Barb introduces me. I sit down so that I have eye to eye contact and begin with some small talk. I then invite Barb to tell me what she has observed about this patient. Her observations will not be all about dentistry but will also include the patient's expectations, hobbies, likes and dislikes, and the like. Barb is using her relationship with this new person to help him/her become comfortable with me before I invade his/her comfort zone or touch him/her.

Once I feel that the patient is comfortable with me, I begin my clinical examination. As I examine the patient's mouth, Barb will tell me about any of her observations as well as possible solutions. I want the patient to know that Barb is a trusted ally and that we work together as a team. We will talk about my clinical findings in patient language across the patient and answer any questions as they arise. I do not think it is necessary for me to describe the clinical examination in minute detail, because you all know how to do one. We take lots of photos to use later in our treatment conference. My part of the exam usually does not last more than 10 to 15 minutes. I finish by telling Barb what other diagnostic materials we need, and then I tell the patient that I will look at all the information we gathered today including his/her preferences and expectations, putting together a treatment plan that will save his/her teeth for the rest of his/her life.

Barb finishes by getting whatever diagnostic materials we need and by answering any further questions the new patient might have about anything that was said or has happened during the process of introducing him/her to the practice. Barb will go to the computer in the treatment room and make the next appointment for the patient. She will give the patient her business card with instructions to call her if there are any questions.

Our goal in treatment planning is to tell the patient about the conditions present in his or her mouth today and which of these conditions threatens the balance of good oral health. Barb and I plan the treatment necessary to correct these conditions together. Barb has seen and heard things that I have not, and the reverse is true. Two heads are better than one. Generally, dentistry can be planned and does not have to be done all at one time. I am a great advocate of quadrant dentistry and present this concept to the patient. It is great to have a number of patients with a number of quadrants stored in our "bank." Start time on these quadrants may be controlled by the calendar, by insurance payments, by money, or whatever.

During the next appointment, Barb and I will have a treatment conference with the new patient. I talk about the conditions present and the benefits to the patient in correcting these conditions. I do not specifically talk about materials (except in a case with allergy problems) during the conference. I try to sell the sizzle and not the steak. I feel that we have been selling piecemeal products (crowns, fillings, and dentures) for too many years. We need to break out of that box and talk about how doing dentistry will benefit the patient! I will quote the fee and then ask if the patient has any further questions. Usually, they don't. They will ask Barb. The financial coordinator then comes in to show the patient how he/she can afford this fine dentistry. It is extremely important that you have several ways to help the patient afford your dentistry. Care Credit and Dental Fee Plan are two great patient finance companies. Once the financial arrangements have been agreed upon, the clinical appointment is made.

I am not going to tell you that my acceptance rate is 100%—you wouldn't believe it anyway! But I have found that this "relationship selling" has greatly increased the number of patients that say yes! Probably the number one reason that people turn down treatment is money. Perhaps they don't perceive value in what you have recommended. Perhaps they have five kids in college and just can't afford it right now. Perhaps they are totally insurance driven and you need to find them a new home. We can work with insurance as long as the patients understand that their insurance plan should not dictate the type of care. The point is that sometimes dentistry has to be delayed. I put my patients in a holding program to maintain what they have. If some teeth are broken down, I will place temporary crowns. I can make temporary crowns with materials available today that will last years instead of a few months. Tight financial situations are going to change, and I want that patient to be in my practice when he/she is ready to proceed with the treatment I have outlined for him/her.

I mentioned before that many of my patients choose to restore their teeth a quadrant at a time. If this is the case, it is important to have some type of tracking system that will remind the staff that it is time to treat the next quadrant. Most often, this reminder is presented in the hygiene department.

In order to have stress-free days in your practice, follow the treatment plans that you have outlined. Your clinical staff has set up the treatment room for a certain procedure. If you change this procedure, then, in all likelihood, a new setup will be necessary. According to your clinical staff, this is a number one cause of stress in the office.

Active Hygiene Program

I have never seen a successful dental practice without an effective hygiene department. In order for this to happen, we have to quit low-balling hygiene fees and running the hygiene program as a "loss leader!" The hygiene area should be as carefully monitored as your entire practice. In your computer system, set up your hygienists as providers and carefully track their production and expenses. Set your fees so that your patients will value the hygiene service. Begin this by breaking out your hygiene fees instead of lumping your entire hygiene visit under one fee. Your hygiene department will quickly become the profit center that it should be.

One of the biggest problems in hygiene is staying on time. The first step to solving this problem is to improve your scheduling system. Go to a 10-minute scheduler rather than a 15-minute scheduler. This allows for greater freedom in scheduling the hygiene visits, particularly when you have implemented a perio-driven hygiene department. Keeping the hygiene schedule on time requires timely checks by the doctor. Nothing can frustrate the hygienist and the patient more than waiting for the doctor to come to do his/her part of the visit. One of the hardest things that I must do in the office is to break away from what I am doing clinically to check a hygiene patient. It is very hard for me to quickly change hats and focus on another patient when my mind is still back in the treatment room deciding what I will do next on my clinical case.

The hygienist's dilemma is different. She knows that if she finds too many problems, the doctor will spend an inordinate amount of time presenting dentistry to that patient, resulting in a schedule problem. I have solved that in my practice by allowing the hygienist to reschedule a patient who requires more than a simple filling or a single crown. When I sit down to check that patient, the hygienist will present her findings and concerns. I will ask a few questions for clarification and check some of the areas that she is concerned with. I will then sit the patient up, look them in the eye and say, "Jim, during your visit today, Pam has observed a number of areas that we are concerned about. I need to put you in my schedule so that I can diagnose some of these conditions, and, together, you and I can discuss the treatment options, keeping in mind that our goal is for you to keep your teeth the rest of your life." I have never had a patient say no to this. Jim is then scheduled with me, and basically we put him through the new patient process and co-develop a treatment plan for him. Our hygienists love this process, which we have developed to help them to stay on time.

Why is it that the hygienists always seem to get the hand-me-down equipment? Why is it that they are told to "make do" with this or that? There are some great new pieces of equipment in the hygiene market today that can enhance your practice and help your hygienists to be more effective and efficient. Things like the Diagnodent from Kavo, Seal & Protect from Dentsply Caulk, pezioelectric scaler from Pro-Dentec, SE Bond from Kuraray, and the great lightweight disposable prophy hand pieces from Preventech. So keep your hygiene equipment up to date. Another area to check—be sure that your hygienists have enough instruments so that they are not waiting around for the bell to ring on the autoclave. What a time waster that is!

I feel that it is important to start a periodontal therapy program in your hygiene department. This is key to helping your patients keep their teeth for the rest of their lives. Just remember that some of your patients will leave the practice simply because they only want to have their teeth cleaned. They don't want to have their gums stuck! However, that exodus will free up some time in your hygiene schedule so that you can begin scheduling in patients for periodontal therapy. This includes root planing and scaling, treatment with the new antimicrobial therapies, and laser treatment. Don't forget to follow these patients closely and to stress the importance of restorative dentistry in the recovery of gingival tissues.

Teach your hygienists to observe and to educate their patients about the options that are available today in restorative dentistry. Be certain that your hygienists are aware of all the possibilities that are available today. Show them the cases that you are treating, both before and after. I want my hygienists to present and sell undone dentistry. That's all those "watches" that are in your patients records. Many of you are "file cabinet" millionaires. In terms of numbers, I expect two things from my hygienists:

- I want 30% of the practice production to come from hygiene
- I want my hygienists to be referring 35% of my production from the hygiene department

That means that I want them to be able to sell dentistry. This needs to be a team effort!

Great Scheduling System

Time management is the heartbeat of the practice, and scheduling is nothing more than managing your time effectively! It is important for you to recognize time as a commodity that cannot be restored. Scheduling problems are probably the cause of more stress in the dental office than any other one thing. When times for appointments are set by somebody's guesstimate, everyone in the office is upset! The back blames the front, and the lines of battle are drawn. It is impossible to please everyone since our patients know when they want to come in, the clinical assistants have another idea, and the doctor probably has his/her opinions as well. If the hygienist is working on commission, she can be extremely frustrated if she is unable to complete procedures because not enough time was allotted.

We are all looking for a number of things when it comes to scheduling. Does anybody have an "ideal" scheduler out there? There are some great ones, but we could never find software that had everything. Oh, you don't schedule on a computer? Then you can design your own scheduler. For years we had our personalized appointment book pages that we had designed printed by a local printer. If you have computer software with a scheduler, then you have probably had to compromise something because none of them have everything that I want. The main benefit of a great scheduler is a stress-free practice where everyone enjoys coming to the office to work. Side benefits include profitability, effective and efficient use of time, much better service to your patients, and I believe that it allows us to do a higher quality of dentistry.

Good scheduling requires a good system. Set up a system to streamline the clinical side of your practice. This is easily said, but is a big undertaking. I'm talking about looking at everything you do in your treatment rooms and brainstorming with your clinical staff on how to make it better. I'll illustrate with another story. In my practice, we started on this course a few years ago when my clinical assistants rebelled because we had so many dental instruments. Years ago, we had begun using the cassette systems for our instruments. We had eight cassettes for eight different procedures, all with different color codes and with every instrument color-coded. Each cassette contained an average of 24 instruments. We were out of control.

At a Friday staff meeting, my clinical assistants brought all of the instruments and set them on the table. When we finished the regular business of the day, the three of us met over the instruments. Here was their plan—they would open an individual cassette, lay out all of the instruments and pick them up one at a time and hand them to me. I had 15 seconds to look at the instrument and tell them what I used it for. If I couldn't, they took that instrument out of the cassette. By the end of the day, we had reduced the number of cassettes to four and the average instruments to 15. We did this exercise four more times during the year and were able to come up with one cassette of 14 instruments that I can use for any procedure. No more color-coding. No more searching for instruments. We have simplified the instrument systems in our office and we love it! After our first success, we began looking for other areas that we could improve. That's what I would urge you to do in your practice.

Do you know how long it takes you to prep a single crown? Do you usually prep it in that amount of time, or do you often run over or have time left over? Who decided how long it takes you to prep a crown? Did anyone ever time 10 single crowns and then average the time it took? Does it take you longer to prep a molar crown than a bicuspid? What if you need a buildup? What if you were able to do quadrants? More time or less time? You should be able to answer these questions and so should everyone on your staff. Now come up with times for all the procedures that you do in the office. Do the same for the hygienists.

Most dentists set goals in their offices, but sometimes they are unrealistic. It is discouraging for the staff if the goals are set so high that they are never reached. In our practice, we set an hourly goal simply because the hours that we work per day vary. So, it is easier simply to multiply our hourly goal to get the goal for that particular day. Now, if we have set our goal at $150.00 per hour and we are working 10 hours, then our daily goal for that day is $1,500.00. You must monitor your production and collection daily, because they tend to vary. For instance, if we produced $1,000.00 on the day I just described, then we were $500.00 under goal. Tomorrow, our hourly goal will have to be higher in order to make up the difference for the month. This is something that should be reported at the morning huddle so that every one is aware. The huddle is also the time to discuss what the team can do to help improve the day. If everyone is engaged in this process, many times a slight adjustment can be made in the schedule that can make the day easier for everyone.

Please don't just fill the appointment book! Put appointments in certain time slots for a reason. Determine when you are at your best. If you don't know, ask your team—they do! I am a morning person. We start early in the morning because I want to have my daily goal done by one o'clock when we go to lunch. I want the afternoon to be easy—some new patient exams, treatment conferences, a denture adjustment, or maybe some occlusal composites. Not too long after we had put this system into place, we all experienced a terrific day. On a Tuesday by noon, we had produced close to $10,000.00 and the afternoon was easy so we all walked out the door together on time with high fives all around. We had set a record one-day production total with no stress, and we all had a good time doing it.

The following Friday, a team meeting was scheduled with a full agenda. We were so excited about what had happened Tuesday that we agreed to set the agenda aside while we discussed what happened and why. We totally dissected the day. We had some great patients who really valued what we were doing for them. We had some people that we really liked. We had selected cases that were a challenge and because we had prepared for them, we actually finished ahead of schedule. In every case, we had paid attention to the details and it paid off. Everyone was very focused that day with no outside problems causing us to forget our purpose. Someone threw out a challenge. Hey, we were able to do this once—can we do it again? Yes! We answered as a group! So, we decided to model on what we now call "perfect day," and soon we were having one or two of them a month. Now we have one or two a week.

Have you ever had a perfect day? I hope so! I know from experience that if you have had one, you can certainly model to have more. Dr. Omer Reed was fond of saying, "If its already been done, it's probably possible." If your teams "buys in" to the concept of a perfect day, then begin by brainstorming what you enjoy doing the most. That should be the type of case you focus on first. I hope that you all understand the process of "brainstorming." I will give a quick explanation here and if you are interested, there are some great resources to help you to implement the process. Brainstorming is a process to let ideas surface in an open environment. Someone is designated as secretary to record the ideas—preferably on a flip chart. Everyone begins giving their ideas no matter how crazy, because no ideas are wrong—the quicker the better and no one is limited to a certain number. Keep going until there are no more. Go back and discuss each idea. Talk about how it could be implemented. Some will stay; some will go by mutual consent. It's fun and amazing how many great ideas come out of this process.

One of the first objections to perfect day is that there is no room in the appointment book! The keeper of the book generally voices this opinion. She is probably right! The solution to this dilemma is to preblock time in the appointment book for the types of procedures you have decided to do. This time is set aside for these procedures only, and it must be protected from poachers who would steal time for their own purposes—like squeezing in Mary Smith for a two-surface composite. These time slots must be respected, or you will be right back where you started. So, what happens if you look ahead to next week, and there are all these blocks of time with nobody in them? You must set a time limit on holding the blocks open. That time limit varies by practice, but it depends on how long it takes the appointment book person to fill the time that is open. If that is one week, then one week is the time limit. If it takes three days, then three days is the cut off point. Each practice will be different. Start off with one day a week, and when you can easily fill that one day with great cases, preblock another day per week. You will be surprised how quickly your system will reap results.

In my perfect day scenario, I do not want to do any heavy-duty procedures in the afternoon. So, we no longer do crowns in the afternoon. Since I perceive cementing veneers to be a heavy-duty procedure, none of those either. I will seat a single crown in the afternoon since that is pretty straightforward and easy. My patients were accustomed to coming most any time. Now the team had to turn them around. My team has been with me for a number of years, so they know me well. One clinical assistant has been with me for 20 years, another for 15, and my hygienist for 12. They can look a patient right in the eye and tell them something like; "We have known Dr. Blaes for a long time. We have seen him at his best and sometimes at his worst. He comes in to the office in the morning ready to get to work. It is interesting that the very best work that he has ever done is done in the morning. Yes, the most beautiful cases are definitely done in the morning. Now would you like to have a morning or an afternoon appointment?"

You may be chuckling at this story, but this is the script that we used to let the patients know that we no longer even considered doing that kind of procedure in the afternoon. In a fairly short time, we had won over our patients to a whole new system of scheduling. Take some time to brainstorm the objections, and then put together some scripts to answer those objections. In a few weeks, the scripts become part of everyone's vocabulary, and they don't seem like a foreign language anymore. The team then becomes enthusiastic and confident with the new system. When questions are answered with enthusiasm and confidence, it is tough to argue or object.

The last piece of the scheduling puzzle is the emergency patient. I am sure that I have tried every emergency system that has ever been presented. Then we came up with our own. This is how it works. We have cross trained everyone in the office to be able to get the needed information on the emergency patient. After all, most emergencies are not rocket science, since the patient usually is able to tell you enough symptoms to diagnose the case. When the patient calls with a toothache, whoever answers the phone says, "I am sorry you are experiencing a problem, how soon can you be here?" This is a screening question. If it is Monday and the patient answers that he/she can make it in on Thursday afternoon—that is not an emergency. However, it is a different story if he/she can be there in 15 minutes. This is the true emergency. The person answering the phone then gives the caller some important information. "We are going to work you into our busy schedule this morning, and you may have to wait for a treatment room to become available. However, we will do whatever is needed to get you comfortable before you leave." We have told the caller two things—he/she may have to wait and he/she will be comfortable.

When the patient arrives, the first available member of the team will get him/her into the first available treatment room. Then the team member begins to gather the information needed to find out the cause of the problem. X-rays are taken and processed, diagnostic tests are performed. If it is an obvious root canal, our endodontist is called and an emergency time is arranged for the patient. The team member comes to me with the information and her observations. I go to the patient and confirm the diagnosis and the proposed treatment. At this time, we only perform palliative treatment. Remember our promise was to get the patient comfortable. If a cusp has broken off, the assistant can replace it with some composite material very quickly and easily. (Composite is our temporary material of choice.) This is the time to restrain the dentist to keep him/her from trying to do more for the patient on this visit. Many dentists want to do the full treatment. Don't let them! Always reappoint the emergency patient for further treatment even if you have had a cancellation and have the time. My experience is that these are the cases that never go the way you expect, and you ruin the day's schedule by squeezing this patient in. This causes stress between you and the rest of the team, because you then throw the whole office off schedule, including the hygienist.

If the emergency was a patient of record who is fully restored and making regular hygiene visits, he/she can usually be reappointed for the procedure. If he/she is a patient of record who has ignored your treatment recommendations, then he/she is reappointed into the new patient process so that his/her mouth can be reevaluated and a new treatment plan presented. If it is a new patient emergency, then certainly we want that patient appointed for the new patient process. This emergency system has worked extremely well for us for a number of years.

The key to scheduling is for everybody in the practice to support the scheduling system. This means that the doctor, in particular, should stay out of the process. My experience has been that I was always trying to please the patient and putting him/her anywhere in the schedule. That way, I was always Mr. Nice Guy! Doctor, keep your hands out of the appointment book. Trust your team to do the job that you have delegated to them.

The Pivotal Role of the Clinical Assistant

By incorporating these five keys into your practice, you will begin to see a practice that you never thought was possible. Expect a practice where everyone pulls together for a common cause. There was a reason why communication was in the leadoff position—it is simply the most important player. Without a great understanding of the way we use words, you and your team are doomed to failure. So, do whatever it takes to learn great communication skills. A good place to learn is to take a course form Sandy Roth, Terry Goss, or Dr. Paul Homoly. They are all excellent teachers of the skills you need to both communicate and relate with the people that we all call patients.

The clinical assistant is my favorite person in the office. She, more than any other one person, has her finger on the pulse of the practice. She knows what is happening in the dental office, and why. If the doctor is behind, she knows the source of the problem. If the doctor is in a bad mood, who is the first to know? If the patient is uncooperative, she probably could have told you it would happen. If the impression material doesn't deliver an excellent impression, who's to blame? You guessed it: One of the most misunderstood, unappreciated, under-rated, under-utilized, and underpaid people in the dental practice.

In more than 35 years of dental practice, I have made many mistakes along the way. But I quickly learned that the person who sits across from me at the dental chair is the most important person in the dental practice. I learned that I could either do it all by myself or I could have a highly trained person at the chair. I chose to have the partner. Over the years, I have had many fine clinical assistants. Two of the best were Barb Lammert and Rhonda Hunt. These two people have helped me to fulfill my vision and I could not have done it without them.

Traditionally, the dental chairside assistant has been little more than a "go-for" and a "spit-sucker." She is quite often hired with no training and receives limited training in the office. The training usually consists of watching the other "girls" and being told by them what is expected of them. So, the new "girl" is expected to rise to the same level of mediocrity that already exists. Without any formal training or positive feedback or performance reviews, she rather quickly reaches that level. Based on her own self-esteem and self-motivation, she will both quickly discover she is in the wrong place and quit, or she will last a couple of years and finally become burned out and will quit or be fired. Many years ago, Avrom King described this person and aptly named her a "twit." Twits are usually attractive young people who are easily controlled, have low self-esteem, and can be hired at a low salary.

In every successful dental office that I have surveyed or visited or met at a seminar, I have found a highly motivated and committed group of people that I would call a "team." The leader of the team must be the dentist who has a vision that has been shared with that group of people. Everyone has "bought" into that vision and is motivated by it. The size of the group depends very much on the vision, and the number can vary significantly. There are no twits on these teams. These people are all self-starters and are willing to accept responsibility, be accountable, and the leader has empowered them.

In these successful practices, I would prefer to call the chairside assistant a *clinical* assistant because I think it more aptly describes their responsibilities. So, what does this clinical assistant do for me that makes her the most important person in the office? To answer that, let me first point out five attributes that I feel this individual must possess.

- She must be a highly organized person. There are many parts that come together to make any procedure in dentistry a success. She must be able to organize these parts in such a way that the office will be able to produce a quality product consistently. She must be able to organize these parts into systems that become part of an office operations manual.

- In dealing with these parts on a daily basis, she must be able to anticipate what the doctor will need next and what direction the procedure is going.

- The dentist is the "star of the show" in the office. The clinical assistant must be able to live daily with that aura and yet still let her own personality shine through. A very difficult job! In my opinion, she must be empowered to be a partner, to provide another set of eyes.

- In my office, the patients are assigned to the clinical assistants. She becomes responsible for building the patient relationship, which is so essential in a successful practice. She must be a student of the behavioral sciences and learn to build strong trust relationships with patients.

- The clinical assistant must also be prepared to be an enthusiastic, committed member of the team. There must be a commitment to building and enhancing her relationship with the rest of the members.

Please understand that this is more than simple delegation of duties to a chairside assistant. The clinical assistant has been empowered to make decisions on her own, based on the systems that have been established for the practice. She becomes the primary connection to the practice for her patients. It is she who educates her patients and makes suggestions about the possibility of treatment options open to the patient. She and the patient become friends and look forward to seeing each other.

Successful practices all have clinical assistants who have assumed a tremendous amount of responsibility in the practice. They are the key to a clinical practice that is a reflection of the vision of the leader. In my clinical practice, this means that we enrich the lives of our patients by providing them with world-class products with a passion for legendary service. My clinical assistants know that the systems that they have designed are not static rules but ever-changing guidelines for providing consistent quality-of-life experiences for our customers.

Barb, Rhonda, and I have worked together so long that there is little need for me to ask for anything. Long ago, I empowered them to be my partners. For example, during a crown preparation, they may see something that I have missed and simply ask me to look at that area of the tooth. I approve of this because it's certainly easier to make a correction now than later on. In order for this to happen, the clinical assistant must be properly positioned at the chair to see the procedure. Sometimes the modern dental chair makes this difficult. Chair manufacturers have made the chair backs extremely wide in order to make them more comfortable for patients. Because the chair is so wide, it is difficult to get the assistant into proper position. My point is that you will have to work with getting the clinical assistant into the proper position so she can see the procedure and truly become another set of eyes. In my opinion, the DentalEz J Chair is the only chair that allows you to do this.

I visited a practice located in a suburb of Chicago. The one thing that impressed me the most was the enthusiasm and commitment of the team. Everyone was upbeat and doing their jobs and obviously enjoying it. This was a fun office to visit. I think that they were feeling that they were making a difference in the lives of the people they were serving. It is no wonder that the production of the practice has grown tremendously. This team has obviously been empowered.

The labor pool is shrinking in the service industry. It is becoming more difficult to find qualified people to hire for the jobs that are available. As dentists, we must be aware of this trend and strive to find people who enjoy serving others. Once we find them and train them for dentistry, we must strive to keep them. The tactic of saving money by hiring twits to suck spit hardly makes sense in today's successful dental practice.

I listen to some dentists complaining how hard it is to change things in their offices. They are probably right, but change is really not all that difficult unless you accept that it is. In order to change anything, all you have to do is decide to change. When I stopped smoking, I attended Smoke Enders for five weeks while I prepared to stop. But at one point after those five weeks, I had to throw away the cigarettes and stop in one instant. I have worked hard ever since to stay off, but began the change quickly. I maintain that to change something in your practice, all you have to do is decide to change. Sure, you will have lots of things to do to make the change permanent, but it begins with a decision.

What are the benefits to the dentist when you empower staff? Is it worth the hassle? Yes, it is! You will notice an increase in production, your procedures will be more efficient and consistent, your days will be more stress-free, and the practice will actually become enjoyable.

Enjoy the journey!

Chapter 3

Children, Parents, Dentists: Dilemmas and Solutions

By Marvin H. Berman, D.D.S.

Years pass. Times change. Cultural differences vary. Economic conditions fluctuate. Stress and challenge are forever present. It is no simple matter to build and sustain a vital and thriving dental practice. It requires a combination of clinical competence, a strong work ethic, and a sense of caring about your fellow human beings. Dentists who exhibit the most versatility in these areas will consistently be the most successful and derive the greatest professional and personal satisfaction.

The Vision

Child patients are the seeds of a new practice and the lifeblood of an existing one. Yet many dentists are uncomfortable treating children and coping with their parents. As a result, they overlook or neglect a valuable practice resource that brings with it substantial personal, professional, and financial rewards.

Caring for children requires patience, emotional strength, and clinical skills. The anticipation of the arrival of a child patient strikes a note of fear and dread in the hearts of many dentists and their auxiliary team.

What is needed most of all is an inspirational dose of self-confidence...the kind of confidence that enables us to view all patients and their treatment with equanimity.

For the most part, the majority of general practitioners are involved in every aspect of dentistry from periodontia, endodontia, and oral surgery to cosmetic dentistry and orthodontia. We all reach a comfort or confidence level, hopefully motivated by our ability to perform a particular dental procedure to the best of our ability and in the best interests of our patients. Most general practitioners will confess that they would just as soon undertake the extraction of an impacted third molar or an implant procedure on an adult patient rather than attempt a simple prophylaxis and examination on an apprehensive or reluctant crying child. So treatment is often delayed, or the reluctant child patient is automatically referred to a pediatric specialist.

When questioned as to their motivations, some dentists will simply state that they can't tolerate the noise. Others will rationalize that the time spent working with a child is not financially rewarding when compared with a similar amount of time spent with an adult. In the short term, this assessment may have some validity. If, however, you are a family dentist striving for practice growth and stability, bear in mind that parents, almost without exception, place a higher priority on their child's well being than their own. If you can provide competent treatment for their baby in a relatively pleasant manner, you've taken a giant step in establishing a positive image with the parent, who will then most certainly not hesitate to place his/her own dental care in your capable hands. If you establish this pattern of patient care, your practice will take on a life of its own. Your competency with pediatric dentistry will be a magnet for the adults. Moreover, as your patients mature, your practice will become multi-generational and self-perpetuating.

There is no question that, as with every aspect of clinical dentistry, there are situations where in the best interest of all concerned, a patient should be referred to a specialist. Never worry that a patient will think less of you because you refer them for specialty care. It indicates that you have his/her best interests in mind. But, referring children out of the practice merely because they are children is ignoring a golden opportunity to expand your horizons.

Developing the ability to work competently with children is a learned skill much like any other that we are required to master. The difference is that treating children involves not only clinical expertise, but psychological and social acumen as well. There are those who maintain that possessing people skills is inborn, and to some degree that may be true. But, hopefully, all of us have the capacity to improve our social grace, smile more, walk straighter, and communicate better...if there is a willingness to open ourselves to the learning experience. This particular discussion is meant to be perspective on why children are the way they are, the trials and tribulations of being a parent, and then how we as professionals can maximize the successful interrelationship between the child, the parent, and the dentist. Obviously, the sum and substance of clinical pediatric dentistry in its entirety can be gleaned from any one of several excellent textbooks available.[1-3]

It is imperative that before we consider specific clinical dental treatment for a child, we have a working knowledge of child development and the child-parent relationship. This family unit is what we encounter each and every day in our offices. Using this information as a baseline, we can then become more skillful in assessing the challenge that any particular child or parent presents and become more adept at managing whatever may arise during the visit to the dentist. Just imagine you were to receive a box in the mail without a label or a gift without a card. Just imagine a blank sheet of paper with an invisible message on it...a combination lock with no combination. Who is this package of protoplasm in your chair? Where did he come from? What is she made of? Why are children the way they are?

Heredity vs. environment

To what degree is the personality of a child determined by hereditary factors, and to what extent could these hereditary factors be modified positively or negatively by environmental influences—specifically parenting? Gesell, Ilg, and Ames[4] came to certain conclusions in their research, and they had a major impact upon psychologists and family counselors.

"Understanding that there are basic, deep-seated physical and psychological differences in people will help parents understand their children. These differences are not merely a result of the way an individual has been treated by his parents or by the world around him."

They go on to elaborate on this premise. "This means that the body structure provides the raw material out of which personality is formed. That is the instrument upon which life forces—internal and external—play. Tendencies to behave in certain ways are to a large extent pre-determined and those tendencies are either reinforced or modified by the environment. So a boy might develop along very different lines in contrasting environments...but certain behaviors would be more or less possible for him than for others because of predisposing hereditary influences. Hereditary endowment is an inner environmental factor."

In even more practical terms, each of us is dealt a hand in the "card game" of life. Each of the cards contains a set of characteristics with which we've been endowed. One child may have a king, jack, eight, and six. Another is dealt an ace, queen, nine, and three. Just as we know that children are destined to be short or tall, have blue eyes or brown eyes, we also know that some children possess a special talent in music and others exhibit an extraordinary ability in visual arts. Some are gifted in mathematics and reasoning, and others are endowed with athletic prowess.

Carrying these premises a step further, the hereditary contribution to personality cannot be ignored. One child from the very beginning likes to be held and cuddled; the other is constantly on the move. One child tends to be optimistic and happy even when life doesn't go smoothly, and others tend to be moody and depressed and have temper tantrums when life is less than perfect. These kinds of personality characteristics surface early in infancy and portend what a parent can expect in the future.

Whether children behave the way they do as a result of hereditary or environmental influences or a combination of both is a moot point. Those kinds of debates only confuse the issue when attempting in retrospect to give praise or place blame for parenting skills or the lack thereof. It makes little difference once your child reaches adulthood. Hindsight is 20-20. But the key to being a good parent is to recognize at the outset your child's nature and his/her pattern of behavior. I strongly advise dealing with problems that surface early on before the negative behavior gets so ingrained it's impossible to unlearn. Emphasize and maximize the positives, but at the same time, point out the negatives before they become part of the child's "normal" behavior.[5]

Parents today tend to make a myriad of excuses for their child's negative behavior. Typical among them is "He's probably had too much sugar. He's allergic to the red dyes and he had a hot dog. He can't help it, that's the way he is, he's always had a bad temper." Are they addressing that issue with their child? Or is that exhibition of temper going to become more magnified and eventually lead to violence, physical abuse, or criminal behavior? What can parents do about it? Is there a solution?

The dilemma

There is so much confusing information given to parents that they have become impotent when it comes to setting parameters of behavior. No spanking! No yelling! Don't lower self esteem! Always be positive! Children are people too! Give children choices and they'll make the correct one! Ask the child what he/she thinks! Not surprisingly, the child grows up assuming that he/she always gets what he/she wants in real life situations. Parents even apply this thought process to the child's physician, dentist, or teacher as well. The inability of the parents to assert themselves with their children causes them to over-compensate. The epitome of parental impotence for me is clearly evident when a mother will ask her three-year-old right in front of me, "Do you like this doctor? Do you want to come back? Should we do your cavities today?" This over-compensation serves to immobilize the whole host of professionals who deal with children on a daily basis, often preventing them from performing to the best of their ability. What ever happened to blind faith? "Do it because I said so! I'm your mother! That's why! Listen to your teacher! Hold my hand! We're crossing the street! Time for a nap...you'll be tired later. Wash your hands...they're dirty. Make on the toilet...we're not stopping again. Don't forget to say 'thank you and please.'" There is no reason that a parent or some other authority figure should not be able to give a direct order and expect to get blind obedience from a toddler. There should be no need to justify a reasonable request.

In 1964, Dreikurs[6] stated, "Children are particularly sensitive to social climate. They have been quick to latch on to the idea that they share in the equal rights of everyone. They sense their equality with adults and no longer tolerate an autocratic dominant-submissive relationship. Parents, in turn, vaguely realize that their children have become their equals and have lessened the pressures of the you-do-as-I-say form of child raising. Thus we are faced with a dilemma. How to find the middle ground or comfort level for all concerned." He elucidates the problem further when he writes "To so many, democracy means freedom to do as you please, but if everyone did as they pleased we would have anarchy, friction and conflict. With freedom comes responsibility. With no sense of responsibility the children become tyrants and the enslaved parents are left with all the responsibility."

Perhaps this parental subservience had its beginnings in the "I'm OK. You're OK" turmoil that grew out of the 1960s, but that mood permeates child rearing even as we speak. Parents bombarded by advice from books on everything from potty training to hyperactivity to planning the future career of their pre-school child are paralyzed and confused. Whatever birds and bees instincts we should have as parents have been dulled. We've gone from family-based child guidance to a philosophy that "the world or the village will raise a child." Nothing could be further from the truth. If we accept the fact that the child is a bundle of joy, containing all the inherited ingredients that two parents have supplied, then we must realize that we as parents must begin immediately to help that child utilize those ingredients in a positive and productive manner.

The Learning Begins

Most of us think of learning in terms of the learning we do in school—reading, writing, and arithmetic. In fact, in recent years the controversy ebbs and flows in regard to windows of learning opportunity as children develop. Will listening to Mozart in the womb, practicing the alphabet at 18 months old, memorizing the multiplication table flash cards, or reading the newspaper at 3 years old signify that you're raising a "super child?" Will that child be more intelligent and be an automatic Harvard or Yale candidate? Sarles,[7] in his chapter on psychological development in the Forrester textbook, points out that psychological development proceeds in a logical, sequential order, with each period relying upon the foundation and the stability of the preceding phase. "Give us a child for the first five years of his life and his thoughts are ours forever."

Bruer[8] in his work with the McDonnell Foundation refers to the magical first three years as a "myth." He takes issue with the conclusions of others who describe a crisis in which children are deprived of early-accelerated learning experiences...especially in the case of dual career families. To paraphrase, "pressured parents mean unnecessarily pressured kids who may show brilliance early on but other children with innate intelligence catch up later anyway. Parents spend a lot of time today making certain that their children get music and dance lessons, learn some words in French, etc., (*Note:* you don't learn to speak a second language unless that language is used every day at home) take a class in karate, and play Little League baseball. Everything is planned and programmed even to the extent that mothers have to set up "play-dates" for their two year-old toddlers. Children have very little time for serendipitous fun.

On the other hand, parents need to understand that there is such a thing as social intelligence and unlike being "book smart," social skills should be taught and learned from the time a child is born. The emphasis should be on human interaction. Parent-child playtime provides important human facial expression and physical interaction. Cuddling, laughing and crying, sharing food and toys give the child a chance to develop emotionally. Teachers will tell you that they don't care if a child knows how to spell or add when they start kindergarten or first grade. That's what school is for. But they do care that the child can follow instructions, show good manners, and be considerate of their contemporaries... all social skills that should have been taught to them by their parents.

Unfortunately, with many families today, both parents are pursuing careers and they're not spending as much one on one time with their children. The kids are in day care or even if they're home, they spend much more time indoors on a computer, playing with an electronic toy, or watching television. Pediatricians and psychologists bemoan the fact that children don't play "catch" outside in the yard, draw pictures, color with crayons, build with Legos or Lincoln Logs, read books out loud, or make up stories...activities that call for imagination and creativity. Instead parents take the easy way out and permit and encourage the children to play video games or read books on the computer, with artificially enhanced sounds and images.

How early do babies show evidence of learning and understanding? A six-month old infant has been fed. His diaper has been changed and we put him down to sleep in the crib. He begins to scream and cry. We pick him up and rock him in our arms and he stops crying. In a couple of minutes, his eyes are closed so we carefully place him in the crib again. Lo and behold, he begins to cry again. Does that little infant know that if he cries he gets picked up? How early does a baby recognize his mother's smell or his father's voice? How early do they understand the meaning of the word...NO!

There are child experts advising parents about childproofing their houses so their children will be safe. This concept, although well intentioned, flies in the face of everything we know about the learning process in even the very young child. Lock up all the sharp knives, put gates up at the basement stairs, tape over all electrical outlets. Don't buy any furniture with sharp corners. Do your cooking while the child is napping. Don't leave your pens and pencils out on your desk—and so forth. What happened to the magical words No! Don't touch! Daddy's desk! Mommy's books! Sharp! What about the ever popular HOT! It is impossible to protect a child from every possible life situation. Much more important is teaching the child how to get along in the real world. You're not going to go into a store with your baby and tell the store owner to move everything that's sharp or hot. Your baby has to learn not to touch those things. Even the mother tiger said to her baby "honey, be careful, it's a jungle out there."

Small issues...big issues

Psychologists tend to say things like don't make a big issue out of something inconsequential. Don't make a mountain out of a molehill. Just address the important issues. What exactly is an important issue for a two year old? The presidential election? Who will win the World Series? What kind of car to buy? Important issues for a two year old are mundane items such as "make on the toilet, don't hit your sister, eat your vegetables, don't throw the book, and it's time for bed." Parental advisors might question the importance of a parent insisting that a child perform these basic behavioral tasks on command. What difference will it make 50 years from now? The point is that if your baby doesn't pay attention to you about these seemingly superficial items now, what makes you think the child will suddenly listen to your instruction or advice in regard to more important issues such as smoking, drinking, drugs, dating, or studying when he/she becomes a teenager? Perhaps if the continuity between infancy and adolescence would be better maintained, we wouldn't have as many teens "searching for their identity" or labeled "troubled teens."

The pattern of the parent-child relationship is established early in infancy. Good manners, consideration for others, and the sense of right and wrong are first learned as a toddler from a parent. The learning experience is then reinforced by teachers, clergy, and even by physicians and dentists who come in contact with young patients. Once you've reached adulthood, it is very difficult for a leopard to change its spots or for a dog to learn new tricks.

Parental discipline... yelling, spanking, and time out

This particular subject is a sensitive one for children, parents, and professionals alike. The image of a child being hit with a stick or beaten with a belt by their parents is vivid in the minds of many of us. In my case, I can still feel the sting of my mother's disciplinary methods. But in those days, spanking was not an issue because it almost always was associated with a parent's love and their desire to make you a better person. Moreover, if you had any sense at all, you thought twice about misbehaving the next time.

There is no doubt that in many cases the physical punishment was a little over the top and perhaps too frequent, but ironically even with the prevalence of sometimes excessive physical discipline, the love and respect that children had for their parents were much more evident than they are today. To clarify, punishment meted out by a parent to a child that knows what he's done wrong, if administered with love in mind and not out of frustration and not with the intent to hurt, can be very effective as an adjunct to other avenues of discipline.

Yelling, screaming, ranting, and raving are common avenues of expression for parents whose kids carry them to the edge. If the screaming is not constant where the children just say to themselves "that's mom just blowing off steam again," a sudden rise in the decibels can bring a child who has not been paying attention back into the real world. If your goal is to teach a child right from wrong, he/she has to focus on what you're saying. That means direct eye contact…the look your mother gave you when you crossed the line. "Look at me when I'm talking to you" was a phrase I was very familiar with. All of these approaches have validity, but none of them work all of the time.

Time out

The term "time out" is a familiar one in sports where it means a break in the action…a break to allow those involved in the competition to rest or reconsider their options. We all need a time out once in a while to take stock of our situation and make adjustments in our behavior. But the world doesn't wait indefinitely for you, and the number of timeouts is limited.

If a child is misbehaving, the mother or father with the encouragement of some psychologists will say "If you don't stop, honey, we'll have to do a time out!" or "That's it, we're going to have a time out in your room!" or, the threat "Are you asking for a time out?" Whatever happened to that "look" your mother or father would give you? That stare with the finger pointed at you was all you needed to remind you that you had crossed the line and you'd better shape up—NOW!

Time out for me as a child was long enough to duck. Recourse was instant. You didn't have all day to shape up and get with the program. If the behavior problem occurs in a public place like the supermarket or restaurant, where do you execute the time out procedure? The produce section, the meat locker, or at the salad bar?

Crying

The fact that a child is crying does not necessarily equate with fear or pain or apprehension. Babies cry a lot for any number of reasons. Newborns cry. Toddlers and preschool children often cry because they're tired or out of frustration, anger, or reluctance. If they cry enough and scream loudly, they won't have to perform the task at hand. At home, this pattern is the way of life. It begins with the whining, then the crying, then the all-out tantrum. This behavior is precipitated by a demand for a toy or candy they want or for the bath or toothbrushing they don't want. In our distant memories are the voices of our mom and dad saying, "If you want to cry I'll give you something to cry about." This was a reference to the story of the boy who cried "wolf." Today, parents respond to that crying by giving in or backing off because they don't like to hear their baby cry...for whatever reason.

Many parents will say to me, "I hope he doesn't cry!" as if that's the measure of our skills. They look upon the visit to the dentist as an unpleasant and painful experience and they transfer that same feeling to their child. One of the unspoken parental prejudices is that if the visit to the dentist doesn't proceed perfectly and their child has any negative reaction, that we're the problem—not the child. They do that with teachers as well and refer to it as "bad vibes" or "poor chemistry." The reason we're changing dentists is that the chemistry was poor at the other place. Of course, if things don't go smoothly it's not the child's fault in today's confused world. The majority of children are better behaved, more outgoing, and more respectful and certainly more fun in the absence of the parents.

The basis for this observation is the unequivocal testimony from fellow grandparents all over the world who attest to the fact that their grandchildren are perfect angels, happy and cooperative until mom and dad come on the scene. Then, like a virus, the whining begins anew.

49

Feelings and Self Esteem

Feelings and self esteem—two buzzwords that are thrown about with abandon by psychologists and social workers have stymied those of us that live and work with children every day. It goes without saying that all of us should be sensitive to the feelings of others. It's certainly not nice to hurt someone's feelings. We should always be kind and not hurtful. Each and every one of us has "feelings," and when our feelings our hurt, we sometimes react. When children are in the toddler stage, they often react inappropriately. Sometimes, it's a crying spell or a temper tantrum. Sometimes they'll hit or kick or swear.

When feelings are hurt, frustration may take over and with frustration comes anger. Correcting a child, by showing him/her an easier way to do something or helping him/her control emotions does not constitute hurting feelings. It's not *what* you say. It's *how* you say it. You cannot always speak about positives when explaining to a child that he/she can't hit his/her sister or that two plus two is not five. A mistake is a mistake. Correct it and move on and don't make a federal case out of it. It doesn't mean the child is bad. The child just did something bad and shouldn't do it again.

Moreover, a child must learn that it's not just *his/her* feelings that are important but the feelings of *others* as well. The balance between individual rights versus the welfare of society as a whole comes into play here. Children today are very self-centered. They think the world revolves around them and will adjust to accommodate them. As adults, we know that doesn't happen. You must learn that early on, otherwise you're in for a rude awakening.

Self esteem comes from within and cannot be bestowed upon you. Your mother or father telling you that you're the smartest or the prettiest or the most handsome or the best athlete does not give you self esteem. Accomplishing something like learning how to make on the toilet, tying your own shoes, riding your bike without training wheels, scoring a goal in soccer, and going to the dentist and getting a shot without freaking out will give you that elusive sense of self-worth.

Drugs for a Population that Can't Pay Attention

Many parents experience a great deal of difficulty and are repeatedly frustrated in dealing with the reluctant and willful behavior of their children. Unfortunately, they don't always share this information with us when completing the medical history form. They probably feel that it's not relevant or perhaps they're embarrassed or defensive about the problems they've been experiencing. The situation is exacerbated when school officials complain that the children are a disturbance in school, and finally they're forced to seek professional help—and rightfully so.

In searching for answers for the child's inability or unwillingness to go with the flow of life, the possibilities can range from A to Z and back again. Hopefully a psychologist, psychiatrist, or social worker with insight will put the child and the family back on a good track, but often, instead of eliminating the obvious causes first, the family and professional get bogged down in a sea of syndromes. The parents are anxiously looking for answers that will identify entities like hyperactivity, attention deficit, manic depression, schizophrenia, explosive disorder, or one of my favorites…"obedience deficit disorder." They need something to hang their hats on so they can say to themselves "no wonder my child is the way he is, he's sick! " Frequently the family counselor is willing to oblige them.

There is no doubt that there are children who have inherent psychological problems or hormonal irregularities, rendering them certainly incapable of responding properly in everyday situations, but not in the numbers and to the degree that is being reported. As a result, children are being treated for hyperactivity, attention deficit, and other disorders arbitrarily with Ritalin, Zoloft, Prozac, and other drugs with varying results. Most importantly, the children are being labeled "different" or "mental cases" instead of children in need of a stronger parental presence with more definitive attention at an earlier age. And now, of course, the child has a built in excuse for his inappropriate behavior. For example, "manic depressive disorder" and "bi-polar" behavior has become a more common diagnosis in the pre-school age group, with a corresponding increase in the prescription of antidepressants. How can you tell if a three year old is depressed? A three year old often exhibits extreme "ups" when they're happy and excited or prolonged "downs" when they're frustrated or sad.

The point is that parents and professionals working with children should exhaust every behavioral approach to child management before resorting to mind-altering drug therapy. We shouldn't be prescribing these drugs without a more definitive diagnosis.

Diet and Nutrition for Newborns, Infants, and Toddlers

The subject of diet and nutrition gets very little attention in medical school or dental school. We hear and talk a lot about too many sweets and eating a balanced diet and healthy foods, but we need to translate this information into a concrete and usable form for parents of newborns, infants, toddlers, and preschool children in general. Even before the child is born, an expectant mom and dad should be in possession of certain vital information about diet and nutrition that will prevent dental disease and enhance the health and development of the primary and permanent dentitions. We as dentists need to be more knowledgeable about this subject because we are often prime advice givers when it comes to food consumption and dietary supplements and restrictions.

As we know, the primary teeth are developing and calcifying during the mother's pregnancy. What she eats, the overall state of her own health, and the viability of the connection between her and her baby reflect positively or negatively on the symbiotic relationship between mother and child. These factors have a major impact on the morphologic and histologic integrity of the baby's bones and teeth (*i.e.*, mottling, enamel hypoplasia, and hypo-calcification) and even aberrations in the tooth eruption patterns.

We are well aware of the role that trauma can play during the differentiation and calcification stages of fetal dental development with the resulting atypical tooth morphology and defects in tooth enamel integrity. Schour and Massler[9] described the etiology of the neo-natal hypoplastic ring and its relationship to birth trauma and the transition of the fetus from intra-uterine to extra-uterine life.

We are just beginning to understand the impact that smoking, alcohol, and drugs can have on a developing fetus, but there are also subtle effects that the expectant mother's well being or lack thereof will have on her child's development. When we encounter children with severe enamel and dentin anomalies in the primary dentition, it should provoke a series of delicate questions pertaining to the mother's pregnancy experience and family history.

A question that parents will often pose is whether or not the permanent teeth will be affected. As we know, defects in the primary teeth relate to intra-uterine problems, whereas similar defects in permanent teeth relate to problems during the early infancy stage. Sometimes there's an overlapping and you can't predict with certainty which teeth will or will not be affected. In any case, offer your best educated guess and assure the parent that the end result will be positive for the child, one way or another.

Breast-feeding

Breast-feeding is an activity that runs in cycles with new mothers. Today, expectant moms in general are imbued with the desire to breast-feed if they can. Mother's milk has a well-deserved reputation for providing the best nutrition for a newborn baby without the downside of allergic reactions from substances found in various formula preparations. In addition to the nutritive value of breast-feeding, there is a bonding between mother and child for which there is no substitute.[10]

Increasingly common is the phenomenon of women marrying at a more advanced age because they're acquiring more advanced education and building careers. Young couples are waiting longer to have children. Many more women today are encountering difficulties in achieving pregnancy and subsequently carrying their fetus through the nine-month cycle. As a result, when their bundle of joy arrives, the excitement, the anticipation, and the accompanying anxieties are heightened. There is a need among young working mothers today to make up for the time they're not spending with their children by indulging their babies a little bit more. We therefore see more moms sleeping with their infants in bed and nursing intermittently throughout the night. The teeth are constantly bathed in the mother's milk with the resulting decalcification and caries very similar in pattern and severity to excessive baby-bottle feeding.[11]

As with all other activities in life, moderation is the byword. Mothers should set a reasonable goal for themselves as to how long they're going to breast-feed, but be aware that the constant nighttime exposure to their milk may be doing as much damage as good.

Baby bottle-feeding

Along with the more laissez faire attitude about breast-feeding, we have a more permissive attitude in regard to bottle-feeding as well.[12] Despite all the warnings, it is still very common for parents to let the baby lie in bed, the buggy, the stroller, or the playpen or walk around sucking on a bottle filled with milk or juice (Fig. 3-1). If the baby cries in the middle of the night, the parent refills the bottle and the first thing you know the maxillary primary incisors are decayed into the pulp, requiring crown restorations, pulp therapy, and sometimes even extraction (Fig. 3-2).

It is important to get the message across to parents of newborns that they should never start the "bottle in bed" routine. The baby should be fed in the high chair or in their arms. The gums or teeth should be wiped with a damp cloth or gauze after the baby is fed and the baby should be put in the bed to sleep. If you want to feed him/her again, take the baby out of bed, or give him/her the bottle, wipe the teeth and gums, kiss the baby, and then "back into bed you go." Eating and sleeping should not be confused. The baby bottle is not an object of love; so don't allow the child to become so significantly attached to it.

The associated habit of dragging a blanket around the house and through the supermarket can also be short circuited by making the baby aware early on that blankets belong in bed "so you can be nice and warm when you're sleeping. We don't drag your clean blanket on the floor. It will get dirty."

Just as in the case of breast-feeding, if the child is walking around the house sucking on a bottle, the teeth become easy targets for the rampant decay phenomenon known as baby bottle syndrome or nursing caries.

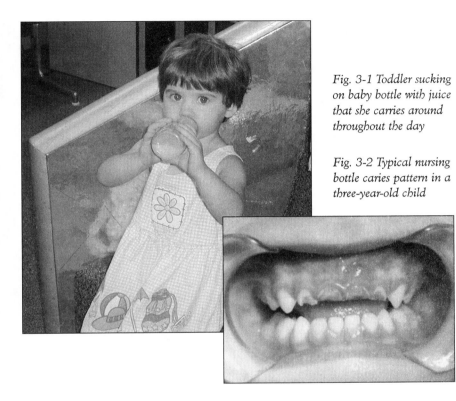

Fig. 3-1 Toddler sucking on baby bottle with juice that she carries around throughout the day

Fig. 3-2 Typical nursing bottle caries pattern in a three-year-old child

Moreover, it sets up a vicious cycle where the child sucks on a bottle all day and then comes to the dinner table with no appetite. Then he/she's hungry later, has another bottle, and is not hungry for the meal again. The parents are unhappy because the child is not eating normally, but they continue the bottle because "at least he/she's eating something." The advice to parents that have a child still using the bottle is to take the bottle away and begin using a sippy cup with the intent that the child will graduate to a normal glass or cup. Weaning a child from the bottle, in my experience, works best using the "cold turkey" approach. "No more bottle. You're such a big boy/girl. You can drink from the glass. Yeah!" It's not a punishment. It's simply time for a transition.

Special note. The "sippy" cup with juice or milk will cause damage to the maxillary incisors as well, if used frequently throughout the day as a pacifier. As children progress through toddler-hood, parents indulge them with "sippy" cups filled with juice and a little container of either breakfast cereal or some empty calorie, fermentable carbohydrate food. This habit not only leads to a greater likelihood of developing caries, but it keeps the child in a constant state of a satiated, "filled-up" feeling. So when he/she comes to the dinner table, the sight of food does not excite him/her. The child resists eating meat or chicken and vegetables and potatoes and salad, etc.—foods that are good for him/her, so it's back to the snack foods between meals.

Moreover, with all that in-between meal eating there is no way you can brush after each eating episode, since the eating is constant. Prohibiting candy and other sweets is not the answer to preventing dental decay. Sugar is not the chief culprit. It's the frequency of eating fermentable carbohydrates that causes most of the problems[13] (Fig. 3-3). Parents are always amazed when I tell them that their child can have two or three cookies with very little caries risk if he/she eats them at one sitting and then rinse the mouth or brush the teeth.

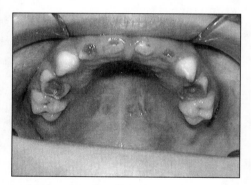

Fig. 3-3 Rampant neglected caries due to excessive between-meal snacking

But if the child eats the same three cookies, one at a time, at separate intervals, the chances of getting cavities are much greater. I go on, of course, to explain how the acid level ebbs and flows with the ingestion of food and how the bacteria participate in the whole process. If children would just eat their regular meals and have a snack or two, the danger of dental caries could be substantially avoided. Moreover, there are so many foods like fresh fruit, popcorn, peanuts, and others that are not implicated in the decay process that the child could have instead.

Mealtime at the zoo

Many parents face mealtime with their young children with apprehension. There was a time when your mother prepared lunch or dinner and that was *it*. I'm reminded of the cartoon picturing the mother anteater and the baby anteater and the beleaguered mother is saying to her baby, "What do you mean you don't like ants?"

You might not have been crazy about what was on your plate, but you ate it or you made believe you ate it. I am besieged by parents who are desperate to solve the mealtime meltdowns with their fussy eating children. They don't like meat. They won't eat their vegetables. They don't like big pieces. They don't like mushy stuff. You name it.

It all begins with the systematic introduction of various foods in your baby's diet. First it's breast milk or formula, then rice cereal with milk, and then strained carrots, peas, and green beans, and then strained meats in a jar. Often when parents are spoon-feeding their babies, the infant seems like he/she doesn't want to eat. You put the spoon to his/her lips. He/she shakes his/her head and spits it out. You try again in greater earnest using your best show business voice. "Here's one for Uncle Joe! Here comes another one for Aunt Bessie! Ooh we can't forget one spoon for the doggy...and then the kitty...and here comes the Choo Choo train! Choo! Choo!" We did everything we could, including stand on our head, to get our babies to eat.

Then the transition is made to junior food that's more solid and then to table food, cut up in small pieces. The object is to expose the child to as many different foods and tastes as possible (Fig. 3-4). The child should grow up knowing that he/she has to partake of a variety of foods. "You only have to have one spoon of peas...just two

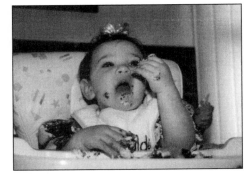

Fig. 3-4 Infant food-tasting test

asparagus. OK the two small ones." There's a fine line between coaxing and trickery and forcing the issue, but the child *will* learn to enjoy a wider variety of foods.

A major mistake parents make is allowing their children to have between meal snacks, at will. Moms and dads should be able to say to their children, "Don't eat that now, wait until dinner." But instead, a parent will tell me, "I can't help it, she's smart. She knows where everything is and she gets it herself." My response is "If she's smart enough to go into the cabinet, then she's smart enough to know that she's not supposed to go into the cabinet without permission." Children should not have carte blanche access to the kitchen cabinets.

As with everything else, children are given too many choices when it comes to food. It's not about always catering to what a child likes or doesn't like. He/she might love pizza and ice cream and hotdogs, and sometimes we have that. But today we're having meat loaf. It's a mistake for mothers to give their children the impression that they're running a restaurant or cafeteria where each child and dad can eat something different. This pattern begins when the child is an infant, where the mother and the father allow the child to gravitate to "what she likes" rather than helping the child acquire a taste for a broader spectrum of foods.

You don't feel like chicken, you can have a bologna sandwich. You don't want pork chops, well then here's a peanut butter and jelly sandwich. Dinner is served. You eat it or you don't eat it. Next meal is breakfast. Don't allow the child to manipulate you into a snack an hour later on the pretense that he/she's hungry. "You're hungry? Next time eat your dinner." It's very simple. No arguing, no yelling, and no screaming. He/she won't starve. If he/she's hungry, he/she'll eat.

The subject of diet and nutrition could obviously fill an entire book. For our purposes, let's focus on the basic information that we must make certain parents have to in order to maximize their children's oral health. We've already mentioned that children in this day and age tend to eat excessively between meals. From my experience in doing diet surveys with parents, at least 25% of a child's calories are ingested between meals and not at mealtime. The factors influencing this statistic are:

- Busy families with their heavily programmed children and parents don't sit down for their meals together, but rather eat individually or in groups as their schedules allow. The old breakfast, lunch, and dinner regimen with a couple of snacks in-between is practically non-existent

- Parents today are less likely to insist that children eat the balanced meal at mealtime. The meat or chicken, vegetable, starch standards go by the wayside, because parents indulge their children's' finicky tastes

- Since the child doesn't eat his/her fill at the scheduled mealtime, he/she expresses feelings of hunger (real or not) shortly after the meal and the parent usually gives in. The frequent feeding or eating begins in infancy where a mom will breastfeed or bottle-feed on demand and even without the demand. Then, as a toddler, the child is allowed and even encouraged to carry a "sippy" cup and a container of some kind of carbohydrate snack around (sugar coated cereals, chips, etc.) to keep him/her happy or quiet. So the child grows into his/her pre-school years accustomed to eating small amounts frequently, rather than larger amounts on a more orderly schedule

A reminder. As dentists, the quality of the foods eaten by developing children is of concern to us as well. We are quite aware of how important vitamins and minerals are for children, especially in the formative years. For example, a lot of families today don't drink milk in deference to juices, sports drinks, and soda pop. Not only is this tendency damaging to the teeth, but the empty calories comprised almost entirely of sugar and acids have no nutritional value. Children have to be told that they can have the occasional juice or soda, but milk should be their basic drink during the formative years. First make the rules and then decide on the exceptions. It should not be a laissez faire policy.

Oral hygiene advice

Rather than reciting the litany of advice that is generically communicated to patients in regard to oral hygiene and home care, I've chosen to concentrate on the specific areas that are relevant to young children:

- Parental counseling in regard to caring for their baby's mouth should be user-friendly. Avoid technicalities and deal with practicality. A parent should be directly or indirectly involved with cleaning a child's teeth and gums until the child can do it effectively on his/her own (usually not before 8-10 years old). Even afterwards, the parent should monitor the child's oral hygiene activities

- From the time that a child is born and is being breast or bottle fed, the gums of the baby should be wiped with a soft cloth or gauze after the feeding. A by-product of the cleansing procedure is the familiarization of the infants with someone being in their mouths. This serves as a prelude for future visits to the dentist

- A soft toothbrush with an easy to grasp handle should be introduced at the first sign of erupting primary teeth (usually 6-8 months of age). The baby can be allowed to grasp the brush, but the parent should be in complete control of the brush's movement so as not to cause injury[14]

- The pre-school child (3-5 years) is feeling more independent and should be allowed a little more freedom to do his/her thing. But the parent should be right there doing the "final touchup." Let the child have the feeling that he/she did it, but you're involved

- There should be no controversy in regard to using a manual toothbrush or an electric one. There is a time and place for both.[15] Very young children need to develop the manual dexterity of moving the toothbrush around. Moreover, if given an electric brush, they tend to let it rest in one spot for too, long resulting in excessive abrasion of the soft tissues

A toddler is simply not ready to operate an electric brush safely and effectively. However, there is nothing wrong with the parent using the electric brush with the child in order to stimulate enthusiasm for brushing.

Don't use excessive amounts of toothpaste on the brush. Just a smear on the surface should be sufficient. The excessive paste ends up being swallowed because that child doesn't rinse well or on the mirror or the walls of the bathroom. A fluoridated paste with ADA approval is suggested.

- Toothbrushing experts place a lot of emphasis on the method of brushing the teeth, *i.e.*, circular, vertically, sulcular, etc.[16] Certainly, in the case of the mature dentition of teenagers and adults, these details are pertinent. But for the infant and toddler and pre-school child, the object is to get in there and get the debris off the teeth and soft tissues in a speedy, efficient, and gentle manner. Fun is of the essence. The parent should sit down on a chair or stool with the child's back to them as if giving a loving hug. This positioning also provides the maximum control and visualization (Fig. 3-5)

- Don't hesitate to sing and be playful. Brushing should be a fun, bonding experience between parent and child and not an unpleasant chore

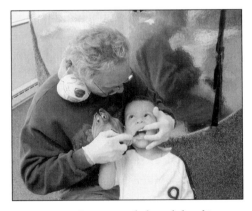

Fig. 3-5 Recommended tooth brushing position for maximum control and fun

- Try to brush the child's teeth in correlation with the eating habits. Since you don't want to be brushing several times a day, the between-meal snacks should be limited. After breakfast and following dinner would be a good regimen. In addition, if the child has a bed-time snack other than fresh fruit, there should be a bedtime brushing right before the bedtime story

- Flossing becomes more relevant as the primary dentition matures and interproximal spaces are difficult to negotiate with the toothbrush. Again the pre-school age and younger child needs direct supervision to accomplish the task. Certainly, once the permanent have erupted into position, flossing should become part and parcel of the total home care hygiene experience

- Mouth rinses and mouthwashes are not recommended for the very young child who does not have good rinsing skills

What Parents Should Tell Children Before the First Visit

One of the most frequent questions asked by parents concerns the preparation of their child for the first visit to the dentist. My advice to most parents is to say as little as possible because whatever they say tends to create fear instead of allaying it. "Don't worry! It's just a pinch! I'll be right there! I won't let anyone hurt you! We'll get you a toy afterwards if you're good!"

Undoubtedly, mom and dad mean well. But all they're doing is transferring their anxiety and apprehension to the child. Anytime somebody says "don't worry" to me, I start to worry. Parental anxiety is the single most influential factor affecting a child's behavior at the first dental visit.[17] Unknowingly, they get their child so worked up that by the time they arrive for their appointment, the parent and child are on the verge of a breakdown. The parent would do well to say "we're going to a fun place today. We're going to have such a good time." But most parents don't believe or can't imagine how enjoyable a visit to the dentist can be if they had a more positive attitude. Instead, they are apologetic with their children as if to say " I'm so sorry I'm putting you through this, I know how you feel. I hate it too!" And with that, negativity is perpetuated and implanted in the minds of another generation.

Formal Parental Consent

Your written office policy that every parent receives should contain the basic philosophy of life in your office—the way you do things and the reason why. The treatment consent form is part of that office policy. Every consent form should be individualized for your practice.[18] As the years go by, it seems that there is an ever-increasing need to clarify what we do and how we do it with the parent. The reality is, however, that the longer you're in practice, the more confidence you should have in yourself. Subsequently, there is less need to use aversive techniques involving drugs, sedation, hospitalization, pre-medication, and papoose restraints...all requiring specific permission from the parent. Even the use of local anesthesia should be cleared with mom and dad.[19]

Cautionary note. Do not use hand over the mouth because it's an aversive technique that is easily mishandled and misinterpreted. There are other, less intrusive methods of minimizing the crying and screaming, and remember, if the child is safe and you are behaving properly, don't sweat the crying. Don't mask the noise. Anticipate it and prepare the parents to deal with it.

If, by the way, the scenario changes to a more physical or violent mood on the part of the child, make certain that either the doctor or a dental assistant goes out to the waiting room to inform the parent of the turn of events. Put the burden on the child and perhaps even bring the child out to the mom so she can set things straight. When things don't go smoothly, there is the tendency for the parent to lay blame on the dentist for their child's lack of cooperation. If a child has sufficient linguistic skills to understand the meaning of your request for his/her cooperation, especially if there's no discomfort involved, then he/she should be willing to promise cooperation.[20]

By the same token, the doctor and the dental auxiliaries are responsible for keeping the child safe from harm under any circumstances. If you feel uncomfortable with the whole situation, there is no reason why you can't refer the patient to a pediatric specialist. Don't lose your temper. The children are not yours. Don't get tangled up emotionally in a battle with the child. Don't call names "You brat! You're a spoiled little girl. Bad boy! Bad girl." The children will tell the parent you were mean to them...that you called them names. Don't give a parent any excuse to accuse you of unprofessional behavior.

Chambers[21] refers to the choices for behavior management for pediatric dentists as "an embarrassment of riches," but as with any dental procedure, you must be comfortable and confident with what you are doing. The bottom line as stated by Pinkham[22] is "communication with the parents and the children. Articulate the options for the parent and develop a clear understanding of everyone's intentions to maximize satisfaction." Working with children affords many benefits when it comes to the vitality of your practice. By trying harder and learning as much as you can, you can improve your technique and increase your comfort level. Working with children affords many benefits when it comes to building a practice. Don't give up easily.

The Medical History

In addition to the psychological assessment of the child, it goes without saying that a thorough medical history is mandatory. The design of your medical history information form is very individual (Fig. 3-6). However, there are certain pertinent bits of information that have a direct affect on proposed treatment. The routine questions about immunizations, etc. tell us very little about what's in store for us. More to the point is the pregnancy experience and birth history that relate directly to tooth development and calcification. Difficulties in these areas may have a direct connection to what you observe in the mouth. Inquiries about drug reactions and allergies are certainly relevant before you do anything with the child. Latex allergies are becoming increasingly common. With

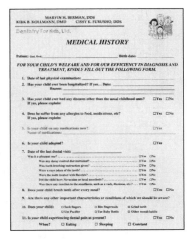

Fig. 3-6 An example of a simple medical history form

so many children suffering from all sorts of viral and bacterial infections, they are frequently treated with various antibiotics, cough medicines, and decongestants, and allergies and drug tolerances are more common.

Coincidentally, with the increase in behavioral problems, there has been a corresponding increase in the frequency of behavior-altering drugs such as Prozac, Valium, Zoloft, Phenobarbital, and Ritalin. Ask the question as you would any other.

Inquiries about oral hygiene and dietary patterns at home are obviously important when it comes to conversations concerning caries prevention. Do the parents brush their toddler's teeth every day? Is it a hassle for them? Do they use toothpaste?

Another important question would be the previous dental experience, if any. Pleasant? Unpleasant? This will give you a heads-up to the approach you might take in managing the child and the parent.

Parents in the Operatory—Yes or No?

Perhaps no issue precipitates more controversy among pediatric specialists than whether the parent should be in the treatment room with the child. This issue is not about right or wrong, but about what is in the best interest of the doctor, the patient, and the parent.[23] Given a situation where a child is content, happy, and well behaved, the presence of a parent in the treatment room might make little difference (Fig. 3-7). But given an apprehensive and reluctant child coupled with a nervous and anxious parent, it's best for all concerned that the parent waits in the waiting room during the treatment.

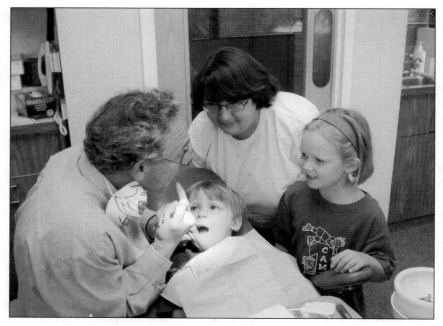

Fig. 3-7 Chairside communication with mother and children

The separation of the child from the parent is the essential part of successful management of children (Fig. 3-8). In most cases, it is beneficial to interrupt the pattern of behavior between parent and child that is sometimes confrontational, but most often hazy, nebulous, or non-existent. The father or mother has his/her own misgivings or hang-ups about dentists, and these feelings are easily absorbed and transferred to the child. The more conflicted the relationship, the greater the chance the parent will object to the child going into the operatory on their own with a dental assistant. So it requires a little more effort to ease the process.

After more than four decades of practice and as a father of four and a grandfather of seven, I can say with certainty that the most reliable prediction of a child's behavior at the first visit is the overt or underlying parental anxiety. The same pattern of behavior that dominates the family relationships at home, the questioning, the whining, the temper tantrums on the part of the child, coupled with the anxious coaxing, cajoling, and hand wringing by the parent can be short circuited by doing a gentle, planned, and informed "parentectomy" at the earliest possible convenience.

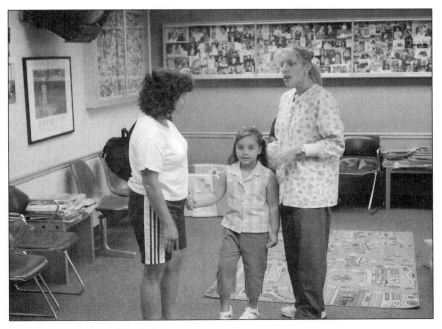

Fig. 3-8 Dental assistant preparing parent
for temporary separation from child

Accomplishing the separation begins at the moment that your office receives the telephone call for the appointment, as depicted in my video-tapes.[24] The front desk personnel should obtain all the usual pertinent information requested from new patients, followed by a short exposition describing the methodologies used in your office. Within this exposition, the principle of the doctor and child meeting each other in the absence of the parent is broached with a thorough description of the reasons that this choice is the preferred one. Don't speak apologetically. You're stating your policy, in a friendly manner, but very matter of fact. The issue is not negotiable. Following this conversation, a copy of the office policy statement is sent to the prospective family (if time allows) or else this office policy brochure is given to the mother or father when he/she arrives for the appointment.

When the family arrives, they're greeted and welcomed with the utmost friendliness (Fig. 3-9). Most of the attention should be lavished on the child. "Hi Judy! We've been waiting for you? Are you ready to have fun with Dr. Berman? I see you brought your mommy! Hi Mom!" The people at the front desk reiterate the policy, so there's a clear understanding that while mom completes all the boring paperwork, the dental assistant will bring the child into the operatory area to meet Dr. Berman, after which the doctor and parent will sit down for a conversation. Should the parent voice objection to the separation procedure, the doctor should meet with the parent and child in the private office in order to discuss the issues and confirm the policy in an amicable manner (Fig. 3-10). As with all relationships between people, it's never what you say but rather how you say it that carries the day.

If it is necessary for the doctor to re-confirm the no-parent rule, personally, do so in the private office. Walk into the office with a smile on your face. Don't be on the defensive. The first words out of your mouth should be directed at the child, something like "Hi Billy, I'm Dr. Berman. We have a beautiful new toothbrush for you, so you can show me how you brush, but I'm going to talk with Mommy for a minute." Then "Hi Mrs. Smith, I understand there's a problem!" Interestingly, experience has shown that the most frequent response to that statement is "No, there's no problem!" This sign of them backing off should not be accepted at face value. "Well, there must be a problem, because Barbara (lady at front desk) said you were unhappy about something." Continue the conversation in a calm and reassuring tone.

Don't forget, the child is in the room and listening to the conversation that he/she may very well interpret as adversarial. The mother is being protective of him/her and, *you*, the *doctor* are placed in the position of being the intruder. Turn the tables on them.

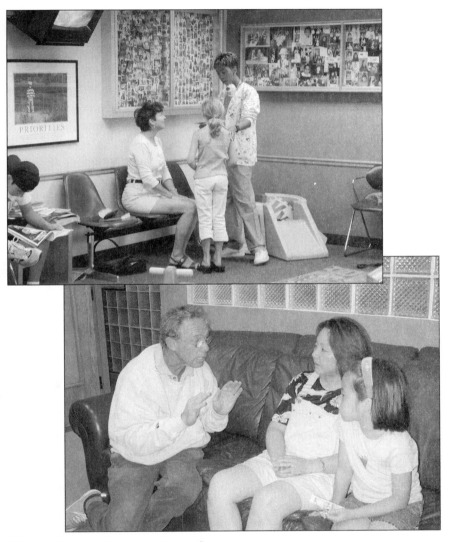

Fig. 3-9 Dental assistant greeting mother and child and explaining the system

Fig. 3-10 Doctor meeting with mother and child in response to her refusal to allow her child to enter operatory on her own

Remember! Why does a parent want to be with the child? Because he/she needs to go through this "terrible" experience with the child! That's why! This is about trust. Does he/she trust you alone with his/her baby? To inspire that trust, the conversation should evolve in this manner. "I understand how you feel Mrs. Smith. But imagine you're at a cocktail party and you're meeting lots of people and talking but not really getting to know anybody. Billy is the most important person at this visit (turn to Billy)...right Billy? We'll get your toothbrush in just a minute Billy. (Back to the mom.) So you see Mrs. Smith I need to be with Billy, one on one...so we can really get to know each other and have fun together. If you let us do our thing he'll have a wonderful experience." In other words you are letting her know that she's interfering with the normal sequence of events that has been your successful modus operandi in the past. Almost invariably, the parent will consent to go with the flow. I emphasize again that reluctance and crying do not necessarily mean the child is having a negative experience.

There are those who would say if the child or the parent is reluctant that perhaps we should wait for a better day when everyone is more in the mood. I strongly disagree, because you're just postponing the inevitable challenge of dealing with the child and the parent. If the parent speaks about the child missing a nap or having a cold or didn't get to wear new shoes or a million other excuses, put those alibis aside. Whatever the purpose was for the dental visit—whatever you intended to accomplish—*now is the hour...do it*. Otherwise, the reluctance or the apprehension becomes more magnified, and the manipulation goes on and on. Somebody has to be willing to go to the wall, so to speak. It may as well be you.

The only exception I make to the "no parent rule" is during an examination or consultation with new infants. Mom comes in with the baby, but I immediately take the baby from here onto my lap and do the examination in that position. It doesn't matter if the baby cries either. Just speak nicely as you would to your own baby. Be playful and fun even as the crying persists. Let the mother or father see just how patient and skillful you are despite the child's negative behavior. If treatment is necessary, the mother goes out to the waiting room to wait, and a dental assistant gets into the chair and holds the baby in the papoose position while you complete the treatment aided by your other assistants.

Premedication

One alternative that dentists choose to alter a child's behavior is the prescription of tranquilizing or sedating drugs to be taken orally prior to the dental appointment. If you knew the definitive dose or the combination of drugs that would be most effective with any given child, this avenue might be more useful. It sometimes requires two or three visits to decide on the most effective drug and establish the most effective therapeutic level. Determining the dosage by weight may not be the most accurate. A thinner child with a high anxiety level may require a higher dosage than the larger, more lethargic child. In order for these drugs to be effective, the dose has to be high enough and you have to allow enough time for them to work (approximately one hour). Moreover, you are often relying on the parent to administer the drug correctly. Often the child is uncooperative and then the appointment has to be cancelled or the child has to be sent home with nothing accomplished. The parents will not be happy campers.

Again, drugs should never be the first choice if you can gain a child's confidence using the behavioral approach. I'm always emphasizing the educational aspects of the dentist-child relationship, which suffers when we introduce the drug factor. Combinations of Demerol, Atarax, Chloral Hydrate, Valium, etc. can all serve the purpose if you're determined to use premedicating drugs. The publications issued by the American Academy of Pediatric Dentistry defining policy and outlining the use of various drugs for the management of child behavior should serve as a definitive resource.[25]

The child may still cry or squirm and be reluctant to open his mouth or keep his hands down, etc. but his/her ability to resist will be diminished. By the same token, remember his/her ability to comprehend and learn from the experience will also certainly be limited. So at the next visit, you'll be starting from ground zero. At best, the outcome is unpredictable.

Sedation and General Anesthesia

The skill level of a general dentist or a pediatric specialist should not be measured by the ability to administer drugs to modify the child's behavior. There is a great emphasis today on sedation, general anesthesia, and premedication within the profession because there is an apprehension about dealing with children in general. Sedation—who needs it—the child or the dentist?

My philosophy and methodology for working with children are not an arbitrary dismissal of sedation or general anesthesia. There is a time and place for these techniques when all else fails. They should not be the first choice or the only way of dealing with reluctant child patients. The polarization within the profession on this issue does a disservice to dentists and patients alike. This is not about pro-life or pro-choice or Republican or Democratic issues. This is about the welfare of children and the joy of caring for them. Flying on a trapeze without a net can be an exhilarating experience for you and the child. It's about educating children and their parents so they'll be less fearful of and more knowledgeable about dentistry. When a general practitioner refers a patient to our office, it should not be about putting a child to sleep. You would assume that the pediatric specialist has special behavioral skills that enable him to better manage the child.

The fact is that the more confidence you have in yourself as a dental practitioner, the less you will rely on drugs to manage children or adults. Surveys conducted frequently amongst pediatric specialists reveal that the longer a dentist has been in practice, the less likely he is to hospitalize or sedate a child to perform routine operative dentistry. Moreover, one of the important goals we set when treating children is to educate and inform. Meaningful communication is hampered when the child is under the influence of mind-altering medication. It's like speaking with a person under the influence of alcohol.

One of the excuses offered for employing these drugs is the patient's fear of the dentist. Going to sleep during your dental treatment does not abolish the fear. It masks it. It ignores it. But it does not deal with it. It's comparable to an unhappy person who gets drunk to forget his/her problems. Unfortunately, when he/she's sober again, his/her problems are still there.

If you do choose to utilize the in-office IV sedation technique, education, training, and experience for the dentist and the auxiliary personnel who are assisting during the procedure are essential to maximize a child's safety. Sedation or hospitalization for general anesthesia should not be the first alternatives. The behavioral approach offers the maximum opportunity to educate the mind while treating the teeth.

A Note About Restraint

Papoose boards, Velcro straps, and other artificial restraints are abhorrent to me and unpleasant for a child as well. That does not mean that you can't restrain a child or that some form of restraint may not be necessary. One very gentle and effective approach especially with children three years old and under is for a dental assistant (not the parent...too much anxiety) to sit in the chair and the child is placed in her lap. The dental assistant gently wraps her arms around the baby and her legs lightly around the baby's legs, like a human papoose board, resembling a mother hugging her baby (Fig. 3-11). There is a playfulness about the atmosphere with lots of active conversation. The dentist has free access to the head and the mouth. Although the child may be crying or reluctant, he/she is physically comfortable and safe, which is the important thing. Let the parents look from some vantage point without the child being aware of their presence. This visit also serves as a visual parental consent.

Auxiliary personnel

It is impossible to manage children and parents in the dental environment without the skill and enthusiasm of dental assistants, hygienists, and front desk personnel. From the moment a parent contacts the office for an appointment until the child patient leaves after the appointment, the auxiliary personnel are essential to assure a positive experience for everyone concerned. In the operatory, it is the responsibility of the den-

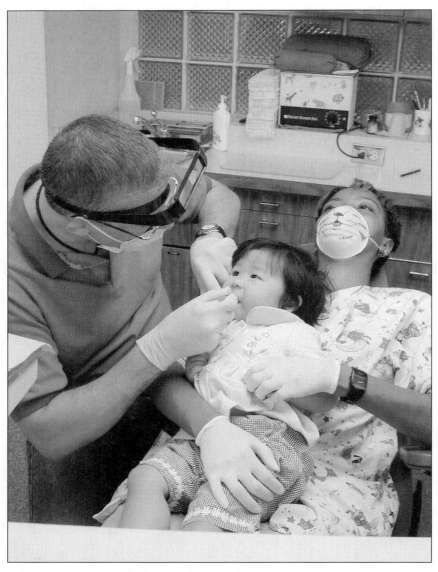

Fig. 3-11 Baby comfortably nestled in dental assistant embrace

tal assistants to not merely set instruments and assist the doctor in the dental procedure, they must take an active role in potentiating the positive behavior of the child by talking, laughing, playing, and hugging or anything else it takes to make the parent and child feel comfortable and happy (Fig. 3-12). The more fun the ambience of the encounter, the less the need for drugs.

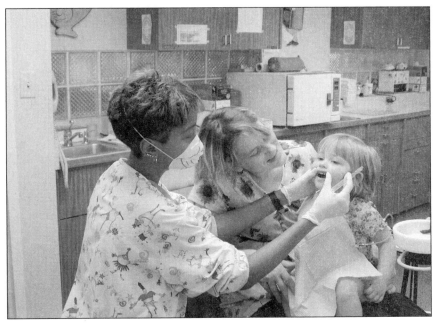

Fig. 3-12 Dental assistant exhibiting the chairside manner essential for establishing rapport with patients

Note: In states where expanded duties for auxiliaries are part of the dental practice act, there is an increased responsibility borne by the doctor and the auxiliary. The allocation of certain procedures to hygienists and dental assistants with the supervision of the dentist has been and will continue to be most beneficial to dentists and patients alike. However, as the doctor, you are ultimately responsible for everything. Don't abdicate that function.

When Dentist and Child Meet

Once you, the dentist and/or the dental assistant and the child are face to face in the operatory in the absence of a parent, it is incumbent upon you to make every effort to enhance the success of the encounter. Whether you're dealing with a youngster that's apprehensive, belligerent, or reluctant or one that's sweet and compliant, remember that this first visit could be the one that defines this child's attitude toward dentists and dentistry forever. The following are some tips that will elucidate my methodology:[26]

Initial impressions are everything

When meeting a new person, body language and the verbal communication both have to convey confidence, authority, and most importantly, warmth. It's all about chairside manners. It's not what you say as much as how you say it. Begin with a smile and make sure that you address the patient using the first name. Don't ask "So what's your name sweetheart?" or "Hi, big guy!" Those kinds of greetings are too generic. Instead, with a big smile say something like "Hi Laurie! We're so glad you came today. I'm Dr. Berman and I picked out my favorite color toothbrush for you. Show me how you brush."

Show, tell, and do

Make sure you take the child from the familiar to the unfamiliar...from what she knows to what she doesn't know. For example, before you even place the child in the dental chair give her a toothbrush (which she's already seen at home). "Oh did you bring toothpaste? No? Well I have the best tasting toothpaste." Let her begin to brush and then "we need some water!" (something else that she recognizes). Of course the cup of water is at the cuspidor of the unit. Lift the child onto the chair so she can reach the cup of water. "But wait, we don't want to spill the water on your beautiful dress, let's put this napkin on!" When the rinse is finished, you say, "let's see if you got the teeth clean!" But then "wait a minute, you don't have a mirror to see! Here's a mirror!" Hand her the mirror and then "it's too dark, we need a light." Turn on the dental light. "This is your toothbrush. This is my toothbrush. We brush my finger first, then yours. Here's your big mirror and here's my little one." With this kind of rational progression, each item or procedure you add has a motivational purpose. Don't rush! Each step leads to the next (Fig. 3-13a and Fig. 3-13b). At some point, the parent gets to watch for a few minutes without the child being aware he/she's there so we don't break the spell.

Remember the first visit with a young patient is more about education and acclimation than the dental treatment itself. You're setting a long-term pattern of behavior.

No elective dentistry at the first visit

This should be the rule unless the child is in pain or if it's necessary to perform an emergency procedure (*e.g.*, bond a fractured incisor, etc.). Don't rush things. Let the child absorb the sights and sounds of the dental office if possible. Should you encounter a situation where the first visit requires immediate invasive treatment (*e.g.*, local anesthesia, extraction, operative dentistry, etc.) start from scratch just like any other patient (show, tell, do) and ease into the more involved treatment.

Never lose your temper

You're always in control of yourself, regardless of how negative the child's behavior may become. You are the professional.

Crying and whining

They are part and parcel of working with children. Rather than say "stop crying!" it may be more effective to simply ask the child why he/she's crying. He/she often says, "I want my mommy!" and you're response will be "of course, your mommy brought you! Show me how you brush and let's go to mommy!" In other words, first you do what I want and then we'll do what you want, a principle that the child needs to learn to survive in life.

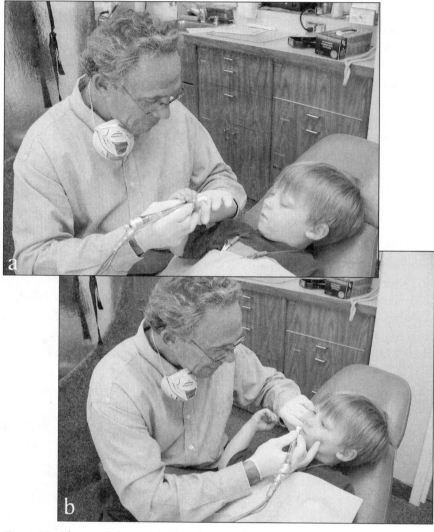

Fig. 3-13a *The art of show-tell-do, acclimating the child to the feel of the prophy cup on the fingers first*

3-13b *Repeating the introduction on the teeth*

A child who is screaming hysterically is certainly not capable of listening to you, so either the parent can calm his/her child down or, in the absence of the parent, you can. My experience has taught me that the hysteria ends more quickly without parental assistance. If you're dealing with an infant, ignore the crying and simply proceed with the treatment quickly and efficiently. Don't let the crying deter you from your task as long as the child can be controlled safely. Don't let the child's behavior compromise your choice of treatment.

Important tip: Don't try to stop the crying of an older child by saying things like, "You're acting like a two year old. Don't be a baby. Act your age." Definitely don't call names "You brat! Whiny girl! Horrible child!" Instead, when a crying child is capable of understanding language and thought, ask the question, "What do you want? What would you like? Why are you crying?" Listen for the answer and respond appropriately.

In other words, don't buy into the child's agenda. Whether he/she is afraid, or if the child is just being manipulative, you've taken the most effective and least inflammatory approach. Don't back off. Call their bluff.

Chair position should be more upright

You and your patient need to look at each other, eye to eye. Communication is enhanced because of the more direct eye contact, and the child does not feel so overpowered with you towering over him/her.

Many dentists prefer the horizontal working position because it enables them to lay their head down over the patient and try to use direct vision. In dental school, we were forced to learn to operate in a more upright position, using the mouth mirror, with everything backwards of course. The "lying down flat in the chair" position may be more comfortable for the dentist, but very disconcerting for the child patient. The child feels more vulnerable and helpless with the dentist hovering above...and the view up the nose is not particularly pleasant. With or without a rubber dam there is a feeling of choking and problems breathing (real or imagined) and the saliva welling up in the throat, even with suction. The more upright position allows the best control of the head and access to the mouth.

Eyes open during all treatment

When your eyes are closed, your imagination takes over and all fears and emotions are magnified. Moreover, when the eyes are closed, the other senses become more acute and intense. In addition, with the eyes open, the treatment becomes a learning experience in addition to merely fixing the teeth.

Talk! Talk! Silence is deadly

Very young children have a very short span of attention. They need the vocal or visual stimulation to keep them occupied, content, and happy. Maintain a constant line of talk appropriate to the age of the child. If the patient is two years old, your subject matter is certainly different than with a seven year old. Don't leave the child alone with his/her thoughts. He/she'll start to think bad things.

Dental assistant

A child needs full attention to ensure safety and comfort for all concerned. This means an assistant should be present for all operative dentistry.

Compromise not confrontation

Try to make the visit end on a positive note. You and the child and the parent should part on good terms, no matter what happened in the middle.

The Dreaded Shot

Local anesthesia alias...the shot...is the one clinical procedure on which I'll focus because the shot represents the defining moment in the establishment of the patient-doctor relationship. If you can give a painless injection, the trust between you and the child or the adult will be boundless.[27] The fear of the needle has its roots in the fear of the unknown and, once engrained in your mind as a child, it becomes the dominant point of apprehension throughout adulthood. Even dentists themselves are sometimes queasy about the thought of giving the injection. This lack of comfort level and the stress factor cross the doctor-patient placental barrier and in effect destroy the mutual trust.

This lack of confidence in their ability to administer a painless injection causes many dentists to avoid giving the shot altogether or to try and mask the fears with mind-altering drugs. This anxiety is reflected in the noble and endless search for the panacea that avoids shots and drilling, and no doubt sometime in the future, the technology will be there. But for now, trying to circumvent the inevitable through various means is meeting with a wide range of dissatisfaction. The fact is that the limitations on medical and dental technology for pain control means that a patient is going to get stuck with a needle sometime, somewhere, someplace, so let's make it as pleasant as we possible can—*and we can.*

"Points" to consider

If you feel that the procedure you're about to perform will cause discomfort for the patient, do not hesitate to use local anesthesia. The caries may look superficial, but if you approach the dento-enamel junction, it's going to hurt. Don't say to the child "hold on it's just another second. I'm almost done." Stop and administer the injection. Once you've hurt a child, it's very difficult to re-establish a good rapport.

- Any patient who has the linguistic skills to comprehend the situation should actually see the shot (the needle) before, after, during, and/or all three. Even a three year old should leave the office knowing that he/she's had a shot and it didn't hurt. If the child is a first time patient with no previous experience, we administer the injection and then show them the needle. If we're dealing with a child who's had previous experience but is frightened, we'll show the shot first, explain everything, and then do the injection

- Since the whole anesthetizing procedure is a learning experience, I administer the total dose of the anesthetic in steps. On the first thrust I express a small amount of anesthesia and then take the needle out to show the patient "Look what we did! I gave you a shot! Didn't you love it?" Then "now I'm going to show you again." The patient often says "not again!" I answer "of course, we need the practice!" Don't rush! Let the eyes focus on the needle and call it by name. Then validate the moment by saying "wasn't that the best shot ever?" Be animated and enthusiastic. This is important stuff

- The infiltration, the mandibular block, and even the palatal injection should be pain free if you take the time and make the effort, if you take heed of the following (refer to "Oh No! Not the Shot" video for complete description of details):

    1. Make sure the patient is not lying down, but sitting semi-upright in the chair with a dental assistant standing on the opposite side of the chair

    2. The dental assistant should have one hand over the patient's hands that are folded in his/her lap. Her other arm is resting lightly on the patient's shoulder and snugly placed against the neck (Fig. 3-14)

    3. Child's eyes should be open and not closed. When your eyes are closed, the imagination becomes more vivid and the feedback from the other senses (hearing, smell, and touch) is exaggerated. You want the patient completely involved with you, not drifting off in a sea of negative thoughts

    4. *Silence is deadly.* It's mandatory that, along with eye contact, the dentist maintain a constant flow of words on some subject or other directed to the child. It doesn't have to be about teeth. Maintain a conversational tone about any subject that pertains to the child's life experience at that particular age. A three year old and a nine year old require a different mind-set. Age appropriate is the guideline

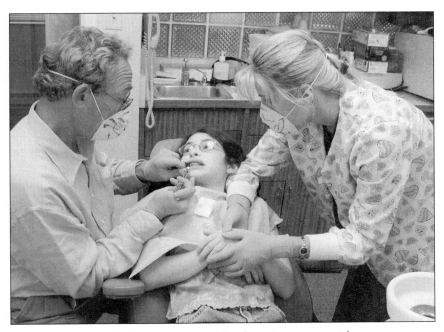

Fig. 3-14 The "battle station position" with patient more upright, eyes open, hands across stomach. Dental assistant right arm resting on patient's shoulder next to head. Her left hand resting lightly over the patient's hands. Dentist and patient eye to eye. Good finger rests. Note the working triangle formed by the dental assistant, the dentist, and the patient

The painless injection

It's one thing to make a promise. It's another to keep that promise. If you tell the child that nothing is going to hurt, then you have to make sure that you don't.

- Apply topical anesthetic with a Q-tip on the area to be injected. This procedure serves the purpose of making the point of injection less sensitive, but more importantly it gives the dentist the opportunity to introduce a non-invasive procedure and assess the response of the child (Fig. 3-15)

- When performing an infiltration in the maxillary arch, ask the patient to bite the teeth together in order to loosen the buccal or labial tissues. This allows you with a wiggling motion to pull the tissue into the needle instead of poking the needle into the tissues (Fig. 3-16)

- All patients who are capable of absorbing the concept should be shown the needle before, after, or during. Don't be afraid to inject a little anesthetic, come out for a look, and then back in again

- Don't overdo the local anesthesia. With young children, we're not with dealing with multiple carpules. We're using fractions of carpules. It's not the amount of anesthesia, it's location...location

- The ideal local anesthetic for a young child would be one that doesn't contain epinephrine (*e.g.*, mepivicaine 3%...no epinephrine). Bear in mind that the three elements of the local anesthesia experience for the patient and the doctor, after the shot has been administered, are the time of onset, the duration of working anesthesia, and the time the numbness disappears. In the case of a dental student or a dentist who is more deliberate, a more long lasting anesthesia is preferable, one with epinephrine (*e.g.*, lidocaine 2% 1:100,000), because you need more working time. The advantage of the quick acting anesthetic is the more rapid disappearance of the numbness so as to lessen the chance that the child will bite or chew on his soft tissues

- Do not leave the child alone following the injection. Either the doctor or a dental assistant should keep the child company, explaining what's happening (the weird feeling). Show the child in the mirror that although the lip feels likes it's blowing up like a balloon, it still looks normal. Make certain you are very specific about the post-operative instructions to the parent in regard to eating, etc. Written instructions are fine, but a verbal version is essential (Fig. 3-17)

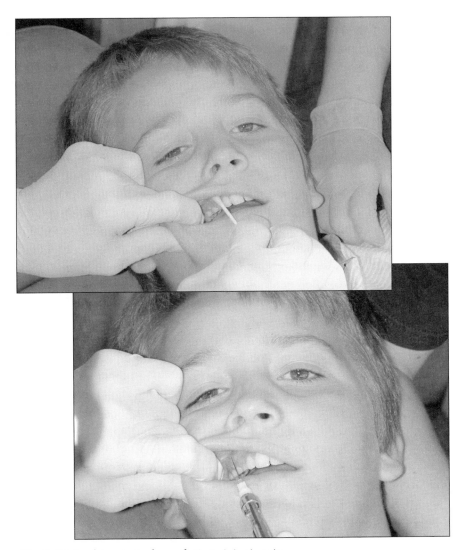

Fig. 3-15 Applying topical anesthetic to injection site

Fig. 3-16 Administering local anesthesia (infiltration). Note patient's eyes open, teeth biting together, soft tissues relaxed

Drs. Berman, Kollmann, & Furusho
Dentistry For Kids, Ltd
4801 W. PETERSON AVE.
CHICAGO, ILLINOIS 60646
PHONE: 773.764.0007

HOME CARE FOLLOWING EXTRACTIONS

1. CAUTION: Don't let child chew or pick on cheeks, lips or tongue until effects of local anesthetic are over. (At least 1 hour).

2. Bleeding: Bite firmly on guaze for at least 30 minutes. Repeat if necessary. Call us if bleeding persists.

3. Eating Drink plenty of fluids (not from straw), but don't rinse mouth for at least 2 hours. Do not eat for 1 hour. Soft, bland foods e.g. Soup, bread, pasta for 12 hours thereafter. Avoid crunchy foods (potato chips, hard candy, etc.).

4. Pain: Slight discomfort is normal. Use pain reliever as directed if necessary.

5. Activity: Limit physical exertion (no gymnastics, swimming or rough play for 6-8 hours).

IF YOU ARE WORRIED ABOUT ANYTHING...
PLEASE CALL

DR. BERMAN
DR. KOLLMANN
DR. FURUSHO

Fig. 3-17 Post-operative extraction instructions should be specific and geared to your particular practice. Details should be repeated verbally

Voice Control

Voice control or voice modulation is often mentioned in reference to controlling or modifying a child's negative behavior in the dental chair.[28] A discussion of this valuable modality is often vague and circumspect and necessarily anecdotal. It's difficult to describe in words, but you know it when you see it being used effectively. The educational videotapes, "Excellent Adventures With Children" and "Winning Friends and Influencing People," both previously referenced, clearly illustrate how effective voice modulation can work to control or modify a reluctant child's behavior.

To put it simply, you must gain the patient's attention if you hope to communicate. There must be a focus. When you're dealing with a toddler with minimal language skills, gesture and eye contact are most important. Eye contact! Eye contact! The patient needs to focus on you. Many children diagnosed with attention deficit are not deficient in anything. They're just not listening and paying attention.

Once a child has some language skill and is capable of understanding the basic words and their meaning, then those words become the key to overcoming a child's resistance. Most importantly, it's not what you say! It's how you say it. It's about raising your voice and then lowering your voice to a whisper. It's about speaking very excitedly and quickly and then changing to a more controlled purposeful pace and tone where you *emphasize each word* and space the words so they sound important. "Open your mouth now, please!" is fine. But "open...your...mouth...now...please!" is much better.

A calm, firm voice with good eye contact carries a lot of weight. If you're nervous, angry, impatient, or frustrated, the patient picks up on that immediately and whatever you say doesn't matter. Direct eye contact is mandatory. "Look at me. I'm speaking to you!" Go eye to eye with the patient so there's no mistaking your intent.

Facial expression tells it all, from the smile, to the frown, and back again—that look your mother or father gave you when you did something good and the other look when you did something wrong. The quiet stare, with nothing spoken can be most persuasive.

Prizes and Rewards

Everyone likes to get a prize or to be given a gift. Presenting a gift to a child for performing the basic minimum tasks that are part of getting through each day is a bad habit parents fall into early on in the child rearing process. Putting on your pajamas, watching your baby sister, getting good grades in school, making your bed, and keeping your room clean should all be the basic behavior requirements that should be expected by parents from their children. Instead parents feel the pressure of having to bribe or reward their kids to perform the daily tasks essential to survival. It's all part of the requests and promises idea that Pinkham suggests.

This particular parental pattern continues in conjunction with the dental visit in the form of incentives for "being good." The promise of special toys or money or a trip somewhere if the child behaves is among his/her many offerings.

My recommendation is that everybody gets a prize or reward after the dental treatment regardless of his/her behavior (Fig. 3-18). Don't threaten to withhold a prize from a child in hopes that he/she'll be good. If he/she was good...wonderful! If he/she was not so cooperative, maybe he/she'll improve next time. Besides, in today's world you couldn't give a prize valuable enough to seduce a child because he/she is overindulged in so many ways with material possessions that far exceed anything you could realistically offer. Pencils, rings, bracelets, stickers, sports cards are all appropriate prizes that represent a gesture and not a bribe.

Reinforcement and Review

An essential adjunct to the traditional "show—tell—do" methodology is the principle of reviewing with the child and parent the events of the day and what is in store for them at the next visit. At the end of any given

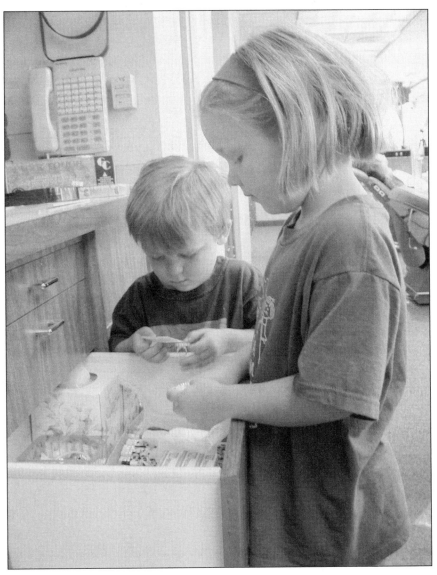

Fig. 3-18 Children choosing prizes after dental treatment

operative visit, especially if it involved extensive operative dentistry, say to the child "So today we put those nice crowns on these two teeth (show in mirror) and next time we're going to put another crown on this tooth over here. But first I'll give you the shot, just like today so everything feels nice and nothing hurts you."

When the child arrives the next visit, the dental assistant or the doctor goes through the drill again, "What did we do last time? Remember we gave you the shot and it felt funny and then we did those beautiful crowns. Let me see! Oh they look great! And today we'll do the other side." Don't assume that the child or the parent remembers. The parents don't keep the details of the treatment plan in their head, so the reminder keeps them in the flow.

Those Nasty Habits—Bottles, Pacifiers, and Thumbs

The discussion of oral habits in children is perhaps at the epicenter of the dentist-parent-child interaction. Without going into the minute details of the effect excessive sucking can have on the development of the dental arches, suffice it to say that oral habits are a melding of clinical and psychological considerations (Fig. 3-19). You can't simply say to a child, "Stop that!" and expect that the matter be settled.

That little toddler loves his/her bottle, his/her blanket, his/her pacifier (Fig. 3-20), better known as "binky" or the thumb (Fig. 3-21). During the night and in the quiet moments during the day, he/she indulges in one or more of these habits with enthusiasm. As with an alcoholic or a smoker or a drug abuser, we have to find the key to interrupting a pattern that has become engrained. Parents are often frustrated because their emotional involvement with the child over the "habit" issue creates unpleasant conflict. The dentist, on the other hand can be more objective, and the attention the child gets from someone other than a parent often yields positive results. Some general principles to keep in mind in regard to controlling or eliminating undesirable oral habits:[29-30]

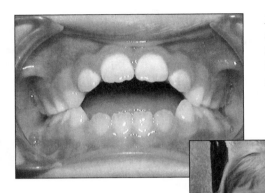

Fig. 3-19 Anterior open bite and constricted arches, caused by ongoing thumbsucking and potentiated by the subsequent thrusting of the tongue into the already open space

Fig. 3-20 Toddler enjoying her pacifier and her fragment of blanket

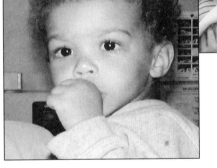

Fig. 3-21 Two year old sucking thumb

- *Punitive measures are not appropriate under any circumstances*
- Offering incentives or bribery will not work unless the child is capable of postponing immediate gratification for eventual pleasure. Is the child old enough to understand that if he/she does something now it will mean something else later? Some children are more mature than others so results can vary
- Always begin with a short-term achievable goal. "Can you stop for one day? How about for two days? Call me tomorrow and tell me the good news. Then come in and pick up

your special surprise." This approach should be intimate and quiet to establish a strong connection between you and the child. You're not lecturing or berating. You're empathizing and encouraging

- The transaction should be between you and the child...the parent should be eliminated from the equation. The child is usually very impressed that a "total stranger" is interested in him/her and therefore is more likely to want to please that person

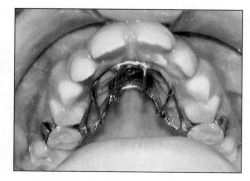

Fig. 3-22 Thumbsucking crib in place. Note curved wires that serve as a distraction and not a punishment

Appliances are a last resort and reserved for a child who can understand the intent of the appliance...namely to be a reminder about not sucking the finger and not an instrument of torture (Fig. 3-22).

Some Thoughts about the Special Child

In the not so distant past, some children were described in terms like gifted or genius. Others were called handicapped, crippled, or retarded. In this age of enlightenment, all children who are not in the so-called "normal" category are labeled "special" to indicate they are different. For the purposes of this discussion, we're speaking about children who are physically or mentally compromised.

What makes these children "special" is the dedication, the courage, and the superhuman effort exerted by the children and their parents to achieve beyond anyone's expectations. As dentists, we must understand that there is no special place for these children. In fact, every parent of one of these children will tell you that you that his/her fervent wish is that the child be included in the mainstream of society in as many ways as possible. Separate but equal does not apply here. This is not a civil rights issue.

The point is that when encountering a special child or when being asked if you treat them, don't think initially in terms of referring them to a specialist. This child is part of a symbiotic life experience. You need the child and the child needs you. Furthermore, it is most important for that youngster to be exposed in an open situation to other children and for the other children to be exposed to him/her so he/she can develop an empathy and a tolerance for those that are different.

So in the waiting room we'll find an array of children of assorted colors, religions, shapes, sizes, and intelligence levels. There are crutches and wheel chairs and endotracheal tubes and oxygen tanks. This is how children learn the meaning of diversity, not from a book.

Continuing with this theme, the dentist and the auxiliaries must make every effort to treat these children as much like others as possible. The following are some of the basics and for a more comprehensive coverage of the subject:[31]

- Make certain your office is accessible to wheelchairs or other accoutrements. If the child can walk with support, no matter how hesitatingly, take the time to walk with him/her from the waiting room to the operatory (Fig. 3-23a). The physical closeness enhances the relationship with the child and is a prelude to your laying hands on when you go into the oral cavity

- In the case of a wheelchair-bound child, be flexible about treating him/her in the wheelchair or moving onto the dental chair (Fig. 3-23b). The decision should be made based on the comfort of the child. Sometimes the dentist has to be the one that's inconvenienced

- Don't compromise the course of treatment because of the child's shortcomings, over which we have no control. His/her dental health and the enhancement of his/her abili-

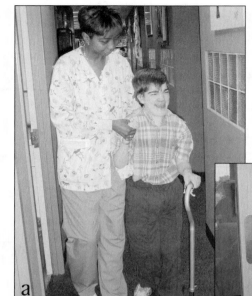

Fig. 3-23a *Young boy with cane making his way down the hall accompanied by a dental assistant*

Fig. 3-23b *Dental assistant working with special child in his wheel chair*

ty to enjoy eating are things we can influence positively. Establish a comfort level for yourself

- Speak directly to the child...not about him/her. Don't use the third person as in "He/she's got a lot of cavities! Who's here with him/her today! They're not brushing his/her teeth!" Use the first person, *e.g.*, "Bobby, why aren't you brushing your teeth? You have two loose teeth over here, Bobby, but here come the new teeth. Aren't you excited?" (Act excited)

- There are some patients that, because of their size, or lack of cooperation, or medical conditions, are more appropriately treated in a hospital environment where you have access to all of the emergency equipment and medical expertise to guarantee their safety. Use your best judgment and don't forget to consult and advise the parents accordingly

Case Presentation

When the "one on one" with the child is complete, it is now time to devote the same kind of attention, enthusiasm, and energy to the parent during the so-called private consultation or case presentation.[32]

The treatment plan should be specific and in written form following the examination of the child. The treatment plan should be discussed thoroughly with the parent, emphasizing all of the clinical aspects of the plan. Make certain you devote the necessary amount of time for the parent to ask any questions he/she may have. It's their turn to be with you, so don't rush.

As I explain and illustrate in the "Winning Friends and Influencing Patients" videotape (Part 1—Case Presentation), the doctor is the storyteller...so tell the story. Remember you're educating and not selling. The goal is to make the parent an educated consumer who will now be in a position to make an informed decision in regard to your treatment proposal. Be upfront and personal. Don't sit behind your desk. It becomes a barrier to communication (Fig. 3-24). Use terminology that a layman can understand. Avoid terms like caries, gingival, extraction, and pulpotomy. Don't be afraid to let your hair down and talk about decay, cavities, gums, and nerve treatment. What do you mean...nerve treatment?...Explain!

Don't discuss specific fees. Speak about the child and the importance of the treatment you're recommending. Leave the financial discussion to the people at your front desk. You are the doctor.

The most difficult concept for parents to accept and understand is prevention.[33] When you point to cavities on an x-ray or a discolored tooth or a swelling on the gums or a cold sore on the lip, they can relate. But the more abstract benefits of fluoride treatments, sealants, restoring baby teeth, or saving space are more elusive. When I speak to parents about weaning the child away from the bottle or throwing away the pacifier or brushing the teeth more frequently, or eliminating some of the between meal treats, there is often an air of condescension. "Yeh! Yeh! I know. Whatever!" People in general don't put a lot of value on what might happen if you don't do something. It's much easier to understand after the damage occurs. Then it's too late for prevention. It's time for guilt

It is not uncommon for me to expend much more energy explaining the circumstances to the parents than working with their children. But then again, you are an educator. You are coaching and encouraging the parents to take a stronger hand with their kids to ensure a better outcome for them in the future.

Saying goodbye at the front desk

The private office session is followed up by the front desk person who will reiterate the treatment plan and discuss the financial considerations. I prefer not to get directly involved with the financial or payment details because I'm focusing on the welfare of the child. So I leave the money talk as well as the other administrative matters to the front desk personnel. I recommend a watchful, but not interfering style of management on the part of the dentist. Delegate responsibility, but maintain your awareness of everything.[34]

In addition, the front desk people are responsible for setting the next appointments whether they are for treatment or checkups and clarifying any questions or verifying the parent's understanding of what's in store for his/her child. A pleasant and friendly demeanor punctuates the theme that has already been created (Fig. 3-25). The family's experience at the front desk is the first and last contact with the office. Keep in mind that your goal is a long-term, mutually beneficial relationship with your patients.

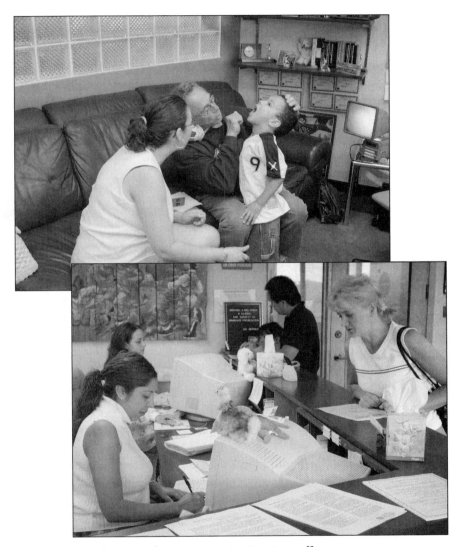

Fig. 3-24 Consultation and case presentation in private office with parent and child. Note up-close and personal approach

Fig. 3-25 Front desk personnel pleasantly attending to business details

Conclusion

Parents, children, and dentists…a brave new world

When we view the big picture as if from a vantage point in the sky, it comes down to the fact that many parents today have not taught their children the basic lessons of life. When these children accompanied by their parents arrive at our offices for dental care, we must be prepared to deal with more than the mouth, the teeth, and the gums. Before we can address the dental concerns, we must be able to evaluate the human behavior aspect of the situation and deal with the patients and their parents as people. This task is by far more time consuming and difficult than merely fixing teeth.

Parents can be anxious, nervous, even hostile, perhaps stemming from their own pre-conditioned feeling about dentists. The children may be apprehensive or even belligerent…yes and crying. The parents don't want any hassle because they're accustomed to backing off when their children act up. The children are accustomed to having their own way, not required to do anything they don't want to do. Over-indulged, spoiled, and self-centered are terms that could easily be applied.

Many moms and dads are on the defensive because they're often worried or embarrassed about how their child is going to behave since the rapport is on the edge at home. No parameters of behavior have been set and the line hasn't been drawn in the sand by the parent at home, so it will be up to you, the dentist, for the length of the dental appointment to set the house rules and regulations that will enable you to accomplish the treatment effectively and instill a positive attitude at the same time. Whatever behavior management techniques you employ, the object is to achieve a positive outcome.[35]

Strive to develop a cooperative relationship between you, the child, and the parent—a relationship that's built on trust. Look upon the child and the dental visit as a defining moment in time that becomes a marketing tool for the future of your practice as well. It's not far fetched to believe that when that child grows up, he/she remains your patient and should he/she marry and have children of his/her own, they'll become your patients as well.

When it's all said and done, the grateful smile of an anxious parent and the warmth of a hug from a happy child will make your life as a dentist rich and fulfilling as no other area of dentistry can (Fig. 3-26). Working with children represents the upside of dentistry. In your dental chair is a brand new child, with new teeth and a new long-term outlook on life. The dawn of a new life...an empty canvas on which you can paint a picture. Make it a beautiful one.

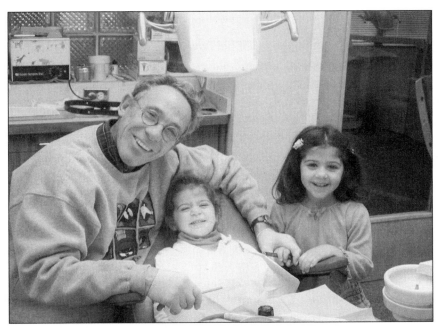

Fig. 3-26 Reaping the rewards that are derived from working with children

Notes

1 McDonald, R.E. and Avery D.R. *Dentistry for the Child and Adolescent*, 6th ed., St. Louis: Mosby, 1994

2 Forrester, D.J. *Pediatric Dental Medicine*, Philadelphia: Lea & Febiger, 1981

3 Pinkham, J.B., et al. *Pediatric Dentistry: Infancy Through Adolescence*, 2nd ed., Philadelphia: Saunders, 1994

4 Ilg, F.L. and Ames, L.B. *Child Behavior*, Gesell Institute, Dell, 1963

5 Rosemond, J. *Because I Said So!* www.linearpublishing.com, 2000

6 Dreikurs, R. and Soltz, V. *Children The Challenge*, New York: Hawthorn Books, 1964

7 Sarles, R., Forrester, D.J. *Pediatric Dental Medicine Psychologic Growth and Development*, Philadelphia: Lea & Febiger, chap. 3, 1981

8 Bruer, J.T. *The Window of Opportunity: The Myth of the First Three Years*, www.jsmf.org

9 Schour, I. and Massler, M. Studies in Tooth Development: The Growth Pattern of Human Teeth, *JADA* 27 (11): 1778-1793 and 1918-1931, 1940

10 McDonald, R.E. and Avery, D.R. *Dentistry for the Child and Adolescent*, 6th ed., St. Louis: Mosby, pp. 290-291, 1994

11 Gardner, D.E., et al. At Will Breast Feeding and Dental Caries. 4 Case Reports, *J.Dent., Child* 44: 186-191, 1977

[12] Dilley, C.G., et al. Prolonged Nursing Habit: A Profile of Parents and Their Families, *J.Dent Child* 47: 102-108, 1980

[13] Weiss, R.L. and Trithart, A.H. Between Meal Eating Habits and Dental Caries Experience in Pre-School Experience, *Am. Jour Public Health*, 50: 1,097-1,104

[14] Nowak, A.J. Toothbrush Selection for Children 1-5 years old. *AAPD Research Abstract*, AAPD Session, 1992

[15] Walsh, M., et al. Comparison of Manual and Power Toothbrushing with and without Adjunctive Oral Irrigation for Controlling Plaque and Gingivitis, *J. Clinical Periodont*, 16:419-427, 1989

[16] Mescher, K.D. Ability of elementary school children to perform sulcular toothbrushing as related to hand function ability, *Pediatric Dent.* 2 (1): 33-36, 1980

[17] Wright, G.Z., Alpern, G.D., and Leake, J.L. The modifiability of maternal anxiety as it relates to children's cooperative behavior, *J. Dent. Child* 40:265-271, 1973

[18] Pinkham, J.B. *Pediatric Dentistry: Infancy Through Adolescence*, 2nd ed., Philadelphia: Saunders, 1994, p. 347

[19] American Academy of Pediatric Dentistry: *Guidelines for behavior management* Chicago, 1991 revised 2000, pp. 47-51

[20] Pinkham, J. The role of requests and promises in child patient management, *J. Dent Child* May, June, 1993

[21] Chambers, D.W. Behavior management for pediatric dentists: an embarrassment of riches, *J. Dent. Child* 44: 30-34, 1977

[22] Pinkham, J., et al. *Pediatric Dentistry: Infancy Through Adolescence* 2nd ed., Philadelphia: Saunders, 1994, p. 352

[23] Wright, G.Z. *Behavior Management in Dentistry for Children*, Philadelphia: Saunders, 1975

[24] Berman, M.H. Videotape: *Winning Friends and Influencing Patients: Chairside Manners*, Part III, 2000

[25] American Academy of Pediatric Dentistry. Guidelines for the elective use of conscious sedation, deep sedation and general anesthesia in pediatric patients, *Pediatric Dent*, 7:334-337, 1985 revised 1998

[26] Berman, M.H. Videotape: *Excellent Adventures With Children*, 1992

[27] Berman, M.H. Videotape: *Oh No! Not The Shot!*, 1995

[28] Greenbaum, P.E., et al. Dentist's voice control: effect on children's disruptive behavior, *Health Psychology* 5, pp. 546-558, 1990

[29] Haryett, R.D., Hansen, F.C., and Davidson P.O. Chronic thumb-sucking: A second report on treatment and its psychological effects, *Am. J. Orthod*, 57: 167-17, 1970

[30] Christensen, J.R., Fields, Jr., H.W., Pinkham, J., et al. *Pediatric Dentistry: Infancy through adolescence*, chap. 26, Philadelphia: Saunders, 1994, pp. 366-380

[31] Weddell, J.A., McDonald R.E., and Avery D.R. *Dentistry For the Child and Adolescent*, 6th ed., Mosby, 1994, chap. 23, pp. 592-652

[32] Berman, M.H. Videotape: *Winning Friends and Influencing Patients. Case Presentation*, Part I, 1999

[33] Berman, M.H. Ask The Expert: How dentists and parents can communicate effectively about children's dental health needs, *JADA*, vol.32, June, 2001, pp. 797-796

[34] Berman, M.H. Videotape: *Winning Friends and Influencing Patients. It's What's Up Front That Counts*, Part II, 1999

[35] Quality Assurance Criteria For Pediatric Dentistry: Behavior Management, *J. Amer. Acad. Ped. Dent Reference Manual*, vol.22 #7, 2000, p.107

Chapter 4

Esthetic Posterior Restorations: A Problem-Solving Guide

By George Freedman, D.D.S.

The scientific development of esthetic restorations has posed a number of problems for the dental practitioner—whether to get involved in this area of dentistry, how to approach patients, what position to take on amalgam, which adhesives to use, how to avoid postoperative sensitivity, which techniques to use for the greatest efficiency, and how to polish the restoration (Fig. 4-1).

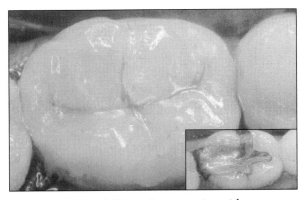

Fig. 4-1 Composite restoration with inset of previous amalgam filling

Getting Involved

The first problem that many dentists face with esthetic posterior restorations is whether to offer these fillings at all. This dilemma involves not only new skills and new materials, but a series of scientific and ethical questions as well. The question of costs to the patient must also be considered. Our patients, of course, do not ask any of these questions; their concerns are rather straightforward. Patients simply want to know if the restorations will:

- Look like their natural teeth
- Last a long time
- Cause any pain
- Cost more

These questions are understandable. The first and foremost issue is that of appearance.[1] In fact, many of today's patients assume that any restoration they are given will be indistinguishable from their natural teeth. For many patients, the demand for esthetic materials is the one and only general parameter they place upon their dentist.

The question of longevity also arises, but since both traditional and more recent filling materials are relatively successful in the difficult environment of the human mouth, and routinely last for longer than a decade, this is more of a rote issue than a real concern. The ultimate success of any restoration is far more likely to depend on the patient's oral hygiene than on the selection of the filling material.

Dentistry has largely answered the issue of pain during dental procedures. Local anesthesia is routinely used, and technologies such as The Wand (Milestone Scientific, Deerfield, IL) (Fig. 4-2) and the Comfort Control (Dentsply/Midwest, Des Plaines, IL) make even this innocuous procedure less threatening. The advent of techniques such as Fissurotomy (SSWhite, Piscataway, NJ) (Fig. 4-3) and CariSolv (Biodenix Technologies Inc., Richmond, BC) permit the preparation and restoration of small cavities without the need for dental injections or anesthetic.

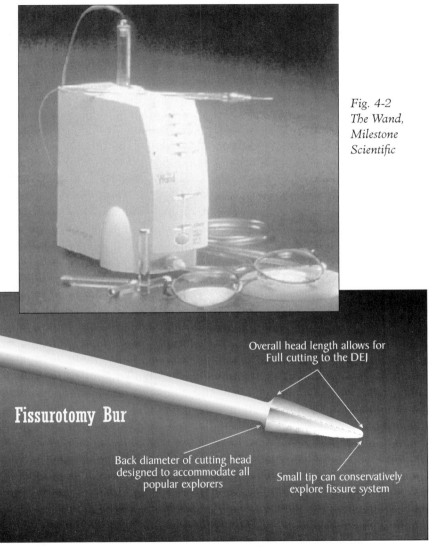

*Fig. 4-2
The Wand,
Milestone
Scientific*

Fissurotomy Bur

Overall head length allows for
Full cutting to the DEJ

Back diameter of cutting head
designed to accommodate all
popular explorers

Small tip can conservatively
explore fissure system

Fig. 4-3 Fissurotomy bur

Much is made of the cost issue by some dentists. Patients are far less sanguine about the matter. For most patients, the esthetic issue is the paramount one. In addition, some or all of the cost of most basic restorations is covered by dental insurance. When one considers the cost of a dental restoration in relation to its longevity and function, the difference of a few dollars at the initial placement is rather inconsequential.

The professional issues faced by the dentist are real ones. Each and every practitioner would like to deliver optimal care to his or her patients. Fortunately, the scientific evidence is there in abundance; adhesive (esthetic) restorations last at least as long, or longer than, similar amalgam restorations.[2-3] The margins of adhesive restorations are better adapted to the remaining tooth structure,[4] and are less likely to be involved in redecay or breakdown. In terms of continuing function, microhybrid composites wear considerably less than amalgams and approximately at the same rate as human enamel.

The new skills that are required to place posterior esthetic restorations are not greatly removed from the old skills that were required for posterior amalgam restorations.[5] Any dentist who can successfully place an amalgam can readily reorient to successful composites.

One question remaining is that of the increased cost for posterior esthetic fillings. The usual recommendation is that the fee for esthetic restorations be one and one half to two times the fee for similar amalgam restorations. This is simply a function of the additional time required to place, contour, define, and polish an esthetic restoration. It does not imply that dentists are altering their fees or that patients are being overcharged. Esthetic restorations, very simply, take somewhat longer to do, and cost somewhat more.

Approaching the Patient

This is probably one of the most difficult barriers to esthetic posterior restorations for many dentists. Most practitioners are uncomfortable proposing techniques and materials to their patients that may be more expensive (but longer lasting and better) than current treatment options.

We as dentists are afraid that this may make us look greedy and less professional in the eyes of our patients. As well, few dentists have been trained in patient management—this is not one of the courses offered at dental schools.

Some of the dentist discomfort is brought about by the aggressive marketing that is often recommended and taught by practice management courses. While this kind of marketing suits some practitioners, it makes others uncomfortable.

I prefer to *educate* rather than *market*. A careful analysis of these two terms reveals that they are actually quite similar. The underlying purpose of both processes involves the transmission of information. In order to be successful, both education and marketing have to be interesting, purposeful, focused, clear, and effective. Thus, education and marketing can be seen as two sides of the same coin.

As a dentist, I have a professional obligation to educate and inform my patients about the new materials and techniques that may have an impact on their well-being. This means that I have a duty to compare the various treatment options available and to recommend that which I consider the best, and which I would use for my own teeth. If I am to be successful at educating my patients, my transmission of dental information must be interesting, focused, clear, and effective. The process of patient education is the most effective and least aggressive form of marketing. It presents the available options to the patient and lets the patient decide the course of their own treatment. There is absolutely no reason that either the dentist or patient should be uncomfortable with dental education in the dental office.

For posterior esthetic restorations, both education and marketing are a moot point. Many of our patients have progressed well beyond *need dentistry* and position themselves and their dentists in the era of *want dentistry*. They are aware of the importance of appearance,[6] are well-informed about the latest developments in dental materials, and have specific dental demands. Today, most new patients will begin by ascertaining that the dentist does "tooth colored" fillings. For these patients, composite posterior restorations are not an option—they are a basic requirement.

Position on Amalgam

The controversy surrounding amalgam is unfortunately mired in parallel but unrelated dentist/patient issues. While dentists defend mercury amalgam based upon the profession's experience with this material over more than 100 years, the lack of evidence of deleterious effects, and its ease-of-use, the public has largely dismissed it on the basis of appearance, misinformation, and media hysteria. Since dentistry is a service industry, the profession should make itself familiar with the trends developing among consumers. Ultimately, it is they who will make the long-term decisions about amalgam use. There are three simple criteria that can be used to choose adhesive restorations over amalgam fillings:

1. Composite restorations can be bonded to tooth structure, both dentin and enamel, very effectively. The strengths of these bonds are high enough to resist fracture, redecay, and other forms of catastrophic failure. Adhesives seal the interface between the tooth and restoration continuously such that eventual marginal breakdown can be easily repaired without replacing the entire restoration.

   On the other hand, amalgams are placed in the tooth with a non-adhesive base or liner. Even bonded amalgams have bond strengths to tooth structure that are pitifully weak and deteriorate rapidly. The interface between the amalgam and tooth, at any given time after the restoration is placed, can be viewed as a four-lane superhighway for bacteria and oral fluids, allowing microleakage and subsequent redecay. (Fig. 4-4).

2. Micro-hybrid composites are designed to wear in the range of 10-15 microns per year. This, not accidentally, is the same as the wear rate of human enamel. Most amalgams, on the other hand, wear in the range of 30-50 microns per year. Amalgam wears more quickly than natural tooth structure and can contribute to occlusal and masticatory dysfunction.

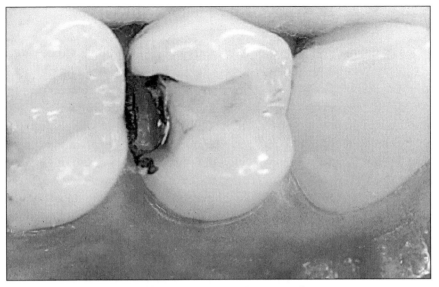

Fig. 4-4 Microleakage under an amalgam

3. Composite restorations look like natural tooth structure. Amalgams do not (see Fig. 4-1).

Leaving aside all the other concerns that one may have with amalgam (such as wedge-fracturing of cusp tips, permanent staining of dentin and enamel by the metals in amalgam, amalgam tattooing of the gingiva, etc.), the three points listed above should be enough to lead most dentists and patients in the direction of adhesive restorations.

A number of countries (Sweden, Germany, and others) around the world have banned or placed restrictions on amalgam use in children and women of childbearing age. Others have restricted amalgam use due to environmental safety concerns.

Which Adhesives to Use

Esthetic posterior restorations require the use of dental adhesives to bond the composite filling materials to tooth structures. The dentist is faced with a plethora of adhesive resin choices that have evolved through a series of "generations." (Fig. 4-5) The most recent materials are differentiated by bond strengths, solvents, and mode of cure. Every material will claim a certain range of bond strengths to dentin and enamel. Although it is difficult to evaluate all the numbers presented, it is known that 17 MPa of bond strength is required to resist the polymerization contraction of composite resin.[7-8] (If the bond strength of the adhesive is less than 17 MPa, the adhesive will be pulled away from the dentinal surfaces of the tooth as the composite is being light cured.) While it is not difficult to bond to enamel (we have been able to bond effectively to its crystalline structures for more than 30 years), dentin is altogether a different material. The organic components of dentin complicate the mechanism of adhesion. The various generations of adhesives have all sought to address the difficulty of bonding to dentin.[9]

The first generation of dentin adhesives was developed in the late 1970s, and while they bonded effectively to enamel, their bond to dentin was in the range of 2-3 MPa. This weakness resulted in a 50% failure rate for Class V restorations at six months.

The second generation, in the early 1980s, was a series of phosphate-ester bonding agents that adhered to the smear layer through ionic bonds to calcium. The bond strengths were better, in the range of 2-8 MPa, but still not strong enough to provide an effective dentin bond. In addition, the ionic bonds to calcium underwent hydrolysis, and the adhesion weakened with time.

In the late 1980s, the third generation of adhesives offered 8-15 MPa, a markedly improved bonding strength, but still not enough to resist the contractive forces of light-cured composite. This group of adhesives was characterized by spaghetti-like projections of resin into the dentinal tubules.

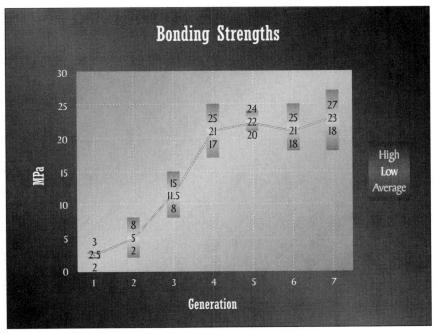

Fig. 4-5 Advances in bonding through the generations

It was in the fourth generation, in the early 1990s, that adhesive dentistry finally came into its own. For the first time, bond strength to the dentin (17-25 MPa) was able to resist the curing of composite. The concept of etching the dentin as well as the enamel, based upon Japanese research and practice in the 1980s, was introduced.[10-12] The dentin-etch step removed the entire smear layer, and left the dentinal tubules open to provide additional mechanical attention. Fourth-generation adhesives bond to enamel, dentin, ceramic, and metal. The one drawback of this generation of adhesives, and a major one at that, is the requirement to mix these materials chairside. It is difficult to measure accurately the amount of each component that is being dispensed into the mixing well. Given that all the research studies to establish bond strength values were done in laboratory settings, with precise measurements and controlled conditions, it is easy to see how chairside bonding values may differ greatly from (and may be much lower than) the academic ones. This makes fourth-generation adhesives less reliable in real practice conditions than one would like.

In the mid-1990s, the fifth-generation adhesives were introduced. These materials are very similar to fourth-generation bonding agents except for one major improvement—they are provided to the dentist in a single bottle. Thus, there is no chairside mixing required and none of the uncertainty that this process can introduce into the chemistry of the adhesive. The bonding range of early fifth-generation materials to dentin is narrower, 20-24 MPa, but of course, more predictable. Fifth generation adhesives bond to enamel, dentin, metal, and ceramic. The ease-of-use and predictability of these bonding agents, in addition to their virtually universal applicability, accounts for their tremendous popularity today.

Some dentists would prefer to omit the etching step. Certainly, eliminating one step is time beneficial. And for those dentists who are still concerned about the etching of dentin, this is a welcome development. In 1999, the so-called sixth-generation of adhesives was introduced. (The distinct nature, and thus the separate generation for these bonding agents, has not been universally accepted.) As a class, these products eliminated the etching step by including the enamel and dentin conditioner within the adhesive chemistry; the activity of the etch was self-limiting, and the post-etching compounds were integrated into the adhesive layer between the tooth and the restoration. Generally, bond strengths with the sixth-generation adhesives were slightly, but insignificantly, lower. Post-operative sensitivity was decreased even further from the fifth-generation. The key drawback of the sixth-generation adhesives is their multi-step, multi-component chemistry, and the likely introduction of incorrect mixing and/or incorrect sequencing. This is a step back from the ease-of-use and chairside predictability of the previous generation of adhesives.

The year 2003 saw the introduction of the first seventh-generation dental adhesives. These products combine the advantages of eliminating the etching step with the predictability of a single bottle application. The entire range of products required for the adhesive process has been packaged into a single bottle; the chemistry of the adhesive performs all the necessary steps for the dentist. There is no more etching and no more rinsing. A simple application of the adhesive to the tooth surface is all that is required to ensure successful and predictable adhesion and minimal post-operative sensitivity. The bond strengths of this generation are in the same range as the previous three generations, and their utilization is simpler, faster, and easier.

Dental adhesives are provided in one of three *solvents* (Fig. 4-6):

Acetone

This is the most common solvent for bonding agents today.[13] Its advantages include rapid volatility

Adhesive Solvents

Acetone
- iBond
- Prime & Bond NT
- Gluma Comfort Bond
- One-Step
- Bond 1
- Tenure Quick w Fl

Water
- One Coat Bond

Ethanol
- Excite
- Single Bond
- PQ1
- Optibond Solo

Fig. 4-6 Table of adhesive solvents

and its aggressive displacement of water, a major advantage in current moist bonding techniques.[14] Acetone's volatility is also its major disadvantage. It evaporates into air very readily (the method by which it removes moisture from the dentinal tubules and the intertubular dentin), but if it is left in the dispensing well for more than a few seconds, it volatilizes. It is best to dropper acetone-based bonding agents onto the applicator brush directly, without contact, and to immediately place the bonding agent onto the prepared tooth. This assures maximum moisture scavenging of the bonding agent in the preparation and minimal evaporation of the acetone into the air.

Ethanol

This is also a very common solvent for bonding agents. It displaces moisture less aggressively than acetone inside the dental tubule and in the intertubular dentin, but it is less volatile and to that extent less technique-sensitive. Ethanol-based bonding agents can be dispensed into wells, and allowed to remain there for a number of seconds prior to use. With these materials, the need for a moist dentinal environment is less critical.

Water

Water is another bonding agents solvent. Water, of course, is not at all volatile in the same sense that acetone and ethanol are, and thus there is no technique sensitivity. Water-based bonding agents can be used on moist or dry dentin, and they work with an alternative chemistry that is not dependent on the elimination of moisture from the dentin.

Postoperative Sensitivity

The most common reason that dentists give for not using adhesive restorations is that of postoperative sensitivity. While some postoperative sensitivity exists with composite restorations, it must be remembered that post-treatment sensitivity was far more prevalent with amalgam fillings. In fact, adhesive restorations in posterior teeth, without liners or bases, have a reported postoperative sensitivity rate of 1-3%. Posterior amalgams, with liners and bases, were typically expected to produce postoperative discomfort in 5-10% of cases.

The two most common reasons for postoperative sensitivity with composite materials are using a curing light that is too weak and not following instructions precisely. The former is easy remedied. An up-to-date halogen, plasma arc, or LED curing light should be the mainstay of every dental practice. It is important to remember that halogen lights require regular monitoring of the light output and occasional replacement of the bulb. If the curing light is not emitting enough power, then the deeper layers of composite and adhesive are not being effectively cured and this, in turn, can cause postoperative sensitivity.

Researchers develop instructions for use of a material with a particular interest in making the material both effective and efficient. There is usually an important reason for every step in the instructions. Eliminating some of these steps, taking shortcuts, and ignoring the sequence is risking the success of the entire operation. It must be remembered that the chemistries of different adhesives may be different. Therefore, the steps in the procedure may be different as well. While most fifth-generation adhesives offer similar instructions, there are enough product-to-product differences so that it is imperative that the dentist or the assistant familiarize the practice with the particular nuances of each material. Most of today's adhesives, when used according to their instructions, will routinely provide a sensitivity-free, and stress-free, postoperative environment.

One of the current concepts of dentinal sensitivity is that it results from the negative pressures on the odontoblastic process inside the dentinal tubule.[15] If at any time during or after the treatment there is a shrinkage of materials inside the dentinal tubule away from the odontoblast, this creates a local vacuum or negative pressure on the process. In turn, this is interpreted by the odontoblast as pain. In earlier years, when the process of adhesion did not guarantee the polymerization of the bonding agents within the dentinal tubule, this fluid could move and cause the negative pressure. The curing (and shrinkage) of a composite layer over an uncured adhesive resin can suck the liquid resin away from the odontoblast inside the dentinal tubule, creating a microlocal vacuum and postoperative sensitivity. An ineffective curing light can similarly leave the deeper portions of a restoration unhardened, allowing for fluid movement of the resin, thus creating postoperative sensitivity.

The simple solutions for eliminating postoperative sensitivity are the following:

- Follow instructions precisely
- Use an effective curing light (monitored regularly if a halogen curing light)
- Cure the adhesive resin prior to placing the first layer of composite

Technique Tips

The preparation of the tooth for an esthetic posterior restoration is similar to that of an amalgam, but more conservative and less angular. A typical composite restoration can occupy 80% less surface and volume than a corresponding amalgam restoration (Fig 4-7). With composites, there is no need to extend for retention (the restoration is micromechanically self-retentive) nor to extend for prevention (small, remote occlusal caries are better treated with fissurotomy and/or microabrasion without connection to the main restoration). The Class II box does not have to be flared out gingivally, a process that may further weaken the overlying cusps.

Amalgams require line angles and point angles to improve the retention of the restoration. The sharp angles where metal meets tooth have often been implicated in crack propagation and tooth fracture. Composite restorations require rounded internal anatomy (both ceramics and composites perform best in situations where interfaces are rounded rather than sharp and pointy). The rounded internal anatomy, best provided by burs such as the Great White (SSWhite, Piscataway, NJ) tends to protect the remaining structures of the tooth (Fig. 4-8). The bonded composite will support the remaining portions of the tooth much as the healthy intact dentin did originally.

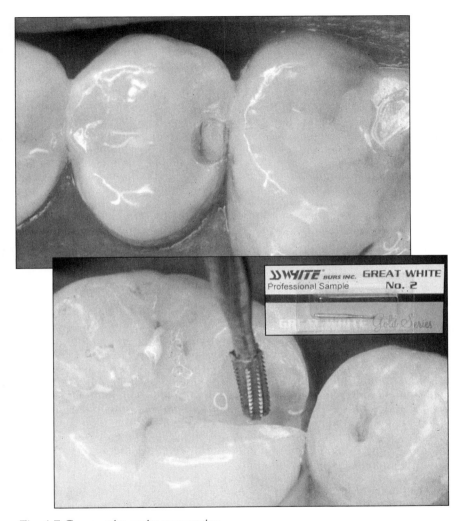

Fig. 4-7 Conservative cavity preparation

Fig. 4-8 Creating the rounded internal anatomy

It is important to keep the width of the occlusal portion as conservative responsible (Fig. 4-9); the greater the width of the preparation, the weaker the coronal sections and the entire tooth.[16] Slot preparations, if possible, are far better for long-term prognosis of the tooth.[17] Box only Class II restorations require greater loads for failure than traditional preparations.[18]

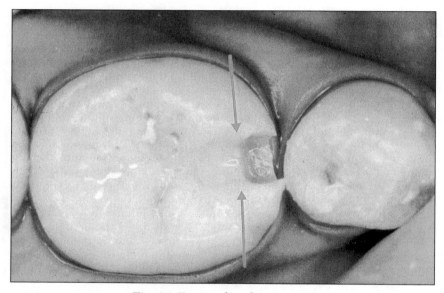

Fig. 4-9 Keeping the isthmus narrow

The wedging of the matrix band against the margins of the preparation is a very critical step. If there is an open space at the gingival margin of the box, the resulting overhanging composite will be very difficult to remove without damaging the tooth, the gingiva, or both. Traditional wedges, designed for amalgam, have not addressed this issue completely (Fig. 4-10b). Flexiwedges (Common Sense Dental, Nunica, MI) are plastic wedges that have to be squeezed in order to enter into the interdental space. They have a memory that re-expands the plastic towards its original shape immediately, pushing the matrix into an intimate contact with margins of the preparation (Fig. 4-10a). The sides of the anatomically-shaped Flexiwedge are contoured to approximate tooth shape (as opposed to the flatness of wooden wedges), and the gingival surface is indented to provide a space for the papilla, minimizing tissue irritation (Fig. 4-11).

Fig. 4-10a Matrix in intimate
contact with margin (flexiwedge)

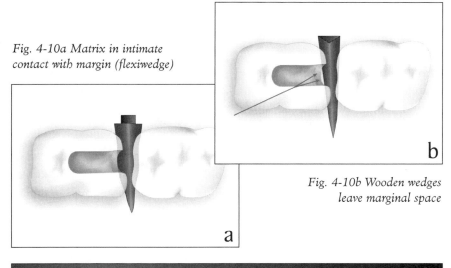

Fig. 4-10b Wooden wedges
leave marginal space

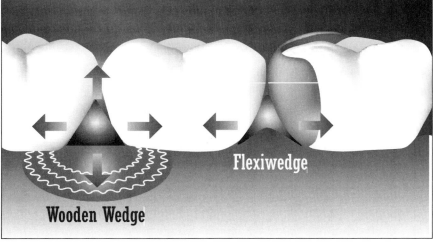

Fig 4-11 Anatomically-contoured wedge compared to wooden wedge

When using a moist bonding technique, ensure the ongoing success of the bonding process by monitoring the appearance of the dentin throughout the procedure. The dentin should be glossy or moist with water (not saliva) prior to the application of the dentin adhesive (Fig. 4-12). It should be glossy again after the even and complete application of the adhesive (Fig. 4-13). The third time to look for the glossy appearance on both the dentin the enamel is after the bonding agent is cured, prior to the application of the first layer of composite (Fig. 4-14).

The interproximal contact is created actively by the contact cure instrument (CCI) (Hu-Fredy, Chicago, IL). The dentist establishes the interproximal contact manually (Fig. 4-15) and maintains its stability through the early stage of curing with the metal CCI (Fig. 4-16). The metal CCI does not transmit light, and therefore, the composite immediately adjacent to this instrument will *not* cure. (If the resin did cure without the presence of air, an oxygen-inhibiting layer would *not* develop,

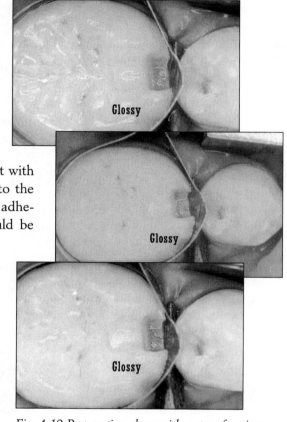

Fig. 4-12 Preparation glossy with water after rinse

Fig. 4-13 Preparation glossy with adhesive

Fig. 4-14 Preparation glossy with light-cured adhesive

making it unbondable to the subsequent composite layers.) Once the interproximal contact has been established—typically, one-half of the layer curing time—the CCI is removed and the restoration is cured again and continued layer by layer until the occlusal surface is reached.

Polishing of composite restorations takes inordinately long. It is not necessary to over-build the occlusal surface extensively with composite materials. The shrinkage of the last one millimeter layer of surface composite may be as little as 20 microns. It makes more sense, and saves more time, to establish the general shape of the occlusal anatomy *prior* to curing the final layer of composite. The occlusal surface of molars and bicuspids includes cusp ridges and troughs. Cusp ridges are convex in three dimensions, but unfortunately, the instruments previously available to contour this surface were either straight or convex themselves. The introduction of the "duckhead" contouring instrument (Fig. 4-17) (Hu Fredy Manufacturing, Chicago, IL), has simplified the shaping of the occlusal surface. This instrument is concave, shaped and sized to accurately impart a cusp ridge form to composite prior to curing. The "duckhead" uses existing anatomical landmarks to recreate the missing ones, leaving surfaces smooth and grooves and troughs rounded and cleansible (Fig. 4-18). The recreation of

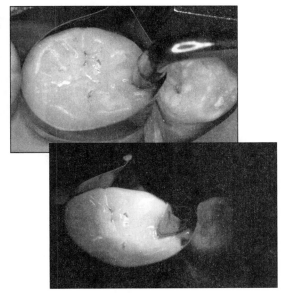

Fig. 4-15 CCI instrument making tactile interproximal contact

Fig. 4-16 Partial light cure with CCI in composite

Creating Occlusal Anatomy

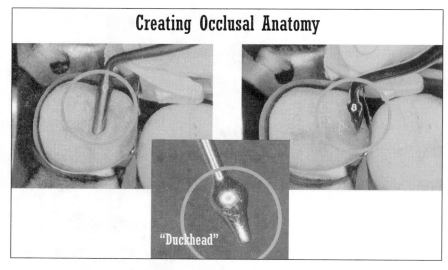

"Duckhead"

Fig. 4-17 Progression of instruments

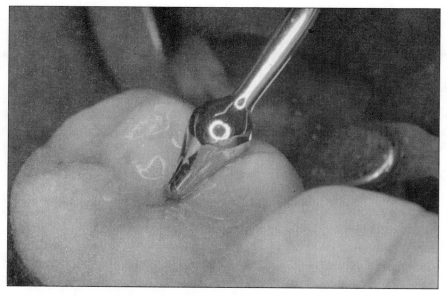

Fig. 4-18 Duckhead and its adaptation to the occlusal surface

the anatomy prior to curing leaves the composite in an almost finished state, one that requires minor occlusal adjustment and polishing.

Polishing

There are many polishing tips, points, burs, and pastes available. Some are more efficient than others, but all systems require a final paste polish. The guidelines for polishing are simple. The polishing paste, whether in a tube or impregnated into a wheel, cup, or point, should have particle sizes that are smaller than the particle sizes of the composite that is to be polished. If the particle size of the polisher is larger than the particle size of composite, the surface will be roughened by process. If the particle size of the polisher is too small, little or no overall surface polishing will be accomplished. The ideal particle size for the polisher is approximately one half that of the filler particles to be polished (Fig. 4-19). Therefore, after having placed a microhybrid composite where the majority of the filler particles are in the one micron range, the suitable polishing material will have a half micron as its mean size. Given the proper creation of the occlusal anatomy prior to curing, the adjustment and polishing steps should take no more than one or two minutes. The completed restoration will often encourage the patient to more comprehensive dentistry and better home care and maintenance (Fig. 4-20).

How to Begin

As with any new procedure, esthetic posterior composites involve the decision to begin and the fortitude to stick with the decision throughout the learning curve. Given the parameters of the materials, easy techniques, worldwide trends, and our patients' increasingly esthetic demands, the decision to offer (perhaps exclusively) esthetic posterior restorations is really a very simple one. Any dentist who does *not* offer this procedure runs the risk of losing patients to those dentists who do.

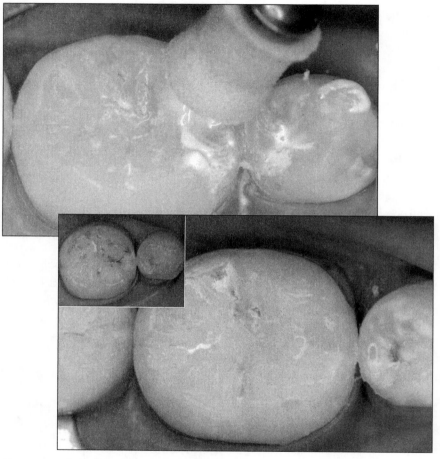

Fig. 4-19 Polishing with paste   Fig. 4-20 Finished restoration

It is important to remember that the task of learning involves frustrations and mistakes. In the long run, however, both patients and dentists benefit from the incorporation of newer and better techniques and materials into the practice.

Notes

1 *Does your smile say it all? Survey*, American Academy of Cosmetic Dentistry, Madison, WI, 1994

2 Hugo, B., Stassinakis, A., Hofmann, N., Hoffmann, O., and Klaiber, B. Vergleich verschiedener Präparationstechniken und Kavitätengestaltungen zur approximalen Erstversorgung. *Dtsch Zahnärztl Z*, 1998, 53: 441-447

3 Mair, L.H. Ten-year clinical assessment of three posterior resin composites and two amalgams. *Quintessence Int* 29, 483-490, 1998

4 Fukushima, M., Setcos, J.C., and Phillips, R.W. Marginal fracture of posterior composite resins, *JADA*, 1988, 117(5):577-83

5 Freedman, G., and Goldstep, F., Fifth Generation Bonding Systems: State of the Art in Adhesive Dentistry, *J Canadian Dental Assoc.*, June, 1997, 63:6 347-350

6 Freedman, G., and McLaughlin, G. *The Color Atlas of Porcelain Laminate Veneers*, Ishiyaku EuroAmerica, St Louis, MO, 1989

7 Munksgaard, E.C., Irie, M., and Asmussen, E. Dentin-polymer bond promoted by GLUMA and various resins. *J Dent Res*, 1985, 64: 1409-1411

8 Retief, H., Mandras, R.S., and Russel, C.M. Shear bond strength required to prevent microleakage at the dentin/restoration interface. *Am J Dent*, 7: 43-44, 1994

9 Freedman G. 5th Generation Bonding Systems Buyers Guide - *Dentistry Today*, 16:3, 106-111, March, 1997

[10] Fusayama, T. *New concept in operative dentistry*. Chicago: Quintessence Pub. Co., 1980

[11] Nakabayashi, N., Kojima, K., and Masuhara, E. The promotion of adhesion by the infiltration of monomers into tooth substrates. *J Biomed Mater Res*, 16/3/265-273, 1982, 55

[12] Nakabayashi, N., Nakamura, M., and Yasuda, N. Hybrid layer as a dentin-bonding mechanism. *J Esthet Dent*, 3/4/133-138, 1991, 44

[13] Kugel, G., and Ferrari, M. The science of bonding: from first to sixth generation. *J Am Dent Assoc.*, June, 2000, 131, Suppl:20S-25S[1]

[14] Tay, F.R., Gwinnett, A.J., and Wei, S.H. Micromorphological spectrum of acid-conditioned dentin following the application of a water-based adhesive. *Dent Mater*, September, 1998, 14(5):329-38

[15] Ciucchi, B., Bouillaguet, S., Holz, J., and Pashley, D. Dentinal fluid dynamics in human teeth, in vivo. *J Endod*, April, 1995, 21(4):191-4

[16] Larson, T.D., Douglas, W.H., and Geistfeld, R.E. Effect of prepared cavities on the strength of teeth. *Oper Dent.*, 1981, 6(1):2-5

[17] Oddera, M. Conservative amalgam restoration of Class II lesions—the "slot" restoration: a case report. *Quintessence Int.*, July, 1994, 25(7):493-8

[18] Sturdevant, J.R., Taylor, D.F., Leonard, R.H., Straka, W.F., Roberson, T.M., and Wilder, A.D. Conservative preparation designs for Class II amalgam restorations. *Dent Mater.*, June, 1987, 3(3):144-8

Chapter 5

Endodontics

By Joe H. Camp, D.D.S., M.S.D.

Diagnosis

The establishment of a correct diagnosis is essential in order to arrive at appropriate treatment. The clinician should formulate a systematic protocol of data gathering that is synthesized to reach the proper diagnosis. It is critical that all pertinent information be obtained by questioning the patient and that necessary tests be performed. By carefully evaluating the medical history, dental history including signs and symptoms, and test results, the clinician will be able to arrive at a diagnosis and institute procedures to correct the problem.

Endodontic treatment should be undertaken only in cases in which it is certain that a pulpal problem exists. Teeth should never be treated when the diagnosis is questionable. Initiation of root canal treatment only further clouds an uncertain situation and make determination of a correct diagnosis much harder, especially in cases of nonodontogenic origin. Referral to dental specialists or physicians may be necessary.

Medical History

A current medical history must be taken before any diagnosis, treatment planning, or emergency treatment to relieve pain is undertaken. The pertinent information is gathered on a preprinted medical history form. This will make the clinician aware of any systemic medical conditions that might influence treatment, the need for prophylactic antibiotics, and possible drug interactions. Certain conditions such as communicable diseases or anticoagulation therapy may require consultation with physicians before any treatment is initiated. Any consultations with other health personnel are recorded and become a part of the patient record.

Dental History

The patient is questioned in detail about the problem, and all data is recorded. Many prefer a preprinted form that the patient is asked to complete. This is then expanded by discussion with the patient. The clinician must carefully listen to the patient and ask leading questions to develop the patient's chief complaint. Following is a list of commonly asked questions:

- Tell me about the problem.
- How long have you had the pain?
- Is the pain mild, moderate, or severe?
- Is the pain a throbbing sensation or a constant pain?
- Is the pain spontaneous or is it provoked by anything such as hot, cold, biting, or eating?
- How long does the pain last when provoked?
- Does anything relieve the pain such as hot, cold, lying down, bending over, or sitting up?
- How often has the pain occurred?
- Have you had any recent dental treatment?

- If medication is being taken—How long have you been on medication and when was it last taken?

- Is there anything else you would like to tell me about the problem?

The clinician must listen carefully and assimilate the information to begin the diagnosis. The patient is asked to pinpoint the area or tooth that hurts. Often, the problem is quite obvious, such as a badly decayed or fractured tooth. However, it must not be assumed that the obvious is the problem until the remaining steps of the diagnosis are completed. It is common to see long-standing decayed or fractured teeth that are asymptomatic, while a hidden carious lesion or pulpal abscess is the cause of the pain.

Referral of dental pain is common and most often manifest in adjacent teeth or in the opposing quadrant.[1] Pain is commonly referred to the ear, temple, and down the neck. It rarely crosses the midline. Never accept the diagnosis of the patient related to the specific tooth, as the information is often wrong (Fig. 5-1).

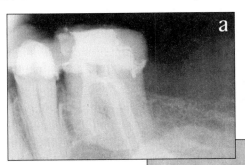

Fig. 5-1 (a, b) Referred pain to opposing arch. Patient presented with complaint of hot and cold sensitivity and identified area as maxillary molar. a) radiograph of maxillary molar shows incomplete treatment of mesio-facial root and temporary crown. Hot and cold testing of maxillary arch was negative. b) Radiograph of mandibular molars showing carious pulpal exposure on the second molar (first molar missing). Tooth tested positive to temperature showing pulpal inflammation.

Examination and Testing

Examination of the patient includes a visual inspection both extra- and intraorally, palpation, and percussion of any suspected teeth. The external observation should include areas of facial asymmetry that might indicate swelling of odontogenic origin. The intraoral visual examination should note discolored or fractured teeth, areas of caries, defective restorations, areas of abrasion, attrition, cervical erosion, developmental defects, tissue lesions or swellings, and sinus tracts.

If a sinus tract is present, it must be traced out by placing a gutta-percha cone to the source and exposing a radiograph (Fig.5-2). Sinus tracts generally indicate pulpal necrosis and periapical involvement but may be of periodontal origin. As a rule, abscessed teeth generally drain to the facial. Notable exceptions are the maxillary lateral incisor and palatal roots of maxillary molars, which may drain lingually. Most lingual sinus tracts are of periodontal origin.

The occlusion should be checked in both centric and eccentric positions to detect any gross abnormalities. Teeth that are in traumatic occlu-

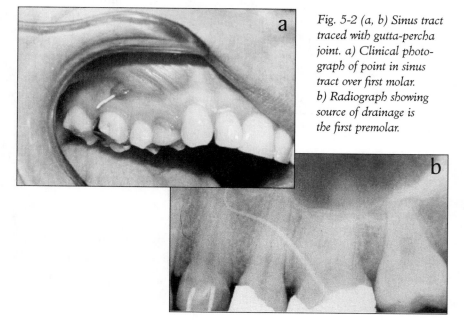

a

Fig. 5-2 (a, b) Sinus tract traced with gutta-percha joint. a) Clinical photograph of point in sinus tract over first molar. b) Radiograph showing source of drainage is the first premolar.

b

sion often exhibit symptoms that can mimic pulpal involvement. These symptoms may include percussion and cold sensitivity as well as low-grade chronic pain. Tooth mobility may aid in the diagnosis.

Palpation has both an extraoral and intraoral aspect. By gently palpating beneath the inferior border of the mandible and into the neck, enlarged lymph nodes or other tissue masses may be identified. The muscles of mastication should be palpated to reveal any soreness, as myofacial pain may often mimic pulpal pain.

Intraorally, the index finger is used to palpate the gingival tissues and mucosa on the facial and lingual sides of the alveolar ridges. The mucosa is pressed against the underlying cortical bone, and any tenderness or distension of tissues is noted. Frequently, periapical involvement of a tooth is discovered by palpation over the apical end of the root.

The percussion test is an invaluable aid in diagnosis. While it will not indicate pulpal status, it reveals inflammation of the periodontal and/or periapical tissues. Thus, it is essential that any tooth with positive percussion sensitivity be probed to rule out periodontal involvement. As a routine, all suspicious teeth should be periodontally probed and any abnormalities noted. Since percussive pain from periodontal or periapical abscess is indistinguishable, it is essential that any tooth with positive results be probed to rule out periodontal involvement. A positive response to percussion can be judged to be periapical if the periodontal tissues are healthy and the tooth is in normal occlusion.

Open contacts with resultant food pack may cause inflammation at the marginal gingiva, with resultant percussion sensitivity that is easily confused with pulpal symptoms. Flossing of suspected areas to determine open contacts and bleeding of interproximal tissues will aid in diagnosis, and other pulp tests will be normal.

Before beginning the percussion test, the patient should receive an explanation of the procedure and asked to respond if any differences are noted as individual teeth are percussed. Unsuspected contralateral teeth should be tested prior to suspected teeth to allow the patient to perceive normal results. The blunt end of a mirror handle is the usual tool to perform the percussion test. The teeth are gently tapped, and the response of the patient is recorded.

Radiographs

At this stage, appropriate radiographs are exposed of all areas in question. Long cone techniques taken perpendicular to the long axis of the tooth provide the best information. If possible, multiple angles are extremely beneficial. The first film is exposed straight on to allow visualization of the mesiodistal anatomy. The horizontal angulation is altered by 10 degrees to 15 degrees either mesial or distal to produce a second film that will help visualize the faciolingual anatomy. In addition to periapical films, bitewings are very helpful in diagnosing early caries, previous pulp treatments, and the depth of previous restorations.

Exposures of contralateral teeth may add valuable information related to anatomy. When a radiolucency or opacity is detected, radiographs must include all borders of the area.

The use of radiovisiography is beneficial, and radiation is kept to a minimum. The magnification of computer images and changes in contrast and brightness are often helpful in detecting lesions. If viewing conventional films, the use of a bright background light and magnification will greatly aid in interpretation.

Although pulpal health cannot be diagnosed from radiographs alone, valuable information is gained from the presence of caries, deep restorations, previous pulp treatments, calcifications, resorptions, radiolucencies, periodontal disease, or fractures.

Radiographic interpretation is highly variable among dentists and even with the same individuals at different times.[2] Anatomical structures and other areas may be easily misdiagnosed as pulpal involvement (Fig. 5-3). Pulpal status is determined in these cases by appropriate pulp tests to determine vitality. A diagnosis must never be made based solely upon radiographic evidence (Fig. 5-4).

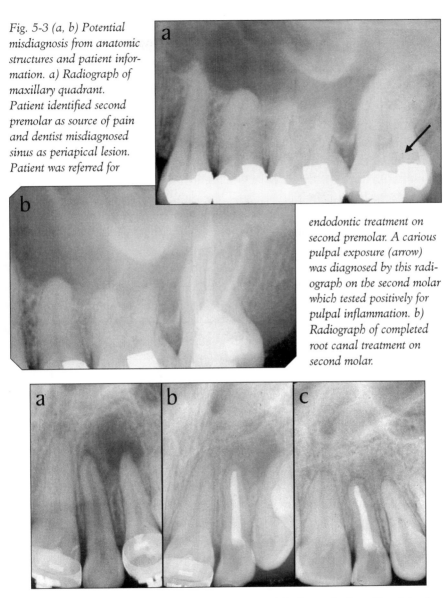

Fig. 5-3 (a, b) Potential misdiagnosis from anatomic structures and patient information. a) Radiograph of maxillary quadrant. Patient identified second premolar as source of pain and dentist misdiagnosed sinus as periapical lesion. Patient was referred for endodontic treatment on second premolar. A carious pulpal exposure (arrow) was diagnosed by this radiograph on the second molar which tested positively for pulpal inflammation. b) Radiograph of completed root canal treatment on second molar.

Fig. 5-4 (a, b, c) Deceptive radiographic appearance. a) Radiograph of maxillary lateral incisor and canine. Canine appears to have a radiographic endodontic lesion at the apex. Test proved the canine normal. The lateral incisor has overly large canal and tests negative to vitality test. b) Completed endodontic treatment of lateral incisor. Note in this view the canine does not appear to be involved. c) Radiograph of healed lesion.

Thermal Tests

With certain types of pulpal inflammation, symptoms may be elicited or relieved by the application of cold or hot stimulus. This is often the chief complaint of individuals with a toothache. If the patient reports sensitivity to thermal changes, the dentist should be able to clinically duplicate the symptoms to aid in the diagnosis. While thermal tests are quite reliable, interpretation of the results may depend upon the skill of the dentist to correctly access the patient response. A thorough explanation of the test to the patient is necessary to avoid erroneous responses that may lead to misdiagnosis. Responses of young or apprehensive patients are often unreliable.

The presence of moisture on the teeth or pooled at the cervical margins will alter the response. Therefore, all pulp tests should be conducted with the teeth dry and isolated with cotton rolls or sponges. The area of application of the stimulus is also important as large restoration or exposed dentin may give aggravated responses. Thermal tests should be applied to the crown or enamel if possible. Metals such as amalgam or gold may transfer temperature changes to the gingival tissues or periodontal ligament and give false positive reactions, while porcelains or resinous restoration may delay pulpal response. Normal teeth should always be tested first to allow the patient to judge the reaction while the dentist accesses the patient response.

Cold tests may be used to determine pulpal vitality or to access the extent of pulpal inflammation. For testing pulpal inflammation, the application of cold is best achieved with the use of a refrigerant such as ethyl chloride rather than ice. Because of the body temperature, ice quickly melts and may flow into the cervical areas on adjacent teeth, causing invalid responses. The ethyl chloride is applied to a cotton tipped applicator or a cotton pellet in a plier and applied to the tooth. The cotton is wet again each time before testing another tooth.

Cold testing to determine pulpal vitality is best done with carbon dioxide ice (Fig. 5-5). A cylinder of dry ice is formed in the ice pencil from a tank of carbon dioxide. A positive response usually indicates pul-

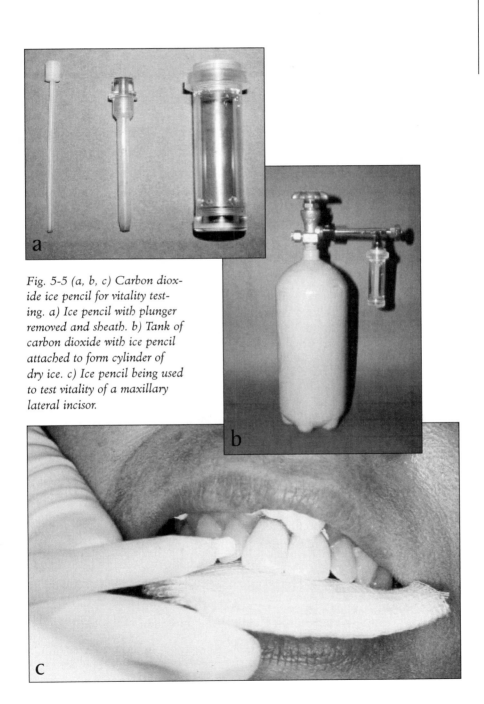

Fig. 5-5 (a, b, c) Carbon dioxide ice pencil for vitality testing. a) Ice pencil with plunger removed and sheath. b) Tank of carbon dioxide with ice pencil attached to form cylinder of dry ice. c) Ice pencil being used to test vitality of a maxillary lateral incisor.

pal vitality. The carbon dioxide ice pencil can be used to pulp test through ceramic metal crowns. Severely calcified teeth may give a false negative. The response of contralateral teeth with similar amounts of calcification should be compared to judge the results.

Isolation of individual teeth with a rubber dam and the application of iced water from a syringe may be necessary to adequately cold test some teeth. While this method requires more time and may elicit some pain with application of the rubber dam, especially in apprehensive and young patients, it is very effective.

Interpretation of results from cold testing is very subjective and depends upon a correct assessment of the patient's response. Providing it is valid, a response to cold indicates pulpal vitality. The determination of the extent of pulpal inflammation is much more difficult. Minor cold-sensitivity is normal following dental restorations, prophylaxis, or periodontal therapy. Areas of gingival recession or root exposure may be cold sensitive and correctable by desensitization or a period of time. Extreme reactions or the presence of prolonged discomfort following cold application are indicative of extensive pulpal inflammation and usually require root canal therapy to alleviate the problem.

Heat testing is achieved by several methods. These include the application of heat via heating temporary stopping in a bunsen burner (Fig. 5-6), the use of a rotating prophy cup to create frictional heat, or a hot water bath with single tooth isolation under a rubber dam. An aggravated response or prolonged discomfort indicates pulpal degeneration and would require root canal therapy. Like cold testing, the assessment of the response is critical to determining the results.

Experiments were conducted to determine the effects of dry ice and heated gutta-percha temporary stopping on human dental pulps. Histologic examination of human teeth subjected to the tests and extracted for orthodontic reasons revealed no evidence of pulpal injury.[3]

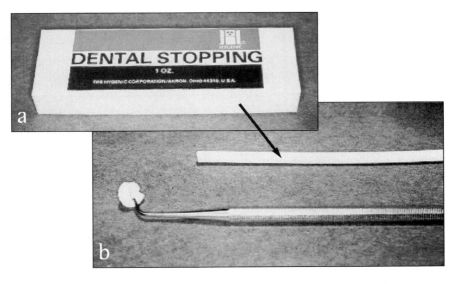

Fig. 5-6 (a, b) Temporary stopping placed on plastic instrument for heat testing. The stick of temporary stopping is heated over a bunsen burner and then applied to the tooth for evaluation.

Electric Pulp Tests

The electric pulp tester elicits a response of the sensory fibers in the pulp, but does not provide information regarding the vascular supply to the pulp.[4] The electric pulp tester has limited use, but may provide valuable information in inconclusive cases, especially those with extensive calcification of the pulp. Treatment is never rendered based solely on the results of electric pulp testing. Normal teeth with similar pulps are always tested for comparison and judging patient response before teeth with suspected pulpal involvement. It must be remembered that some normal teeth do not respond to electrical stimulation, and false negative or positive results are possible.

Primary teeth and teeth with incompletely developed apices do not usually respond to electric pulp testing. Apprehensive and young patients often give erroneous responses. The electric pulp tester is more reliable on single-rooted than multirooted teeth, as vital sensory fibers may remain in one root while others contain only necrotic tissue.

Anesthetic Test

The use of anesthetic to help establish a diagnosis can only be used effectively if the pain has been established to be pulpal and is isolated to opposing arches. The most suspicious arch is anesthetized. If the pain disappears, the diagnosis has been established. If the pain persists, the clinician must be certain of profound anesthesia. The other arch is then anesthetized and should result in cessation of the pain and establishment of the diagnosis. If pain is not relieved by anesthesia, the clinician must consider nonodontogenic sources.

If unable to conclusively establish pain as odontogenic, endodontic treatment should not be instituted. The patient is referred for other dental or medical consultations or brought back in two to three days and retested. The passage of time may lead to further developments that will enable a conclusive diagnosis to be made. Endodontic treatment should not be instituted in patients with pain as part of the diagnostic procedure. If the pain is of nonodontogenic origin and endodontic treatment is begun, the problem is masked and becomes much more difficult to diagnose. It may become impossible to completely rule out the treated tooth short of extraction.

Anesthesia

Profound dental anesthesia is more difficult to achieve in the presence of inflammation, especially acute apical periodontitis. Once inflammation and/or infection has spread into the periapical tissues and the tooth is exquisitely painful to percussion, infiltration techniques are many times ineffective. The use of nerve blocks or intra-osseous injections may be necessary to achieve profound anesthesia. Use of the Stabident system or the X-Tip allows easy intra-osseous injections providing there is space between the tooth roots to allow insertion of the drill. In the maxillary arch, the anesthetic may be injected either mesially or distally intra-osseously and achieve profound anesthesia. For endodontic procedures on the mandibular arch, it has been the experience of the author that the anesthetic must be injected intra-osseously distal to the offending tooth in order to be effective. Injection of anesthetic into a periapical lesion is ineffective and may cause an increase in pain, especially in the presence of acute inflammation.

Intra-osseous anesthesia is of shorter duration than nerve blocks and may need to be repeated in difficult or lengthy procedures. One distinct advantage of the X-Tip is that the cannule may be left in place during treatment making reinjection of more anesthetic solution easy to achieve.

When intra-osseous injection cannot be utilized in the maxillary arch, following facial and lingual infiltration, an infra-orbital block is usually effective in achieving profound anesthesia. This block is easily administered intra-orally by depositing a carpule of anesthetic over the infra-orbital canal located just below the inferior orbital ridge (Fig. 5-7). Following injection, the cheek is palpated for 20-30 seconds to force the anesthetic into the foramen.

Fig. 5-7 Infra-orbital injection. Human skull demonstrating placement of injection syringe with needle near the infra-orbital foramen. Prior to the injection, the sheathed needle is placed over the cheek and aligned with the foramen. A depth reference point is noted on the syringe hub in relation to the teeth. When penetrating with the needle, the reference point is realigned to assure proper position for injection over the foramen.

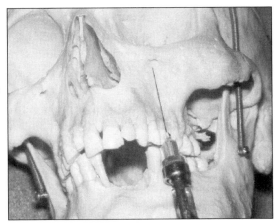

To achieve profound mandibular anesthesia, it may be necessary following a mandibular or Gow-Gates block to anesthetize nerve fibers derived from the cervical chain that come anteriorly and innervate the mandibular molars. This innervation may enter the molars through three different avenues. Fibers passing through the mylohyoid muscle are anesthetized by a small infiltration on the lingual side slightly posterior and inferior to the tooth to be treated. Mental foramen fibers are injected facially at the level of and slightly distal to the foramen. Fibers passing through the periodontal membrane are anesthetized by injecting into the membrane at each corner of the tooth.

Access and Rubber Dam Isolation

It is absolutely essential that endodontic procedures be performed under rubber dam isolation. However, the rubber dam should not be applied to anterior and premolar teeth until after the endodontic access has been achieved. Placement of the dam prior to access in these teeth obscures visibility and leads to more iatrogenic mishaps. Visualization of the long axis of the tooth and the mesio-distal and facio-lingual planes allow easier access with conservation of tooth structure and less likelihood of perforation. Once the pulp chamber is exposed, the canals are identified with a DG-16 explorer. The access is completed and the rubber dam applied before endodontic files are used to negotiate the canals.

In molar teeth, the rubber dam is usually applied before access is made. If orientation becomes a problem, the dam should be removed to allow visualization of the crown and reorientation to the long axis of the tooth.

Access should be made to allow straight-line approach into the canals. This can be achieved without sacrificing marginal ridges. It is a common mistake by general dentists to remove inadequate tooth structure and attempt to perform endodontic therapy through too small an access. Conversely, unnecessary removal of tooth structure should be avoided. Remove only that which is necessary to achieve straight-line access into the canals.

Rubber dam isolation can be achieved in most teeth with very few rubber dam clamps. Commonly utilized clamps include the following:

Old Style #'s		Serrated Jaw (Tiger) #'s
90 N	Anteriors and Premolars	9-T
W-2A	Premolars	2-T
26		
3	Molar	12-AT
7		13-AT
200		
27	Prepared Molars	2-AT
		1-T

Cleaning and Shaping of Root Canals

According to West and Roane, the longevity of a tooth is based upon a healthy attachment apparatus. If a contaminated canal system is cleaned, shaped, and sealed, resolution of the infection and healing will occur. Therefore, treatment must be based on thoroughly cleansing, shaping, and obturating the canal to promote healing.[5]

Frequent, copious irrigation with sodium hypochlorite serves several purposes. It flushes out debris, is an organic solvent that dissolves necrotic tissue, and it kills bacteria. The easiest source of sodium hypochlorite is Clorox, which has a concentration of 5.25%. The solution may be used full strength or diluted with equal amounts of water to form a concentration of approximately 2.5%.

Length Determination

Where to terminate the root canal preparation and filling has been debated for many years without resolution. Some feel that any amount of overfilling will lead to failure, while others have no concern for puffs of sealer into the periodontal spaces. The terminus of the pulp is at the apical constriction, the narrowest point within the canal.[6] Although this point can vary several mm's, it is usually ½ to 1 mm from the radiographic apex. While there are advocates for termination at this point, others vary from the radiographic apex to 2-3 mm shy of the apical constriction. In the latter group, teeth with vital tissue are filled shorter than those with necrotic tissue. Since the inflammatory status of a pulp cannot be determined short of microscopic examination, it is the opinion of the author that the shaping and filling should terminate at the apical constriction in order to remove all pulpal tissue. Also, this point can be precisely determined with the use of an apex locator.

Crown Down Technique

Tremendous technological and metallurgic advancements have radically changed root canal preparation. In the past, because of the limitations of stainless steel (commonly used for endodontic instruments), techniques were oriented toward achieving and maintaining the working length from smaller to larger sizes. Due to the lack of flexibility, using larger files short of the working length in curved canals tended to create ledging. Also, most stainless steel instruments had a cutting tip. As the file returned to its memory position of straight, the tip gouged into the dentinal wall, often leading to ledging or perforation. Filing, which is an up and down motion while rasping the dentinal walls, tended to pack debris apically, compounding problems (Fig. 5-8).

The introduction of safe-tipped instruments reduced the chances of ledging and made the crown down technique possible. The further introduction of nickel titanium endodontic instrumentation provided a method of utilizing the dental hand piece to prepare canals. Increases in the taper of nickel titanium files added the necessary strength to greatly reduce instrument breakage during rotation. Due to the flexibility of nickel titanium, a safe ended rotating file will follow the canal and prevent ledging. Radial lands separate the cutting edges and keep the file centered in the canal. Also the U-blade design spirals debris occlusally

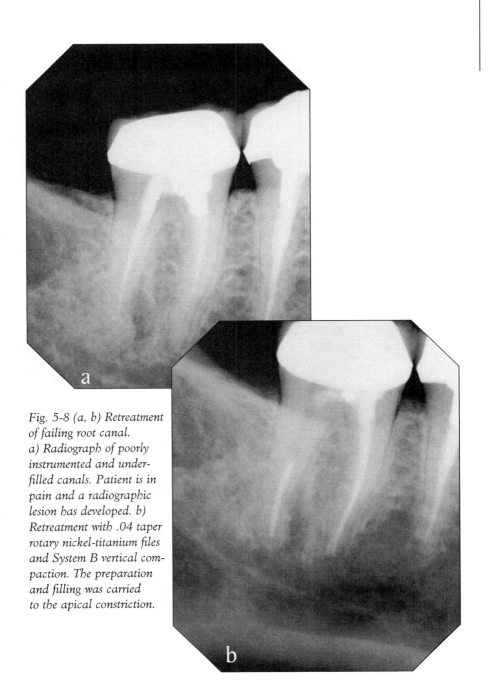

Fig. 5-8 (a, b) Retreatment of failing root canal.
a) Radiograph of poorly instrumented and under-filled canals. Patient is in pain and a radiographic lesion has developed. b) Retreatment with .04 taper rotary nickel-titanium files and System B vertical compaction. The preparation and filling was carried to the apical constriction.

rather than packing it apically. This combination of factors has altered the traditional approach of reaching and maintaining the canal length to a true or modified crown down technique in which the coronal ½ to ⅔ of the canal is opened to allow better access to the apical portion.

In the crown down technique, a small stainless steel hand file, size #10 or #15 with a lubricant such as RC Prep or Glide, is utilized to pathfind and establish patency of the canal. The canal is penetrated until some resistance to insertion is perceived. Usually, this occurs at ½ to ⅔ the canal length. This becomes a temporary working length. Rotary nickel titanium files are then used to open the constriction in the coronal half of the root canal. Working length is not established until the coronal flaring has been achieved. Since canals calcify from the coronal aspect apically, much of the resistance to penetration of the canal is removed following the coronal flaring (Fig. 5-9). Cleansing of the apical canal is facilitated since irrigants reach the working length more freely.

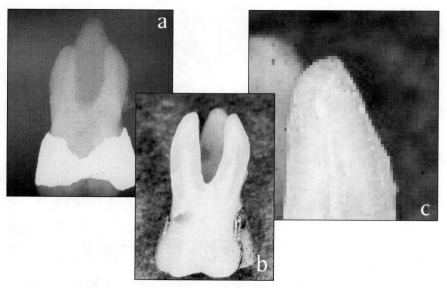

Fig. 5-9 (a, b, c) Coronal calcification of root canal. Coronal calcification of root canal. a) Radiograph of calcified maxillary molar. b) Photograph of tooth with facial of roots ground away to visualize calcification in canal. Note the extreme coronal calcification which tapers out apically. c) Higher magnification of the mesio-facial root showing a dilaceration of the canal mesially.

Following coronal flaring, the working length is established radiographically and with an apex locator. It is important to take a working length radiograph to define the canal anatomy. The apex locator will allow definition of the apical constriction.

Once the working length is determined, instrumentation with different sizes and tapers of nickel titanium rotary instruments are utilized to form the ideal shape, a tapering funnel form orifice to apex, for obturation of the canal with gutta-percha.

A high torque, constant RPM hand piece must be utilized for rotary nickel titanium instrumentation. This requires a special hand piece such as the MM-325 (Medidenta) or a special electric engine with gear reduction hand pieces. Newer electric engines have torque-control features that utilize computer programs to reverse the rotation when a certain stress level is reached (Fig. 5-10). Programs on the engines allow the torque to be set for different sizes of files. With this feature, fracture of files is greatly reduced. The ideal speed for most files is 300 rpm. With extremely large files ,(above size 50) 500 rpm is more effective. The nickel titanium

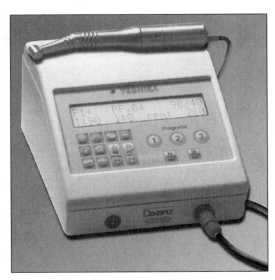

Fig. 5-10 Torque-controlled electric engine and handpiece. The ATR by Tecnika (Dentsply Tulsa Dental) allows torque settings for each rotary nickel-titanium file to be programmed into its computer to greatly reduce instrument breakage.

files may be augmented with the use of Gates-Glidden drills, sonic or ultrasonic instrumentation, and occasionally stainless steel hand files.

Numerous technique sequences have been advocated by different clinicians. While no one technique is good for all teeth, the following file sequence has been used by the author to instrument thousands of canals (Table 5-1). It is especially effective in calcified teeth. With larger canal sizes, larger diameter files are substituted in order to properly instrument the canal.

1. Access tooth and locate canals with DG-16 explorer

2. Pathfind with a #10 or #15 stainless steel (SS) hand file until resistance met (usually 1/2 to 3/4 estimated length of canal). *Constantly irrigate with NaOCL throughout the procedure*

3. Next, use .04 taper rotary nickel-titanium files to go to the length previously penetrated by the SS hand file using the following sequence of .04 taper rotary files:

   a. #25   To stress

   b. #30   To stress

   Note: If not to the depth reached with the SS hand file (step 2), the size #20 and #15 files may be necessary in some cases. Once the desired depth is reached, smaller files are unnecessary. In calcified cases, it may be necessary to repeat the above sequence

4. Establish *working length* with x-ray and/or apex locator

5. Next, coronal flaring of the canal is achieved by one, or a combination of the following methods:

   a. Use MM1500 Sonic for 30 seconds per canal (with #15 shaper) to the working length

   b. Gates-Glidden drills (usually 2, 3, and 4)

   c. Larger taper nickel titanium rotary files or orifice shaper files

6. The preparation is continued using the following sequence of nickel-titanium .04 taper rotary files:

   a. #25 To working length if possible. If achieved, skip to step 7d

   b. #30 To working length if possible

   c. #20 Only when needed to reach working length

   d. #15 Only when needed to reach working length

7. Once working length is reached, the use of smaller files is not necessary. Begin the sequence with first file to reach working length and proceed with the following sequence (a continuation of step 6):

a. (Size 15) (If necessary) To working length

b. (Size 20) (If necessary) To working length

c. #25 — To working length

d. #30 — To working length

e. #35 — Slightly short (1-2 mm) of #30 file

f. #40-#50 — Only in large canals

Note: The last size file carried to the working length is determined by the canal size and is usually #35, but is never less than the #25. All instrumentation is done in wet canals (NaOCL). Never use nickel titanium rotary files until canal has been penetrated by a minimum size #10 hand file

When filling with vertical condensation method (System B), finish prep with an appropriate GT file to achieve deeper flare so plugger will go to desired depth (usually on .08 taper in small canals and a .10 or .12 taper in larger canals)

Table 5-1 Modified crown-down technique utilizing .04 taper rotary nickel-titanium, by Dr. Ben Johnson

The rotary nickel titanium technique, as with any new procedure, has a learning curve. It is advisable to practice on extracted teeth before attempting clinical cases. Begin with easy straight canals rather than difficult ones. Transportation or blockage of canals, ledging, and perforation has virtually been eliminated with nickel titanium. Breakage is the most common iatrogenic hazard.

Too much pressure applied to the file or metal fatigue from over-use are the most common causes of fracture. The files should be marked after each use and discarded after instrumenting 3-4 teeth. In severely curved teeth (60° or more), the files should be discarded after single use

(Fig. 5-11). The use of torque-controlled engines will greatly reduce fracture due to the reversal when too much pressure is applied.

Listed below are the most common causes and ways to minimize nickel-titanium file fracture:

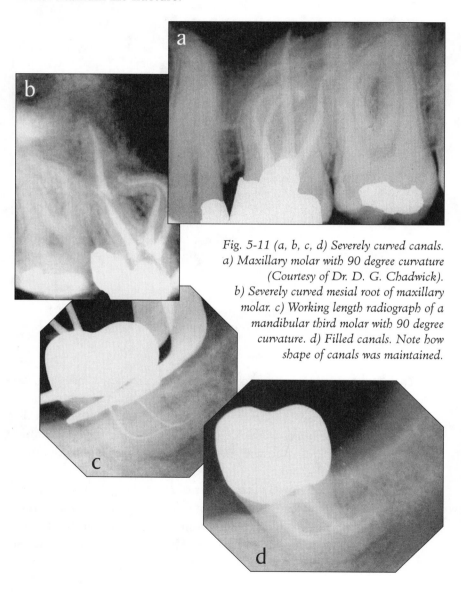

Fig. 5-11 (a, b, c, d) Severely curved canals. a) Maxillary molar with 90 degree curvature (Courtesy of Dr. D. G. Chadwick). b) Severely curved mesial root of maxillary molar. c) Working length radiograph of a mandibular third molar with 90 degree curvature. d) Filled canals. Note how shape of canals was maintained.

Causes of Nickel-Titanium Fracture

- Too much pressure applied on file: failure occurs due to increased torque
- Fatigue of metal from over-use or abuse: cyclic fatigue
- Sudden changes in direction of instrument, i.e., jerky or jabbing movements
- Canals come together abruptly at sharp angle
- Abrupt curvature over a radius of 1-3 mm
- Dilacerated canal—canal abruptly changes directions
- Inadequate coronal flaring prior to apical instrumentation. If the file feels tight throughout length of blade, flare orifice and coronal canal more
- Tooth with an S curve—pressure causes deflection as the file enters the second curve
- Curvature more than 60 degrees with more than 3-4 mm of canal to apex—in this situation, pressure to negotiate causes enough deflection at start of curve to induce fracture
- Extreme curvature over a small radius (elbow-type curve)
- Ledge in canal with space for deflection of file
- Large canal with a shelf close to the apex that stops a hand file as though a solid bottom exists. The stainless hand file can be passed further after a bend is made in the file. Seen frequently in distal of lower molars. The rotary nickel-titanium depends upon a constant opening to guide the tip. As the rotary hits the ledge, if pressure is applied, the file bends or it suddenly deflects into the opening and fractures
- File is progressing easily in canal—then feels like it hits bottom—pressure applied will cause fracture. If this happens, immediately go to a hand file and enlarge slightly, then go back to rotary

- If file starts to chatter—stop immediately and flare coronal more or use hand file to slightly enlarge
- Most fractures occur with sizes #25-#35

How to Minimize Fracture

- Never force file—very minimal pressure. If any resistance is encountered, immediately stop and enlarge slightly with hand file before proceeding
- Flaring of upper half of canal before passing rotaries into the apical half, especially if a curve is present. Flaring achieved with larger rotaries, orifice shapers, sonic, or Gates-Glidden
- Never try to pass a rotary that has not been preceded by a minimum size #10 stainless hand file. This does not preclude the crown-down technique—simply carry the rotaries just short of where the #10 hand file has passed
- Don't get in a hurry
- Action of instrument is touch-retract, each time passing ½ to 2 mm further down the canal. In calcified canals, will progress much slower. Never leave file rotating in a stationary position—this will not enlarge canal further and might cause fracture
- In crown-down prep—if you don't reach apex on the first try as you go through the series, simply repeat sequence until it reaches apex. Always go back with #10 stainless hand file or hand file that reached the apex. Additional coronal flaring with large size or larger tapered files will facilitate sequence
- Remember, you can always do some or all of the prep by hand. There is a tendency to never want to use hand files, but this is impossible, although hand file use is minimal
- Repeatedly remove file and look at blade. Rotate file while removed—if any deflection has occurred, immediately dis-

card file. Remember, nickel-titanium has a perfect memory and if any bend is present, the instrument is about to break

- Have your dental assistant clean file as you go to others and visually inspect each file—any sign of bend or twist—discard

- If you are having trouble passing up series, put out other files and try a different one or change to a different taper or size. Remember, manufacturers have a tolerance and all sizes are not exact, although this occurs less with nickel-titanium than stainless steel

- Remember that all uses of a file are not equal. A calcified canal stresses the file more than an uncalcified canal. A curved canal stresses the file more than a straight canal. Tests have shown breakage after approximately 600 deflections in canals with 90-degree curvature. Each turn around a curve is a deflection. The greater the curvature, the greater the deflection

- All operators have experienced more fracture after files have been used a number of times. All metals reach fatigue and eventually will break

- Consider discarding a file after abusive use in a very calcified or severely curved canal even though it has only been used in one canal or tooth

- Use new files after sterilization in hard cases and use older files in easier cases

- No one knows the maximum or ideal number of times a file can be used. Follow the rule of "better safe than sorry"

- Consider raising fee of root canal to cover cost of files and discarding files after use in one tooth

- Mark shaft of file with tiny notch to keep up with number of uses

- In no circumstances should files be used in more than four to five teeth

- Files sizes #50 and larger do not usually fracture and may be used multiple times (15-20). This size file is usually used only in straight portion of canal and does not undergo deflection

One Appointment Endodontics

Completion of root canal therapy in one appointment has been widely accepted among practicing endodontists and many general dentists. The literature shows similar success rates and incidence of pain when comparing one to multiple visit endodontics. A partial review of the literature is provided by Dorn and Gartner.[7] While the number of appointments is still a controversial subject, most agree that root canals with vital pulp tissue, traumatically exposed healthy pulps, and necrotic teeth with draining sinus tracts are acceptable candidates for one appointment. Most symptomatic teeth, those with acute apical periodontitis, and most retreatments are generally best treated in multiple appointments. The difficulty of the case may be a limiting factor due to the amount of time required to complete therapy. Root canals that cannot be dried after instrumentation should not be completed.

When multiple appointments are required, the canals should be thoroughly cleansed before closing. The canals are medicated with calcium hydroxide before closure. A slurry may be formed with calcium hydroxide powder and water, or commercial preparations such as Calasept, Pulpdent, or Hypo-Cal are acceptable. Care must be taken to thoroughly seal the access cavity and any other areas of leakage under restoration or crowns. Leakage will lead to reinfection and pain.

Obturation of the Root Canal

Obturation is important to eliminate leakage and recontamination of the root canal and to prevent irritants left behind by the cleansing process from reaching the periapical tissues.[8] Probably of equal importance is coronal leakage under faulty restorations or caries that contacts the root canal filling. Bacterial leakage along gutta-percha fillings can penetrate to the apex and cause recontamination of the periapical tissues. This has led to the recommendation that all root canals contaminated coronally for three months should be redone prior to placement of permanent restorations.[9]

All filling techniques require the use of a root canal sealer. The most widely used root canal cements are composed primarily of zinc oxide-eugenol, resins, or calcium hydroxide. Gutmann and Witherspoon list commonly used root canal sealers, their composition, and primary indications.[10]

Removal of the smear layer prior to obturation is advocated by many operators. While studies show more dye leakage to occur if not removed, its clinical significance remains to be established. Removal is achieved by irrigation of the canal prior to obturation with 5 cc of 17% EDTA, followed by rinsing the canal with sodium hypochlorite.

While many materials have been utilized over the years, gutta-percha continues to be the standard. While three-dimensional obturation can be achieved with many different techniques, the ability to achieve this goal is more dependent upon the cleansing and shaping of the canal and the skill of the clinician than the method of filling. Of the widely accepted filling techniques, none have been shown to achieve a significantly higher success rate than others. The two most common techniques are lateral condensation and vertical condensation. Newer methods of thermoplasticized obturation with or without a central carrier have gained popularity.

In the lateral condensation technique, a master gutta-percha cone is fitted slightly short of the working length (½ to 1 mm) with a slight resistance to withdrawal. It is removed and a hand or finger spreader is chosen, which will go to the working length without binding in the canal. The MA-57 spreader is usually satisfactory. For smaller canals, the D-11T works well.

Following selection of the master cone and spreader, the canal is thoroughly dried with paper points. Sealer is applied into the canal and the walls coated utilizing a lentulo spiral, paper point, hand endodontic file, or sonic filler (Medidenta). The master cone is reseated and a radiograph exposed to check the fit. Alterations are made if the length of the master cone is incorrect.

The coronal portion of the master cone is removed with a heated plastic instrument. The spreader is then inserted beside the master cone to within 1-2 mm of the working length, and the canal is backfilled with accessory gutta-percha points. The excess coronal gutta-percha is removed periodically after 3-4 accessory cones are placed. This procedure is repeated until the canal is obliterated (Fig. 5-12).

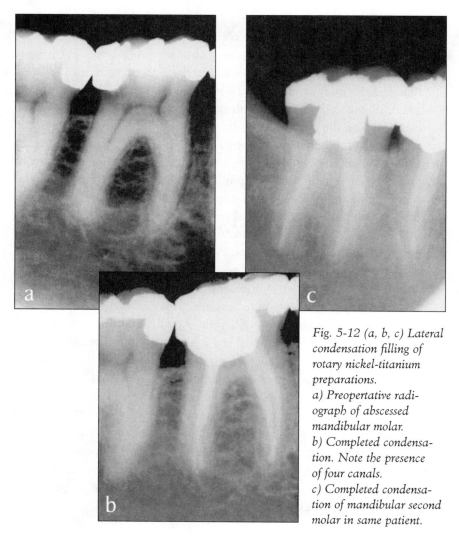

Fig. 5-12 (a, b, c) Lateral condensation filling of rotary nickel-titanium preparations.
a) Preopertative radiograph of abscessed mandibular molar.
b) Completed condensation. Note the presence of four canals.
c) Completed condensation of mandibular second molar in same patient.

Vertical compaction was popularized by Schilder.[11] A series of hand or finger pluggers are prefitted to allow penetration to within several mm of the working length without binding against the canal walls. Sealer and the master cone are fitted and placed in the canal in essentially the same manner as with lateral condensation. A heated instrument is used to sear and transfer heat to the gutta-percha. The cold plugger is used to compact the softened material apically. The process is repeated down the canal until softened gutta-percha reaches the apical 3-4 mm of prepared canal, thus forming an apical plug. Additional segments of gutta-percha are added and compacted to obturate the canal. As the compaction continues coronally, progressively larger pluggers are utilized. Others choose to backfill with thermoplasticized injectable gutta-percha utilizing the Obtura II (Obtura Corp.) or other similar devices.

Heating instruments and techniques have been developed to soften the intracanal gutta-percha. The System B (EIE/Analytic Technology) (Fig. 5-13) compacts the gutta-percha as softening occurs 4-5 mm ahead of the advancing 200° C heated plugger. The heat is deactivated several mm before reaching a predetermined point 4-5 mm from the working length. The plugger is then held under pressure at that point for 10 seconds as the softened mass is molded to the canal configuration, forming the apical plug.

The plugger is momentarily reheated and retracted leaving the apical plug in place. The remaining canal is backfilled with additional gutta-percha and the System B plugger heated to 100° C or an injectable thermoplasticized material. Once the canal is obturated, a large plugger is used to apply apical pressure to the mass as it cools to compensate for shrinkage.

Other methods of obturating canals involve the use of a central carrier such as the Thermafil Plus System (Dentsply Tulsa Dental) or utilize a motorized compactor to deliver the gutta-percha. All of these different methods may require slight modifications in the preparation to accommodate the technique.

Endodontically treated teeth should be restored permanently as soon as feasible. In anterior teeth that will be restored with bonded composite, the final restoration should be placed immediately after obturation to

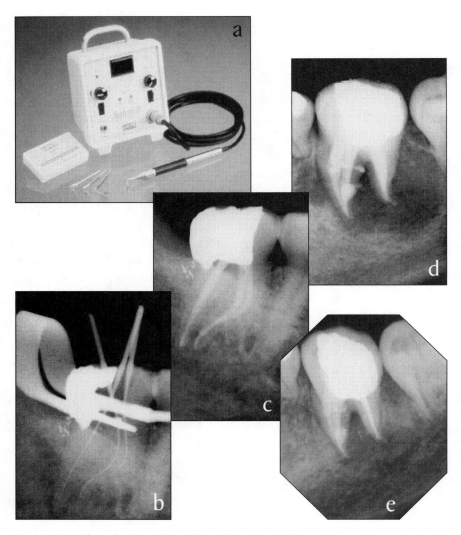

Fig. 5-13 (a, b, c, d, e) Condensation with System B Obturator (analytic technology) of canals prepared with rotary nickel-titanium files. a) System B obturator. Variable sized tips are chosen to fit the canal prior to use. The depth of penetration is set with the rubber stop on the condensor tips. b) Canal length determination radiograph of mandibular molar with "S" curve canals. c) Completed obturation. Canals were shaped with .04 rotary nickel-titanium files. d) Obliterated root canal system of a young mandibular molar with a large periapical lesion. Note the lateral canals filled by the vertical condensation. e) Six month follow-up showing healing of lesion.

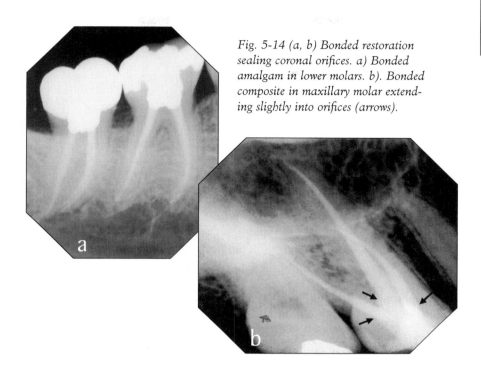

Fig. 5-14 (a, b) Bonded restoration sealing coronal orifices. a) Bonded amalgam in lower molars. b). Bonded composite in maxillary molar extending slightly into orifices (arrows).

assure a coronal seal. In all other teeth except those to receive a post, an acid-etched bonded restoration should be placed over and slightly into the coronal accesses of each canal to prevent occlusal leakage (Fig. 5-14). If a post preparation is prepared, care must be taken to achieve a good occlusal seal, because the depth of remaining gutta-percha is minimal to prevent apical leakage.

References

[1] Cohen, S. and Liewehr, F. Diagnostic procedures. In Cohen, S., and Burns, R.C. *Pathways of the pulp*, 8th ed., St. Louis: Mosby, 2002

[2] Goldman, M., and Pearson, A. Darzenta, N. Reliability of radio-graphic interpretations, *Oral Surg.*, 32:287, 1974

[3] Rickoff, B., et al. Effects of thermal vitality tests on human dental pulp, *J Endod*, 14:482, 1988

[4] Seltzer, S. *Endodontology: biologic consideration in endodontic procedures*, 2nd ed., Philadelphia: Lea & Febiger, 1988

[5] West, J.D., and Roane, J.B. Cleaning and shaping the root canal system. In Cohen, S., and Burns, R.C. *Pathways of the pulp*, 7th ed., St. Louis: Mosby, 1998

[6] Kuttler, Y. Microscopic investigation of root apexes, *JADA*, 50:544, 1955

[7] Dorn, S.O., Gartner, A.H. Case selection and treatment planning. In Cohen, S., and Burns, R.C. *Pathways of the pulp*, 7th ed., St. Louis: Mosby, 1998

[8] Saunders, W.P., and Saunders, E.M. Coronal leakage as a cause of failure in root canal therapy: a review. Endod Dent Traumatol, 10:105, 1994

[9] Khayat, A., Lee, S-J, and Torabinejad, M. Human saliva penetration of coronally unsealed obturated root canals, *J Endod*, 19:458, 1993

[10] Gutmann, J.L., and Witherspoon, D.E. Obturation of the cleaned and shaped root canal system. In Cohen, S., and Burns, R.C. Pathways of the pulp, 8th ed., St. Louis: Mosby, 2002

[11] Schilder, H. Filling root canals in three dimensions, *DentClin North Am*, 11:723, 1967

Chapter 6

Medical Emergencies

By Alan J. Drinnan, M.B., Ch.B., D.D.S.

Although serious medical emergencies occurring in the dental office are relatively uncommon, it is still essential that the dentist and his/her team be aware of the nature of such emergencies, the ways to recognize them, and the methods for their management. In this chapter, there will be no attempt to cover every possible emergency that could arise in the dental setting. For such information, the reader is referred to one of several texts devoted to the topic.

This chapter will start with some general comments, then review some of the more common problems concerning consciousness that might arise in the office. The basic pathology involved in each case will be explained, along with the signs and symptoms of the conditions and the ways to manage them.

Subjects to be discussed include:

- Syncope
- Hyperventilation syndrome
- Diabetic reactions (hypo- and hyperglycemic reactions)
- Seizures

- Cardiovascular system problems, including myocardial infarction and angina
- Hypersensitivity reactions (including latex and drug allergies and anaphylactic shock)

General Considerations

An American Dental Association report on "office and emergency kits" prepared by the, then named, Council on Dental Therapeutics contained the following:

"Dentists should be able to recognize and treat office emergencies. The dental team must be well prepared for any emergency. To this end, the Council on Dental Therapeutics encourages each member of the profession to receive courses in basic and advanced life support. The Council recognizes that the skills acquired through this training must be continually reviewed and practiced because action during an emergency must be taken quickly and confidently."[1]

Each member of the dental team should have a clear understanding of the nature of the common medical emergencies likely to be seen in the office setting. There is a variety of very informative literature available from the American Heart Association concerning such topics as Basic Life Support (BLS) for the health care provider, Pediatric Advanced Life Support (PALS), and Advanced Cardiovascular Life Support (ACLS).[2] It is highly recommended that such literature be available in the dental office.

Each person should be regularly updated on this knowledge, understand his/her own particular role in an emergency situation, and be prepared to participate. For example, a clerical person may be responsible for calling for specialist medical aid, contacting an emergency medical service, or dialing an emergency number such as 911. A particular dental assistant may be charged with maintaining emergency equipment and supplies and making sure that all emergency drugs are current.

An important way to prepare for a possible emergency is to "know" every patient from the medical point of view. A complete medical history for each patient is essential and should be obtained before any dental treatment is begun. Any history of previous medical emergencies occurring in a dental office *must* be elucidated and histories of conditions such as epilepsy, diabetes, and drug use (legal or illegal) must be thoroughly evaluated.

The physical evaluation of a patient before each dental treatment is essential. The dentist should be confident that he/she is able to recognize any changes in a patient's demeanor, undue anxiety, or other evidence of a change in behavioral status. Someone who becomes severely anxious when visiting a dentist might benefit by the dentist making sure that the patient has an early morning appointment and is not kept waiting too long in a waiting room.

The dentist may also use his personal psychotherapy to allay any "dentophobia," reassuring a patient as to what is planned and what the patient should expect. The dentist must be certain that he/she and other members of his/her team are skilled in blood pressure determination and the evaluation of other vital signs. He/she must be certain that any blood pressure determination made in a crisis situation is reliable and that the person taking a blood pressure and other vital signs is practiced and confident.

A discussion about medical emergency supplies, equipment, and drugs will be given at the end of the chapter. One matter to be discussed later is the need for the practitioner to be aware of any manufacturers' recommendations concerning the use of a medication. A "package insert" often provides important warnings. For example, a well-known and widely used local anesthetic agent containing a vasoconstrictor comes with a package insert that warns:

Dental practitioners who employ local anesthetic agents should be well versed in diagnosis and management of emergencies which may arise from their use. Resuscitative equipment, oxygen and other resuscitative drugs should be available for immediate use.

The insert goes on to discuss *overdosage* and comments on the methods of dealing with such events. It states that certain medications such as thiopental or a benzodiazepine (such as diazepam) may be administered. The statement is made that the clinician should be familiar, prior to *the use of local anesthetics, with these anticonvulsant drugs.*

Another manufacturer's insert for a different local anesthetic agent states *resuscitative equipment and drugs should be immediately available* and states that its product *should be used with extreme caution for patients whose medical history and physical examination suggest the existence of hypertension, arteriosclerotic heart disease, cerebrovascular insufficiency, heart block, thyrotoxicosis and diabetes, etc.*

It is realized that many dental practitioners who may be using local anesthetic agents on a frequent and regular basis may not be as well prepared as they might feel they should be, but it is considered most prudent that they at least be *aware* of the product manufacturer's recommendations!

Some Basic Physiology

Although the exact nature of consciousness, unconsciousness, and sleep are not fully understood, there are some basic principles that should always be remembered. Effective brain function depends on a number of factors that include—

- An adequate supply of oxygen
- An adequate supply of glucose
- A pH range that varies only slightly
- An electrical equilibrium that is consistent

Oxygen

The oxygen supply to the brain depends primarily on—

- Adequate cerebral blood flow (quantity)
- Adequate oxygen-carrying capacity (quality)

Any severe restriction of cerebral blood flow resulting from, say, arteriosclerotic carotid or cerebral arteries may lead to a *quantitative* deficiency of blood. Carbon monoxide poisoning (which interferes with oxygen carriage by the hemoglobin) would lead to a *qualitative* deficiency.

Cerebral Blood Flow

The cerebral blood flow depends on two main factors:

- Patency of the cerebral blood vessels and
- Blood pressure

Arteriosclerotic disease is quite common, and some patients may advise the dentist that they suffer from some feeling of dizziness should they move their head in a particular way, *e.g.*, a person may have severe carotid artery disease so that a movement of the neck may be just sufficient to kink a narrowed artery, reduce or occlude its lumen, and compromise the cerebral blood flow.

Blood Pressure

There are complicated mechanisms for controlling the blood pressure that depend on many factors including—

- The cardiac output (blood volume pumped per unit time)
- Patency of the blood vessels, postural considerations

and whether there are other factors affecting normal BP regulation (use of certain hypotensive agents).

Cardiac output

The cardiac output depends principally on the amount of blood pumped with each contraction and the number of beats per unit time, so an irregular heart beat may lead to a significant drop in cardiac output. Myocardial attacks might lead to serious cardiac output problems with poor cardiac contraction and/or abnormal rhythm.

Patency of blood vessels and postural considerations

Many of the medications used to treat hypertension have a side effect of postural hypotension. These include the beta-blockers. Patients taking such medications may experience dizziness or may even become unconscious if they change position quickly, e.g., patients who have been reclining in dental chairs, perhaps, for more than an hour may need several minutes to regain blood pressure if they sit or stand suddenly.

Glucose

Brain function depends on an adequate level of blood glucose. Blood sugar control is mediated through several mechanisms, and the blood glucose level is normally maintained in a fairly narrow range throughout the day. The fasting blood sugar (FBS) level, normally considered to be that after eight hours of fasting, is of the order of 70-110 milligrams of glucose. It rises after a meal and then, in the normal person, returns to the fasting level within a few hours. In diabetic patients, the FBS level may be within the normal range or higher, but after food intake the glucose level rises abnormally high and it might be several hours before it falls back to the previous normal levels. Glucose levels may be higher than normal (hyperglycemia) or lower than normal (hypoglycemia). An "out of control" diabetic with a very high blood sugar may also have an abnormal blood pH as a result of the development of acidic metabolic products such as ketone bodies, oxybutyric acid, and acetone. Prolonged hyperglycemia with diabetic acidosis may lead to changes in consciousness, but usually such changes only develop over a period of hours or days.

On the other hand, hypoglycemia, which might result from the use of insulin or other hypoglycemic agents (medications frequently used in the treatment of diabetic patients), may develop quite quickly and could occur in the dental office setting. The appearance of a hypoglycemic reaction may resemble that of a syncopal attack and, thus, it is very important for a dentist to know before dental treatment whether a patient is diabetic, whether he/she is taking any medications to treat the disease, and whether he/she has ever experienced any hypoglycemic reactions.

pH range of the blood

It is necessary for the pH of the blood to be maintained within a fairly narrow range, being neither too acid nor too alkaline. The normal pH ranges between 7.35 and 7.45. Respiratory and metabolic processes affect the pH, *e.g.*, in severe obstructive respiratory disease an *acidosis* may develop because of the excessive retention of CO_2 in the blood. If there is a significant increase in the respiratory rate, such as occurs in the so-called hyperventilation syndrome, excess CO_2 is expelled and there results a respiratory *alkalosis*. Either state—acidosis or alkalosis—whether a result of respiratory or metabolic causes—could lead to a change in consciousness.

Electrical equilibrium

There are several conditions in which a disturbance in the electrical stability of the brain is a feature. The most common of these diseases is epilepsy. Seizures may result from a variety of diseases, including cerebral vascular disturbances, brain injury, or neoplasms. A seizure may be thought of as a sudden discharge of abnormal electrical impulses within the brain that can lead to a wide spectrum of symptoms varying from mood changes, to abnormal sensations, to partial or even complete loss of consciousness.

Clinically Important Conditions
That Can Lead to Changes in Consciousness or Other Significant Medical Changes

Syncope

Syncope has been defined as a transient loss of consciousness that is usually a result of cerebral ischemia. There are a number of synonyms used to describe these attacks including neurogenic or psychogenic syncope, fainting, atrial bradycardia, and several others. Cerebral blood flow may be reduced in a variety of states, *e.g.*, a drop in blood pressure (with reduced cerebral blood flow) may result from a swift posture change (especially occurring in patients who are taking medications that might interfere with normal compensating mechanisms). A pregnant patient in the later stages of pregnancy lying back in a dental chair may have the fetus impede the return of venous blood to the heart, thus reducing the cardiac output and provoking a syncope.

The most common reason for a dental office syncope is a vasovagal or vasodepressor attack. This type of syncope is best thought of as being due to a breakdown in one of the mechanisms for controlling cardiac output and blood pressure. Much of the nervous control of the cardiovascular system is mediated through the vagus nerve (X^{th} cranial nerve), hence the term vasovagal attack. Some have suggested that the effect of an overwhelming output of higher central nervous system activity (such as might be generated in a state of severe anxiety, fear, pain, emotional stress, etc.) may depress the cardiovascular system by stimulating the vagus nerve. Regardless of the actual mechanism by which a syncopal event is caused, the condition is normally self-limiting. It has been suggested, teleologically, that nature takes care of a faint by the patient falling to the ground. This assists by removing any gravitational factor that might have been involved in lowering the blood pressure and consequent reduction of cerebral blood flow.

Body's response to syncope

It might be helpful to think of the body's natural response to a "fearful" situation. Let us assume that there is some stimulation of the vagus—the heart is "depressed" and a bradycardia develops, leading to a reduced cardiac output, fall in blood pressure, and a reduction in cerebral blood flow. The patient starts to feel slightly lightheaded. The body responds to this "unpleasant state" by activating its "fear, fright, and flight" response that involves the release of catecholamines (epinephrine and norepinephrine). These have many effects on the body. They include helping restore the blood pressure by stimulating the heart rate and preparing the body for a stressful situation in several ways. Blood flow through the skin may be considered a less important need than blood flow through vital organs so the skin pales, noticeably in the hands and the skin of the face. There is an increase in sweat gland activity (perhaps to anticipate a need for the body to dissipate more heat than usual following an expected increase in metabolism). Perspiration is noted around the face, forehead, and lips, and the hands may be quite clammy.

Signs of syncope (objective indications)

- Paleness, especially hands, lips, and face
- Sweating of hands, forehead, face—especially circumorally (lips)
- A slow pulse in the early stages of the attack—later the pulse rate usually increases
- The eyes may roll and the patient presents a wandering or "out of it" look
- Looks "sick" and may vomit
- If these signs are followed by a loss of consciousness, there may well be a loss of sphincter control and the patient may wet or soil him/herself

Symptoms of syncope (subjective indications)

- The patient feels light-headed and may black out
- He/she may comment on feeling unduly warm
- Feels that he/she needs to breathe more deeply (may try to loosen his/her tie or shirt collar)
- Notes he/she is sweating more
- The patient may feel nauseous and in some cases may vomit

It is important to know that sometimes a patient may demonstrate uncontrolled muscular twitching. These movements may resemble those seen in an epileptic seizure, but should *not* be construed to indicate that a patient has *necessarily* had a true epileptic event. These involuntary movements are attributed to the transient cerebral anoxia that occurs in a syncope. (See later text under "seizures" for further comment on this.)

Management of syncope

This starts before any dental work is begun in that the dentist should have identified any patient with a history of previous syncopal episodes, especially if these had occurred in a dental situation. Such patients should be carefully monitored and steps taken to reduce any anxiety that could precipitate a syncopal event.

If a syncope should start to occur, then all dental work should be stopped. All materials and instruments, including any rubber dam, must be removed from the mouth, the patency of the airway established, and the patient be permitted to recline with head back as soon as possible. The vital signs should be monitored, bearing in mind that, in the early stages of a syncope, the radial pulse may be difficult to appreciate. If it is not palpable easily, then a pulse should be looked for in the temporal or carotid arteries. As soon as the situation begins to resolve naturally, the pulse should not be too difficult to find. If there is any vomiting, then it is important to be certain that the vomitus is fully evacuated from the mouth and that there is no possibility of any being aspirated.

In the majority of syncopal events, the patient starts to recover within a few minutes. Any decision about continuing dental treatment will depend on whether the patient feels better, whether the dental work can be safely left for completion at another appointment, and often, other factors. There is seldom a need to use any specific medication when managing a syncope. The use of a medullary stimulus such as aromatic spirits of ammonia is sometime advocated. A capsule of the pungent smelling medication, broken open and place under the nose, acts as a noxious challenge to the respiratory mucosa, resulting in a stimulus to the vital centers in the medulla of the brainstem. Increased cardiac vascular activity and respiration result. The need for oxygen is debatable. Certainly, the general public expects it to be used in emergency situations, and there is little doubt that the recovering syncopal patient may have an important psychological boost from having an oxygen mask available through which he/she can breathe deeply. However, it must be remembered that the basic physiological problem in a syncope is *not* a *qualitative* deficiency in the oxygenation of the blood but rather a *quantitative* deficiency resulting from poor cerebral flow—a consequence of the drop in blood pressure. Nevertheless, oxygen *should* be available in the dental office and its use be determined by the dentist under the particular circumstances of the event.

There is frequently a question as to whether an unaccompanied patient who has suffered a syncopal episode should be allowed to return home without an escort. Particularly worrisome is whether a patient may drive home alone especially if he/she has shown some involuntary movements during the syncope suggesting that he/she may have had a seizure (see earlier discussion). If a syncopal patient is unaccompanied, he/she should be allowed to recover fully in the waiting room or in some other quiet place and then be evaluated by the dentist. If the patient feels better and the blood pressure and pulse rate are within the normal range then there should be no difficulty in letting the patient travel alone. If there is any doubt about a patient's recovery, then an escort should be used or, if available, medical advice be sought. It is important to fully document any syncopal episode in the patient's record, including the patient's blood pressure and pulse rate at the time of leaving the office.

Hyperventilation Syndrome

An increased respiratory rate that is sustained over a prolonged period may lead to an unnatural loss of CO_2 and a subsequent change in the blood pH to the alkaline side (respiratory alkalosis). The condition probably occurs more frequently in dental patients than is recognized. An apprehensive patient kept waiting for an unduly long time and one who is very anxious about dental treatment may slowly start to develop a respiratory alkalosis. The condition itself seldom would lead to any loss of consciousness, but the body's response to the change in pH coupled with a "fear, flight, and fright" reaction to the symptoms may cause the patient to be very concerned. The more the patient experiences the symptoms, the more likely he/she is to become anxious and hyperventilate even more.

Signs

- The patient appears anxious and restless
- Respiratory rate increased (normal rate is about 15 per minute—may increase to 25 or so)
- The patient may perspire a little and feel lightheaded
- There may some twitching of the facial muscles (attributed to a reduction in CA ions due to the change in the blood pH and an increased neuromuscular sensitivity)

Symptoms

- The patient may complain of the heart "thumping" or "pounding" or complain of an "extra beat." (These palpitations are probably a result of the adrenaline response)
- The patient may state that he/she feels "odd" or on edge and may say he/she can't relax
- There may be some paresthesia of the fingers, toes, and around the lips
- Epigastric discomfort may be experienced

Management of hyperventilation syndrome

The most important element of proper management of this condition is to be aware of the possibility of it happening in the dental office and, especially, the possibility of it occurring in a patient with a previous history of some sort of dental office reaction. Prior episodes may be attributed to a "reaction to an injection" or something similar. However, anyone who reports having a strange reaction during a previous dental visit should be monitored careful and all steps taken to avoid stress, using "psychosedation" techniques and in some cases pharmacologic stress reducers to prevent hyperventilation syndrome from occurring.

The definitive steps to be taken are those that will help the patient reduce the respiratory rate and, if possible, rebreathe some of their expired air in order to restore the pH to normal as soon as possible. The patient may be persuaded to breathe his/her expired air into a paper bag and re-breathe it or to place his/her cupped hands under his/her mouth. This helps keep the expired air in the region of the mouth and assists in the restoring of the pH.

The author has found the following technique to be quite beneficial. The patient is reassured and told to relax and to breathe in only when told by the dentist—"Breathe in...one...breathe in...two, etc." If the dentist sets a rate that is much slower than the rate at which the patient was previously breathing, it is generally easier to reduce the patient's respiratory rate that way than by just asking the patient to breathe more slowly.

When the reaction has settled, it is usually in order for the dental treatment to be continued, unless of course, in the judgment of the dentist, it might be better postponed.

Diabetic Reactions

A diabetic patient may suffer from any one of the other medical emergencies that might befall a dental patient. In this section, we shall review those reactions specific to the diabetic state. Any patient with a history of diabetes should be questioned further about the nature of his/her diabetes. Is it controlled by diet and/or weight control only? Does the patient receive any drug therapy? Is the therapy by mouth or by injection? Does the patient take insulin? If so, in what dosage? Daily? Twice daily? More frequently? Answers to these questions will give some idea as to the likelihood of an untoward reaction occurring. The lability of the diabetes is important, and any patients taking hypoglycemic drugs, including insulin, should be asked if they have ever suffered from a hypoglycemic (insulin) reaction and what steps they have been advised to take should one start to develop. Obviously, if a patient reports that he/she is susceptible to hypoglycemic reactions, then the dentist should establish at what time such a reaction is likely to occur, *e.g.*, mornings, evenings, or nighttime and be prepared to adjust appointments to the times least likely to coincide with a reaction.

A *hyperglycemic reaction* (*i.e.*, one in which the blood sugar regulation has gone out of control and the patient develops extremely high blood sugar levels) is often accompanied by the formation of acid products. This reaction is unlikely to occur suddenly. It is usually a slower process and takes hours or even days to develop and therefore is extremely unlikely to develop in the dental office setting.

Symptoms of hyperglycemia include:

- Polyuria, polydipsia, and polyphagia
- Visual disturbances
- Tiredness and excessive fatigue
- Paresthesias

Signs include:

- Florid appearance of the face
- Deep and irregular breathing (Kussmaul's respiration—a type of altered respiration seen in diabetic patients that results from the body's attempt to adjust an altered pH state by changing the respiratory rate and altering the rate of CO_2 loss)

- Dry skin
- "Fruity" acetone odor to the breath

Management is to correct the blood sugar levels and reverse any metabolic acidosis. There is no immediate treatment that would normally be given in the dental office. The patient should be referred to an appropriate medical facility for definitive treatment. As mentioned earlier, such a state is very unlikely to develop in the dental office.

However, a *hypoglycemic* reaction could well occur. When the blood sugar level falls to a level of around 40 mgs of glucose per 100 ml of blood, then a person may start to feel "peculiar." The level of blood glucose at which a patient may fall into an unconscious state is variable. In some patients, it may be in the 40-mg range, in others the level might drop to the 30s or lower before the patient loses consciousness. In others, the unconscious state might develop with levels in the "normal range." It is clear that a careful history should be taken in any circumstance in which a patient reports an "insulin" reaction. It should also be remembered that hypoglycemic reactions may occur in patients who have never been identified as diabetics and who, occasionally, usually after a heavy carbohydrate meal, simply develop a hypoglycemic state.

Symptoms

There is a blunting of consciousness that may manifest as something like an inability to "think clearly," to be unable to carry on a simple conversation, or to lose the ability to perform a simple calculation.

The patient may not lose consciousness, but the mood alters—he/she may be surly or uncooperative. Malamed summarizes such changes as "altered consciousness."[3]

There may be a feeling of lightheadedness and the patient may black out.

Signs

- A "fear, fright, and flight" response develops, and there may sweating, increased pulse rate, and other signs suggesting an adrenaline response
- Patients may appear confused
- If the patient relapses into the unconscious state, then there may be some involuntary muscle movements

Management of hypoglycemia

Because so many of the signs of hypoglycemia resemble a syncopal episode, it is important for the dentist to appreciate the importance of determining whether a "syncope" is, in fact, a hypoglycemic reaction. The placing of a person in the supine position will not do much to correct the blood sugar level. The key to treatment is to restore the blood glucose. This can be done, for example, by the use of an oral glucose preparation if the patient is responsive, by the use of glucose paste introduced into the mouth, or by the use of agents such as a glucose solution or glucagon (intramuscularly or intravenously) that raise the blood sugar level. It is recommended that any change in consciousness that develops suddenly in a diabetic patient should be considered to be a hypoglycemic reaction rather than a hyperglycemic reaction and treated quickly by the raising of the glucose level. If a fall in glucose to a significantly low level is not reversed quickly, then it might result in some permanent cerebral damage. In the event that an episode was indeed due to hyperglycemia, then is very unlikely that an attempt to raise the blood sugar level (i.e., one, which it was believed, in error, was too low) would have any significant effect on the patient. Management of a diabetic patient should include the usual monitoring of the vital signs—blood pressure, pulse rate, and respirations.

Seizures

Epilepsy has been defined as "a recurrent paroxysmal disorder of cerebral function characterized by sudden brief attacks of altered consciousness, motor activity, sensory phenomena, or inappropriate behavior caused by abnormal excessive discharge of cerebral neurons."

There are a number of conditions in which seizures are a feature, and they include systemic disorders such as high temperatures, infections and anaphylactic reactions, and metabolic disorders such as hypoglycemia and other endocrine abnormalities. Cerebral trauma, tumors, and other brain injuries frequently give rise to seizures, and many are classified as "idiopathic" when no specific explanation of the seizures can be given. Up to about 75% of young adults with seizures were considered to have idiopathic seizures, but with the increasing availability (and use) of sophisticated techniques such as electroencephalography and PET (positron emission tomography) scanning, there has been a great improvement in the understanding of seizures and a very detailed and expanded classification of seizure disorders has been developed.

From the dental point of view, it still seems reasonable to consider the two main groups of seizure disorders under the headings—

- Petit mal—(little malady)
- Grand mal—the "great" malady

In the former, there may a very limited loss of consciousness sometimes referred to as an "absence" attack. Patients may seem "out of it" for a period of between 15 and 30 seconds. They stop what they are doing and seem to be dreaming and then as quickly resume what they were doing before. These attacks are most usually seen in children and may be noticed initially by an observant teacher, who sees a child who seems to "drift" or "day dream" for a few seconds. From a practical point of view, these attacks should not present any problems for the dentist, although he/she should be aware of any child for whom this diagnosis has been made.

The grand mal episode (or tonic-clonic) episode can be much more dramatic. A patient may be aware of its onset by experiencing an aura—a strange smell, a particular sound, or some epigastric discomfort. The aura is then usually followed by a cry and the patient loses consciousness, falls, and starts tonic contractions of the muscles of the head, neck, trunk, and extremities. During this phase, the patient may demonstrate some dyspnea and there may even be a degree of cyanosis. There may be some oral bleeding from teeth-gnashing movements abrading soft tissues. These tonic contractions, which usually last little more than 20–30 seconds, are followed by clonic (intermittent) contractions. There may be incontinence (fecal and/or urinary). After the attack subsides (usually within 2-5 minutes), the patient may pass into a postictal state as if sleeping deeply—recovering eventually, often with muscle soreness and a headache. Full recovery from a grand mal seizure may take up to 2 hours, but there are clearly variations in the severity of seizures.

The dental management of a patient who has a history of seizures necessitates a full understanding of the frequency of the seizures, of any events that seem to predispose the patient to developing an attack and whether the patient is under medical care, what medications are being used to control the condition, and, most importantly, whether the patient has been compliant with his/her medications [common ones include dilantin (phenytoin), tegretol (carbamazepine), phenobaritone]. If a patient who is compliant with his/her medications reports no seizures for several years, then the risk of an untoward event occurring in the dental office during routine procedures is minimal. On the other hand, a non-compliant patient with a history of frequent seizures would need to be evaluated carefully, and it may well be advisable to seek advice from the patient's physician before a course of dental treatment is started.

Apart from recognizing the nature of the seizures, there is little that can be done for patients except to protect them from hurting themselves against sharp or protruding objects and ensuring that there is a good clear airway with adequate respiration. In most circumstances, the patient should be allowed to sleep comfortably until consciousness is regained. It must not be forgotten that, in some circumstances, a patient may develop the serious condition of status epilepticus—a continuous seizure or recurrent seizures that occur so closely together that there is virtually no recovery phase discernible between episodes. Any seizure that lasts for five minutes or longer should be regarded with great caution and emergency medical care sought. Vital signs of the patient should be monitored, as the blood pressure may rise dramatically in a sustained seizure and this knowledge may be important when communicating with emergency medical personnel.

Differential Diagnosis—Syncope v. Epilepsy

Mention was made earlier concerning the occasional involuntary muscle movements seen in some cases of syncope. It was noted that these movements should not necessarily be interpreted as an indication that an epileptic event has occurred. Clearly, it is important to distinguish between a syncopal v. an epileptic event, as such a distinction would be needed when deciding whether a patient who had suffered an event in the dental office should be allowed to travel home alone or whether an escort would be needed.

The following summarizes some of the differences between the two events:

Vasovagal syncope	Epilepsy
May be sudden	Usually there is a prodrome
Onset may be recalled	Retrograde amnesia may occur
Injury sometimes occurs	Injury often occurs
Tongue biting is unusual	Tongue biting is more common
Continence is usually preserved	Incontinence frequently occurs
Recovery is often rapid	Usually a longer and more confused recovery

Cardiovascular conditions

There are a large number of clinical conditions that can develop as a result of disease of the cardiovascular system. These include diseases of the heart muscle, of the conducting system (arrhythmias, dysrhythmias), etc. In this chapter, we shall deal with several important problems associated with such conditions that the dental practitioner may encounter. We believe that, if there is any doubt about a cardiovascular patient's ability to withstand any dental operative procedure, it is incumbent on the dentist to seek a consultation with the patient's physician.

Angina pectoris

This term is used to describe the discomfort that is experienced by a patient who suffers from a relative deficiency of cardiac circulation (usually arteriosclerotic coronary artery disease) and who, at times when there is a call for increased cardiac muscle activity, may develop some uncomfortable feeling. The increased cardiac muscle activity is not always a result of physical activity, but may be brought on by emotional stress, increased tension, or even by a heavy meal. The discomfort may manifest as frank pain, perhaps as a feeling of a tight band around the chest, some pain in the shoulder or down one of the arms, or epigastric discomfort. It is important to know that very occasionally an angina pain is experienced significantly in the jaw or even in a tooth, and a patient may seek the advice of a dentist for a "tooth or jaw ache" that is, in fact, a pain caused by myocardial insufficiency! The pain usually resolves spontaneously after a few minutes of rest or if a vasodilator such as nitroglycerin is administered. The medication is most usually administered by the use of sublinqual nitroglycerin tablets, but may be delivered by a nitroglycerin absorption skin patch. In acute cases of cardiac pain, such as may occur in a heart attack, the nitroglycerin may be given intravenously.

Many patients may report that they have suffered from angina pectoris for many months or even years, and in such cases the dentist should determine the severity of the condition.

- Does the patient carry nitroglycerin tablets for use as needed?
- Does he/she wear a nitroglycerin skin absorption patch daily?
- Under what circumstances does he/she need to take a nitroglycerin tablet?
- Is it likely that the stress of a dental procedure might induce an anginal attack?

After such an evaluation, the dentist should be able to determine whether a particular patient might present a problem during treatment. Patients who are considered likely to need nitroglycerin during a dental visit should be advised to bring their medications with them to the office. The usual steps to reduce stress should be taken, *e.g.* waiting time should be kept to a minimum, possible use of anxiolytic drugs, etc. If an "angina" pain or discomfort does not resolve after nitroglycerin, then the possibility of a more severe heart problem such as a myocardial event must be considered.

Myocardial infarction

Although myocardial infarction or a heart attack is a relatively common event, its occurrence in the dental office setting is, fortunately, rather uncommon. However, cases have been reported, and the dental team should be prepared to deal with such an event. The usual cause is an acute deficiency of blood to the heart muscle that leads to muscle death and necrosis. The effects of a heart attack are highly variable. Everyone has heard of cases in which evidence of a previous heart attack is discovered at a routine physical examination, and yet the patient denies any knowledge of ever having experienced any symptoms suggesting one. On the other hand, some heart attacks are massive and lead to death almost immediately. No attempt will be made here to review all of the salient aspects of heart attacks except to summarize as follows.

Sudden damage to heart muscle such as may develop after a myocardial infarction could lead to:

- A minimal clinical effect
- Such a severe loss of "pumping" effectiveness that the patient goes into acute heart failure
- Intense pain associated with shock
- Development of an abnormal rhythm that leads to impaired functioning of the heart
- In the worse case scenario, to ventricular fibrillation—a state in which the ventricle no longer is coordinating its pumping

action and, from a functional point of view, fails to work as a pump. Such a situation requires immediate care. For a fuller understanding and explanation of what can be done, including the possible use of external defibrillators, the reader is referred to one of the American Heart Association texts mentioned earlier[4]

Myocardial infarction (signs and symptoms)

The patient may experience intense crushing or choking pain across the chest. This pain may radiate across the chest, through to the back, up into the neck or jaw, into the shoulder, or down one of the arms to the hand. There may be severe nausea, weakness, a feeling that the person is going to faint, that he/she is perspiring, and the heart is beating irregularly. The signs of an infarction may be severe restlessness, an appearance of extreme anxiety, paleness, and perspiration. The pulse rate may be irregular and may be faster or slower than normal. As discussed earlier, some of the characteristics of myocardial infarction may resemble the pain of angina pectoris, but it must be remembered that, if a pain does not resolve quickly, then a putative myocardial infarction patient should be referred as soon as possible to emergency medical personnel. The most critical time for the infarction patient is in the first five hours following the onset of the clinical symptoms and signs. The degree of management that can be accomplished in the dental office will depend on the preparedness, skill, and confidence of the members of the dental team. At the very least, BLS measures must be instituted, including the use of oxygen.

Hypersensitivity reactions

Allergy has been defined as a condition in which exposure to a particular substance (an allergen) sensitizes the body so that a subsequent exposure leads to an unusual heightened reaction. These reactions may be immediate or delayed—they may be very mild (such as a transient skin rash) or they may very intense, so severe that the patient may go into shock (anaphylactic shock) and unless aggressive anti-shock treatment is given, may die. Asthma is a form of allergy and such patients experience breathing difficulties when they are exposed to certain substances that vary from types of dust to pollens. There are several substances and medications used frequently in dental practice that are recognized as allergens. These include antibiotics such as penicillin and its derivatives, other antibiotics, and drugs. Latex allergy has become a more significant problem in recent years, and more and more dental patients are reporting reactions from the use of gloves and rubber dam.

Perhaps the most important aspect of managing allergic patients is to identify those patients with a known history of allergic reactions and then to conduct an in-depth evaluation of their particular problem. Each patient at the initial visit should be asked about allergies.

- Have you had any reactions to drugs, medications, or foodstuffs?
- If so, what was the nature of the reaction?
- Was it a transient skin rash or mild urticaria (hives)?
- Did it involve any swelling of the mouth, face, or throat?
- Did you have any breathing difficulty, etc.?

Clearly, any history of previous allergic reaction, even if only trivial, must be taken as a warning *not* to challenge the patient with the same allergen again. True allergic reactions to local anesthetics used in dentistry are considered very, very unusual, and reported reactions may result from the preservatives and stabilizers used rather than the anesthetic solution itself. In the experience of the author, when patients reporting local anesthetic reactions during previous dental appointments are evaluated by an allergist, usually no positive conclusions can be reached. If there is any doubt in the mind of a dentist about the safety of using a local anesthetic, he/she should seek a medical consultation from an allergist.

Allergic reactions to an antibiotic may develop during dental treatment, especially if a patient has been given, for example, a dose of prophylactic antibiotic for a preexisting cardiac condition an hour or so before the treatment. If such a patient complains of developing an itchy skin or starts to develop hives, then he/she should be very carefully monitored to ascertain whether the reaction is progressing to a serious level, e.g., swelling in the mouth, throat, or breathing difficulty or even cardiovascular collapse—shock. In the mild cases, an antihistamine may be considered. Benadryl is often used (by mouth or by intramuscular injection), but it must be remembered that most antihistamines have a side effect of causing drowsiness and, for some patients, this may lead to a degree of sedation that might make driving inadvisable. Anaphylactic shock is the most serious allergic reaction with which the dentist may be faced and, in this condition, definitive drug use may be needed.

Shock has been defined as being like a "prolonged syncope," i.e., there is a collapse of the respiratory and circulatory systems that does not resolve quickly, there is usually a low blood pressure, a rapid and weak pulse. A very dramatic "fear, flight, and fright" reaction is seen with paleness and clamminess of the skin. In such cases, steps should be taken immediately to treat the patient, and the drug of choice recommended by most drug manufacturers is epinephrine. The medication is readily available and is usually packaged as a preloaded 1:1000 solution. The initial dose is normally 0.3 mg given intramuscularly or subcutaneously. A preloaded syringe containing 1 ml of the 1:1000 solution (1 mgm) is available that permits the contents to be given easily in separate 0.3 mg doses. The preparation is made so that the first dose can be easily given, but the syringe plunger cannot deliver more unless it is rotated. After rotation of the plunger, a second 0.3 mg dose may be given, and then on further turning of the plunger, a third dose may be delivered. This arrangement helps prevent the inadvertent injection of a too large initial dose.

It is salutary to note that nearly every package insert concerning local anesthetic use recommends that *epinephrine be readily available at the time of administering a local anesthetic agent.*

Continual monitoring of an anaphylactic patient's vital signs should be maintained until the patient recovers or an emergency team arrives or transports the patient to an emergency facility.

Emergency supplies, equipment, and drugs

Emergency supplies, equipment, and drugs should be readily available in every situation in which surgical treatment involving the use of medications is being rendered.

There is no general agreement among dentists and oral surgeons as to the composition of a dental emergency drug kit.

Some have advocated a minimum number of drugs; others have suggested a "mini pharmacy!" Malamed makes reference to the fact that some years ago, the American Dental Association's Council on Dental Therapeutics issued a statement on emergency drug kits.[4] Although this report was published in 1973, some of the comments are still most relevant. The report included the following comments:

All dentists must be prepared to diagnose and treat expeditiously life threatening emergencies that may arise in their practices. The best way to accomplish this objective is by taking continuing education courses on the subject of emergencies...

The report continued: *Since emergency kits should be individualized to meet the special needs and capabilities of each clinician, no stereotyped kit can be approved by the Council on Dental Therapeutics. Practitioners are encouraged to assemble their own individual kit that will be safe and effective in their hands or to purchase a kit that contains drugs that they are fully trained to administer.*[5]

Malamed comments: *The most desirable approach to emergency drug kits is for the doctor to prepare a kit that is individualized to meet his or her special requirements and capabilities. In the author's experience commercially prepared emergency kits are quickly placed in a cabinet where they will not be touched until they are needed. The doctor and staff do not spend any time familiarizing themselves with the contents of the kit or the indications for the use of these agents and the emergency kit quickly becomes a security blanket.*

There is a variety of medical emergency kits on the market, and these vary from a minimum of supplies to sophisticated kits that include color coded medications, tracheotomy needles, tourniquets, syringes, and automated external defibrillators.

One reasonable approach to the question "What emergency equipment and drugs do I need in the office?" would be to recommend that, at the very least, a dentist should have available those emergency drugs (and resuscitative supplies and equipment) that a drug manufacturer recommends be available at the time of administration of the product.

In my opinion, Malamed has developed an excellent approach to the matter of emergency drugs.[4] He reminds his readers that BLS (basic life support) techniques are essential and then considers several groups (modules) of emergency drugs and equipment.

Module 1

Critical (Essential) Emergency Drugs and Equipment (the minimum—absolutely basic)

This module consists of:

Two injectable drugs:

- Epinephrine
- Antihistamine

Two non-injectable drugs:

- Oxygen
- Vasodilator

Emergency equipment:

- Oxygen delivery system
- Suction and suction tips
- Tourniquets
- Syringes

There is a variety of choices for these differing elements. For example, epinephrine can be obtained in a preloaded syringe, or in ampoules, etc. The practitioner is advised to select the particular method of epinephrine administration with which he/she would be most comfortable and the same for the other elements in Malamed's Module 1.

Module 2

Non-critical (Secondary) Emergency Drugs and Equipment

This module, according to the author, contains drugs and equipment that *though important and valuable in the management of emergency situations, are not considered to be essential or critical elements of the office emergency kit. Doctors who have received training in the use of theses drugs should consider their inclusion in the emergency kit.*

Module 2 consists of categories of injectable drugs such as anticonvulsant, analgesic, vasopressor, antihypoglycemic, corticosteroid, antihypertensive, and anticholinergic. Malamed recommends also noninjectable drugs such as a respiratory stimulus, an antihypoglycemic, and a bronchodilator.

He describes two additional module levels:

Module 3

Advanced life support measures, and

Module 4

Antidotal drugs used to manage the effects of drugs used in anesthetic or sedation practice

Summary

The dental practitioner must know that he/she and his/her team should always be aware of the possibility of a medical emergency arising in the dental office. He/she and his/her team must be prepared for such an eventuality by—

- being aware of the manufacturer's recommendations about the use of a product
- preparing themselves (be familiar with the principles of BLS and ACLS)
- preparing the office (emergency supplies and equipment)
- thoroughly evaluating all patients to determine those most likely to develop a problem

Notes

[1] Office emergencies and emergency kits, an association report, *JADA*, 101(8): 305, 1980

[2] American Heart Association - Authorized Distributor of Publications, Channing L. Bete Company, AHA Fulfillment Center, 200 State Road, South Deerfield, MA 01373-0200 http://aha.channing-bete.com

[3] Malamed, Stanley F. *Medical Emergencies in the Dental Office*, 5th ed., Philadelphia: W.B. Saunders, 1999, p. 540

[4] Op. cit.

[5] Emergency Kits. Council on Dental Therapeutics, *JADA*, 87(4): 909, 1973

Chapter 7

Communicating Financially with Your Patients

By Jennifer de St. Georges

Virtually every consumer product on the market comes with instructions for use and the necessary monitoring and/or maintenance needed to maintain the product in sound working order. Buy a car and receive directions to check the oil. Buy a coffee maker and get tips to keep it perking along.

For a dental practice to be financially solvent, it requires that the owner invest time, money, and training in utilizing and monitoring sound financial/business systems. Yet this knowledge and education are not included in today's dental school curricula.

The following chapter focuses the reader on identifying key components required to successfully communicate financially with your patients while building a strong business foundation. This ensures that the health provider receives payments for services rendered and is financially able to maintain the practice.

An effective financial program consists of seven basic components:

- A well thought out, fair, and firm internal financial policy. This allows doctor and staff to be consistent in their financial communication with patients

- On-going training on systems and the necessary verbal skills needed to communicate with patients
- Written and signed financial agreements to be completed by all patients prior to treatment
- An effective billing system that is user-friendly to both operator and patients
- Installation of strong, reliable financial monitoring systems. Monitoring is required weekly and monthly. This is possible only when quality protected time is scheduled for doctor and staff to actually monitor and take the necessary follow-up action as needed

The Dentist's Financial Responsibilities

- Set fees in a fair and consistent way—Fees are set in relationship to expenses, experience, and a fair return on investment
- Believe in the value of the dental services being provided by dentist and staff
- Maintain these values by hiring to these standards and invest in ongoing continuing education (CE) courses to maintain the clinical and management standards
- Provide a comfortable and private environment for patient, doctor, and staff to fully discuss all treatment approaches, costs, and financial options
- Work with staff to create strong but comfortable communication skills with patients about their financial responsibilities
- Create and maintain an effective record system—logical in design, efficient to run—that captures the maximum clinical, management, and financial information with the least amount of input, work, and stress for the team

- Install and maintain financial monitoring systems to oversee patient's financial responsibility and current payment status

Dentists work long and hard to increase their communication skills so patients can learn more about the exciting procedures being performed in dentistry today and the benefits patients can enjoy. The goal of this chapter is to help the dentist, and thereby the team, create strong communication and management systems in his/her practice, to allow the dentist to enjoy the financial fruits of his/her labors and to gain communication between practice and patient in the area of financial responsibility.

The Consumer's Financial Needs

Inform before you perform—no surprises

In the mid-70's, the California State Dental Board surveyed nearly 800 people. The number one concern of nearly 90% of those polled was, "Tell me, Doctor, how much will the treatment cost and please tell me *before* you do the dentistry." They did not state that they wanted the cheapest price in town. What they said, in no uncertain terms, was that they wanted to be told the cost of the dentistry prior to treatment. This request leads me to believe that many patients have experienced the reverse—only learning about the fees *after* receiving the treatment.

In the United States, the average practice receives approximately 70% of its new dental patients through a direct referral of friends, relatives, neighbors, or co-workers. These referred patients call your office with great expectations about the service. What many practices forget is that these patients probably have also heard about what's expected of them financially. This information can include your fees, how your fees are pegged in the market place, your payment methods, collection attitude, and other personal experiences. The building of confidence and trust in the doctor's clinical expertise and management philosophies has already begun. Financial communication with these referred patients should be relatively easy. They walked through the door already knowing that there are financial guidelines to be followed.

The remaining 30% of new patients, however, will come to you for one of more of a wide range of reasons, often centered around convenience (close to home or work, extended office hours, visible locations, etc.). You haven't had the benefit of one of your patients of record educating these patients as to the ground rules and what is expected of them. Therefore, one needs to slow down and take extra time to reach out and help these patients come up to speed with your financial requirements.

Remember: *A patient who comes to you because it is convenient will leave when it becomes inconvenient, unless you have established a relationship of confidence and trust with him/her and he/she perceives the benefit.*

New Patient Telephone Calls

Effective financial communication begins when your new patient first contacts the practice

The majority of patients' first contact with a dental practice is by phone. My research shows that most offices do not bring up the subject of money on this initial call unless the patient asks for information about fees and payment methods.

My advice to the dental profession is to be proactive, not reactive. Bring up the subject of money on this initial call before the patient has to ask. Take the stress and guesswork out of this first communication. For every patient who asks, there are three that are dying to ask but don't know how to bring up the subject.

This financial discussion, in my opinion, can be extremely positive as long as it is held at the correct point in the conversation. Discussing the patient's financial responsibilities at any place except at the very end of the conversation is a recipe for disaster.

The new patient call is clearly broken down into three specific parts:

- Identifying the patient's clinical and emotional concerns
- Scheduling the patient appropriately
- Opening the lines of financial communication

Closing out the call: "Mrs. Patient, we look forward to seeing you this Wednesday, May 29th at 10:30 a.m." An optional phrase can then be added here: "And we ask that all new patients joining the practice take care of their charges in full on the initial visit." Breaking down this phrase:

- "We ask" is soft, understated, a request versus "you need to," which is not user friendly
- "All" infers you ask the same of everyone calling in—no favorites
- "New" infers that once the patient has established a record, there is a different set of guidelines
- "Joining the practice" tells the patient the practice is making an assumption that the patient will become a permanent client of the practice
- "Take care of the charges in full" is a mouthful—seven words. What one word could be used instead? *Pay.* Pretty tacky, non-health related, and makes it sound as if you are selling a product and not a service

There's another phrase that may—or may not—belong in your optional statement. That is: "We ask that all new patients joining the practice take care of their charges in full on the initial visit *regardless of insurance involvement.*" Whether to use this phrase, or not, has to be your decision. If you're like the majority of dental practices, 70% or more of your patients have insurance coverage of some kind. By making this philosophy statement you accomplish three things. You show the patient—

- You're educating him/her as to his/her responsibility
- You've broken the ice to continue this subject in more detail later
- You're very comfortable with the subject, which means he/she will feel comfortable

If you make the statement of financial policy and don't include the tag line, and the majority of your patients have insurance, patients respond with "I have dental insurance that pays 100% of exam and x-rays." Your staff has now opened Pandora's box. Not only does this call become time consuming, but invariably the practice will be on the losing end as it is both impossible and inappropriate to get into details about the patient insurance on the phone before the patient has even met the doctor and the team. The focus is now on the patient's insurance and not on the patient's clinical and emotional needs. Questions can range from table of allowances and fees schedules to deductibles and maximums. In many cases, I feel that the practice comes out the loser in this situation.

However, there is a potential negative in bringing this phrase "regardless of your insurance involvement" into the conversation. In a minority of cases it will immediately elicit the question "how much is the first visit going to cost?" However, with the correct training (which we cover later in the chapter under Telephone Shoppers), we provide the solution to take care of this potential problem.

If your practice has less than 50% insurance patients, you may well want to consider not including this phrase. A frank discussion and training session with the administrative staff are required to fully explore the pros and cons of utilizing this phrase in your telephone communication for your special practice needs.

Welcome Packets

Practices wanting to raise the level of communication with new patients take the extra effort to mail a welcome packet prior to the first visit to the office. The packet consists of a minimum of five items.

Welcome letter—a kind, soft, caring letter. It both welcomes the patient to the practice as well as informing him/her briefly of procedures to be performed on the first visit. If your initial examination appointment is unusually long (in some practices, this appointment can run to two hours), this letter would be a good place to advise the patient of your schedule.

A welcome letter is *not* the place to make policy statements relating either to money or insurance processing. It is absolutely not the place to make such pompous time-keeping statements as I see in many welcome letters… "Except for emergencies, we usually run on time and we expect the same of you." I would advise to take this type of language out of your written communication. Also, no reference should ever be made in this letter to your no show policy and charges for missed appointments.

Practice brochure—A professionally written and printed brochure outlines details of the doctor and his/her philosophy to treating teeth and what services are available in the practice. Any mention of your financial policies need to be discreet and take a positive approach. The patient has not yet met the doctor. The relationship has yet to be established. Inappropriate emphasis on the cost of treatment, methods of payment, and non-treatment costs (*i.e.*, no shows) is inappropriate.

The heading for this financial section is "Your Financial Investment"—We're banning the following three words, which are greatly overused in most dental practices.

Fee, cost, and price—The phrase "The financial investment" that replaces these non-benefit words still conveys financial responsibility, but makes the point in an understated and professional manner.

However, three financial areas of concern need to be quietly covered. They support the initial phone call and allow the patient to feel that this is an office that truly "informs before they perform, no surprises."

"We're happy to provide a written estimate prior to any needed treatment being performed."

Remember, 90% of consumers told the California State Board that they wanted to know how much the treatment would cost before the treatment was rendered. This phrase now takes care of their number one concern.

"Our administrative staff will be happy to discuss with you our range of financial options."

- By replacing the term "receptionist" with "administrative" we acknowledge the authority of the business administrative staff to discuss and collect fees
- The word "happy" denotes that the practice is both comfortable discussing fees and happy to work with the patient in this area
- The phrase "our range of financial options" conveys an organized practice with a menu of prepared payment options from which the patient can choose
- The phrase "financial arrangements" is eliminated. I believe that it leaves the door open for patients to feel that they can negotiate *how* they will pay

Most offices talk within the team and even to patients about financial arrangements (FAs). I would recommend that we retire the term financial arrangements and replace it with financial agreement. "Arrangement" relates to the process—"Agreement" infers that the patient is indeed agreeing to the arrangement.

"We ask that all new patients joining the practice take care of the charges in full at the initial appointment"

This is a reconfirmation of the statement made on the initial phone call. It both confirms your financial policy and shows management consistency.

Dental, medical, and personal history forms are also included in the packet. Forms filled out in the reception room are generally 30% incomplete. Forms mailed to patients prior to their initial visit will result in completely filled-out forms.

The patient, medical, and dental history forms should be used for fact gathering only. It is not appropriate on the patient history form to include statements that the practice runs credit checks or that the cost of turning over a delinquent account to an attorney will be borne by the patient, or that past-due accounts can be required to be brought current on demand.

A reminder to the reader: The patient has not yet met the doctor. There is no relationship. In fact, the patient may not like the doctor. Such statements infer that the patient is going to go ahead with any needed treatment. It also conveys that so many patients (unhappy ones?) get behind on their account, that there are three policy statements about past due accounts for the patient to sign off on before even meeting the doctor.

So, am I suggesting that we forego commenting on these areas of concern? Absolutely not. Running credit checks, advising patients of the cost of collecting past due accounts, and "calling in" past accounts is very appropriate. As in life, timing is everything. These subjects, along with others, need to be included in the financial agreement form that both the patient and staff will sign after the exam, but before treatment commences.

Legally, it is required to have patients sign an informed consent prior to examination. If emergency care were needed, the patient would then sign a more extensive informed consent after the diagnosis, but prior to treatment.

Two business cards should be included in the packet—one to keep at home and one for the wallet/office.

One appointment card also needs to be included. The following financial policy statement is found on most appointment cards: "There will be a charge unless we receive at least 24 hours notice." In my opinion, this is a most negative approach to the subject of scheduling changes. I recommend the following line instead: "There will be absolutely no charge as long as we receive at least 48 hours notice of your need to change your appointment." We achieve two goals with this approach:

- We have replaced the negative approach with a positive one

- By increasing 24 to 48 hours, hopefully you will get 24 hours notice. Ask for 24 and you will be lucky to get it by midnight the night before

There is a trend for the more sophisticated dental practices to direct patients to their web sites and to eliminate the welcome packet "hard copy." I think that a web site can be a very nice vehicle by which a practice can share practice information with the new patients. However, when I talk to marketing gurus outside dentistry, the feedback I'm getting is that both choices should be made available to the consumer. The vast majority of successful web sites are the ones that support their "bricks and mortar" locations rather than replacing it. I still believe in the welcome packet being mailed out, so include information about your web site in it. If your web site has a "virtual tour" feature, direct your patients to use it.

Reception Room Signs

The ideal number of signs to post in your reception room is none at all! A reception room cluttered with signs gives your patients the impression that your practice is unable to effectively communicate with its patients, face to face. However, there are a few signs that we need to consider for legal, logistical, and efficiency reasons.

"Thank You for Not Smoking" replaces "No Smoking." The positive versus negative approach.

Mission Statement—Patients appreciate a nicely mounted and framed notice of your dental team's intention to provide excellent dental care and exemplary patient service.

Logistical signs—"Exit" above the reception room door is a legal requirement in many counties to keep the fire marshal happy. Other appropriate signs might be "Mind the Step," "Bathroom Around the Corner," etc.

Financial signs—There are two kinds of financial signs posted in dental receptions rooms—professional signs and a group of signs that are not only unprofessional, but send very confusing messages to patients.

Limit your professional financial signs to the following:

- Retail credit cards—MasterCard, Visa, American Express, Discover
- Dental credit card (Healthcare outside patient financing)
- Financial signs sending out "mixed messages" are to be eliminated.

A sign saying, *"Payment is expected the day that services are rendered, unless previous arrangements have been made,"* shows the patient two diametrically opposing policies. On one hand it states that patients are required to pay for services on the day they are rendered. But it immediately goes on to say that, if the patient makes alternate arrangements, that is not necessarily the case. Thus, this sign actually encourages patients to think that there is a whole set of financial options available that they were not made privy to before coming to the office.

No show charge policy sign—Displaying a sign stating your no show policy tells new patients that there are so many patients missing their appointments that the practice has had to put up a sign. What, thinks the new patient, have these other patients experienced that causes them to miss so many appointments that this sign is necessary? Take the sign down and cover how patients need to change an appointment in your signed financial agreement form.

Offering percentage discount for prepaying sign—The word "discount" is inappropriate in a dental practice. Dentists don't discount their quality of dentistry. This word has a low-quality connotation. Offering a "bookkeeping courtesy for prepayment" should also be covered in your signed financial agreement form.

$15 returned check charge sign—The law is quite strict on this subject. When a practice levies a charge for a bounced check, a sign advising consumers of this fact, and the amount involved, must be posted in the facility. The reception room however, is not the place. Place a small sign on the counter, at the area where your patients write their checks at the end of their visit. Again, this potential charge needs to be covered in your signed financial agreement form, as well as legally displaying the sign.

Insurance patients are asked to pay a 30% co-payment 'sign'— Remember, *it is harder to collect money from patients with insurance than patients without.* So, this sign is fraught with problems. It implies that patients' dental insurance coverage will pick up the balance of treatment cost. There is no such guarantee. It also hinders your education of patients being responsible for 100% of the bill, even when you take the assignment of benefits and their coverage is well below your usual, customary, and reasonable (UCR) schedule. Instead, you'll need a detailed paragraph in the signed financial agreement form detailing your dental insurance processing policies. If taking the assignment of benefits, define what procedures you need the patient to follow and fully outline his/her responsibilities.

Scheduling the consultation appointment

Many dentists, consultants, and speakers call this meeting a "case presentation." It is a phrase that I am personally very uncomfortable with using. "Case" infers that the patient is being seen as a "bunch of teeth, a case number." "Presentation" gives the impression that the patient is in the driver's seat to clinically make decisions, to accept or deny treatment that affects his/her oral health. There is an inference that the dentistry is elective, not necessarily needed.

"Consultation" is a meeting between doctor and patient to discuss (consult) together on the patient's dental needs and to make joint decisions about the current status of the patient's mouth and future needs and benefits of the proposed treatment.

Patients only question the fee when they question the quality of the service, as they perceive it

> *Until the patient has bought the problem, they cannot buy*
> *the solution.*   —Dr. Clyde Schultz of San Francisco

I have espoused this philosophy for years. As Dr. Schultz says in his wonderful seminar program, "Once the patient understands the benefits of having the dentistry, and says 'yes,' money becomes a non-issue."

Dr. Schultz accompanies the saying above with a second adage, "An educated patient can't say no." Making this into a positive statement becomes "an educated patient can only say yes."

Bottom line—when a patient informs doctor/staff that he/she is not accepting the doctor's treatment recommendations, the patient, in essence, is declaring that he/she doesn't understand the benefits of receiving the treatment and the potential problems of delaying/refusing treatment. At this point, any fee quoted will be considered too high.

Dentists, as left-brain, scientific-based, and trained professionals, tend to approach the consultation appointment as a place to give the patient a lesson in clinical dentistry. The patient, unfortunately, did not go to dental school. He/she does not understand dentistry. However, what is understood is bottom line, non-clinical explanations.

In the consumer marketplace, we're told that the public buys 95% on emotion and 5% on product knowledge. The discussion of fees and how they are to be paid can only be held after the patient has bought into the problem.

Creating an Effective Consultation Program

There are five key aspects to consider when designing a consultation program:

- *Which* patients receive a consultation?
- *When* is the consultation appointment scheduled?
- *Where* is the consultation held?
- Is the patient's *spouse* invited?
- Are *staff* involved in the meeting?

Which patients receive a consultation?

All patients, regardless of the how simple the treatment, should be given the opportunity to meet the doctor and be educated on the benefits of their needed dentistry. To me, it is part of the price of the examination. It is also a wonderful opportunity to expand and build on the doctor/patient relationship.

Information to be shared with each patient falls into four specific areas:

- Clinical—current findings and future needs
- Financial cost of proposed treatment
- Financial options available
- Key internal financial policies that could come into play during treatment:
  - ◊ returned check policy
  - ◊ finance charges on past due accounts
  - ◊ confirmation of appointment policy
  - ◊ changing an appointment requirements
  - ◊ handling minors in general and for emergencies specifically
  - ◊ a patient's responsibility when covered by dental insurance

When is the consultation appointment scheduled?

Ideally, it is part of the first appointment. Logically, this is the best time to educate the patient as to the clinical findings and proposed solutions. However, the vast majority of dentists feel much more comfortable scheduling the consultation appointment on a subsequent visit. A second visit has several advantages:

- The doctor has quality time to prepare a written treatment plan
- Staff prepares fees, totals, insurance involvement, financial options, etc.
- Spouse can be invited to join patient (the benefits of which are discussed below)

However, when the consultation is scheduled as a second appointment, it needs to be scheduled promptly after the examination appointment. The more time left between the exam and the consultation, the more time needed at the consultation to bring the patient up to speed regarding the findings/information discussed during the initial appointment.

Where is the consultation held?

Ideally, it is scheduled in a separate consultation room. However, if facility limitations make this impossible, the dentist's private office is a second option. While I do not like to see money discussed in the clinical area, there can be a really positive reason for doing so. Some dentists have been found to be far superior communicators when working in the clinical area, a place they feel most comfortable, and therefore most productive. Taken out of this environment to a separate consultation room, they "freeze up," losing that spark and passion about dentistry. If you fall into this category, turn your consultation room into a hygiene room and return your consultations to the treatment room.

Caution: Ensure that your patient feels he/she has privacy from being overheard by the patient in the next room.

Should the patient's spouse be invited?

The answer to this question is a resounding "yes." It is particularly important to include the patient's spouse when treatment is extensive. Extensive, by the way, is relative. To an elderly patient on a fixed income, $500 treatment can be "extensive." It is all relative to a patient's overall standard of living.

Marketing research shows that American couples make joint decisions on expensive purchases. Extensive dentistry falls into this category. When the partner is excluded, the consultation outcome is in doubt. The patient returns home and usually has a really hard time describing to their spouse/partner the dental problems currently being experienced and the benefits to be enjoyed by the proposed treatment. However, the patient seems to have absolutely no problem remembering the cost involved. Thus, the spouse hears the fee but not the benefits. The spouse, not having all the facts, or in some cases, the incorrect facts, often will "un-sell" the patient.

Solution: Extend an invitation to the spouse. "Mr. Patient, many of our patients have asked that we include their spouse in the consultation process. Would you like to schedule a time where both you and your wife can come in to talk to the doctor?" If the answer is "yes," you have just learned that this is a "joint decision" family. If the answer is "no," you learn that the patient makes his/her own decisions.

Note: At the consultation, if this same patient then says "I need to go home and talk to my wife about it" you have a patient who has just sent you mixed messages. (i.e., a smoke screen). What they really meant to say was "I've not bought into the problem" but hide behind "I need to talk to my wife."

Does a staff member join the doctor in the consultation?

The answer to this question is another resounding "yes."

Problem: Historically, most dentists do not involve the financial staff member in the consultation. The exclusion of the team member creates huge communication and financial problems. So often, a patient gives the dentist all the "buying" signs. Doctor is quite sure that the patient has accepted treatment, is ready to schedule appointments, and make financial arrangements. Doctor escorts the patient to the front desk area and moves on to the next patient. Instead of making an appointment as the staff was lead to believe; the patient now asks the staff a question for which they have no answer. "Why is Doctor extracting tooth number three?" Staff doesn't know. Doctor has moved on to the next patient. Patient leaves, confused. Staff tries to get the answer from Doctor later and then call patient. In most cases, you will find these patients put a hold on the treatment. They are not emotionally tied into the treatment and don't have enough information on which to make a decision.

Solution: Allow the business staff member to sit in during the consultation. This allows the employee to learn about the patient's specific needs and proposed treatment. It allows staff to hear the patient's questions to Doctor and the answers Doctor gives. What a wonderful way for the employee to learn more about dentistry in general, and the Doctor's clinical philosophy specifically, and a patient's proposed treatment details first-hand. The sequence would follow the following format:

- Doctor educates patients as to the clinical findings, explains the benefits of the proposed treatment and potential downside of delaying treatment
- Doctor handles any questions
- Doctor obtains patient acceptance of treatment plan
- Doctor excuses him/herself from room
- Staff answers any questions, often reducing the clinical explanation to a non-clinical explanation

- Scheduling times are discussed, appointment openings are identified
- Patient is offered the range of financial options
- Patient reads and signs detailed financial arrangement form, covering financial option chosen and overall financial policies and procedures
- Financial option chosen is entered into computer and patient records

Note: In some practices, the doctor chooses not to be involved in the consultation process at all. Doctor discusses the treatment plan fully with the staff members, who then handle the whole process with the patient themselves. Dentists choosing to take this approach tell me that they have a much higher patient acceptance rate than when they were directly involved. This approach is very much each doctor's call as to what works best for him/her.

Financial Options

The most effective way to get a financial commitment from the patient is to reduce the process to a very simple and fully disclosed method. (Fig. 7-1)

"Mrs. Patient, in our practice, we have three financial options available for our patients. Option #1 is...Option #2 is...Option #3 is...Which one best suits your needs?"

The options that I recommend in my seminars are as follows:

Prepay

"We are happy to offer a 5% bookkeeping courtesy to patients who bring in the full treatment amount to the practice five working days prior to the first scheduled appointment. Your saving on this treatment would be $X."

Financial In-Office Worksheet

Patient: Account #:

Estimated Total Treatment $________

Estimated Insurance Benefit $________

Estimated Patient Portion $________

Available Financial Options   Details

1. Prepayment $________ ________
2. Retail Credit Card $________ ________
3. Dental Financing $________ ________

Patient Acceptance

Patient Signature: ________________ Date: ________

Staff Signature: ________________ Date: ________

P.O. Box 35640, Monte Sereno, California 95030 USA • 800-366-7004 • Fax 408-354-1931 • Email:info@jdsg.com

Fig. 7-1 Financial in-office worksheet

If you do not build in a time buffer between when the payment is due and the first treatment appointment, you may well experience the following scenario. At the end of the visit, the patient comes to the front desk and informs the business staff that he/she forgot to bring a checkbook. When payment is finally received (after several telephone calls), it is usually for the "adjusted" amount, because that was the amount noted by the patient. The ability to offer the prepayment courtesy is based on the fact that staff doesn't have to make collection calls and worry about payment. Building in a five-day buffer takes care of this problem.

Note for insurance patients: Be sure to state on the insurance claim form as to the adjustment % and amount. Full disclosure prevents you being guilty of insurance fraud and usually still delivers the full-expected dollar amount.

Benefits of prepayment:

- Schedule long appointments, rather than shorter ones—better for patient and dentist
- Reduce no shows and cancel short notice—It is amazing how patients remember their appointments when their money is already in your bank account

Retail credit card—Master Card, Visa, American Express, Discover

Visa research shows that nearly 80% of the American public is happy to pay their dental bills by credit card, when the service is made available to them.

Benefits of using credit cards:

- Instant guaranteed cash flow
- No collection problems

Negatives:

- The "discount" charged back to the dentist by the bank is seen by some dentists as being a negative. Actually, bankcard discounts should not be seen as a negative. It is the cost of doing business and should be included in the overhead

- According to Bank One of Ohio, the average American consumer has $450 of available credit on his/her Master Card or Visa at any one time. Thus, even one crown can't be charged on a credit card for the majority of times. So, why have a retail credit card? It is used for payment of the minor treatment, such as initial exam, emergencies, and minor treatment

Dental financing

The latest 2000 statistics show that the average American owes more than $7,000 to $8,000 on his/her credit cards. Remember he/she only has $450 available credit at any one time. To help patients finance their dentistry, it is essential that a practice have outside dental financing provided by a well-run, reputable finance company offering non-recourse financing, great training, and follow-up service. Americans purchasing large ticket items break down the total cost into a manageable monthly commitment in order to see if the amount will fit into their budget. Analyze how the auto industry sells cars. The ads focus on "so much a month for so many months" rather than the total cost of the car.

Financing allows patients to make small monthly payments, over several months, choosing an amount that fits into their monthly budget. The practice receives the money in their bank account 24-48 hours after treatment has been provided. The loan goes bad? The dentist keeps the payments and the finance company does the collecting and absorbs any bad loans.

Benefits:

- Instant guaranteed cash flow
- Increased patient acceptance
- Ability to schedule long appointments
- No collection problems
- Reduced no shows and cancel short notice

Negatives:

- The "discount" charged the dentist by the finance company? See earlier discussion

- Patients can be refused credit. Absolutely true. However, let me make this into a positive rather than a negative. You have just received a free credit check

Forewarned is forearmed. I see this, in fact, as a positive

Custom plan. Most practices have an under-the-counter plan that they offer good patients of record on a case-by-case basis.

Financial options having some potential problems for doctor

A majority of practices still offer patients four financial options, which I think are fraught with potential problems.

Pay as you go

Benefits:

- Doctor does not do any dentistry for which he/she does not get paid

Negatives:

- Increases no shows, cancel short notice. When patients run out of money, on a good day they call and cancel, on a bad day they are so embarrassed, they are a no show

- Limits length of appointment (more small appointments rather than fewer longer appointments will be scheduled)

- Treatment takes longer (shorter versus longer appointments)

- Practice incurs more room set up costs due to more shorter appointments

Half down at prep appointment, balance at cement/delivery appointment

Benefits:

- You get majority of your overhead cost as a down payment. True, but…

Negatives:

- If patient turns up for cement/delivery appointment without the balance, legally you must deliver the crown/bridge/partial/denture. By withholding delivery, a dentist is legally guilty of abandonment, and you now have a potential collection problem.

Half down and three equal payments method

Benefits:

- Practice gets majority of overhead cost as a down payment. True, but…

Negatives:

- Bank One of Ohio says that 93% of American consumers renege on their commitment to creditors for paying off a loan within the 90-day limit. Ninety-three percent! That means only 7% of people keep their word. Does this statistic mean that 93% of consumers lied when they made their 90-day commitment? No! I believe the majority genuinely planned on keeping their promises. However, within the 90 days, they experienced a financial emergency, i.e., a car stopped operating, etc. By the way, the true name for this option is "90-day interest-free financing by Doctor!"

Mail statements and pray method

Benefits:

- Unless the practice is in an established area, where there's a history of families belonging to the practice for years/generations, who have been shown to send in their payments in full upon immediate receipt of a statement, I'm hard pressed to think of any benefits for using this method

Negatives:

- You have no control over whether the patient will send you the money due or go out and buy a new car

Telephone Shoppers

Most practices do not look favorably on these potential patients, feeling that they are looking for the cheapest "prices" in town. While a small percentage of patients do indeed fall into this category, I believe that the majority of these patients have the potential of becoming good regular patients. Usually what is needed are a few minutes of quality staff time on the phone to offer the caller a professional service.

Three golden rules for handling telephone shoppers:

- Don't quote fees over the telephone
- Don't tell the patient that you don't quote fees over the telephone
- Show your helpful attitude by immediately asking an open-ended question

Patient: "How much does Doctor charge for a crown?"
Staff: "It will be our pleasure to help you, Mrs. Patient. May I ask what kind of crown you have in mind...a porcelain to metal crown, full gold crown, etc.?"

The classic patient answer is "I don't know." The power is now back with the practice and the team member.

Staff: "Well, Mrs. Patient, that creates a problem because we can't tell, without seeing the tooth, whether a crown is needed, and if so, what kind of crown is needed for your particular situation. But...I have a solution to this problem."

There are five options available—always start with the ideal

Ideal—An initial new patient exam and range of necessary x-rays. However, do not be disappointed if the patient refuses. In fact, rarely do telephone shoppers accept this offer. But, it is part of patient education to offer the patient first what is the best for the patient.

Compromise—A brief, no-charge observation visit. I find that a well-trained staff is able to motivate about 80% of callers to accept this appointment option. If the patient refuses the offer of this appointment...go immediately into Option Three:

Educate and refer out—"May we suggest that you call your friends, neighbors, relatives, and co-workers and see which dentist they use? You may feel very comfortable going to one of those dentists." We're now educating the patient as to how the referral system works. For staff proud of the doctor they work for, the next comment just flows "In fact, Mrs. Patient, you may find the majority of your friends and neighbors come here."

The final two options, in my opinion, create more problems than they solve. However, offices routinely use them so we need to address the potential hazards of using them:

"We don't quote over the telephone."—Patients now perceive that your fees are so high that staff is uncomfortable discussing them. In fact, this approach reinforces, for the telephone shopper, the importance of making these shopping calls. This patient is saying to him/herself. "Look, this practice's fees are so high, they don't feel comfortable telling me what they are. Wow, a good thing I called and asked first. I think I just saved myself going to a very expensive dentist."

"The fee for a crown is $X."—The problem here is that instead of raising the patient's dental IQ to appreciate that price should not be the main factor used to find a quality dentist, the practice has now lowered itself to the patient's level and confirmed that this is indeed the criterion the practice endorses for a patient to choose a dentist.

Other telephone shoppers questions are handled with the same philosophy:

> **Question:** "How much does Doctor charge for a filling?"
>
> **Answer:** "What kind of filling did you have in mind? One surface, two surface, brands, etc.?"
>
> **Question:** "How much does Doctor charge to pull a tooth?"
>
> **Answer:** "What kind of extraction did you have in mind? Surgical extraction, impaction, etc.?"

Exception to not quoting fees over the phone

There are three clinical procedures for which the fee can and should be easily quotable to any patient calling your practice. A simple phrase begins each quote. "Our standard fee on file for a...

- New patient examination is $X"
- A series of necessary x-rays can range from $X to $Y to any figure in between, depending on each patient's specific needs"
- Maintenance cleaning, which is a cleaning for patients who receive regular cleanings, on an ongoing basis, through our Continuing Care program, is $X. For a new patient, once

Doctor has examined the patient and determined his/her specific cleaning/perio needs, we'll be happy to quote the fee in advance of any required treatment"

Second Opinion

Problem: When the patient actually has the answer to your question.

Staff: "What kind of crown did you have in mind?"
Patient: "A porcelain to metal crown on tooth number four with a dowel pin."
Staff: "Ah, it sounds as if you are looking for a second opinion. Let me share with you how we handle second opinion requests in this practice."

Each dentist needs to decide how he/she wishes to handle second opinions in his/her practice. I found that second opinion patients usually become excellent patients. They've already visited another dentist and been educated about the dentistry that they need. They've been told the benefits of receiving the treatment and the cost involved. In my personal opinion, the majority of these patients are not shopping for price. They're calling around because of a lack of confidence and trust with the first doctor and/or practice that they visited.

You have two choices:

- An initial new patient exam (requesting prior x-rays before the visit) or

- An observation visit (no x-rays are on hand or taken), it is literally a get-acquainted 10-minute meeting

Remember why the patient is calling around. Money is usually not the issue. A lack of confidence and trust is the issue. Having x-rays in hand is not needed for the patient to have a brief visit with doctor, feel the confidence and trust they were looking for, and be happy to return for another visit for a full exam, x-rays, etc.

Emergencies and Money

Emergency patients fall into two categories:

- Being new to the practice or
- Having established a credit history with you

Staff should make a statement of financial policy to all new emergency patients along the same lines as for new patient exams. "We ask all new patients joining the practice to take care of the charges in full on the initial visit" (regarding of any insurance involvement).

However, in the case of emergencies, this statement many times elicits the question, "How much is that going to be?" We have discussed the negatives of quoting fees over the phone. In the case of emergencies, you genuinely are unable to quote a fee until Doctor ascertains what treatment is specifically needed.

You can, however, promise this patient that he/she will receive no treatment without being fully informed of both the clinical diagnosis and financial costs involved *before* any treatment is undertaken.

"I can't pay today"

When a new patient states his/her inability to pay for any emergency treatment today, my recommendation is to thank them for their honesty and offer some practical solutions.

Staff: "Mrs. Patient, we appreciate you being so upfront about your inability to take care of any charges today, should treatment be required. Thank you, you did not have to tell me. Your honesty is very much appreciated. Let me offer some solutions."

- Offer the ability to use a post-dated check
- Offer a retail credit card, Master Card, Visa, American Express

My experience tells me that there is a very good chance the patient may have neither a checking account nor a credit card. We, therefore, go to option three:

- Offer to let the patient return later that week, no later than Friday, with the money

The majority of patients will return on Friday, with the money, and be grateful for your kindness. Potentially, these patients will not only book an exam and become patients of records, but also will expand your referral base with words about your kindness and understanding in their time of need. It is a tiny, tiny minority of patients who'll abuse your kind nature by not returning by Friday to pay you. Sleep well and let it go. You made a gift to humanity.

Note for new practices: When starting a new practice from scratch, realize that you could lose more money in the first three to four months of practice than you'll probably lose in all the following years. If word gets out in town that you have non-existent or extremely lax credit policies, the practice has the potential of attracting a host of emergency patients who heard on the grapevine of the practice's lack of financial communication.

Minors and Money

In most states, a minor becomes an adult and liable for his/her own bills when he/she reaches the age of 18. There are exceptions. For instance, in California, a 15-year-old or older teenage, living permanently away from home and totally financially independent, is considered an adult.

Minors can only be treated after the dentist has received signed medical, dental history, and informed consent release forms from a parent/guardian. For a minor requiring emergency treatment, not accompanied by an adult, staff needs to telephone a parent or legal guardian to get verbal permission to render treatment and confirm financial responsibility. An even better plan would be to design a standard form to fax to the parent/guardian for authorization. This system ensures your records reflect written permission to treat the minor. A dentist potentially could be sued for battery if rendering treatment to a minor without parent/guardian permission.

No Show Charge

Historically, most practices don't have a formal policy for no shows (also called missed appointments (MA), failed appointments (FA) or did not arrive (DNA). When good patients miss an appointment, they usually get re-appointed without being charged a no show fee or having the whole issue of missing the appointment addressed. However, when the patient missing the appointment is not particularly a practice favorite, we find that the patient's account is often charged, after the fact and with no notice, for a no show charge.

The result is usually an upset patient on the phone. To pacify the patient, the charge is then removed. The patient, however, usually remains upset, often going elsewhere. While that might have been the goal of the practice, the result creates several negatives for the practice:

- You have created a poor practice image for this patient
- You can't control what the patient says in town (bad news travels 15 times faster than good news)
- You have two policies for two kinds of patients, which creates stress and havoc at the administrative staff

The positive way to handle this situation is to be proactive rather than reactive—Inform before you perform, no surprises.

- Advise all new patients during the financial consultation what you require of them, should they have a need to change an appointment. "As long as we receive at least 48 hours notice of your need to change an appointment, there will be absolutely no charge. Should something prevent you from calling us, there will be a charge of $X for each half hour missed. However, we are sure that this will not be an issue"

An effective no show policy could include:

- $50 for each half hour missed
- Three consecutive no shows and patient is asked to seek dental care elsewhere
- The first no show is always waived

What is the goal of your no show charge? It is not to create a profit center or an income source. It is to encourage patients to take responsibility for their appointments. We want patients to either keep their appointment or to telephone well in advance to change the appointment. We don't want their money!

Charging Interest

When talking to patients or billing out this charge on your statements, be sure to refer to these charges not as interest, but as finance charges. This will keep you from running afoul of strict federal credit laws. Computers make finance charges a very easy procedure. (Noncomputerized practices should not charge this fee. The labor of processing the charges would exceed the income generated.) The majority of dental practices today charge their patients 1½% per month, 18% per annum on their overdue accounts. This charge is incurred after the accounts are 60 days past due. Do not charge Delta or any other provider for which you have signed a waiver stating that patients will not be charged finance charges.

A word of warning. Wholesale financing of your patient's dental care in-house is fraught with problems. I recommend referring all financing out where possible to a good dental financing company such as

CareCredit as discussed earlier in this chapter. Your in-house finance charge on monthly statements needs to be at the maximum percentage allowed in your state. The quickest way to stop patients from signing up for outside financing (which guarantees money directly into your bank account) is to offer patients interest-free in-house financing!

Summary

For a dentist to be financially successful in today's market place, doctor and team must design, implement, and maintain a very high level of quality financial communication with their patients. Such a level of communication is wasted if not supported and backed up by strong financial internal management systems. Management systems, once in place, however, cannot be ignored. Daily, weekly, and monthly monitoring is essential for the financial health of the practice.

One out of four dental practices is, has, or will be embezzled. Only the veterinary profession experiences more embezzlement and fraud than dentistry (one out of two vet practices). For the majority of dentists, the joy of their day is spent with patients providing quality care. The business side of the practice is not what attracted them to dentistry. However, to be able to provide quality care to patients, a practice must be solvent. All I ask is that someone, whether it be you, your spouse, or an outside supervisor be designated to help you, the dentist, protect your financial assets in the practice so that you may continue to enjoy what you brought you into dentistry to begin with—working with your patients to provide them with quality dental care.

From a patient's perspective, 85% of dentistry is elective and is paid for from discretionary income. The competition for this discretionary income is the Caribbean cruise, the new TV, a Hawaiian vacation. None of these perks give the patient the lasting value of a well-made crown or replacing missing teeth with an outstanding bridge. An educated patient says "yes" to the needed treatment and accompanying financial responsibility. Patients are buying confidence and trust. When a patient believes in a dentist and the service he/she provides, more often than not, the financial cost of treatment becomes a non-issue. We buy emotionally, then justify our decision with logic, reason, and fact. That is the market place today. Hopefully, this chapter will help you both increase your treatment acceptance rate and increase and protect your cash protect.

To Do Check List

- Educate patients, from their initial contact to the practice, as to what your expectations are of their need to fulfill their financial responsibilities
- Include staff in your consultation process
- Offer a range of financial options to the patient
- Ensure that your signed financial agreement form covers the fees, total cost of treatment, financial option chosen, and your internal financial polices on a wide range of issues as outlined in this chapter
- Monitor the financial aspect of the practice on a consistent, ongoing basis

Chapter 8

Informed Consent: An Overview

By Debra S. Reiser, Esq.

Introduction

The intention of this chapter is to aid the dental practitioner in common sense and cost-effective methods of avoiding a malpractice lawsuit based upon a cause of action in lack of informed consent. I will provide suggestions for successfully setting up your office procedures in a more risk-conscious fashion, so that such a claim can be effectively defended should the unfortunate situation arise. I hope to accomplish these goals by presenting actual cases that illustrate the requirements of patient notification in dental treatment, which the general dentist or specialist may confront on a daily basis, and practical, inexpensive tips to aid in obtaining a definitive informed consent. While a dentist friend of mine quipped that reading such materials usually provokes the desire to immediately seek a career change, a more pragmatic approach may be preferable.

Historical Background of Informed Consent

Elements of the cause of action

The doctrine of informed consent is grounded in the traditional common law intentional torts of assault and battery. The 1914 decision in *Schloendorff v. Society of New York Hospital*,[1] is viewed by many legal scholars as the first case addressing the issue of a physician's requirement to obtain an informed consent.[2] In the view of Justice Cardozo, "[e]very human being of adult years and sound mind has a right to determine what shall be done with his own body;" consequently, "[a] surgeon who performs an operation without his patient's consent, commits an assault, for which he is liable in damages."[3]

In 1957, informed consent was revisited in the case of *Salgo v. Leland Stanford University Board of Trustees*, where that court established the legal duty of the treating provider to disclose all the facts necessary for the patient to provide an informed consent.[4] The duty to disclose was eventually phrased with the judgment of the provider in mind; *i.e.*, the decision regarding what information should be disclosed was primarily a medically-based conclusion.[5] This concept essentially limited the duty of disclosure to that which a reasonable health care provider would make under similar circumstances. The failure to do so was viewed the same as any other act of professional malpractice.[6]

The *Canterbury v. Spence* decision dramatically altered the yardstick by which the physician or dentist must be measured. The D.C. circuit opined in 1972 that a standard should be set by law for physicians rather than set by the physicians themselves, and concluded that the touchstone should be conduct that is reasonable under the circumstances.[7]

The *Canterbury* court also modified the scope of disclosure to a more patient-oriented approach, focusing on the informational needs of the average reasonable patient. Simultaneously, the court acknowledged that many situations provided exceptions to the disclosure requirement, including the well-known inherent risks in almost any procedure; to wit, infection, emergencies, and risks already known to the patient.[8] A therapeutic privilege was separately recognized to allow for limited disclosure with severely ill or emotionally distraught individuals.

To summarize, the failure to properly obtain the consent of an individual prior to treatment by fully disclosing the risks and alternatives of the procedures to be undertaken is now viewed as "a form of medical malpractice based upon negligence."[9] Along those lines, the *Canterbury* decision concluded that in addition to negligence or breach of duty, a causal connection had to exist between the failure to disclose and a cognizable injury to the patient. Again, an objective standard was utilized, the question being what a reasonably prudent person in the patient's position would have decided if properly informed of all the risks.[10]

The more modern view is favorable to the health care provider, since the patient's burden to prove negligence or medical malpractice under the law is much more difficult than proving a simple battery, which is merely an unlawful touching without the patient's consent. On the other hand, proof of malpractice in most states requires that the dentist departed from the standards of care of another dentist practicing in his or her community and, further, that the departure was a substantial factor in causing injury to the patient.

Codification of informed consent cause of action

Many states have seen fit to specifically codify the elements necessary to maintain an informed consent action by statute. In 1972, apparently based on the *Canterbury* decision, the New York State Legislature codified and limited a plaintiff's action based upon informed consent. Indeed, the defenses delineated in section 4 below mirror those set out by the court in *Canterbury*.[11]

Three years later, Section 2805-d, entitled "Limitation of medical, dental or podiatric malpractice action based on lack of informed consent" was enacted. The statute reads as follows:

1. Lack of informed consent means the failure of the person providing the professional treatment or diagnosis to disclose to the patient such alternatives thereto and the reasonably foreseeable risks and benefits involved as a reasonable med-

ical, dental or podiatric practitioner under similar circumstances would have disclosed, in a manner permitting the patient to make a knowledgeable evaluation

2. The right of action to recover for medical, dental or podiatric malpractice based on a lack of informed consent is limited to those cases involving either (a) non-emergency treatment, procedure or surgery, or (b) a diagnostic procedure which involved invasion or disruption of the integrity of the body

3. For a cause of action therefore it must also be established that a reasonably prudent person in the patient's position would not have undergone the treatment or diagnosis if he had been fully informed and that the lack of informed consent is a proximate cause of the injury or condition for which recovery is sought

The statute denotes the specific defenses that may be raised by the treating practitioner:

4. It shall be a defense to any action for medical, dental or podiatric malpractice based upon an alleged failure to obtain such an informed consent that—

   a) the risk not disclosed is too commonly known to warrant disclosure; or

   b) the patient assured the medical, dental or podiatric practitioner he would undergo the treatment, procedure or diagnosis regardless of the risk involved, or the patient assured the medical, dental or podiatric practitioner that he did not want to be informed of the matters to which he would be entitled to be informed; or

   c) consent by or on behalf of the patient was not reasonably possible; or

   d) the medical, dental or podiatric practitioner, after considering all of the attendant facts and circumstances, used reasonable discretion as to the manner and extent to which such alternatives and risks were disclosed to the patient because he reasonably believed that the manner and extent of such disclosure could reasonably be expected to adversely and substantially affect the patient's condition[12]

The legislature outlined the elements of an informed consent that must be satisfied in order to demonstrate an unassailable consent. The statutory language does not require full disclosure of all possible risks and alternatives; neither does it permit the individual treating dentist to determine the extent of disclosure. Rather, the scope of disclosure is governed by what a reasonable practitioner would have disclosed to a patient under similar circumstances.

Whether viewed as a malpractice action based on negligence or as a malpractice action based on common-law principles of assault and battery, it is nonetheless an action in tort requiring proof of causation between the medical provider's conduct and the resulting injury to the patient.[13]

To be sure, the battery cause of action is still viable in certain circumstances and may inure to the defendant's benefit even though the elements of proof are less formidable. In *Messina v. Matarasso*, the court held that because plaintiff's action sounded in battery, the applicable Statute of Limitations was only one year as opposed to the two and one-half year Statute of Limitations for claims involving medical malpractice.[14] The plaintiff's claims (admittedly brought after the year expired), were dismissed as untimely, where the defendant allegedly performed unanticipated cosmetic surgery upon the plaintiff's breasts without her consent, during consented-to cosmetic facial surgery. The *Messina* court observed:

"Plaintiff does not claim that defendant Matarasso failed to inform her of the risks of the procedure or that he rendered medical treatment beyond the scope of her consent [...] Her claim, rather, is that he performed a procedure on her with no consent at all. This is clearly an allegation of intentional conduct rather than conduct that can be construed as a deviation from the reasonable care standard"[15]

Necessity of pleading separate cause of action

The cause of action for lack of informed consent is differentiated from the cause of action in malpractice, because it must be separately pleaded.[16] If not initially pleaded, the courts are generally liberal in allowing plaintiff to amend the pleadings to add informed consent as a separate cause of action. However, in the dental malpractice case of *Evans v. Kringstein*, the court rejected plaintiff's last minute effort on the eve of trial to amend the pleadings and add the claim.[17] It was likely in this case that plaintiff's expert witness brought the issue up with plaintiff's attorney during trial preparation. Naturally, the patient's attorney was hoping to cure the defect and give the client an added basis for recovery, which the court did not allow.

Requirement of expert testimony

The seminal decision of *Canterbury v. Spence,* initially followed in many states, adhered to the common law rule that no expert testimony was mandated to prove the informed consent cause of action.[18] The theory was that since the patient was making the decision for treatment, a general standard of conduct reasonable under the circumstances should be the gauge by which to measure the provider's conduct, without the necessity to specifically designate professional standards of care.[19]

Prior to 1975, New York courts followed the *Canterbury* decision in permitting an informed consent action to go to the jury without the benefit of expert testimony.[20] This standard is still utilized in some states where, for example, the requirement of an expert affidavit is specifically excluded from informed consent cases.[21]

Most jurisdictions now require expert testimony to establish "the qualitative insufficiency of his [the patient's] consent."[22] This requirement, enacted in 1975 in conjunction with the Medical Malpractice Act, is found in New York CPLR Section 4401-a Motion for Judgment:

A motion for judgment at the end of the plaintiff's case must be granted as to any cause of action for medical malpractice based solely on lack of informed consent if the plaintiff has failed to adduce expert medical testimony in support of the alleged qualitative insufficiency of the consent.[23]

By statutory mandate, the proof regarding the nature and extent of the disclosure required must be presented through expert testimony. The failure of the plaintiff-patient to introduce such testimony requires dismissal of the cause of action at the conclusion of the plaintiff's case.[24] In a dental malpractice case, the expert must specifically address the adequacy of the information provided to the patient by the defendant dentist and must opine that, to a reasonable degree of certainty, the risks and alternatives provided by that dentist were not on par with a fellow dentist practicing in the community.[25]

Some courts in my jurisdiction have now expanded the requirement of Section 4401-a to not only include the insufficiency of the consent, but also the question of whether a "reasonably prudent person" in the patient's position would have undergone the treatment if adequately informed.[26] Other courts have disagreed and maintained that the plaintiff's testimony that he or she would not have submitted to the treatment satisfies the "reasonably prudent person" standard.[27] The latter approach seems more reasonable, while the former places the dental expert in the patient's position, which seems a bit unwieldy.

Jury instructions

In a jury trial where the issue of informed consent is being litigated, the jury considering such an issue in the state of New York is given the following instruction:

PJI 2:150A Malpractice-Informed Consent:
Before obtaining the patient's consent to an operation or invasive diagnostic procedure or the use of medication, a dentist has the duty to provide certain information as to the proposed

treatment alternatives to the operation, procedure, or medication, and the reasonably foreseeable risks of such operation, procedure, or medication. It is the dentist's duty to explain, in words that are understandable to the patient, all the facts that would be explained by a reasonable medical practitioner so that when the patient does, in fact, consent, the consent is given with an awareness of (1) the patient's existing physical condition; (2) the purposes and advantages of the operation, procedure or medication; (3) the reasonably foreseeable risks to the patient's health or life which the operation, procedure or medication may impose; (4) the risks involved to the patient if there is no operation, procedure or use of medication; and (5) the available alternatives and the risks and advantages of those alternatives. The first question on this issue that you will be called upon to answer is whether the defendant, before obtaining plaintiff's consent, provided appropriate information.

The question reads as follows:

(3) Did the defendant before obtaining plaintiff's consent to the (operation, procedure, medication) provide appropriate information?

Plaintiff maintains that the answer to this question is "No", contending that [set forth the specific risks and alternatives that plaintiff claims were not disclosed]. Defendant maintains that the answer is "Yes" and contends that (the information was in fact provided, or a reasonable medical practitioner would not provide such information to the patient in a case such as this)

If you answer "No" to the question, the next question you must decide is whether a reasonably prudent person in the plaintiff's position would have decided not to undergo the operation or procedure or take the medication if given appropriate information concerning the risks and alternatives.

The question reads as follows:

(2) Would a reasonably prudent person in plaintiff's position at the time consent was given have given such consent if given appropriate information?

Plaintiff maintains that the answer to this question is "No", contending that considering the nature of plaintiff's condition at the time and the risks involved in the (operation, procedure, use of medication) and the available alternatives, a reasonably prudent person would not have consented to the (operation, procedure, use of medication). Defendant maintains that the answer to this question is "Yes", contending that considering plaintiff's condition and the need for the (operation, procedure, use of medication) the omitted information would not have caused a reasonably prudent person to refuse to consent to the (operation, procedure, use of medication)

In answering this question, it is important that you consider only plaintiff's condition at the time consent was given and the facts and circumstances that existed at that time and not events that occurred or knowledge that was obtained at a later time.

If you answer "No" to question two, the next and last question to be resolved on this issue is whether the (operation, procedure, medication) was a substantial factor in causing injury to plaintiff.

The question reads as follows:

(3) Was the (operation, procedure, medication) a substantial factor in causing injury to the plaintiff?[28]

As is evident from the jury interrogatories, the courts are specifically addressing the plaintiff's tendency to be a "Monday-morning quarterback" where a bad result is obtained, not necessarily due to malpractice. It is notable that the patient need not prove negligence in the performance of the dental procedure to recover for malpractice pursuant to a lack of informed consent cause of action.[29]

In the recent case of *Foote v. Rajadhyax*, the plaintiff suffered an injured mandibular nerve resulting in permanent paresthesia; the court was found to be in error for failing to have the jury consider the informed consent issue after determining that the defendant did not commit malpractice in the performance of the root canal procedure that resulted in the injury. Despite the finding, the jury should have been allowed to consider whether the patient should have been advised that permanent paresthesia could result from the root canal, whether the patient should have been informed that she could have been referred to an endodontist, and whether the patient was informed regarding alternative treatments.[30]

Case Law on Informed Consent Issues in Dental Malpractice Actions

No cause of action for failure to treat

In *Iazetta v. Vicenzi*,[31] the court ruled that plaintiff *cannot* establish a cause of action based upon the defendant dentist's total failure to treat her periodontal disease, since there was no affirmative violation of her physical integrity; to wit, no treatment. However, plaintiff's allegations that unnecessarily extracted teeth resulted in permanent injuries to her teeth, gums, and mouth, could form the basis for a cause of action in lack of informed consent if the proof satisfied the requirements of Public Health Law 2805(d)(3).

Specifically, plaintiff alleged that during the course of her treatment with defendants, which extended over a 22-year period beginning in October 1966, defendants failed to perform various dental procedures that caused permanent injuries to plaintiff, including "abscesses, breakdown of endodontic structures, and periodontal disease." The evidence established that plaintiff visited defendants about 180 times. The treatment by defendants included cleanings, fillings, crowns, bridges, root canals, and extraction of a number of teeth. The court found for plain-tiff on the claim of unnecessary tooth extractions, concluding that plaintiff met the requirements set forth in Public Health Law §2805-d(3).[32] Accordingly, in order to state a cause of action for lack of informed consent, plaintiff must allege that the wrong complained of arose out of some affirmative violation of plaintiff's physical being, not a lack of treatment.[33]

The same result was obtained in *Smith v. Fields*, where the patient unsuccessfully argued that the defendant's failure to inform her of "the risks and consequences of prescribed treatment, and of the destructive nature of the progressive periodontal disease and the availability of spe-cialists" over a course of 32 years of treatment met the requirements of an action grounded in informed consent.[34] In reaffirming the *Iazetta* decision, the *Smith* court determined that "[s]ince the plaintiff's lack of informed consent claim essentially seeks to recover damages for defen-dant's failure to inform her of the risks of allowing periodontal disease to go untreated, it fails to state a viable cause of action for recovery."[35]

Custom and practice

Experience dictates that lingual or alveolar inferior nerve damage causing permanent paresthesia, usually the result of a tooth extraction, is the dental injury most likely to be the subject of a cause of action in informed consent. By its very nature, it is also one of the most serious dental injuries, often resulting in substantial monetary awards.

Since it is highly unlikely that a dentist will remember exactly what was told to an individual patient prior to an extraction performed years before any litigation, it is wise to follow the same procedure each and every time without exception, which should involve a hygienist or assis-tant, who may then act as a witness. This form of evidence is quite con-vincing to a jury if definitive.

The sagacity of this type of risk management is best illustrated in the case of *Rigie v. Goldman*, where the defendant dentist's typical practice was admissible as circumstantial evidence that he acted in accordance with that practice on the date in question.[36] The court properly allowed evidence of the defendant oral surgeon's habitual custom and practice of advising patients of the risks attendant with the removal of an impacted wisdom tooth. This testimony was admissible as circumstantial evidence that the surgeon acted in conformity with his routine practice with respect to the treatment being considered by the jury in the plaintiff's case. While the dentist admittedly had no independent recollection of what he had specifically told the plaintiff, the court permitted the dentist to recount "his routine practice developed over 19 years of practice in the specialized area of oral and maxillofacial surgery and followed *in every instance* of the thousands of extractions of wisdom teeth he had performed in his career." Testimony from the dentist's assistant was also permitted regarding the dentist's consistent practice that included a warning that temporary or permanent paresthesia of the lip, chin, or tongue could result. The court reasoned that the testimony fit squarely within the evidentiary rule permitting circumstantial evidence of habit.[37]

Consent—written vs. oral

In *Cooper v. U.S.*,[38] the patient, a retired Air Force sergeant, brought a dental malpractice action in South Carolina, after a wisdom tooth extraction resulted in permanent damage to the inferior alveolar nerve. The plaintiff alleged that the defendant general dentist did not obtain an informed consent, or alternatively, if he did so, it was not in writing. The court, applying South Carolina law, found that the state did not require that the consent be in any particular written form; instead "the [informed consent] doctrine focuses on the content of the information conveyed to the patient and not on the form in which it is provided."[39]

A lower court justice in New York affirmed a jury verdict in favor of a defendant dentist, where a patient suffered a permanent lingual nerve paresthesia after an extraction by a general dentist and the defendant specifically acknowledged that he failed to present the plaintiff with a consent form to either read or sign.[40] The court emphasized that the practitioner testified credibly that he discussed the risk of nerve damage with the patient, as well as an alternative to the procedure, even though he did not specifically address the issue of lingual nerve damage.[41]

Significantly, experts for both parties suing and defendant in the case testified that the risk to the lingual nerve during this procedure was exceptionally rare.

This section should in no way suggest to the reader that a consent form is optional. Once there is an absence of an executed consent form, it is fair to say that the defendant's attorney's task to show informed consent is much more difficult and is reduced to a strict credibility contest between the dentist and the patient. In the *Bota* case, the court commented in detail on this issue:

> "Dr. Kaminsky was an extremely likeable man. He came across as a modest, caring professional. He communicated sincere regret as to what had happened to his patient as a result of the procedure, to Ms. Bota whom he genuinely liked. However, he believed he was not negligent and that he communicated what was necessary before the procedure.The jury obviously believed him and agreed with his assessment. This, despite Ms. Bota's testimony that no risks were told to her and the defendant's failure to note the warnings in his chart."[42]

While kudos are certainly in order for the dentist's trial attorney for the painstaking preparation of the client, this case tells us what the dental practitioner should studiously avoid doing as a risk management tool. Indeed, in addition to an executed form, the dentist should also separately note on his/her chart what warnings and alternative treatments were discussed with the patient. While convincing demeanor on the witness stand doesn't hurt, a paper trail that defeats plaintiff's claims that no information was given is documentary evidence that the jury can examine and review.

On the other hand, the fact that a consent form is signed is not dispositive on the issue. It is the form in conjunction with what is told to the patient, (optimally with a witness present), what appears in the dental chart and, most significantly, what the patient testifies to regarding the information communicated and understood. The mere fact that a patient claims that he/she was not advised of the risks and alternatives, even with a signed form, is enough to create an issue of fact for the jury; a motion to dismiss by the defendant in that scenario will thereby be denied.[43]

Individual patient factors

The dentist should always bear in mind the patient's familiarity with the English language, age, dental experience, and educational level, all of which may come into play in assessing the merits of the claim of informed consent. With a patient who is not fluent in English, the most prudent course of action is to request that the patient is accompanied by a friend or relative who will translate the written materials in front of a member of the support staff in the dental office. The fact that the translation was done should be noted on the dental chart. If many of the patients in one's practice are more comfortable in a language such as Russian or Spanish, the office must employ staff fluent in the language and provide translated consent forms. If this suggestion seems like overkill, the unattractive alternative may well be a number of viable claims against your office for lack of informed consent.

Factors such as age, background, and lack of dental experience are also germane to the informed consent analysis. I recently reviewed and accepted a case in which my client, high-school educated and 28 years of age, went to a dentist who recommended and performed a tooth extraction on the lower left third molar, resulting in permanent damage to the inferior alveolar nerve with accompanying paresthesia. The client had very little dental experience beyond a few fillings and had never had a tooth extraction. Not only was there no consent form executed and no notation on the dental chart of any warnings given, the client explained that she had neither been told why the extraction was necessary (the tooth had not been bothering her), nor what the risks entailed.

Timing of the execution of the consent

Another issue relating to informed consent not specifically addressed in the case studies, but nonetheless extremely important, is the timing of the execution of the form and the concomitant discussion of risks and alternatives with the patient. Harkening back again to Justice Cardozo's evocative opinion in the *Schloendorff* case, the court opined that "[t]here may be cases where a patient ought not to be advised of a contemplated operation until shortly before the appointed hour. To discuss such a subject ... might cause needless or even harmful agitation."[44] As a litigator who has both represented dentists and prosecuted cases on behalf of patients, I respectfully differ with the learned Justice Cardozo.

It cannot be overemphasized that no matter how voluminous and detailed a consent form the practitioner utilizes for a dental procedure, if the consent is executed while the patient is in the chair awaiting treatment, that consent is likely to be vitiated and useless. The patient is nervous, apprehensive, and consequently not apt to read or understand what is put before him/her. Even if the patient had the wherewithal to fully comprehend the contents of the document at the time, it is dubious that the patient will admit to it at the deposition or when testifying before a jury, the members of which will certainly place themselves in the patient's shoes.

A tenable alternative, utilized with success by one of the co-authors of this book, is to give the form to the patient at the consultation when the procedure is discussed and have him/her take it home to read at leisure. (As an added precaution, I would suggest that the patient should sign a dated receipt for the form.) When the patient returns for the treatment and the practitioner ensures that the document has been read and reviewed, the document may be signed in front of a witness.

Use of brochures and printed materials

While not a major aspect of the informed consent issue, the types of materials available in the dentist's waiting room addressing potential procedures to be performed can help the practitioner supply additional evidence of what the patient was aware of at the time of the procedure. These booklets should also be kept at the reception desk, where a member of the support staff can personally ensure that the patient has a copy of the applicable brochure. These materials should be updated regularly, and copies of the older informational materials should be retained by the practitioner for at least five to seven years. Should a lawsuit be commenced for allegedly failing to provide appropriate information in years past, the party being sued can merely retrieve what was given to the patients in that particular year for the questioned procedure.

A better practice is to staple a copy of what was actually given to the individual patient in the chart with a notation of the date those informational items were delivered by hand. These materials provide compelling evidence to a jury that the information booklets were read and understood.

Referrals to specialists, consultants, and second opinions— who obtains consent?

Whether the general dentist has an ongoing obligation to inform the patient of the risks and alternatives of prescribed treatment that will be referred to and performed by a dental specialist is a concern that arises frequently. Generally, both the practitioner who prescribes the treatment and the one who performs it are charged with the duty of obtaining an informed consent. There is, however, no need for both the generalist and the specialist to duplicate the consent; once either one obtains an acceptable informed consent, there will be no liability assessed to the other for the failure to do so.[45]

Many jurisdictions such as Connecticut, Louisiana, New Jersey, Pennsylvania, and Texas that have addressed this issue have held that a referring physician does not have a duty to obtain the patient's informed consent.[46] Other jurisdictions, such as New York, approach the issue in a more patient-friendly fashion.

The obligations of the respective health care providers involved in a patient's care in New York are initially addressed by Justice Kassal in the 1980 case of *Prooth v. Walsh*,[47] a medical malpractice action in which the patient sued the hospital, his internist (the generalist), the chief cardiac surgeon, the assistant surgeon, and a private consulting cardiologist, all for damages based upon a lack of informed consent claim. There, the court stated:

"A patient's personal physician bears the responsibility to assure the welfare of his patient in all phases of his treatment. Such treatment must, of necessity, include diagnosis and the prescription of a course of treatment by others, such as specialists. To the degree the physician provides such treatment directly, he obviously bears a duty to advise his patients of the risk. Further, if he refers his patient to another physician and retains a degree of participation, by way of control, consultation or otherwise, his responsibility continues to properly advise his patient with respect to the treatment to be performed by the referred physician [...] on the same basis, once the patient is referred to another physician for treatment, the second physician also has a duty to inform the patient."[48]

The rather strict standard in holding the generalist responsible for treatment performed by another was relaxed in *Nisenholtz v. Mount Sinai Hospital* four years later.[49] The patient brought an action in lack of informed consent against his referring physician who had solely treated plaintiff's condition non-surgically. That physician then referred the patient to a surgeon for a surgical procedure that resulted in impotence. The *Nisenholtz* court limits the physician's responsibility to obtaining informed consent to those procedures that the physician actually prescribes or performs. Here, during the 10-year treatment period, the physician had only treated the patient's condition non-surgically and made the referral merely stating that surgery should seriously be considered. Since the doctor neither performed nor recommended surgery, he was under no duty to obtain his informed consent. The court maintained:

"For liability to arise, the referring physician must do more than retain 'a degree of participation' as described in *Prooth*. The referring physician should be held liable only when that physician has ordered a procedure or actually participates in the treatment or procedure."[50]

In 1989, the New York courts returned to the stricter criteria in *Prooth*, where the plaintiff sued his treating physician who referred and scheduled him for a diagnostic surgical procedure, partly because the physician failed to inform him of the risks of the invasive diagnostic procedure.[51] The court in *Kashkin v. Mt. Sinai Medical Center* relied on *Prooth*, holding that a physician who formally orders a procedure has a duty to obtain the patient's informed consent even though he does not personally perform or assist in the procedure.[52]

The *Prooth* and *Kashkin* rationale, which imposes a fairly stringent disclosure requirement for the referring doctor, was adopted in a dental malpractice action against an orthodontist and an oral surgeon in Hawaii in *O'Neal v. Hammer*, where the patient initially consulted with an orthodontist for treatment of jaw problems.[53] After the consult, the orthodontist presented plaintiff with two alternative treatments: (1) orthodontics, tooth extraction, and mandibular advancement surgery by an oral surgeon and (2) orthodontic treatment only. It was further established that the doctor presented the patient with the *orthodontic* risks of the two plans and the *general risks of surgery*, although he did not inform the patient of the *specific risks of mandibular advancement surgery*. Plaintiff did undergo the extractions and had the mandibular advancement surgery with the co-defendant oral surgeon. Following the reasoning in the strict New York line of cases, the court in *O'Neal* held that the orthodontist's degree of participation and retention of control obligated the defendant to secure an informed consent for the mandibular advancement surgery. The court stated:

"In the instant case, the mandibular advancement surgery was just one phase of Dr. Hammer's four-step treatment plan, which consisted of the extraction of O'Neal's lower bicuspids, orthodontics to prepare her for the surgery, the surgery and follow-up orthodontic treatment. Dr. Hammer prepared the dental molds, took the photographs, ordered the x-rays, rendered the tracings, diagnosed O'Neal's jaw problem, and recommended orthodontics, extractions and surgery [...] Most importantly, Dr. Hammer initiated the first irrevocable step in the treatment plan—the removal of O'Neal's bicuspids. Therefore, Dr. Hammer, like the physicians in *Kashkin* and *Prooth*, retained a degree of participation, by way of control, consultation or otherwise that placed upon him a continuing responsibility to properly advise O'Neal of the risks and alternatives to the proposed surgery."[54]

This portion of the court's ruling is not surprising given the extent of the orthodontist's involvement in the treatment. However, the court went further in considering the question of whether the consulting or second opinion dentist—who does not propose, coordinate, or render treatment—nevertheless has a duty to obtain informed consent from the patient. The *O'Neal* court made a clear distinction between the two: (1) The consulting dentist is to advise and make recommendations to the treating dentist, who will then make the ultimate decision about the extent of information given to the patient, and (2) the "second opinion" dentist, called in directly by the patient to advise the patient whether to undergo the procedure, who clearly has a duty to inform.[55] The court opined:

"[...] an integral function of the second opinion physician is to advise patients of the nature of the proposed treatment, its risks and alternatives. It would be illogical to hold that the second opinion physician does not owe a duty to perform his or her primary duty—to advise of the risks and alternatives of the proposed treatment or surgery.[56]

The determination of who bears the responsibility of informing the patient of relevant information appears to be an exercise in semantics depends on whether the dentist is viewed as the referring doctor, the consult, or the second opinion. The old adage "better safe than sorry" comes to mind. Whether you are the primary dentist making the referral, the specialist called in as a consultant, or the dentist from whom the patient seeks a second opinion, advising that patient of the known risks and alternatives to the treatments being considered can only inure to your benefit.

Emerging Issues

As dentistry progresses into the areas of non-vital cosmetic treatments, and restorative work through implants becomes commonplace, some issues have emerged for the modern practitioner. These often optional treatments are frequently performed on patients who may be unreasonably dissatisfied with results for a number of factors, not the least of which may be their own unrealistic expectations regarding their appearance.

Capacity to consent

A rather frightening case recently litigated in New York involved a patient alleging that she was unable to give an informed consent to plastic surgery because she suffered from a psychiatric condition known as Body Dysmorphic Disorder (BDD), which is an unreasonable preoccupation or obsession with imagined or very minor physical imperfections. Certainly, this type of preoccupation is easily analogous to those patients obsessed with having "perfect teeth." In *Lynn G. v. Hugo*,[57] the patient had visited the plastic surgeon 51 times within 6 years for various cosmetic procedures, and had disclosed her psychiatric history with regard to anxiety and depression. The patient underwent a "tummy tuck" and was unhappy with the resulting abdominal scar. The dual basis for the lack of informed consent, which was eventually rejected by the state's highest court, was that (1) her mental disorder vitiated her consent to the surgery; and (2) her consent was not informed since plaintiff was not advised of less invasive alternatives. In dismissing the claim, the court noted that the affidavits submitted by plaintiff's psychiatrists did not definitively state that she suffered from BDD and was thereby unsubstantiated.[58] It is difficult to say what result would have been obtained should the medical proof regarding the psychiatric disorder been more unequivocal through expert evidence.[59]

Comparing providers

The evolution of informed consent and the corresponding availability of information through the Internet have resulted in the patient's entitlement to more and more information regarding both the procedures he/she plans to undergo and the providers of those procedures. A question has now arisen about the necessity of furnishing information about the relative risks associated with the medical providers performing the procedures. Simply put, the question is—would the patient have consented to the procedure to be performed by one provider with less experience and a higher level of risk and failure, as opposed to being performed by another provider with more expertise and a lower level of risk?[60] The obvious forum for the development of these kinds of cases in dentistry is in the areas of implant placement and related oral surgery such as bone grafting and sinus lifts.

The authors of a 1999 law journal review argue that this type of informed consent case would be easier to prove since "[d]ecision causation is more easily established [...] because it is highly credible that a patient would have opted for a medical provider whose performance was demonstrably better. In addition, injury causation is more directly analyzable..."[61]

Illustrative is the case of *Johnson v. Kokemoor*,[62] where the plaintiff agreed to undergo surgery for a brain aneurysm with her treating doctor and was rendered an incomplete quadriplegic as a result. In bringing an action for informed consent, the injured patient alleged that the doctor had failed to disclose his lack of experience and relative competence, failed to compare morbidity and mortality rates for this kind of surgery with experienced and inexperienced surgeons, and failed to disclose the existence of more experienced surgeons in a nearby care center. The Wisconsin court ruled that the above information was highly relevant to the patient's ability to make an informed choice.[63]

In a more recent decision in May of 2001 addressing the same issue, the Supreme Court of Pennsylvania specifically rejected this broadening of the informed consent doctrine, holding that information personal to the provider, including his experience, is irrelevant to the doctrine of informed consent.[64] The court in *Duttry v. Patterson*, while declining to expand informed consent, instead set out other possible causes of action that could be alleged under those circumstances:

"Our holding should not, however, be read to stand for the proposition that a physician who misleads a patient is immune from suit. Rather, we are merely stating that the doctrine of informed consent is not the legal panacea for all damages arising out of any type of malfeasance by a physician. Nor do we see a need to expand this doctrine into a catchall theory of recovery since other causes of action provide avenues for redress of the injured patient. For example, it is conceivable that a physician's lack of experience in performing an operation would support a plaintiff's case in negligence [...] in situations [...] in which the physician allegedly provides inaccurate information regarding his experience in performing a procedure, the plaintiff may have a cause of action in misrepresentation."[65]

As a rule of thumb, it certainly is not wise to overstate one's skills. However, the courts have not yet ruled that it is necessary to send a copy of your dental school transcript to prospective patients. If pointed questions are asked about your experience (or lack thereof), tell the truth in the most positive light without garnishment. The patient can then form his/her own opinion.

Conclusion

The doctrine of informed consent encompasses a broad continuum of risk management problems. When in doubt, always err on the side of caution and overstatement. Above all, make sure to document relevant conversations, have a signed consent form, and follow the same thorough procedure in each instance. While many of the suggestions contained herein may seem burdensome, most are inexpensive and simple to implement. Once the routine is in place, it will provide the practitioner with both peace of mind and viable defenses to a lawsuit for failure to disclose.

Notes

[1] *Schloendorff v. Society of New York Hospital*, 211 N.Y. 125, 105 N.E. 92 (N.Y. 1914)

[2] Bussey, George D. "Case Note: *Keomaka v. Zakaib*, The Physician's Affirmative Duty to Protect Patient Autonomy Through the Process of Informed Consent," *University of Hawaii Law Review*, Fall 1992, 14 UIHLR 801(1992)

[3] *Schloendorff v. Society of New York Hospital*, 211 N.Y. at 129-30, 105 N.E. 92 (N.Y. 1914)

[4] *Salgo v. Leland Stanford Jr. University Board of Trustees*, 317 P.2nd 170 (Cal. 1957)

[5] *Natanson v. Kline*, 350 P. 2nd 1093 (Kan. 1960)

[6] Bussey, George D. "Case Note: *Keomaka v. Zakaib*, The Physician's Affirmative Duty to Protect Patient Autonomy Through the Process of Informed Consent," *University of Hawaii Law Review*, Fall 1992, 14 UIHLR 801(1992)

[7] *Canterbury v. Spence*, 464 F. 2d 772 (D.C. Cir.), cert. den. 409 U.S. 1064, 93 S. Ct. 560 (1972)

[8] *Id.* at 788-789

[9] *Spinosa v. Weinstein*, 168 A.D. 2d 32, 41, 541 N.Y.S. 2d 747 (2d Dept. 1991), citing, e.g., *Rigie v. Goldman*, 148 A.D. 2d 23, 28, 543 N.Y.S. 2d 983 (2d Dept 1989)

[10] *Canterbury v. Spence*, 464 F. 2d 772 (D.C. Cir.), cert. den. 409 U.S. 1064, 93 S. Ct. 560 (1972)

[11] *Canterbury v. Spence*, 464 F. 2d 772 (D.C. Cir.), cert. den. 409 U.S. 1064, 93 S. Ct. 560 (1972)

[12] New York State Public Health Law Section 2805-d, *McKinney's Consolidated Laws of New York*

[13] *Alberti v. St. John's Hospital-Smithtown*, 116 A.D. 2d 612, 497 N.Y.S. 2d 701 (2d Dept. 1986); *Lipsius v. White*, 91 AD2d 271, 458 N.Y.S. 2d 928 (2d Dept. 1983)

[14] *Messina v. Matarasso*, 729 N.Y.S. 2d 4, 2001 N.Y. Slip. Op. 06398 (1st Dept. 2001)

[15] *Id.* at 7

[16] Silber, Marian E. and Maria Elyse Rabar. "Informed Consent: Evolution and Erosion, Part I, 9/4/98 *New York Law Journal*, vol. 220, no. 47, p.3, col.1; Jolly v. Russell, 203 A.D. 2d 527, 611 N.Y.S. 2d 232 (2d Dept. 1994)

[17] *Evans v. Kringstein*, 193 A.D. 2d 714, 598 N.Y.S. 2d 64 (2d Dept. 1993)

[18] *Canterbury v. Spence*, 464 F. 2d 772 (D.C. Cir.), cert. den. 409 U.S. 1064, 93 S. Ct. 560 (1972)

[19] Moore, Thomas A. "Informed Consent, Part I." 9/5/95 *New York Law Journal*, vol. 214, no. 45, p.3, col. 1

[20] See e.g., *Garone v. Roberts Technical & Trade School, Inc.*, 47 A.D. 2d 306 (1st Dept. 1975); *Zeleznik v. Jewish Chronic Disease Hospital*, 47 A.D. 2d 199 (2d Dept. 1975)

[21] See Hubbard ex rel *Hubbard v. Reed*, 774 A.2d 495, 500 168 N.J. 387, 395 (N.J. 2001) quoting N.D. Cent. Code Section 28-01-46 (1999)

[22] *Gershberg v. Wood-Smith*, 279 A.D. 2d 424, 719 N.Y.S. 2d 846 (1st Dept.2001) *Evans v. Hollaran*, 198 AD 2d 472, 604 NYS 2d 958 (2d Dept. 1993)

[23] *New York Civil Practice Law and Rules* Section 4401-a (2000)

[24] *Berger v. Becker*, 272 A.D. 2d 565, 709 N.Y.S. 2d 418 (2d Dept. 2000); *Lopez v. Sheskier*, 262 A.D. 2d 536, 691 N.Y.S. 2d 794 (2d Dept. 1999)

[25] *Sohn v. Sand*, 180 A.D. 2d 789, 580 N.Y.S. 2d 458 (2d Dept.1992)

[26] *Berger v. Becker*, 272 A.D. 2d 565, 709 N.Y.S. 2d 418 (2d Dept. 2000); *Evans v. Hollaran*, 198 AD 2d 472, 604 NYS 2d 958 (2d Dept. 1993)

[27] *Anderson v. Delaney*, 269 A.D. 2d 193, 703 N.Y.S. 2d 714 (1st Dept.2000) *Santilli v. CHP, Inc.*, 274 A.D. 2d 905, 711 N.Y.S. 2d 249 (3rd Dept. 2000); Thomas A. Moore and Matthew Gaier, "Update on Informed Consent," 6/5/01, *New York Law Journal*, vol. 225, no. 107, p.3, col. 1

[28] *New York Pattern Jury Instructions*, Section 2:150A, 3rd ed., 2001, 1 NY PJI3d 729 (2001)

[29] *Foote v. Rajadhyax*, 268 A.D.2d 745, 702 N.Y.S. 2d 153 (3d Dept. 2000)

[30] *Id.* at 745

[31] *Iazetta v. Vicenzi*, 200 A.D. 2d 209, 613 N.Y.S. 2d 750 (3d Dept. 1994)

[32] *Id.* at 213

[33] *Id.* at 213

[34] *Smith v. Fields*, 268 A.D. 2d 579, 702 N.Y.S. 2d 364 (2d Dept. 2000)

[35] *Id.* at 580

[36] *Rigie v. Goldman*, 148 A.D. 2d 23, 543 N.Y.S. 2d 983 (2d Dept. 1989)

[37] *Id.*; *New York Pattern Jury Instructions*, Section 1:71, 3rd Ed., 2001, 1 N.Y. PJI3d 95 (2001)

[38] *Cooper v. U.S.*, 903 F. Supp. 953 (D.S.C. 1995)

[39] *Id.* at 956, citing *Hook v. Rothstein*, 281 S.C. 541, 316 S.E.2d 690 (Ct. App. 1984)

[40] *Bota v. Kaminsky*, Index No. 115882/98, Sup. Ct. N.Y. Co., (J. Schlesinger, 7/13/01)

[41] *Id.* at pp. 2-3

[42] *Id.* At p. 4

[43] Sec., e.g. *Eppel v Fredericks* 203 A.D. 2nd. 152, 610 N.Y.S. 2nd 254 (1st Dept. 1994)

[44] *Schloendorff v. Society of New York Hospital*, 211 N.Y. at 134, 105 N.E. 92 (N.Y. 1914)

45 *Spinosa v. Weinstein*, 168 A.D. 2d 32, 41, 541 N.Y.S. 2d 747 (2d. Dept. 1991); *Prooth v. Walsh*, 105 Misc. 2d 603, 432 N.Y.S. 2d 663 (N.Y. Sup. Ct. 1980); *Nisenholtz v. Mount Sinai Hospital*, 126 Misc. 2d 658, 483 N.Y.S. 2d 568 (N.Y. Sup. Ct. 1984)

46 See *Davis v. St. Charles General Hospital*, 598 So. 2d 1244 (La. Ct. App. 1992); *Logan v. Greenwich Hospital Ass'n.*, 191 Conn. 282, 465 A. 2d 294 (1983); *Herrera v. Atlantic City Surgical Group*, 277 N.J. Super. 260, 649 A. 2d 637 (Law. Dir. 1994); *Shaw v. Kirschbaum*, 439 Pa. Super. 24, 653 A. 2d 12 (1994); *Johnson v. Whitehurst*, 652 S.W. 2d 441 (Tex. Ct. App. 1983)

47 *Prooth v. Walsh*, 105 Misc. 2d 603, 432 N.Y.S. 2d 663 (N.Y. Sup. Ct. 1980)

48 *Id.* at 605

49 *Nisenholtz v. Mount Sinai Hospital*, 126 Misc. 2d 658, 483 N.Y.S. 2d 568 (N.Y. Sup. Ct. 1984)

50 *Id.* at 664

51 *Kashkin v. Mount Sinai Medical Center*, 142 Misc. 2d 863, 538 N.Y.S. 2d 686 (N.Y. Sup. Ct. 1989)

52 *Id.*

53 *O'Neal v. Hammer*, 87 Hawaii 183, 953 P. 2d 561(Sup. Ct. Hawaii 1998)

54 *Id.* at 188

55 *Id.* at 190; see also *Prooth v. Walsh*, 105 Misc. 2d 603, 432 N.Y.S. 2d 663 (N.Y. Sup. Ct. 1980)

[56] *Id.* at 190

[57] *Lynn v. Hugo*, 96 N.Y. 2d 306, 728 N.Y.S. 2d 121 (2001)

[58] *Id.* at 310

[59] Moore, Thomas A., and Matthew Gaier. "Update on Informed Consent-Part II," 8/7/01 *New York Law Journal*, vol. 226, no. 26, p. 3, col. 1

[60] Twerski, Aaron D., and Neil B. Cohen. "The Second Revolution in Informed Consent: Comparing Physicians to Each Other," *Northwestern University Law Review*, Fall 1999, 94 NWULR 1, 5

[61] Twerski, Aaron D., and Neil B. Cohen. "The Second Revolution in Informed Consent: Comparing Physicians to Each Other," *Northwestern University Law Review*, Fall 1999, 94 NWULR 1, 9

[62] *Johnson v. Kokemoor*, 199 Wis. 2d 615, 545 N.W. 2d 495 (1996)

[63] *Id.*

[64] *Duttry v. Patterson*, 771 A.2d 1255 (Pennsylvania Sup. Ct. 2001)

[65] *Id.* at 1259

Chapter 9

Temporomandibular Disorders

By Henry A. Gremillion, D.D.S., M.A.G.D.

Introduction

The masticatory system is plagued by a number of acute, chronic, and recurrent pain conditions. Data suggest that almost one-fourth of the U.S. population experiences orofacial pain on more than one occasion in a six-month period.[1] Pain involving the teeth and the periodontal structures is the most common presenting concern in dental practice. However, non-odontogenic pain such as temporomandibular disorders (TMD) also occur frequently. Recent scientific investigation has provided an explosion of knowledge with regard to pain mechanisms, pain pathways, and an enhanced understanding of the complexities of the many ramifications of the total pain experience. Therefore, it is mandatory for the dental professional to develop the necessary clinical and scientific expertise on which he/she may base diagnostic and management approaches. Optimum management can only be achieved by determining an accurate and complete diagnosis and identifying all of the factors associated with the underlying pathosis on a case-specific basis. A thorough understanding of the epidemiologic and etiologic aspects of TMD is essential to the practice of evidence-based dentistry/medicine.

Defining Temporomandibular Disorders

Temporomandibular disorders (TMD), a subcategory of orofacial pain, refer to a number of conditions involving the masticatory system. TMD is the most commonly occurring non-odontogenic pain experienced in the masticatory system.[1] TMD has been defined as "a collective term referring to a number of clinical problems involving the masticatory musculature, the temporomandibular joint(s), and/or the associated structures."[2] Recent studies indicate the prevalence of TMD-related pain to be 12%.[3] Other studies indicate that as many as 10 million Americans suffer from TMD-related complaints each year.[4-5]

Clinical features of TMDs

Characteristic signs and symptoms of TMD include:

- Pain in the temporomandibular region
- Limitation or disturbance in mandibular movement and/or masticatory functional ability
- Temporomandibular joint sounds[6]

Features such as onset, location, temporal pattern, and aggravating and relieving factors may provide valuable clues related to the patient's condition. The clinician must appreciate the fact that the response to pain differs from person to person, and one must rely on the patient's subjective assessment of pain.[7] Our current understanding of the complexity of innervation in the head and neck region reveals the dynamic interaction between a number of cranial and cervical nerves, to include the trigeminal system. This complex neural system may make the true source of pain difficult to identify.[8] It is important for the clinician to remember that the area in which the patient perceives his/her pain (site) may not truly represent the area of tissue injury or pathology (source). Confusion with regard to diagnostic and clinical decision-making is compounded by the fact that signs associated with TMD occur quite commonly in the general population. Seventy-five percent of those evaluated in one study exhibited at least one sign such as joint noise or palpation tenderness, and 33% of this non-patient population exhibited at least one symptom.[9] Signs and symptoms in the general population have been found to occur in females only slightly more frequently than males, at a ratio of approximately 2:1.[10-14]

Associated features

TMD is commonly associated with the concomitant occurrence of signs and symptoms affecting other areas of the head and neck. For example, headache is a frequent complaint of TMD patients. A recent publication reported that 75% of a TMD patient population also reported neck pain.[15] Seventy-two percent of this study group indicated that they were experiencing pain in areas of the head other than the masticatory region. Ear-related signs and symptoms including diminished hearing acuity, tinnitus, and dizziness are frequently reported by TMD patients.

Epidemiology of TMD

Epidemiologic study of patient populations reveals that, unlike many other musculoskeletal conditions, TMD has not been found to increase in incidence or prevalence with age.[10,14,16] The most common age group affected is between 15 and 45 years of age, with an average of approximately 33.9 years.[16] Demographic data from clinically-based studies indicate that TMD symptoms are least prevalent in the young and seem to decrease after the age of 45.[17-23] A tremendous female to male gender bias of 6:1 to 9:1 has been found among patient populations.[16,24] The existing literature on experimentally-induced pain indicates that there are sex differences, with females displaying greater sensitivity.[25-26] However, clinical pain differences have not been definitively determined. In epidemiological studies, sex differences are noted with regard to the prevalence of a number of pain syndromes, with females reporting more severe pain, more frequent pain, and pain of longer duration.[26]

History/Clinical Examination

History

The most important part of evaluation of the TMD patient is a detailed history of the chief pain/dysfunction concern. The role of the clinician is to determine a diagnosis from the key pieces of information provided by the patient and to formulate a treatment/management plan that will address all areas of the patient's condition. A questionnaire in the form of simple written questions (Table 9-1), visual analog scale (Fig. 9-1), and diagrams (Fig. 9-2) for patients to fill out prior to their appointment may aid in the accumulation of important baseline data from which a clearer picture of the problem may be more readily obtained.[27-29]

Fig. 9-1 Visual analog scale (VAS)

Fig. 9-2 Patient diagrams for self-reporting their pain

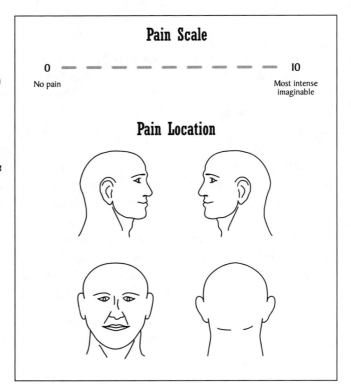

Pain Scale

0 — — — — — — — — — — 10

No pain

Most intense imaginable

Pain Location

Please circle either "YES" or "NO" for each question. If you do not understand the question, please leave it blank and ask the doctor to clarify it during your consultation.

1. Do you have difficulty in opening your mouth? YES NO

   If "YES," is it because of:

      A. Pain? YES NO

      B. Jaw locks or gets stuck? YES NO

2. Do you have pain in your jaw joint(s)? YES NO

3. Do you have pain in the ears, temple, or cheeks? YES NO

4. Is the pain present

      A. All the time? YES NO

      B. Comes and goes? YES NO

5. Do you have difficulty chewing, yawning, or talking? YES NO

6. Does your bite feel uncomfortable or unusual, or has it changed recently? YES NO

7. Do you have noises such as clicking, popping, or grating? YES NO

8. Do you clench or grind your teeth? YES NO

9. How long have you experienced symptoms from your jaw?

10. Have you ever been treated for jaw joint problems before? YES NO

11. Do you suffer from arthritis in any other joint(s)? YES NO

12. Have you had a recent injury to your head or neck? YES NO

13. Do you suffer from any of the following conditions:

      A. Recurrent headaches YES NO

      B. Irritable bowel YES NO

      C. Chronic back/neck pain YES NO

      D. Depression YES NO

14. Do you have difficulty sleeping or constantly wake up during the night? YES NO

15. Do you experience bothersome stress

      A. At work? YES NO

      B. At home? YES NO

16. Have you ever been treated by a psychologist or psychiatrist? YES NO

Table 9-1 Temporomandibular disorder screening questionnaire. These basic questions provide important insight into the history of the patient's chief concern(s).

255

The history of the presenting complaint is in essence a chronological overview of the onset, features (clinical characteristics/temporal aspects), and duration of the symptom complex. This includes a review of the treatment(s) that the patient has undergone for the condition and the response to that care. Key components of a detailed history are listed in Table 9-2. It is essential that the clinician cultivate the important skill of listening and gently directing the evaluation process through simple questioning and an empathetic, caring demeanor. Development of rapport with the patient is key to obtaining important information that may reveal underlying influences such as anxiety, stress, depression, and significant life events that may be related to the case.[27-30]

Chief Pain/Dysfunction Concern(s)
Specific Components of the Chief Concern

History of Chief Concern(s)

- Location
- Onset
- Trauma
- Quality
- Quantity
- Temporal pattern of intensification
- Change or progression over time
- Quality of life changes
- Initiating factors
- Aggravating factors
- Alleviating factors
- Associated symptoms
- Prior evaluations, diagnostic tests and treatment for chief concern(s)
- Most effective treatment to date

Medical History

- Review of systems
- Family members with similar or potentially related conditions
- Allergies/sensitivities
- Prior surgeries/hospitalizations
- Current medications

Dental History
Psychosocial/Behavioral History

- Diet/nutrition/sleep history
- Exercise

Table 9-2 TMD detailed history—key components

Clinical Examination

A comprehensive physical examination of the patient involves observation, palpation, auscultation, and measurement of the mandibular range of motion. Additionally, a thorough evaluation of the patient's occlusal function and masticatory functional ability should be accomplished.

The temporomandibular joint (TMJ) should be evaluated for tenderness to palpation at the lateral and posterolateral aspects, those areas accessible to palpation while at rest and during function. Palpation pressure should be approximately 3-5 lbs/in^2 (just enough to blanch the nail bed). Pain upon loading of the TMJ may be evaluated by gentle manipulation upon gaining neuromuscular release by directing forces to seat the condyle superiorly and anteriorly or by having the patient bite on a tongue blade placed in the most posterior tooth bearing areas unilaterally while closing in the midline. This approach will serve to load the contralateral joint. Joint sounds and their location during opening, closing, and excursive movements of the mandible may be detected with a stethoscope. It must be kept in mind that joint noises such as clicking are a common finding in the general population and may not be related to the patient's chief pain concern. After each aspect of TMJ examination, the patient is asked to rate the level of pain stimulated as—no pain, mild, moderate, or severe. Additionally, the clinician should ask the patient if pain experienced during the evaluation duplicates their chief concern(s). Pain referral patterns should also be noted.

Mandibular range of motion should be assessed. The clinician should note whether the line of vertical opening is straight and smooth or deviates with jerky movements. The range of painless maximal vertical opening (normal range 42-55 mm), protrusive (≥ 7 mm), and lateral excursions (≥ 7 mm) should be recorded. It is essential to determine the cause of the decreased mandibular movements so that the most appropriate course of management may be undertaken.

Examination of the masticatory and cervical musculature may be accomplished by digital palpation. Areas of tenderness, taut bands, myofascial trigger points, and pain referral patterns should be noted. The patient is asked to rate levels of pain as mild, moderate, or severe. Additionally, the patient is asked whether the pain experienced upon palpation is the same as or different than his/her presenting pain concern. Direct palpation of the lateral pterygoid muscle is not possible so provocation testing can be accomplished by having the patient protrude his/her mandible (with the teeth slightly separated) against firm, gentle resistance provided by the clinician's fingers placed against the patient's chin. The clinician is cautioned not to distalize the mandible due to the potential for compression of vascularized, innervated retrodiscal tissue.

Occlusal evaluation is accomplished through static and dynamic assessment. The relationship of the teeth in intercuspal position, wear facets, fracture, mobility patterns, and migration of teeth are noted. Centric relation occlusal relationships, deviations from centric relation occlusion to intercuspal position, and specific occlusal/incisal guidance in excursive movements are also recorded.

Predisposing, initiating, perpetuating factors

There exists a dynamic balance between the various components of the masticatory system including the teeth, periodontium (hard and soft tissue supporting structures), masticatory and cervical musculature, TMJ structures, and the psyche of each individual. This adaptive balance may be disrupted by a number of factors acting alone or in combination resulting in the expression of signs and symptoms associated with TMD. It is essential that the clinician consider predisposing, initiating, and perpetuating factors. Recent scientific investigation has provided an enhanced understanding of pathogenesis, those cellular events and reactions and other pathologic mechanisms occurring in the development and maintenance or recurrence of TMD. Slavkin stated that "Understanding these interrelationships should improve how we promote health, reduce disease and enhance diagnosis and treatment."[5] A model representing factors that may compromise the adaptability of the masticatory system and likely play a role in TMD is represented in Figure 9-3.

Data indicate that there is a significant sexual disparity in the TMD patient population and more globally in the vast majority of human pain conditions.[31] Behavioral factors such as the more stoic nature of males, social conditioning, and car-seeking behaviors have been proposed as being responsible for differences in the pain experience. Studies in which age-matched males and females were exposed to laboratory stressors have found that anxiety impacts on both sexes. However, a significant difference in the levels of various psychophysiologic responses in males and females was revealed.[25] Females demonstrated a greater decrease in pain tolerance and threshold, more disrupted self-control strategies, increased electromyographic activity of the facial and masticatory musculature, and more pain behavior than did the male subjects.[32] Other researchers have also identified sex differences in response to anxiety as well as laboratory-induced pain.[25, 33-35]

Physiologic factors related to sexual structural differences have been reported. Evidence indicates that females tend to exhibit a greater ease of masticatory muscle fatigue.[36-38] A greater concentration of fast twitch, easily fatiguing white fibers versus slower twitch, endurant red fibers may be associated with this phenomenon.[39] Fibromyalgia, a chronic skeletal muscle condition, associated with disruption in pain modulation, is commonly found to coexist with TMD. An increase in the number of red, ragged fibers (a pathologic fiber state) in areas approximating diagnostic tender points is reported to occur in fibromyalgia.[40-41] This finding is also noted in post-exercise muscle soreness and myositis.[42] Class II skeletal subtypes (high angle cases) have been

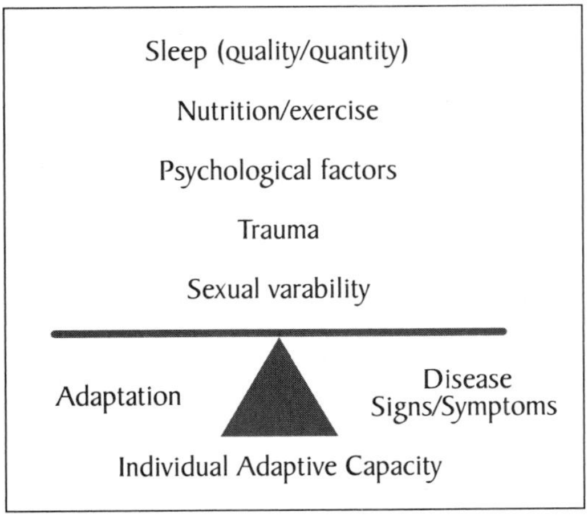

Fig. 9-3 Factors that may compromise the adaptive capacity of the masticatory system leading to the development and/or maintenance of temporomandibular disorder

reported to demonstrate greater propensity for masticatory muscle fatigue.[43] It has been suggested that individuals with a history of systemic joint laxity or certain collagen vascular diseases are predisposed to the development of arthrogenous TMD.[44-45]

Hormonal factors may also be responsible for gender differences in the TMD patient population.[46-47] TMD appears to peak in incidence during the reproductive years, suggesting that either biologic or psychosocial factors unique to women in this period of life could increase the risk of developing and maintaining this condition.[48] Reports have linked female reproductive hormones with the occurrence of migraine in some females.[48] Importantly, migraine is considered to be a form of trigemino-vascular pain. It has been long recognized that females demonstrate greater pain sensitivity during the menstrual cycle, at ovulation, and following menses. The relationship of estrogen, and to a lesser degree prolactin, to pain sensitivity has been elucidated. The use of an estrogen supplement significantly increased the odds of having TMD.[48] Studies have shown that although functional estrogen receptors have been identified in many synovial joints of males and females in equal concentrations, there exists a significant difference in the number of estrogen receptors within the TMJ. Male TMJs have been found to have few, if any estrogen receptors[49] while female TMJs exhibited significant numbers of these receptors.[50-51] Implications regarding hormonal variables relate to their potential to modify the adaptive capacity of the TMJ.[52]

Nerve growth factor (NGF) is expressed during injury of tissue. It is recognized that NGF is capable of activating nociceptive (pain transmitting) nerve endings in the peripheral as well as the central nervous system. NGF levels have also been found to be elevated in synovial fluid from joints of arthritic patients and have been associated with hyperalgesia (exaggerated pain response) in humans. Petty et al. recently reported that when human skeletal muscles were injected with NGF, diffuse myalgia was induced.[53] The onset of myalgia was in six to nine minutes with the peak pain levels reached in four to six hours, and the duration was two to nine days. In some cases, the pain persisted up to seven weeks after a single injection. It was found that women were significantly more sensitive to the effects of NGF than men.

Measurement of TMJ pressure differentials in the superior joint space on patients experiencing several subtypes of internal derangement revealed tremendously elevated pressures.[54] These elevated pressures, which far supercede the end capillary perfusion pressure, can obtund the flow of vital nutrients into the TMJ, resulting in a hypoxic condition. Decreased oxygen saturation with a subsequent reperfusion, the return of flow to the area, has been reported to stimulate the production of tissue-degrading substances such as free radicals and cytokines.[55-56] A trend towards significantly greater TMJ pressures associated with clenching was found to occur in female as contrasted to male subjects.[54] This finding is interesting in light of the fact that males have routinely been found to develop greater biting forces than females.[57] Further study in this area may provide additional explanation with regard to the preponderance of female TMD patients.

Psychological factors

Psychologic factors may be related to the TMD experience. There is little doubt that there is some psychological factor(s) associated with every pain experience. However, the relationship of the psychologic factor(s) either directly or indirectly as a cause must be determined on a case-specific basis. Additionally, the degree of response must be assessed, since psychological response in acute pain states is typically a short-lived, normal reaction. It is well recognized that anxiety, stress, negative affect, and depression may compromise physical and mental well-being. Catastrophizing (thinking the worst) has been identified as a significant impediment to successful management of pain conditions. Pain severity is associated with the degree of life interference and negative affect (depression, anxiety, and anger).[58] A direct relationship between depression and both physical and the psychosocial functioning of facial pain patients has been reported.[59] Additionally, depressed mood is associated with a decrease in the concentration of the central nervous system neurotransmitters norepinephrine and serotonin. Decrease in these neurotransmitters is associated with impairment of endogenous pain inhibition and disrupted sleep patterns. Anxiety and stress have been found to cause compromise in the immune system, thus lowering host resistance.

Studies suggest a relationship between a history of physical and/or sexual abuse and a range of psychological, functional, and physical factors. Abuse history has been identified as a significant feature of TMD chronic pain patient populations as contrasted to non-chronic TMD patients. It has recently been found that an abuse history was likely to increase an individual's tendency to dwell on, amplify, and over-interpret somatic symptoms.[60]

Nutrition and exercise

The importance of quality nutrition and adequate, appropriate exercise cannot be over-emphasized. However, many TMD/orofacial pain patients have withdrawn from normal activities of daily living that may compromise not only their mental well-being, but also their neurophysiological well-being. Exercise on a regular basis boosts the body's natural pain defense mechanisms by enhancing the production of endogenous opioids (enkephlins, dynorphins, endorphins). Likewise, balanced nutrition can enhance the body's pain defense mechanisms by maximizing anti-eicosinoid effects and aiding in the production of antioxidants that limit the damage caused by destructive free radicals in both joint and muscle disorders. Chronic muscle pain disorders such as myofascial pain and fibromyalgia have been associated with a decrease in serum magnesium. Magnesium deficit is associated with an enhanced inflammatory process, an enhanced free radical (superoxide) formation, an enhanced excitatory state in the central nervous system (CNS), and an enhanced calcium-mobilizing potential (abnormal calcium handling). Travell reported that B-vitamin deficiency is a common perpetuating factor of myofascial pain.[61]

Trauma

The role of various types of trauma in the etiology of TMD has been debated for many years. A study of 400 consecutive TMD clinical patients assessed the incidence of jaw injury in relation to onset of symptoms.[62] Only 24.5% of the study population could relate the onset of pain and dysfunction directly to an identifiable macrotraumatic event, primarily extension/flexion injury. Similarly, a study of TMJ degenerative joint disease patients found that only 31.6% reported previous trauma to the head and/or neck.[24] These data indicate that the vast majority of TMD patients experience a more insidious onset of their symptoms, likely related to microtrauma or a repetitive stress response. Microtraumatic factors include bruxing/clenching, postural dysfunction, and other habitual repetitive behaviors.

Occlusal factors

One of the areas of greatest debate relates to the association between occlusal factors and TMD. Although occlusion has been recognized as an important etiologic or perpetuating co-factor, the degree to which it plays a role has not been definitively delineated. Few terms in dentistry are used in the broad context as is malocclusion. *Malocclusion* is defined as any deviation from acceptable contact of opposing dentitions or any deviation from normal occlusion.[63] One must ask, "What is normal occlusion?" An average of the results of 14 studies regarding the prevalence of malocclusion reveals that 42% of the population represented a Class I malocclusion, 23% exhibit Class II malocclusion, and 4% have a Class III malocclusion.[67] Therefore only 31% have what would be termed normal occlusion. One may ask whether or not these occlusal relationships are truly aberrant or are we simply looking at a static relationship?

An association between open bite, posterior crossbite, and deep bite and the occurrence of TMD has been reported.[43] Additionally, a multiple logistic regression analysis to compute the odds ratio for 11 common occlusal features for asymptomatic controls as related to five TMD subgroups found several occlusal factors to demonstrate odds risk ratio of at least 2.[65-66] These occlusal features include anterior open bite, overjet > 6mm, CR/IP slide > 4mm, unilateral lingual crossbite, and five or more missing posterior teeth. Other occlusal schemes were not found to be statistically significant. These studies may not reveal the total story because of the dynamic nature of the masticatory system. While it may be said that the manner in which teeth fit is important, what the individual does with his/her teeth may be more important. Dynamic occlusal function affects multiple interfaces such as:

- Tooth interface
- Tooth/supporting structure interface
- TMJ interface
- Neuromuscular interface

Mechanical stresses at each of these interfaces have been shown to be associated with a compromise in the integrity of tissues. Additionally, we must consider the various case-specific factors that may affect adaptability such as:

- Structural tolerance of the various components of the masticatory system
- Duration of load
- Degree of load
- Variable directions of muscular loading forces
- Host resistance

It may be more appropriate to view TMD cases where occlusal function serves as a significant factor in TMD as a maladaptive occlusion.[64] This term takes into consideration peripheral and central sensory and motor factors involved in masticatory system pathofunction on a case-specific basis.

Postural considerations

Postural imbalances have been suggested as an etiologic variable in TMD.[67] While there is little doubt that craniocervical dysfunction is commonly found in the TMD patient population, a cause and effect relationship has not been definitively established. Studies indicate that a dynamic relationship between the cervical and masticatory musculature exists. Injection of local anesthetic into the trapezius muscle myofascial pain trigger point not only was associated with a decrease in the electromyographic (EMG) activity in the injected muscle, but also with decreased EMG activity in the masseter muscle on the same side.[68] Results from a study of patients in motor vehicular accidents suggest that TMJ or masticatory muscle injury may be associated with various postural relationships.[69] Therefore, it appears that the complex innervation of the head and neck creates an environment in which sensory and motor systems may interact to result in musculoskeletal compromise involving the masticatory and cervical regions.

Sleep disturbances

It is estimated that one in seven Americans suffers from a diagnosable sleep disturbance. Disturbed sleep has significant physiological effects and a number of psychological relationships. It is well recognized that there exist a number of sleep-dependent processes necessary for health maintenance. During the deeper, restorative stage of sleep, growth hormone is produced. Growth hormone is necessary for repair and regeneration of damaged tissues such as joint or muscle. Additionally, T-cell and lymphocyte function is enhanced by quality, restorative sleep. A compromise in the amount of the deeper stage of sleep also results in a decrease in serotonin in the CNS. The ramifications of diminished serotonin levels are widespread, involving altered pain modulation and mood. Unfortunately, disturbed sleep patterns are commonly found among TMD patient populations. Associated with these disrupted sleep cycles may be an increase in nocturnal masticatory system parafunctional activities such as clenching and bruxing. Nocturnal bruxism has been reported to be carried out at levels three to four times more forcefully than during the waking hours due to the reduction in inhibitory controls while sleeping.[70] Due to the significant implications of impaired sleep and nocturnal bruxism, it is essential that a thorough review of each TMD/orofacial pain patient's sleep history be accomplished.

Categorization of TMD

It is generally recognized that two basic categories of TMD exist:

- Extracapsular (myogenous)
- Intracapsular (arthrogenous)

The majority of TMDs are extracapsular in nature; however, it not uncommon for intracapsular and extracapsular conditions to co-exist. Within each of these broad categories, a number of subgroups have been identified (Table 9-3). As we recognize the interrelationships of distinct diagnostic subgroups and better understand neurophysiologic characteristics of the various hard and soft tissue structures involved, improved diagnosis and management will evolve. Figure 9-4 demonstrates the biomechanical relationships in a "normal" TMJ during the opening-closing cycle.

Myogenous TMD

Muscle-related signs and symptoms are also very common in general population and patient-based studies. Masticatory muscle-related conditions are found to be the most common subgroup of TMD.[71-72] Current understanding of the complexity of masticatory muscle function and its dynamic relationship with the cervical musculature provides ample rationale for thorough assessment of these areas in routine TMD patient evaluation. Individual variations in muscle anatomy, biomechanics, and fiber type/composition potentially related to muscle fatigue must be considered. The demands on the musculature in normal function and excessive function while awake or asleep must be appreciated. Importantly, age-related decline of symptomology might not be as great with respect to muscular involvement as that identified with the TMJ.[71]

Recommended diagnostic classification.

11.7 Temporomandibular joint articular disorders

   11.7.1 Congenital or developmental disorders

      11.7.1.1 Aplasia

      11.7.1.2 Hypoplasia

      11.7.1.3 Hyperplasia

      11.7.1.4 Neoplasia

   11.7.2 Disc derangement disorders

      11.7.2.1 Disc displacement with reduction

      11.7.2.2 Disc displacement without reduction

   11.7.3 Temporomandibular joint dislocation

   11.7.4 Inflammatory disorders

      11.7.4.1 Capsulitis/Synovitis

      11.7.4.2 Polyarthritides

   11.7.5 Osteoarthritis (noninflammatory disorders)

      11.7.5.1 Osteoarthritis: primary

      11.7.5.2 Osteoarthritis: secondary

   11.7.6 Ankylosis

   11.7.7 Fracture (condylar process)

11.8 Masticatory muscle disorders

   11.8.1 Myofascial pain

   11.8.2 Myositis

   11.8.3 Myospasm

   11.8.4 Local myalgia—unclassified

   11.8.5 Myofibrotic contracture

   11.8.6 Neoplasia

Table 9-3 Recommended diagnostic classification. Differentiation between arthrogenous and myogenous TMDs, and sub-classifications of each (Adapted from American Academy of Orofacial Pain, Okeson, J.P. (ed). Temporomandibular disorders: Guidelines for Classification, Assessment and Management. *Chicago: Quintessence, 1996)*

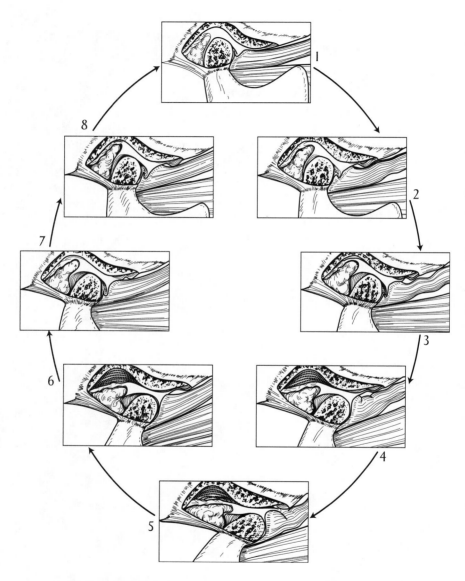

Fig. 9-4 Biomechanics of the temporomandibular joint (From Okeson, J.P. Management of Temporomandibular Disorders and Occlusion, 3rd ed. St Louis: Mosby Year Book, 1993. Used with permission)

Myositis—inflammation of a muscle, usually due to local causes such as infection or injury.

Clinical characteristics (delayed onset muscle soreness)
  increased pain with mandibular movement onset following prolonged or unaccustomed use (up to 48 hours afterward)

Clinical characteristics(generalized myositis)
  • pain, usually acute, in localized area
  • localized tenderness over entire region of the muscle
  • increased pain with mandibular movement
  • moderately to severely limited range of motion due to pain and swelling
  • onset following injury or infection

Management considerations
  • patient education
  • eliminate/minimize cause
  • restrict masticatory function
    ◊ avoid exercise, stretching, muscle injections
  • pharmacotherapy
    ◊ analgesic/anti-inflammatory
    ◊ antibiotic(?)
  • physical therapy
  • control parafunctional behavior(s)
  • stabilization occlusal orthosis

Protective muscle splinting—restricted or guarded mandibular movement due to co-contraction of muscles as a means of avoiding pain caused by movement of the parts.

Clinical characteristics
  • severe pain with function, but not at rest

- marked limited range of motion without significant increase on passive stretch

Management considerations
- patient education
- eliminate/reduce etiologic factor(s)
- restrict masticatory function to within painless limits
- stabilization occlusal orthosis
- pharmacotherapy
  ◊ analgesic/anti-inflammatory
  ◊ muscle relaxant
- control parafunctional behavior(s)
- physical therapy
  ◊ mobilization
  ◊ stretching

Myospasm (acute trismus, cramp)—an involuntary, sudden tonic contraction of a muscle.

Clinical characteristics
- acute pain
- continuous muscle contraction (fasciculation)
- increased EMG activity even at rest

Management considerations
- patient education
- eliminate cause
- restrict function to within painless limits
- pharmacotherapy
  ◊ muscle relaxant
  ◊ analgesic
- behavior modification
- physical therapy
- stabilization occlusal orthosis

Table 9-4 Acute extracapsular disorders

Myofascial pain—a regional, dull, aching pain and presence of localized tender spots (trigger points) in muscle, tendons, or fascia that reproduce pain when palpated and may produce a characteristic pattern of regional referred pain and/or autonomic symptoms on provocation.

Clinical characteristics
- regional pain, usually dull
- localized tenderness in firm bands of muscle and/or fascia
- reduction in pain with local muscle anesthetic injection or vapocoolant spray to trigger point followed by stretch

Management considerations
- patient education
- identify and eliminate etiologic/perpetuating factors
- restrict function to within painless limits
- pharmacotherapy
  ◊ analgesic/anti-inflammatory
  ◊ muscle relaxant
  ◊ sleep aid medication
  ◊ nutritional supplementation
- behavior modification
- physical therapy
  ◊ stretch and spray
  ◊ strengthening/stretching/rehabilitation
  ◊ postural re-education
  ◊ aerobic exercise program
  ◊ ergonomic awareness
- stabilization occlusal occlusal orthosis
- psychotherapy
  ◊ stress management
  ◊ relaxation training

◊ coping skill development
◊ biofeedback therapy
• trigger point injections

Contracture (chronic trismus, muscle fibrosis, muscle scarring)—a chronic resistance of a muscle to passive stretch as a result of fibrosis of the supporting tendons, ligaments, or muscle fibers themselves.

1. Myotatic- reversible condition
2. Myofibrotic- irreversible condition

Clinical characteristics
• limited range of motion
• unyielding firmness on passive stretch
• history of trauma or infection

Management considerations
• patient education
• restrict function to within painless limits
• pharmacotherapy
  ◊ analgesic/anti-inflammatory
  ◊ muscle relaxant
  ◊ nutritional supplementation
• behavior modification
• physical therapy
  ◊ stretch and spray
  ◊ strengthening/stretching/rehabilitation
  ◊ postural re-education
  ◊ ultrasound
• psychotherapy
  ◊ stress management
  ◊ relaxation training
  ◊ coping skill development

Table 9-5 Chronic extracapsular disorders

Arthrogenous TMD

The most common sign of TMD is TMJ clicking. General population based studies have reported clicking to occur in about 50% of those studied.[73] A recent magnetic resonance image study found 33% of non-patient controls to have a displacement of the TMJ articular disc.[74] However, 77% of the patient population in this study demonstrated TMJ discal displacement. Therefore, we must determine whether or not a natural course of TMD exists. Although the concept of natural progression has been suggested, there is currently no convincing evidence that TMJ clicking typically progresses to locking and degeneration, or that arthritic changes must develop in joints that lock.[75-77] It has been reported that most degenerating joints tend to become non-painful with time; however, as many as 16% of these individuals may experience pain long-term.[75-78]

Disc Derangement Disorders

Internal derangement is disturbed arrangement of intracapsular joint parts causing interference with smooth joint movement. In the TM,J it can relate to elongation, tear, or rupture of the capsule or ligaments, causing altered disc position or morphology (Fig. 9-5a and b).

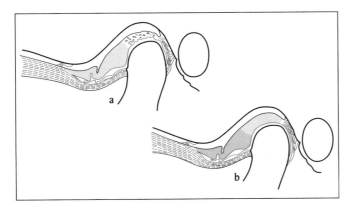

Fig. 9-5 a, b Anteriorly displaced articular disc (From Mahan, P.E., Alling, III, C.C. Facial Pain, 3rd ed. Philadelphia: Lea & Febiger, 1991)

Synovitis/capsulitis/retrodiscitis—an inflammation of the synovial lining, capsular, or retrodiscal tissues of the temporomandibular joint that can be due to infection, an immunologic condition secondary to articular surface degeneration, or trauma.

Diagnostic criteria (mandatory)
- localized TMJ pain exacerbated by function, especially with superior or posterior joint loading and palpation
- no extensive osteoarthritic changes with hard tissue imaging

Additional clinical findings (may exist)
- localized TMJ pain at rest
- limited range of motion secondary to pain
- fluctuating swelling (due to effusion) that decreases ability to occlude on ipsilateral posterior teeth
- ear pain

Management considerations
- patient education
- limit mandibular function
- pharmacotherapy
  - ◊ analgesic/NSAID
  - ◊ muscle relaxant if muscle splinting is determined, physical therapy directed at enhancing reduction of inflammation and ridding the area of inflammatory mediators/by-products control of parafunctional behavioral activities (bruxing/clenching) stabilization occlusal orthotic

Deviation in form—a painless mechanical dysfunction or altered function due to irregularities or aberrations in form of intracapsular soft and hard articular tissues (Fig. 9-6).

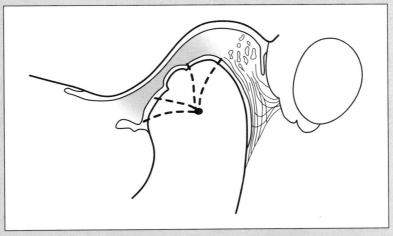

Fig. 9-6 Defect in form (From Mahan, P.E., Alling, III, C.C. Facial Pain, 3rd ed. Philadelphia: Lea & Febiger, 1991)

Diagnostic criteria
- complaint of faulty or compromised joint mechanics (e.g., joint noises, intermittent locking, or dislocation)
- reproducible joint noise usually at same position during opening and closing mandibular movement
- radiographic evidence of mild structural bony abnormality or loss of normal shape may also exist

Management considerations
- establish baseline and monitor over time
- control parafunctional behavior (bruxing/clenching)

Temporomandibular joint dislocation (open lock, subluxation)—a condition in which the condyle is positioned anterior to the articular eminence and is unable to return to a closed position. May be momentary or prolonged (Fig. 9-7).

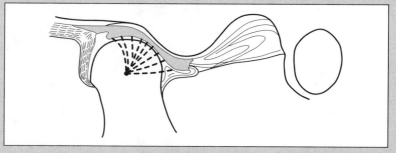

Fig. 9-7 Condylar subluxation/dislocation (From Mahan, P.E., Alling, III, C.C. Facial Pain, 3rd ed. Philadelphia: Lea & Febiger, 1991)

Diagnostic criteria
- inability to close the mouth without a specific manipulative maneuver, radiographic evidence revealing condyle well beyond the eminence, pain may be associated with the dislocation with mild residual pain after the episode

Management considerations
- patient education
- manual reduction
- pharmacotherapy
  ◊ if pain is intolerable, utilize auriculotemporal nerve block to alleviate TMJ pain and reduce muscle splinting
  ◊ muscle relaxant
  ◊ analgesic/NSAID for residual pain
- avoidance training
- surgery
  ◊ sclerosing solution
  ◊ arthroscopic laser cautery
  ◊ eminectomy

Table 9-6 Intracapsular disorders

Disc displacement with reduction—an abrupt alteration or interference of the disc-condyle structural relation during mandibular translation with mouth opening or closing.

Diagnostic criteria
- reproducible joint noise that occurs usually at variable positions during opening and closing mandibular movements
- soft tissue imaging revealing displaced disc that improves its position during jaw opening, and hard tissue imaging showing an absence of extensive degenerative bone changes

Additional clinical findings (may exist)
- pain, when present, precipitated by joint movement
- deviation during movement coinciding with a click
- no restriction in mandibular movement
- episodic and momentary catching of smooth jaw movement during mouth opening (<35 mm) that self-reduces with voluntary mandibular repositioning

Management considerations
- patient education
- restrict mandibular function during painful episodes-pharmacotherapy
  ◊ analgesic/NSAID
  ◊ muscle relaxant if significant muscle involvement identified
- stabilization occlusal orthotic
- control parafunctional behavior(s)
- monitor to assess progression

Disc displacement without reduction—an altered or misaligned disc-condyle structural relation that is maintained during mandibular translation (Fig. 9-8a, b, and c).

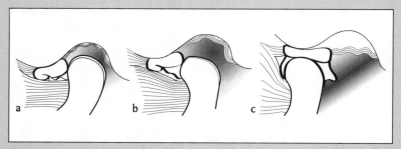

Fig. 9-8 a, b, c Biomechanics of the temporomandibular joint (From Okeson, J.P. Management of Temporomandibular Disorders and Occlusion, *3rd ed. St Louis: Mosby Year Book, 1993. Used with permission)*

Acute
Diagnostic criteria
- persistent marked limited mouth opening (<35 mm) with a history of sudden onset
- mandibular deflection to the affected side on mouth opening
- marked limited movement to the contralateral side (if unilateral disorder)
- soft tissue imaging revealing displaced disc without reduction, and hard tissue imaging revealing no extensive osteoarthritic changes

Additional clinical findings (may exist)
- pain precipitated by forced mouth opening
- history of clicking that ceased with the occurrence of "locking"
- pain with palpation of the affected joint (during acute stage)
- ipsilateral hyperocclusion (during acute stage)
- moderate osteoarthritic changes with hard tissue imaging (chronic stage)

<u>Chronic</u>

Diagnostic criteria
- history of sudden onset of limited mouth opening that occurred at some time in the past
- soft tissue imaging revealing displaced disc without reduction, and hard tissue imaging revealing no extensive osteoarthritic changes

Additional clinical findings (may exist)
- pain, when present, markedly reduced from acute stage, and usually presenting only as a feeling of stiffness
- history of clicking that resolved with sudden onset of locking
- moderate osteoarthritic changes with imaging of hard tissues
- radual resolution of limited mouth opening

Management considerations
- patient education
- manual reduction/mobilization
- pharmacotherapy
  - ◊ local anesthetic (auriculotemporal nerve block) to augment manual reduction
  - ◊ analgesic/NSAID
  - ◊ muscle relaxant if muscle splint identified
- restrict mandibular movement
- control parafunctional behavior(s)
- occlusal orthotic
  - ◊ stabilization orthotic - treatment of first choice
  - ◊ anterior repositioning orthotic- if stabilization orthotic is not effective regarding pain reduction

Table 9-7 Disc derangement disorders

Osteoarthritis (primary)—a degenerative condition of the joint characterized by deterioration and abrasion of the articular tissue and concomitant remodeling of the underlying subchondral bone due to overload on the remodeling mechanism.

Clinical characteristics
- pain with function
- point tenderness with palpation
- limited range of motion with mandibular deviation to the affected side on opening
- crepitus or multiple joint noises

Osteoarthritis (secondary)—a degenerative condition of the joint characterized by deterioration and abrasion of the articular tissue and concomitant remodeling of the underlying subchondral bone due to a prior event or disease that overloaded the remodeling mechanism.

Clinical characteristics
- a clearly documented disease or event associated with osteoarthritis
- pain with function
- point tenderness on palpation
- limited range of mandibular motion with deviation to the affected side on opening
- crepitus or multiple joint sounds

Management considerations
- patient education
- restricted function
- pharmacotherapy
  ◊ analgesic/NSAID
  ◊ muscle relaxant if muscle involvement identified

- control parafunctional behavior(s)
- stabilization occlusal orthotic
- physical therapy
  ◊ gentle range of motion exercises
  ◊ iontophoresis if anti-inflammatory medications not tolerated

Table 9-8 Degenerative joint diseases

Chronic TMD

The orofacial area is frequently associated with recurring or chronic pain. Recent studies reveal that the head and neck region is the most common site of the human body to be involved in a chronic pain condition.[79] Dworkin and Massoth reported that the most prevalent non-odontogenic orofacial pains are musculoskeletal in origin.[80] Currently, TMDs are viewed as a subgroup of commonly recurring musculoskeletal disorders with overlapping signs and symptoms. Importantly, a number of other conditions are frequently expressed concomitantly with TMD. Headache is another commonly occurring pain condition that is many times associated with TMD. Approximately 45 million Americans experience headache pain on a frequently recurring basis.[81] Neuropathic pain expressed in the orofacial region may complicate diagnosis and management of TMD. Although the vast majority of TMDs occur during middle age, there are a number of orofacial pain conditions such as trigeminal neuralgia, post-herpetic neuralgia, and temporal arteritis that are most commonly expressed in the elderly population. Due to the complexity of innervation and clinical presentation similarities, these conditions are at times inaccurately diagnosed and ineffectively managed, and thus become chronic. Von Korff et al. reported that the risks of developing chronic head/facial pain are 24.3% by age 50 and 33.8% by age 70.[82]

Condylar fracture—direct trauma to the mandible may result in fracture of the condylar process. In addition to bony involvement, soft tissues (disc, capsule, synovium, retrodiscal tissue, ligaments, and/or the articular surface) may also be affected. Fractures of the condylar process are typically unilateral and may occur in the condylar neck or within the capsule. Varying degrees of displacement of the proximal portion result. The degree and direction of the displacement are dependent upon the location of the fracture. The lateral pterygoid muscle will typically cause displacement in an anterior-medial-inferior direction.

Clinical characteristics
- associated with trauma
- preauricular pain and swelling
- limited opening
- if condylar fragment is displaced
  ◊ acute occlusal change (hyperocclusion on affected side)
  ◊ mandibular deviation to affected side

Management considerations
- closed or opened reduction
- intermaxillary fixation
- upon removal of intermaxillary fixation
  ◊ physical therapy to improve range of motion and recondition musculature
  ◊ stabilization/compensatory occlusal orthotic during healing phase

Table 9-9 Fractures

TMD represents a multitude of conditions afflicting the masticatory region with implications that transcend anatomic and neurologic boundaries. It must be appreciated that temporomandibular disorders are multifactorial in nature, encompassing both physical and psychosocial domains. There exists a significant variability among patients, indicating that there may be predisposition in some cases. Today's scientific study does suggest that both peripheral and central mechanisms, to include the sympathetic nervous system and compromise in the individual's pain dampening (modulating) system, play a major role in recurrent and chronic cases. Therefore, it is essential that a complete evaluation of the patient from historical, clinical presentation, and physical/psychological perspectives be accomplished. Finding all of the components of TMD/orofacial pain on a case-specific basis is necessary for a complete and accurate diagnosis and effective management.

Management Considerations

The primary goals of treatment of TMD are to reduce or eliminate pain, restore a more normal function, allow for a return to the activities of daily living, and reduce long-term health care needs for the problem. This can be accomplished by development of a diagnosis specific plan of care, utilizing reversible approaches in the vast majority of cases.[2,83-84] It is important to recognize that the natural history of TMD does not reflect a progressive disease process, but rather TMD appears to be a complex disorder that is affected by a multitude of interacting factors serving to maintain the disorder or result in recurrence.[2, 83-86]

There are numerous non-surgical modalities of treatment for TMD. Current understanding of TMD would suggest that treatment regimes frequently involve a multifaceted approach, in some cases necessitating an interdisciplinary team of health care professionals. This team approach not only helps to address the various aspects of the problem, but also enhances the overall potential for treatment success. Key questions in the development of an individualized plan of management include:

- Is intervention necessary?
  ◊ Is condition acute or chronic?
  ◊ Is condition progressive?
  ◊ What is the prognosis with and without treatment?

- To what degree do we intervene?
  ◊ Reversible versus irreversible treatment?
  ◊ Monodisciplinary versus multidisciplinary approach?

Patient Education and Self-Care

After determining a diagnosis, the clinician should explain to the patient the cause and the nature of his/her disorder and offer reassurance of the benign nature of the condition, if appropriate. It is very common for patients to present an emotionally distressed state, many times due to a lack of understanding of the severity and ramifications of their pain problem. Additionally, a significant number of TMD patients have recently experienced a significant life event such as marital conflict or death of a loved one. Suddenly, the patient may focus on the pain and jaw dysfunction he/she had been experiencing and successfully coping with for many years, and may perceive these symptoms as the first signs of a more serious disease.[30] A thorough explanation of the problems may be all that is required to alleviate the fears, emotional stress, and para/pathofunctional behavior such as bruxism or maladaptive posture.

A cornerstone of management is self-care that is based on the patient's knowledge of their pain concern. The aim of a self-care program is to prevent further injury to the musculoskeletal system and to allow for a period of healing to take place. The success of self-care depends on patient motivation, cooperation, and compliance. Self-directed care typically includes:

- Limitation of mandibular function
- Habit awareness and modification
- A home exercise program
- Stress management

Voluntary limitation of mandibular function promotes rest for the injured muscular or articular structures. The patient is advised to maintain a soft diet and to avoid foods that require a great deal of chewing. The patient should avoid wide openings such as associated with yawning or singing, chewing gum, and any other activities that would promote excessive mandibular function. Habits involving excessive jaw function should be identified and eliminated. Clenching, bruxism, or maladaptive tongue-posturing habits must be addressed. However, these habitual behaviors are often difficult to control without clinical intervention, because of the complex psychophysiological factors inherent in these parafunctional activities.[87-88]

A home exercise program will help to reinforce the patient's self-control of his/her TMD. Additionally, an individualized regimen can aid in a more rapid recovery and rehabilitation of the compromised masticatory system. Massage of the affected muscles with application of moist heat will help to soothe aching or fatigued muscles by stimulating relaxation and pain relief. Gentle range of motion exercises are beneficial in both myogenous and arthrogenous disorders. Controlled mandibular movement can encourage the production of a physiologic quality and quantity of synovial fluid, thus enhancing joint lubrication, nutrition, and minimizing the accumulation of metabolic by-products and pain-mediating substances.

Emotional stress often has a significant and adverse influence on the course of TMD. Identification of the source(s) of stress and patient realization of the association between pain and stress are necessary in order that a patient may positively alter his/her lifestyle. Alteration of thought process is not an easy task and may require professional assistance in the nature of a clinical and health psychologist.

The most important aspect of self-care is ongoing encouragement and reinforcement by the clinician during regular follow-up visits. There are many instances where self-care must be supplemented by additional clinical intervention. However, the emphasis on patient self-control and participation in his/her own care must always remain paramount during the course of treatment.[2]

Pharmacotherapy

Medications are often prescribed in conjunction with other forms of treatment for TMD. When utilized as part of a case-specific comprehensive management program, pharmacotherapy can be a valuable adjunct to relief of symptoms.[2, 83-84] No one drug has been proven to be effective for all cases of TMD. Clinicians must be well versed with the different families of drugs that are commonly used to treat musculoskeletal conditions, in particular their potential for interactions with other drugs and their side effects.

Non-steroidal anti-inflammatory drugs (NSAID)

This category of medications is effective in the management of mild to moderate pain and inflammatory conditions, particularly those of musculoskeletal origin. The analgesic effect is typically achieved prior to the anti-inflammatory effect. Common side effects include gastric disturbance, inhibition of platelet aggregation, tinnitus/dizziness, and renal/liver toxicity. A list of those NSAIDs most commonly utilized is provided in Table 9-10. It is important to recognize that NSAIDS differ in formulation, efficacy, and toxicity. If one NSAID is not effective, a clinical trial of one from another chemical class may be warranted.

Steroids

Steroids are typically indicated in cases of non-infectious inflammation such as synovitis when NSAIDs are not effective. Utilization of these medications in injectable form is also indicated in cases of tendonitis or

Category	Generic	Brand	Dose (mg.)
Salicylates	ASA	Bayer	q4h (300)
	salsalate	Disalcid	bid, tid (500)
	diflunisal	Dolobid	bid, tid (500)
Proprionic Acid	ibuprofen	Motrin	tid, qid (600-800)
	Naproxen sodium	Naprosyn	qid (375)
Acetic Acid	indomethacin	Indocin*	tid (25-50)
COX 2 Inhibitors	celecoxib	Celebrex	qd, bid (100-200)
	rofecoxib	Vioxx	qd, bid (12.5-25) (max.- 25 mg/day)
	valdecoxib	Bextra	qd (10-20)

Utilization of Indomethacin for prolonged periods has been associated with accumulation in the sclera of the eye and significant gastrointestinal side effects.

Table 9-10 Non-steroidal anti-inflammatory drugs

tenomyositis where oral medications would provide decreased levels of effectiveness due to the decreased blood flow to these areas. Multiple injections into joints have been demonstrated to exacerbate degenerative processes. Side effects include decreased resistance to infection, fluid retention, weight gain due to redistribution of body fat, painless myopathy, suppression of hypothalamic-pituitary-adrenal axis, osteoporosis, and fixation of mood (euphoria or depression) with only short-term use. Steroidal medications commonly used are listed in Table 9-11.

(methylprednisolone) Medrol Dosepak	4 mg tablets
(betamethasone) Celestone	6 mg/cc
(dexamethasone) Decadron	4 mg/cc

Table 9-11 Steroids

Muscle relaxants

Centrally-acting muscle relaxants are frequently used in the treatment of TMD. It is difficult to ascertain whether the major effect is due to their selective effect on relieving muscle spasm or from their general action as a sedative. Animal studies have shown relief of skeletal muscle spasm only at much higher doses than are prescribed clinically in humans.[86] Primary indications are for muscle spasm and muscle sprain or strain. Side effects include excessive sedation, lightheadedness, and dizziness. Muscle relaxants commonly utilized in TMD are listed in Table 9-12. Note that Diazepam, a benzodiazepine classified as an anxiolytic, is also used as a muscle relaxant when prescribed in low doses and is included in this category. Carisoprodol has recently been found to be associated with significant addiction potential due to the effects of the active metabolite mebrobamate.

Generic	Brand	Dose (mg)
carisoprodol	Soma	350 mg tid
methocarbinol	Robaxin	750 mg tid
cyclobenzaprine*	Flexeril	10 mg tid
diazepam	Valium	2-5 mg tid

*Cyclobenzaprine is chemically related to the tricyclic antidepressant class of drugs. It has been shown to provide significant relief of muscle pain and enhance sleep quality and quantity. The combination of cyclobenzaprine (at bedtime) and a NSAID can be very effective in managing acute TMD. Due to excessive sedation and impaired ambulatory ability, muscle relaxants should be used cautiously during waking hours.

Table 9-12 Muscle relaxants

Antianxiety agents

In the cases where high levels of emotional stress are associated with TMD, anxiolytic agents such as benzodiazepines may be utilized to help the patient cope by helping reduce their perception or reaction to stress.

Agents such as Diazepam can be used as supportive therapy; however, due to the significant potential for dependency and/or addiction, these medications should not be prescribed for more than a consecutive 10-day period when utilized multiple times per day and not longer than 3 weeks when utilized at bedtime as a sleep aid/sleep inducing medication. In many cases, the clinician may desire the assistance of a physician in the management of levels of anxiety requiring pharmacotherapeutic management. Side effects include drowsiness and nausea. These agents are contraindicated in cases of narrow-angle glaucoma. Table 9-13 lists those anxiolytic agents typically utilized in TMD, sleep disturbances to include insomnia, and movement disorders such as bruxism.

Generic	Brand	Dose (mg)
diazepam	Valium	2-5 mg tid
clonazepam	Klonopin	0.5-1 mg tid
lorazepam	Ativan	0.5-1 mg tid
temazepam	Restoril	15-30 mg qhs

Table 9-13 Antianxiety agents

Opioids

Opioids act on specific opioid receptor sites in the central nervous system, conferring a central analgesic effect. This effect is not confined to pain arising from inflammatory processes alone. At usual clinical doses, opioids dampen the patient's emotional response to pain in addition to eliminating or reducing the pain sensation. These medications are best indicated for moderate to severe pain over a short period of time. Typical indications for opioids in the TMD patient population include acute exacerbations of pain, post-operatively, and trauma. Most common side effects are nausea, respiratory depression, and physical dependence. Opioids may be considered in cases of pain refractory to appropriately integrated multidisciplinary care, when properly monitored.

Local anesthetics

Local anesthetics can be of tremendous value as both a diagnostic tool and, in select cases, a therapeutic modality. Indications are as a diagnostic block and in the management of myofascial pain trigger points. The clinician must be aware of the muscle toxicity effects that increase with the profundity of the anesthetic. Injections into skeletal muscle with local anesthetics that contain a vasoconstrictor have an enhanced, undesirable myotoxicity.

The use of diagnostic anesthesia may be an integral component of clinical evaluation of the TMD patient. Diagnostic anesthesia may be as simple as use of a topically applied agent or involve diagnostic injections including somatic blocks (infiltration, field blocks, and division blocks), trigger point injections, temporomandibular joint injections, and/or sympathetic neural blockade. Anesthetic blocks may be utilized to determine if the pain is the result of pathology peripheral to the point of the block. Typically, lidocaine or carbocaine without vasoconstrictor is recommended, especially when injecting into muscle tissue (to minimize myotoxic effects) or anesthetizing the TMJ (to minimize the potential for abuse). Myofascial trigger point injections may result in abolishment of pain at the trigger point as well as at the site(s) of referral.

When utilizing diagnostic anesthesia, several key factors must be kept in mind. First, the procedure should alleviate 100% of that component of the patient's chief complaint. For example, if the complaint is TMJ pain, then anesthetizing via auriculotemporal block should result in resolution of the pain. However, it is quite common for TMJ and masticatory muscle pain to co-exist, therefore, the muscular component of the pain complaint would remain. Second, the relief should last for the expected duration of the anesthetic. Due to the release of endogenous opioids (endorphin, enkephlin) some patients will report a short-term (five to seven minutes) resolution of their pain. The clinician must also be conscious of the potential for a placebo response. Short-term relief of pain following local anesthesia does not always indicate that an irreversible procedure will result in long-lasting relief. Diagnostic anesthesia must be interpreted in context with historical, clinical, and laboratory findings.

Antidepressants

In low doses, tricyclic antidepressants such as amitriptyline, doxepin, and imipramine have been shown to be beneficial in the treatment of chronic musculoskeletal conditions. The analgesic properties of the tricyclic antidepressants are independent of the antidepressant effect, the latter of which requires higher doses. Therapeutically, these drugs are particularly useful for TMD patients with chronic pain, sleep disturbance, and depression. It has also been suggested that these medications are effective in the treatment of certain types of nocturnal bruxism and various oral dysethesias, such as burning mouth/tongue.[89-90] Side effects are mainly related to their anticholinergic activity that induces xerostomia, constipation, fluid retention, and weight gain. One of the most bothersome side effects is sedation upon awakening. This problem may be reduced by having the patient take the medication earlier in the evening. These medications are contraindicated in individuals with cardiac arrhythmias, seizure disorder (controlled and uncontrolled), and those suffering from panic attacks. Table 9-14 lists some commonly utilized drugs in this class. Dosage should begin at the lowest level (10 mg) at bedtime and be increased each week only if needed and tolerated.

Generic	Brand	Dose (mg)
amitriptyline	Elavil	10-75
desipramine	Norpramin	10-50
nortriptyline	Pamelor	10-75
doxepin	Sinequan	10-75

Table 9-14 Antidepressant agents

Physical therapy/physical medicine

The goal of physical therapy/medicine is to restore normal mandibular function. Rehabilitation of the compromised masticatory system may require various physical techniques that serve to relieve musculoskeletal pain and promote healing of tissues.[91] Close cooperation with a physical therapist/physical medicine practitioner who is well versed in the management of musculoskeletal disorders of the head and neck is essential. One or more of the following techniques may be indicated in the management of myogenous and/or arthrogenous TMD:

Massage. Gentle massage over the painful areas is thought to produce an alteration in sensory input that exerts an inhibitory influence on pain. Therapeutic massage is used to temporarily reduce edema and increase local blood flow to the area. The technique is demonstrated by the physiotherapist and the patient is encouraged to gently massage painful muscle areas at regular intervals throughout the day, provided that pain relief is attained.

Joint mobilization. Physical manipulation by gentle, low impact, passive, joint stretching and joint distraction can be used in cases of restricted mouth opening resulting from myofascial pain and/or internal derangement. The goal of this treatment is to passively restore joint motion and improve joint function by repeated digital manipulation of the jaws by the physiotherapist. Prior to manipulation, it is essential that the patient's symptoms of pain and muscle spasm are brought under control by other appropriate means.

Jaw exercises. Jaw exercises are helpful in increasing muscle strength and coordination and increasing stability and range of motion of the TMJs. There are three basic types of exercise, each of which serves a particular purpose. Muscle strength is addressed by isometric exercises. Isotonic exercises are used to increase range of motion. Coordination of muscle function is achieved by repetitive rhythmic exercises. Jaw exercises are helpful in addressing specific problems and should be continually modified as symptoms change. Prior control of symptoms is the key to the success of these exercises, which would otherwise be impossible to undertake on a patient with pain and muscle hypertonicity. Once the patient has attained the goals of treatment, a maintenance program of exercise is advised to ensure long-term resolution of symptoms.

Physical modalities. The most common physical modalities used for the treatment of TMD are superficial heat and cold, ultrasound, short-wave diathermy, trancutaneous electrical nerve stimulation (TENS),[92] and iontophoresis. The use of heat, particularly when applied to areas of muscle spasm, can help relax the muscle and increase blood flow to the compromised muscle. Short-wave diathermy and ultrasound are simply extensions of heat therapy. Short-wave diathermy only provides heat to superficial tissues; whereas, ultrasound can transmit heat through tissues to a depth of 5 cm. The purpose of the use of these modalities is to decrease pain and increase tissue distensibility. TENS uses a low-voltage electrical current that is designed for sensory counterstimulation in painful disorders. It is used to decrease muscle pain and hyperactivity and may also be useful in neuromuscular re-education.[91-92] Iontophoresis utilizes a low-voltage generator to push like-charged ions of therapeutic substances such as dexamethasone or lidocaine into tender, swollen tissues.

Postural re-education. Maladaptive posture (head/neck or mandibular) may result in excessive strain being placed on the masticatory system. Postural re-education is frequently a necessary component of care in the TMD patient. The interdependence of the trigeminal distribution and the upper cervical region is well recognized. Long-term stabilization of the masticatory system may be enhanced through physiotherapist-guided, patient-implemented postural correction through behavior modification/exercises.

Behavioral/psychotherapy

The TMD patient's cognitive, emotional, and behavioral responses to pain are key issues in the overall evaluation and treatment of his/her pain. The patient's perception of and response to the pain may be maladaptive in the nature of somatization, catastrophizing, mood, or subconscious habitual behavior. Failure to identify and address these factors will likely significantly compromise treatment outcomes. Cognitive-behavioral strategies such as behavior modification, life-style counseling, progressive relaxation, guided imagery, hypnosis, and biofeedback may be beneficial.[93-94] A combination of behavioral strategies appears to work better than individual treatments. These approaches can significantly alter the patient's maladaptive behavior and enhance TMD management outcomes. This care would typically be provided by a clinical and health psychologist. It is important for the clinician to realize that psychotherapy is an adjunct to pain management. Psychotherapy does not predictably eliminate the pain unless there is a neuropsychiatric cause for the pain. However, a clear and well-directed thought process can certainly result in enhanced coping mechanisms and elevated tolerance of pain.

Occasionally, TMD may be related to an underlying psychological or psychiatric disorder such as depression or conversion disorder.[93-94] The best indicator of this possibility is when a patient's suffering appears to be excessive or persistent beyond what one would normally expect to see in light of the disorder itself. In such cases, it is important for the clinician to identify the psychological connotations through a careful history and take note of any unusual behavior that may become apparent during the consultation. In these cases, a psychiatric or clinical and health psychology referral would be indicated.

Occlusal appliance therapy

The most common form of treatment for TMD is occlusal appliance therapy. An occlusal appliance is a removable device, usually made of hard acrylic, that is custom made to fit over the occlusal surfaces of the teeth in one arch, either the maxilla or mandible. There are generally two types of occlusal appliances in use—the flat plane (stabilization) appliance (Fig. 9-9) and the anterior repositioning appliance. The effects of appliance therapy include:

- Prevention/reduction in abrasion to the dentition
- Alteration of the motor pattern of the masticatory musculature by altering periodontal ligament proprioception
- Alteration of muscle length
- Enhanced patient awareness of masticatory parafunctional behavior
- Alteration of the number, direction, location, and quality of tooth contacts

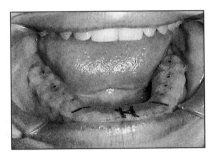

Fig. 9-9 Mandibular stabilization splint adjusted to suggested criteria (From Okeson, J.P. Management of Temporomandibular Disorders and Occlusion, 3rd ed. St Louis: Mosby Year Book, 1993. Used with permission)

The major functions of non-directive, flat plane (stabilization) appliance therapy are muscle relaxation, dispersal of forces, enhanced TMJ stability, and protection of the teeth from abnormal forces such as associated with bruxism.[2,95] The appliance is fabricated to cover all the teeth in the arch. Figure 9-9 provides an example of a mandibular stabilization appliance.

Criteria for optimum treatment effects include:

- Stable and retentive
- Bilateral equal intensity posterior occlusal contacts so that an environment of a stable physiological mandibular posture (typically in centric relation or adapted centric relation) is created

- Canine guidance in lateral and protrusive excursions of the mandible
- Smooth transition from cuspid-guided occlusion to the most anterior tooth available beyond cuspid edge to edge position (crossover)
- No distalizing contacts that would serve to cause compression of vascularized, innervated retrodiscal tissues

Importantly, as pain, muscle activity, and inflammation subside, the resulting changes in maxillo-mandibular relationships must be compensated for by regular adjustments to the appliance. Most patients are advised to utilize the appliance while sleeping or when their activity prohibits conscious awareness of daytime clenching/parafunction. With improvement, the patient is gradually weaned off the appliance if possible. However, many patients experience sleep-related bruxism, a recognized movement disorder associated with disturbed sleep. Long-term wear of an appliance while sleeping may be necessary in selected cases. If there is no improvement within the first two to four weeks, then the patient should be re-evaluated for other factors that may require a partial or complete change in treatment regime.

Anterior repositioning appliances are used less often because repositioning of the mandible over a period of time can result in irreversible changes to the occlusion such as bilateral posterior open bites. The purpose of these appliances is to alter the structural condyle-disc-fossa relationship in an effort to decrease adverse joint loading.[2,96] Although compression of the retrodiscal tissues may be reduced by positioning the mandible forward, the clinician must remember that the TMJ remains loaded when utilizing these devices. Recent studies looking at fluid film pressures within the TMJ in various circumstances raise questions as to the routine utility of this approach.

Complications associated with occlusal appliance therapy arise from poor design/construction and/or excessive or incorrect use of the appliance. Poor design of an occlusal appliance may result in unwanted tooth movement during active treatment. Excessive use of an occlusal appliance may lead to a psychological dependence on the appliance.[2,95] There should be a general time frame within which the appliance should be expected to achieve the desired result.

•

Conclusion

Based upon current understanding of TMD, successful management is dependent upon recognizing several basic principles:

- TMD represents a musculoskeletal disorder that is many times overlaid with psychosocial issues
- Limit the use of invasive and irreversible approaches to care to cases where there is a high probability that the procedure will eliminate or significantly reduce the complaint
- Do not escalate physical treatments without comprehensive re-evaluation to include psychological and behavioral aspects
- Ongoing pain can become a disease in and of itself
- Complete and accurate diagnosis on a case-specific basis will provide for the development of the most efficacious individualized approach to care
- Many cases of TMD will be best managed by a multidisciplinary team involving dentists, physiotherapists, psychologists, and various medical disciplines

Notes

[1] Lipton, J.A., Ship, J.A., and Larach-Robinson, D. Estimated Prevalence and distribution of reported orofacial pain in the United States. *JADA*, 1993,124:115-121

[2] Okeson, J.P., ed. *Orofacial pain: guidelines for assessment, diagnosis and management.* Chicago: Quintessence Publishing Co., Inc., 1996:113-84

[3] Dworkin, S.F., Huggins, K.H., LeResche, L., et al. Epidemiology of signs and symptoms of temporomandibular disorders: clinical signs in cases and controls. *JADA*, 1990; 120:273-81

[4] National Institute of Health Technology and Assessment Conference. *Management of Temporomandibular Disorders.* NIH Technol Assess Statement April 29-May-1 1996; p. 1-31

[5] Slavkin, H.C. Lifetime of Motion: Temporomandibular Joints. *JADA*, 1996,127:1,093-98

[6] McNeill, C, ed. *Temporomandibular disorders: guidelines for classification, assessment, and management.* (2nd ed) Chicago: Quintessence Publishing Co., Inc., 1993

[7] Ohrbach, R., and Gale, E.N. Pressure pain thresholds, clinical assessment and differential diagnosis: reliability and validity in patients with myogenic pain. *Pain* 1989; 39:157-69

[8] Sessle, B.J., Hu, J.W., Amano, N., et al. Convergence of cutaneous, tooth pulp, visceral, neck and muscle afferents onto nocieptive and nonnocieptive neurons in trigeminal subnucleus caudalis (medullary dorsal horn) and its implications for referred pain. *Pain*, 1986; 27:219-35

9 Rugh, J.D., and Solberg, W.K. Oral health status in the United States. *J Dent Educ* 1985; 49:398-404

10 Schiffman, E., and Fricton, J.R. Epidemiology of TMJ and craniofacial pain. In *TMJ and Craniofacial Pain: Diagnosis and Management*, edited by Fricton, J.R., and Kroening, R.J., Hathaway, K.M. St. Louis: Ishiaku Euro American Publ, 1988, p. 1-10

11 Agerberg, G., and Carlsson, G.E. Functional disorders of the masticatory system. I. Distribution of symptoms according to age and sex as judged from investigation by questionnaire. *Acta Odontol Scand*, 1972, 30:597-613

12 Helkimo, M. Studies on function and dysfunction of the masticatory system. I: An epidemiological investigation of symptoms of dysfunction in Lapps in the North of Finland. *Proc Finn Dent Soc*, 1974, 70:37-49

13 Glass, E.G., McGlynn, F.D., Glaros, A.G. et al. Prevalence of temporomandibular disorder symptoms in a major metropolitan area. *J Craniomand Pract*, 1993, 11:217-20

14 Heft, M.W. Prevalence of TMJ signs and symptoms in the elderly. *Gerontology* 1984, 3:125-30

15 Garro, L.C., Stephenson, K.A., and Good, B.J. Chronic Illness of the Temporomandibular Joints as Experienced by Support-group Members. *J Gen Intern Med*, 1994, 9:372-78

16 Howard, J.A. Temporomandibular joint disorders, facial pain and dental problems of performing artists. In *Textbook of Performing Arts Medicine*, edited by Sataloff, R., Brandfonbrener, A., and Lederman, R. New York: Raven Press, 1991:111-69

[17] Von Korff, M., Dworkin, S.F., Le Resche, L., and Kruger, A. An epidemiologic comparison of pain complaints. *Pain*, 1988, 32:173-83

[18] Goulet, J.P., Lavigne, G.J., and Lund, J.P. Jaw pain prevalence among French-speaking Canadians and related symptoms of temporomandibular disorders. *J Dent Res*, 1995, 74:1738-44

[19] Nilner, M., and Lassing, S.A. Prevalence of functional disturbances and diseases of the stomatognathic system in 7-14 year olds. *Swed Dent J*, 1981, 5:173-87

[20] Wanaman, A., and Agerberg, G. Mandibular dysfunction in adolescents. I. Prevalence of signs and symptoms. *Acta Odontal Scand*, 1986, 44:47-54

[21] LeResche, L. Epidemiology of temporomandibular disorders: implications for investigation of etiologic factors. *Crit Rev Oral Biol Med* 1997, 8(3):291-305

[22] Levitt, S.R., and McKinney, M.W. Validating the TMJ scale in a national sample of 10,000 patients: Demographic and epidemiologic characteristics. *J Orofacial Pain*, 1994, 8:25-35

[23] Skeppar, J., and Nilner, M. Treatment of craniomandibular disorders in children and young adults. *J Orofacial Pain*, 1993, 7:362-69

[24] Bates, R.E. Jr., Gremillion, H.A., and Stewart, C.M. Degenerative Joint Disease. Part II: Symptoms and Examination Findings. *J Craniomandib Pract*, 1994, 12(2):88-92

[25] Fillingim, R.B., and Maixner, W. Gender Differences in the Responses to Noxious Stimuli. *Pain Forum*, 1995, 4(4):209-21

26 Robinson, M.E., Riley, J.L., Brown, F.F., and Gremillion, H.A. Sex differences in response to cutaneous anesthesia: a double blind randomized study. *Pain*, 1998, 77(2):143-9

27 Dolwick, M.F. Clinical diagnosis of temporomandibular joint internal derangement and myofascial pain and dysfunction. *Oral Maxillofac Surg Clin North Am*, 1989, 1:1-6

28 Clark, G.T., Seligman, D.A., Solberg, W.K., and Pullinger, A.G. Guidelines for the examination and diagnosis of tempormandibular disorders. *J Craniomandib Disord Facial Oral Pain*, 1989, 3:7-14

29 Ochs, M.W., LaBanc, J.P., and Dolwick, M.F. The diagnosis and management of concomitant dentofacial deformity and temporomandibular disorder *Oral Maxillofac Clin North Am*, 1990, 2:669-90

30 Duinkerke, A.S., Luteijn, F., Bouman, T.K., and de Jong, H.P. Relations between TMJ pain dysfunction syndrome (PDS) and some psychological biographical variables. *Comm Dent Oral Epidemiol*, 1985, 13:185-89

31 Anderson, H.I., Ejlertsson, G., Leden, I., et al. Chronic pain in a geographically defined general population: studies of differences in age, gender, social class, and pain localization. *Clin J Pain*, 1993, 9:174-82

32 Rollman, G.B., and Harris, G. The detectability, discriminability, and perceived magnitude of painful electrical shock. *Percept Psychophys*, 1987, 42:257-68

[33] Biederman, J.J., and Schefft, B.K. Behavioral, physiological, and self-evaluative effects of anxiety on the self-control of pain. *Behav Modif*, 1994, 18:89-105

[34] Cornwall, A., and Donderi, D.C. The effect of experimentally induced anxiety on the experience of pressure pain. *Pain*, 1988, 35:105-113

[35] Cougher, M.J., Goldstein, D., and Leight, K.A. Induced anxiety and pain. *J Anxiety Disord*, 1987, 1:259-64

[36] Clark, G.T., Beemsterboer, P.L., and Jacobson, R. The effect of sustained submaximal clenching on maximum voluntary bite force in myofascial pain dysfunction patients. *J Oral Rehab*, 1984, 11:387

[37] Clark, G.T., and Carter, M.C. Electromyographic study of human and recovery at various isometric force levels. *Arch Oral Biol*, 1985, 30:563

[38] Clark, G.T., Carter, M.C., and Beemsterboer, P.L. Analysis of electromyographic signals in human jaw closing muscles at various isometric force levels. *Arc Oral Biol*, 1988, 33:833

[39] Miller, A. Mandibular Muscle Pain and Craniomandibular Muscle Function. In *Craniomandibular Muscles: Their Role In Function and Form*. Boca Raton: CRC Press, 1991, 181-206

[40] Bengtsson, A., Henriksson, K.G., Jorfeldt, L., et al. Primary fibromyalgia: a clinical and laboratory study of 55 patients. *Scand J Rheumatol*, 1986, 15:340-47

[41] Bengtsson, A., Henriksson, K.G., and Larsson, J. Muscle biopsy in primary fibromyalgia: light microscopical and histochemical findings. *Scand J Rheumatol*, 1986, 15:1-6

[42] Awad, E.A. Interstitial myofibrositis: Hypothesis of the mechanism. *Arch Phys Med Rehabil*, 1973, 54:449

[43] Tanne, K., Tanaka, E., and Sakuda, M. Association between malocclusion and temporomandibular disorders in orthodontic patients before treatment. *J Orofac Pain*, 1993, 7(2):156-62

[44] Dijkstra, P.U., de bont, L.G., Stegenga, B., et al. Temporomandibular joint osteoarthrosis and generalized joint hypermobility. *J Craniomandib Pract*, 1992, 10:221-27

[45] Westling, L. Temporomandibular joint dysfunction and systemic joint laxity. *Swed Dent J*, 1992, Suppl. 81

[46] Covington, P. Women's oral health issues: an exploration of the literature. *Probe* 1996, 30(5):173-77

[47] Zakrzewska, J.M. Women as dental patients: are there gender differences? *Int Dent J*, 1996, 46(6):548-57

[48] Meisler, J.G. Chronic pain conditions in women. *J Women's Health*, 1999, 8(3):313-20

[49] Milam, S.B., Aufdemorte, T.B., Sheridan, P.J., et al. Sexual dimorphism in the distribution of estrogen receptors in the temporomandibular joint complex of the baboon. *Oral Surg Oral Med Oral Path*, 1987, 64:527-32

[50] Aufdemorte, T.B., Van, S.I., Dolwick, M.V., et al. Estrogen receptors in the temporomandibular joint of the baboon (*Papio cynocephalus*): an autoradiographic study. *Oral Surg Oral Med Oral Path*, 1986, 61:307-14

[51] Abubaker, A.O., Raslan, W.F., and Sotereanos, G.C. Estrogen and progesterone receptors in temporomandibular joint discs of symptomatic and asymptomatic persons: a preliminary study. *J Oral Maxillofac Surg*, 1993, 51:1,096-1,100

[52] Haskin, C.L., Milam, S.B., and Cameron, I.L. Pathogenesis of degenerative joint disease in the human temporomandibular joint. *Crit Rev Oral Biol Med*, 1995, 6(3):248-77

[53] Petty, B.G., Cornblath, D.R., Adornato, B.T., et al. The effect of systemically administered recombinant human nerve growth factor in healthy subjects. *Ann Neurol*, 1994, 36(2):244-6

[54] Nitzan, D.W. Intraarticular Pressure in the Functioning Human Temporomandibular Joint and Its Alteration by Uniform Elevation of the Occlusal Plane. *J Oral Maxillofac Surg*, 1994, 52:671-79

[55] Milam, S.B. Articular disk displacements and degenerative temporomandibular joint disease. In *Temporomandibular disorders and related pain conditions*, edited by Sessle, B.J., Bryant, P.S., and Dionne, R.A. Seattle: IASP Press, 1995, 89-112

[56] Milam, S.B., Zardeneta, G., and Schmitz, J.P. Oxidative Stress and Degenerative Temporomandibular Joint Disease: A Proposed Hypothesis. *J Oral Maxillofac Surg*, 1998, 56:214-23

57 Rugh, J.D., and Smith, B.R. Mastication. In *Textbook of Occlusion*, edited by Mohl, N.C., Zarb, G.A., Carlsson, G.E., et al. Chicago: Quintessence, 1988, 143-52

58 Brown, F.F., Robinson, M.E., Riley, J.L., and Gremillion, H.A. Pain severity, negative affect, and microstressors as predictors of life interference in TMD patients. *J Craniomandib Pract*, 1996, 14(1):63-70

59 Holzberg, A.D., Robinson, M.E., Geisser, M.E., and Gremillion, H.A. The effects of depression on psychosocial and physical functioning. *Clin J Pain*, 1996, 12(2):118-125

60 Riley III, J.L., Robinson, M.E., Kvaal, S.A., and Gremillion, H.A. Effects of physical and sexual abuse in facial pain: direct or mediated? *J Craniomandib Pract*, 1998, 16(4):259-66

61 Travell, J.G., and Simons, D.G. *Myofascial Pain and Dysfunction: The trigger point manual*. Vol. 1, Baltimore: Williams and Wilkins, 1983, p. 115

62 DeBoever, J.A., and Keersmaekers, K. Trauma in patients with temporomandibular disorders: frequency and treatment outcome. *J Oral Rehabil*, 1996, 23(2):91-6

63 McGivney, G.P., ed. Glossary of Prosthodontic Terms. *J Prosth Dent*, 1994, 71(1):50-112

64 Gremillion, H.A. TMD and Maladaptive Occlusion: Does a Link Exist? *J Craniomandib Pract*, 1995;13(4):205-6

[65] Pullinger, A.G., Seligman, D.A., and Gornbein, J.A. A Multiple Logistic Regression Analysis of the Risk and Relative Odds of Temporomandibular Disorders as a Function of Common Occlusal Features. *J Dent Res*, 1993, 72(6):968-79

[66] McNamara Jr, J.A., Seligman, D.A., and Okeson, J.P. The relationship of occlusal factors and orthodontic treatment to temporomandibular disorders. In *Temporomandibular Disorders and Related Pain Conditions*, edited by Sessle, B.J., Bryant, P.S., Dionne, R.A. Seattle: IASP Press, 1995: 399-427

[67] Zonnenberg, A.J., Van Maanen, C.J., Oostendorp, R.A., et al. Body posture photographs as a diagnostic aid for musculoskeletal disorders related to temporomandibular disorders (TMD). *J Craniomandib Pract*, 1996, 14(3):225-32

[68] Carlson, C.R., Okeson, J.P., Falace, D.A., et al. Reduction of pain and EMG activity in the masseter region by trapezius trigger point injection. *Pain*, 1993, 155:397-400

[69] Burgess, J.A., Kolbinson, D.A., Lee, P.T., et al. Motor vehicle accidents and TMDS: assessing the relationship. *JADA*, 1996, 127(12):1767-72

[70] Ware, J.C., and Rugh, J.D. Destructive Bruxism: Sleep Stage Relationship. *Sleep*, 1988, 11:172-81

[71] Dworkin, S.F., Huggins, K.H., LeResche, L., et al. Epidemiology of signs and symptoms in temporomandibular disorders: clinical signs in cases and controls. *JADA*, 1990, 120:273-81

[72] Schiffman, E., Fricton, J.R., Haley, D., et al. The prevalence and treatment needs of subjects with temporomandibular disorders. *JADA*, 1990, 120:295-304

73 Wabeke, K.B., and Spruijt, R.J. *On Temporomandibular Joint Sounds: Dental and Psychological Studies* [Thesis]. Amsterdam: University of Amsterdam, 1994, 91-103

74 Ribeiro, R.F., Tallents, R.H., Katzberg, R.W., et al. The prevalence of disc displacement in symptomatic and asymptomatic volunteers aged 6 to 25 years. *J Orofacial Pain*, 1997, 11(1):37-47

75 Nikerson, J.W., and Boering, G. Natural course of osteoarthrosis as it relates to internal derangement of the temporomandibular joint. *Oral Maxillofac Surg Clin North Am*, 1989, 1:1-19

76 de Bont, L.F., Dijkgraaf, L.C., and Stegenga, B. Epidemiology and natural progression of articular temporomandibular disorders. *Oral Surg Oral Med Oral Pathol Oral Radiol Endod*, 1997, 83(1):72-6

77 de Leeuw, R. Boering, G., Stegenga, B., et al. Clinical signs of TMJ osteoarthrosis and internal derangement 30 years after nonsurgical treatment. *J Orofac Pain*, 1994, 8(1):18-24

78 Toller, P.A. Osteoarthritis of the Mandibular Condyle. *Brit Dent J*, 1973, 134:223-31

79 Donaldson, D., and Kroening, R. Recognition and treatment of patients with chronic orofacial pain. *JADA*, 1979, 99:961-66

80 Dworkin, S.F., and Massoth, D.L. New Understanding of the Behavioral and Psychosocial Aspects of Chronic Orofacial Pain. *Dentistry Today*, 1993, 12(10):38-45

81 Sternbach, R.A. Survey of pain in the United States: The Nuprin Pain Report, *Clin J Pain*, 1986, 2:49-53

[82] Von Korff, M., Dworkin, S.F., LeResche, L., et al. An epidemiologic comparison of pain complaints. *Pain*, 1988, 32:173-83

[83] Mejersjo, C., and Carlsson, G.E. Long-term results of treatment of temporomandibular pain dysfunction. *J. Prostht Dent*, 1983, 49:809-15

[84] Okeson, J.P. *Management of Temporomandibular Disorders and Occlusion*, 2nd ed. St Louis: CV Mosby Co., 1989

[85] Nickerson, J.W., and Boering. G. Natural course of osteoarthrosis as it relates to internal derangement of the temporomandibular joint. *Oral and Maxillofac Surg Clin North Am*, 1989, 1:27-46

[86] Greene, C.S., and Marbach, J.J. Epidemiologic studies of mandibular dysfunction. A critical review. *J Prosthet Dent*, 1982, 48:184-90

[87] Rugh, J.D., and Harlan, J. Nocturnal bruxism and temporomandibular disorders. *Adv Neurol*, 1988, 49:329-41

[88] Rugh, J.D., and Johnson, R.W. Temporal analysis of nocturnal bruxism. *J Periodontol*, 1981, 52:263-65

[89] Gangarosa, L.P., and Mahan, P.E. Pharmacologic management of TMD-MPDS. *Ear Nose Throat J*, 1982, 61:30-41

[90] Brown, R.S., and Bottomley, W.K. The utilization and mechanisms of tricyclic antidepressants in the treatment of chronic facial pain. A review of the literature. *Anesth Prog*, 1990, 37:223-9

[91] Clark, G.T., Adachi, N.Y., and Droman, M.R. Physical medicine procedures affect on temporomandibular disorders. A review. *JADA*, 1990, 121:151-61

92 Mohl, N.D., Ohrback, R.K., Crowe, H.C., and Gross, A.J. Devices for the diagnosis and treatment of temporomandibular disorders. Part III. Thermography, ultrasound, electrical stimulation and EMG biofeedback. *J Prosthet Dent*, 1990, 63:472-7

93 Rugh, J.P. Psychological components of pain. *Dent Clin North Am*, 1987, 31:579-94

94 Moss, R.A., and Adams, H.E. The assessment of personality, anxiety and depression in mandibular pain dysfunction subjects. *J Oral Rehabil*, 1984, 11:233-7

95 Clark, G.T. A critical evaluation of orthopedic interocclusal appliance therapy: Design, theory and overall effectiveness. *JADA*, 1984, 108:359-64

96 Maloney, F., and Howard, J.A. Internal derangements of the temporomandibular joint. III. Anterior repositioning splint therapy. *Aust Dent J*, 1986, 311:30-9

Chapter 10

Oral Surgery

By Myer Leonard, D.D.S., M.D.

During the second half of the 20th century, there was an unprecedented and totally unimaginable improvement in the dental health of the American population. This improvement mirrored in whole, or at least in good part, in many Western nations, was in part attributable to public health measures such as water fluoridation. But, whilst of seminal importance, this was not the entire explanation for the improvement—it was the effort of the dental profession to raise the public's sense of oral health and well being through regular checkups, an emphasis on hygiene including making flossing a daily routine amongst millions of people, and a gradual diminution of periodontal disease (though slower than the rate of reduction in caries). Cumulatively, these efforts led to the vast improvement in the individual person's oral health.

One simple statistic captures the era—in 1960, the average 60 to 65 year old person had three of his/her own teeth. In the year 2010, the average 65 year old will possess 25 of his/her own teeth.

In terms of dental education, this transition has meant that the time predoctoral students expend in the oral surgery department or exodontia clinics has been reduced as the demands for that service have fallen. The demands on curriculum time do not allow for the long periods of instruction that once were the norm. As fewer people attend the exodontia clinics, the "student exposure" has withered. Indeed, I know that in some dental schools, some of the students may only get the opportunities to remove impacted third molars, as there is such a paucity of patients for routine or simple extractions.

What this means is that many practitioners have had a very limited teaching and experience in exodontia techniques, and when in practice, may easily find that their skills are not at an optimal level.

Most of us find that we need to perform a procedure a number of times before we begin to appreciate some of the finer points of instruction that we hitherto overlooked or put aside as of little or no importance whilst we were in the early learning phase. A word of caution, if there were only one or two techniques that always and unequivocally gave excellent results and following which a tooth would never break—we'd all be using it! It's because no such techniques exist that we have so many!

This chapter has been written for those who may now be ready to review and relearn some of those "finer points and subtleties" of exodontia technique. Some of the techniques and managements advocated will be new to the reader, but they have been developed by the writer over almost two score of years of teaching and instructing literally hundreds and hundreds of residents. They are based, as far as possible, on the principles of applied anatomy and physiology.

Assessment

The decision whether or not you are to remove a particular tooth/teeth will depend on:

- The history you obtain—you may not be absolutely confident that a pulpitis is the cause of the pain, and the removal of a tooth should not be a therapeutic experiment. One should be very confident that the patient's pain will be relieved by the removal of the tooth

- The patient's medical history may induce you to refer him/her to a specialist colleague
- The clinical exam may include features such as excess anxiety, medical problems, inability to open (trismus), intra- or extraoral swellings; and the state of the tooth/teeth to be removed (instanding or crowded teeth with very limited access to the tooth)

Even if the history and clinical exam are free of incident, the x-ray findings may make you decide to refer the patient. Taking an x-ray of the tooth/teeth to be removed is the standard of care—even more important is to examine that x-ray and to do it before you start! If you positively seek to learn whether the roots are curved, how many there are, what their proximity is to the inferior alveolar nerve or other teeth, whether the roots are conical or not, whether the adjacent teeth have gold/amalgam/porcelain crowns or even periapical lesions, these observations will help you diminish the number of surprises (or shocks) that you will encounter

Part of the importance of this procedure is that it allows you to make an estimate of the time you will need for the extraction. The only way to assure yourself a low-stress, hassle-free, and "peaceful" practice life (and thus create the environment and atmosphere for your employees to enjoy the same "atmosphere") is to so complete your assessment of any procedure—whether it be a crown prep, endodontic treatment, extraction, or whatever—*that you are able to match your performance with your intentions.* To paraphrase Charles Dickens' *Pickwick Papers*—Income a pound, expenditure 19 shillings and sixpence equals happiness. Income a pound, expenditure 20 shillings and sixpence equals unhappiness

If you intend to take 30 minutes and you take one hour, then there is an aura of misery, discontent, unhappiness, and frayed nerves for everyone, with lots of people looking for new jobs. If you estimate something will take 30 minutes and it takes 25 minutes, then the day runs on a seamless even keel, and there is an aura of contentment and happiness, thus job turnover is low. The operator should never fail to realize that all procedures have an added 5 to 10 minutes in clean-up time and preparing for the next patient, and as an air of impertuability is detected by the patient, it adds to the degree of confidence and diminished stress that all of us as patients want so very much

Anesthesia

There are only a couple of points I shall make here. Remember that most studies have shown that the first 8 to 10 hours following an extraction are the most painful hours, and so the use of a long acting anesthetic such as Marcane or Durinest (Bupivicaine or Etidocaine), both of which provide about 8 to 10 hours of anesthesia (in the maxilla it's nearer to 4 hours due to the more rapid dissemination of the solution), is a thoughtful act.

Sometimes, following a lingual block, prior to removal of a mandibular tooth, one can confirm by questioning or testing that the patient's tongue and lip are numb and the gingival tissue around the tooth is also anesthetized, and yet when the forceps are applied the patient reacts in a way that is simply not "too much pressure." In these cases (and in the clinic in which I was employed), after establishing that the lingual block and long buccal injection have succeeded (the tongue, lip, and gingival tissue are numb), we routinely inject a small amount (⅕ of a cc) of local anesthetic solution into each of the four papillae surrounding the tooth to be extracted. This is not done with an intraligament syringe, but just by taking the usual syringe and injecting it into the periodontal membrane at the papillary site and pressing very hard and getting a little more solution into that site. It is salutary how often one gets an "ouch" from the patient. It is a procedure that adds greatly to the degree of anesthesia and does not incur any increase of dry socket.

If these techniques have not added to the degree of anesthesia, one can use the intraosseus anesthesia techniques that are readily described in the literature.[1-3]

One final word—sometimes for seemingly inscrutable reasons, one cannot achieve the depth of anesthesia that permits the patient to allow you to proceed—then, in my opinion, don't. You may win the battle and lose the war. Remember, an unhappy or disconsolate patient will tell 9 to 11 others of the unpleasant experience he/she had with you. Not a good way to build a practice! Don't get your ego involved, just accept and admit that he/she is just too tough today and perhaps refer him/her for a sedation.

It's a point not often emphasized, but worth remembering, that the success of mandibular anesthesia is about 80% in the molars, 65% in the premolars, and approximately 50% with the cuspids and anterior teeth.[4] Thus, although you may use a mandibular block, be prepared to supplement it with long buccal and floor of mouth injections.

For bicuspid and more anterior teeth, I rarely, if ever, use a mandibular block—I inject into the buccal sulcus alongside the apex of the tooth to be extracted and also into the lingual sulcus, again alongside the apex of the tooth to be extracted.

Extraction of Teeth—Some General Observations

With the exception of impacted teeth—third molars, bicuspids, and cuspids, etc.—or an ankylosed tooth, the only real entity that maintains the tooth in its position in the mouth is the periodontal membrane. The periodontal membrane surrounds impacted teeth, but they have an additional physical impediment to their removal. Thus, it is apparent that in order to remove a tooth, it is necessary to separate the periodontal membrane from the tooth. The periodontal membrane is 0.1 to 0.3 mm wide, with the narrowest part being at the apex. There is not an instrument, apart from the scalpel blade that is fine enough to penetrate the periodontal ligament. Thus, the age old instruction that appears to be ubiquitously taught in all dental schools (certainly I was taught in the late 1950s and I've heard it taught at dental schools around the world) that, as a first step, an elevator or straight gouge (Seldin 34S) should be placed

315

between the tooth and the bone in order to separate the periodontal membrane, is vacuous. This elevator is approximately 1.5 mm wide at its operating edge. It is thus impossible for it to be inserted between the bone and the tooth. The elevator is placed between the offending tooth and the adjacent one, provided one bears in mind that the tooth will only obey the laws of physics; and thus if there is a large crown on the adjacent tooth or it has a conical root or is less sturdy (e.g., a lateral being levered against a cuspid in order to dislodge a cuspid), the maneuver of levering against an adjacent tooth does no harm.

The important thing is to realize that one does lean against the adjacent tooth.

Of more recent times, the luxator is an instrument that has come to have a wider use, certainly in the clinic in which I was employed.

Luxators are a width of 0.5 mm or less. In a series of cadaver experiments, I was able to film the action in which the luxator could be inserted into the periodontal space and insinuated down the side of the tooth for about 3 or 4 mm at most. Luxators come in a set of four, two of which are 3 mm wide and one instrument is offset, and two of the instruments are 5 mm wide and again one is offset. The offset angle permits access to the palatal aspect of roots. The instrument can be used not only prior to forceps removal of the tooth, but also, in those cases where a root is remaining, the operator will find that on numerous occasions the luxator can be inserted around the circumference of the root and begin to dislodge it such that one dispenses with the need of making a flap in order to remove the root.

The instrument should be sharpened about once a month, as the sharpness of the edge is an integral part of its efficiency.

Peritomes have recently been developed to provide a similar function, but I have not found them to be as reliable.

At the last count, I found some 40 to 50 forceps on the market and I suspect that there are even a lot more than that. We use very few—the 150 and occasionally the 65 for upper teeth, the Ash 22 for mandibular anterior teeth and bicuspids, and the Ash 33 for mandibular molars. The blades of the forceps should be sharp, and the contour of the forcep is to allow one to push the blades as far towards the apex of the tooth as possible. There will be a fracture of the cervical bone—that's why the socket is squeezed after the extraction. One cannot possibly "squeeze the socket," one can just press in the microfractured bone that is attached to the periostium and mucosa at the neck of the tooth.

Do not lose sight of the fact that in an extraction one has to sever, displace, cut, lacerate, amputate, section, or divorce, or whatever word you will, but you must detach the periodontal membrane from the tooth. Therefore, the further towards the apex that the forcep blades can go then the more periodontal membrane is detached. This can only be for 3 or 4 mm, so how does one detach the remaining periodontal membrane?

By rotating the tooth once the forceps are placed on the tooth and pushed apically for 10 seconds, then, gripping the forceps, the wrist and hand are turned 15 degrees. This is a small amount, but will put a lot of the periodontal membrane on stretch and it will rupture.

This position is held for a further 10 seconds and then the wrist is turned in the opposite direction—stretching previously compressed periodontal membrane, and it, too, will now rupture.

At this juncture, you will feel the tooth to be loose. Continue to repeat the movement and gradually the tooth will loosen up and can be removed. If no visible motion has occurred, then be assured it is taking place—just as the lid of a pickle jar is being loosened despite the fact there is no visible movement when the lid is gripped.

Teeth Are Pushed Out, Not Pulled Out

If you take a tooth bucally, then that becomes a contest between the integrity of the root of the tooth and the integrity of the buccal bone. If the bone wins, then the root breaks. If the root wins then there is frequently a fracture of the buccal plate of bone.

The teaching described previously applies to all teeth in the maxilla except the maxillary molars, which will be described later.

Maxillary Extractions

Chair position

The chair should be angled back at about 145 to 155 degrees. The patient should be seated comfortably with his/her legs on the lower part of the chair and not dangling on either side. His/her head should be in the "sniffing the morning air" position—*i.e.*, with the chin slightly raised up and the neck straight, but not hyperextended. The mouth should be at the height of the operator's elbow (though some authorities recommend 2 to 3" higher).

Operator

The operator should be in a position so that the right leg is in line with the patient's hips to thighs. The left leg should be in advance and somewhat in line with the patient's elbow and the forceps held in the palm of the hand. For extractions on the patient's right, the medial blade of the forceps (150) should be pressed against the base of the thenar eminence of the operator's hand.

The sequence of extractions, if there are to be more than one, is that the painful tooth should be extracted first, then any roots, then anterior teeth prior to posterior teeth. If the incisors and cuspids are to be removed, then it's a good idea to plan for an alveoplasty, which will be explained later.

Once the patient is in position and the operator has confirmed adequate anesthesia, then the luxator can be applied apically alongside the mesial, distal, and palatal aspects of the tooth. The 150 forceps are then applied and for a right maxillary tooth are held in the operator's hand, with the index finger of the left hand holding the mucosa of the palate and the thumb of the left hand against the buccal mucosa. The forcep blades are pushed for 10 seconds as far as possible. The right arm of the operator will be almost straight, though, with a slight bend at the elbow. After 10 seconds, the forceps are rotated 15 degrees and again held for 10 seconds. Then the forceps are turned in the opposite direction. If at this point the tooth is not yielding, then simply repeating the maneuver will continue to disrupt the periodontal membrane and ultimately rend it to make for a loosening of the tooth.

Everyone has had the occasion when the patient is perhaps a very well built individual, and his/her bone seems like concrete. In those cases, I use two hands to rotate the forceps. There will be no adverse sequelae from gripping the forceps with two hands. The patient's head will not move, but the amount of power that can be applied will be increased dramatically. To be sure, in order to extract teeth, one must have a good technique, but that is occasionally not sufficient. An example is simply that technique alone won't enable you to drive a golf ball 300 yards—you need a considerable amount of power too. As soon as the tooth is beginning to move, then the left hand is removed and replaced around the tissues. The tooth is not brought out buccally—that only increases the propensity for fracture (a very common event, 20%, with maxillary first bicuspids because they have two fine roots).

This technique of using a luxator, then apical pressure, and then rotation can be used on all maxillary teeth from the central incisor to the second bicuspid. There are, however, adjustments that are made for the removal of teeth in the left maxilla.

Many people will find it a great help to have the patient turn his/her head to the right when the maxillary left teeth are being extracted. Also, lower the chair some 3 to 4", but do not change the tilt of the chair, nor does the operator change his/her stance. The slight lowering of the chair and the turning of the head compensate for the mechanical advantage that is lost when one has to lean across the patient to address the left maxillary teeth.

The maxillary molars cannot be rotated in the fashion described for the anterior maxillary teeth, because they have two buccal roots and one palatal root, and attempts to rotate the tooth will fail. The technique used is to keep the chair and the patient in the same position as before, and also the operator is in the same position as previously described. The luxator is used against the buccal, distal, and palatal aspect of the tooth, and the 150 forceps is again the forceps of choice. Pressure is used again for 10 seconds as the blades of the forceps are pushed up alongside the root surface of the palatal root. The buccal blade is placed between the two buccal roots, and after 10 seconds the operator's hand is moved buccally with the grip on the tooth maintained. This buccal movement is no more than 10 to 15 degrees and is held for 10 seconds. During that period, the periodontal membrane around the palatal root is rupturing. After the 10 seconds are expended, direct the forceps pressure again in the long axis of the tooth and then return to a buccal movement. Frequently, this is done with a two-handed grip, and the hold of the forceps on the tooth is a very controlled buccal movement. This movement should be slow and deliberate, as a rapid movement will lead to root fracture. Once the tooth is moving, then the left hand can be reapplied to the mucosa around the tooth in order to support it prior to full displacement of the tooth.

On the left side, it is particularly helpful to turn the patient's head and drop the height of the chair, otherwise the operator's right arm is too far out to the side to get a good mechanical advantage.

Generally, maxillary third molars have only a very weak plate of buccal bone, and thus the path of delivery is in an arc from the buccal aspect. Following the removal of the tooth, one should inspect the apex to be sure there is no fracture. A shiny surface and sharp edges on the root usually indicate a fracture, even if one didn't hear it.

Roots that are resorbed are round edged and have a matte finish.

Personally, I don't curette the socket, but we do place ¼" of gel foam coated with tetracycline powder into each socket.

Note: This has reduced the incidence of dry socket (see later for definition) to less than 4%, and there are no cases of reaction to the tetracycline. The dressing, made by dividing a sheet of gel foam (8 cm x 12.5 cm x 1 cm) into 80 pieces and the contents of one 250 mg capsule of tetracycline, is dusted over the segments of gel foam. They are placed in a jar, shaken, and a small cube is placed into each socket. The pieces are kept dry—there is no saline or other liquid added.

After the extraction, the socket should be compressed so that the microfractured cervical bone can be digitally approximated.

Alveoplasty

If one is to make an immediate denture or remove the maxillary teeth from cuspid to cuspid, then the order of extractions should be the cuspid first followed by the lateral and then the incisor. In this way, all the buccal bone that is buttressed around the cuspid is left intact. If one takes the central and lateral first, then one will usually remove a substantial amount of buccal bone with the cuspid.

If, on the other hand, the cuspid is removed first, then the buccal bone is buttressed around the central and lateral and is maintained.

Once one has removed the cuspid and then the lateral and the central and the same teeth on the other side, then one can use a pair of side-cutting Ronguers in order to snip the interseptal bone. Once this has been done on both the palatal and buccal aspect, then with a periosteal elevator, one can outfracture the buccal plate of bone. It would not be possible to fracture in the buccal plate unless it was first fractured out. This maneuver will not lead to the loss of the bone, because the periosteum and mucosa are attached, and so long as they are attached then the bone will remain viable.

Once the buccal plate has been fractured out, then it can be easily infractured and one can be left with a very nice U-shaped ridge upon which the denture can fit without loss of the peripheral seal and without having to remove sections of the buccal acrylic material.[5]

Mandibular Teeth

For mandibular teeth, the chair should be as low as possible and tilted back to approximately 135 degrees. If the chair can't go very low, then it may be necessary to tilt it further back.

For all the right mandibular anterior teeth and bicuspids, I use the Ash 22. I stand behind the patient and his/her head is about the level of my lower abdomen or at the "lap" level. Then the operator has a relatively straight back and can look down on the tooth. The forceps are applied with the right hand. The index finger of the left hand is in the patient's buccal sulcus, and the thumb in the floor of the mouth. The remaining three fingers support the mandible. Again, apply downward pressure for 10 seconds and then the tooth is gripped and the wrist rotated forward 15 degrees and held for 10 seconds and then rotated back for a further 15 degrees and held again for 10 seconds. Again, I emphasize no buccal movement until the tooth is loose and almost at the very point of delivery. A luxator can be used along the buccal and distal aspect of the tooth prior to the application of the forceps.

For the mandibular right molars, I prefer the Ash 33. The reason is from a mechanical viewpoint—the forcep is best applied in the direction of the long axis of the tooth that can be approached by way of the Ash 22 or 33 and not so easily with the cow horn. The latter does have certain advantages of access when the crown is broken down or there is a limited opening of the mouth.

When extracting on the patient's left, then the operator is standing to the front of the patient with the middle finger of the left hand in the floor of the mouth, the index finger of the left hand in the buccal sulcus, and the thumb then supports the mandible. The same movements are made as before.

For removal of the lower anterior teeth prior to a denture, a technique similar to that used for the maxillary alveoplasty cannot be followed, because the mandibular bone is very thin and would not permit the removal of the interceptal bone, subsequent outfracture, and then infracture of the mandibular buccal plate.

Here, it is best to peel back the mandibular gingiva a couple of millimeters and then extract the teeth and gently rasp the buccal edge of the bone. One should then feel the edge with one's finger, after having laid back the mucosa. It's not a good idea to feel the bone directly with one's finger as frequently the bone will feel sharp and there will be a temptation to rasp more of the bone. Remember that when you have finished, nature takes over and there will be even less bone in two or three weeks time.

Instanding Teeth

Typically the most common teeth to be misaligned from the occlusion are the second bicuspid in either the maxilla or the mandible. Although it can affect other teeth (*e.g.*, the maxillary lateral or the maxillary cuspid that can be positioned very buccally), these teeth, if they have to be removed, don't offer quite the challenge that the malaligned bicuspid does.

In the maxilla, the tooth is almost always the second bicuspid and, again, is almost always palatally placed. The difficulty in removing the tooth is in part due to one's inability to put forceps on the tooth that can adequately grasp it. Whether one uses the 150 or the 65 or even the lower Ash forcep, it's difficult to place the blades without traumatizing an adjacent tooth and as soon as one begins any sort of rotation movement it's almost inevitable that the first bicuspid will become mobile. I have found the best success in removing these teeth by using a luxator, pressing it very far up the side of the root, "wiggling" the luxator, and gradually getting the tooth loose so that I am able to pick it out with a pair of 65 when it's very loose.

So far as the mandibular bicuspids are concerned that are outside the occlusion, if the crown faces the tongue, these teeth generally have roots that are fairly short and rather dumpy. The problem again is gaining access. Generally, I have found that the best access is by using the 150 or upper forceps on these lower teeth. The angle of the forcep allows one to approach the tooth and gently begin to rotate it and very soon it comes loose. Again, one must be observant of the status of the adjacent tooth—particularly the first bicuspid.

If the tooth is locked between the first bicuspid and the molar and somewhat submerged, then access is extremely difficult. Furthermore, if this tooth is placed somewhat buccally and the crown breaks off, unless one is careful, it's easy to injure the mental nerve in the course of removing bone and extracting the root. Although most textbooks place the position of the mental inferior to and between the apices of the bicuspids, this is not an absolute. I have seen cases where the mental nerve is still between the roots of the bicuspids, but much higher in position and therefore at much greater risk.

Unless the practitioner feels very comfortable in making a flap and identifying the nerve and confirming that it is protected, then I think the prudent decision would be to refer such a case to an oral and maxillofacial surgeon.

Mouth Prop

Some operators use a mouth prop during the extraction, as they believe it helps to protect the patient's TMJ. I don't think there is any objection to this except insofar as one should not lose sight of the fact that when the patient is biting on a mouth prop, his/her gag reflex has been eliminated. This means that any foreign body, such as part of a tooth or crown or even the tooth itself, can readily pass into either the esophagus or the lungs without the patient being able to gag and occlude the glottis and bring up the foreign object. Thus, the use of the prop without any sort of protecting gauze pad is to be very strongly condemned.

Post Operative Instructions

We encourage our patients to continue to bite on the gauze pad that is placed over the socket for about 30 minutes. We assure them that a small amount of oozing or bleeding over the next 24 hours is not unusual, but if it is more than that, we encourage them to call us and sometimes we will see the patient again.

We tell them if they want to use ice bags to prevent swelling then they should only apply the ice bag for about 20 minutes and then remove it for about 20 and then reapply, and certainly no more than the day of the procedure. We encourage them to rest and eat soft foods and warm liquids, and usually we prescribe Tylenol 3 (acetaminophen 300 mgm with codeine 30 mgm), 2 tablets to be taken every 4 hours for a total of about

16 tablets. If the patient is allergic to Codeine, is in a drug rehabilitation program, or Codeine causes him/her to have constipation, then we usually substitute that with Vicoden (acetaminophen 500 mgm with hydrocodone 5 mgm).

We discourage smoking, the use of a straw, the use of alcohol, hot drinks, and exercise. The day after the extraction, we encourage them to rinse their mouth with a saltwater solution (½ teaspoon of salt in a tumbler of water). We encourage them to return to brushing and flossing the same day.

We tell them that there may be some swelling, and if, in addition, they get a fever of over 100°F, we would certainly like to see them back at the clinic.

Complications

Fracture of the root

When a tooth fractures, the operator should stop and marshal his/her thoughts and assess the situation, intelligently developing a strategy for further action. The first decision is: Do I have to get the remnant? A root remnant *rarely* produces any harm—but the mindless pursuit of such a remnant can give rise to incalculable damage and lead to endless remorse.

There are three sound reasons for removing roots and one lesser reason:

If there is an apical infection at the root, then this root should be removed. This is probably the cause of the pain or swelling that made the patient seek an extraction, and thus to leave this remnant would be to fail to remove the cause of the problem.

A loose fragment of tooth. The reason is because that once a piece of tooth or bone or any tissue is no longer "intimately" linked to the body, it becomes sequestrated. Why this is so is not known with certainty, but the most likely reason is that once it loses its blood supply, it's a foreign body, and in nature's inscrutable way, it is sequestrated from the body. One sees this occasionally with a stitch abscess following a surgery when the piece of silk or gut is slowly exfoliated through the skin. Prior to that, there is usually some swelling and area of tenderness, and when the material is ejected, there might be some purulent flow and the area will subsequently heal up.

Sometimes pieces of bone that no longer have a periosteal attachment will extrude from the socket weeks after the extraction. Similarly, a fragment of tooth will likely be sequestrated, and if it lies under the mucosa in its final stage, that can be discomforting or even painful.

More than ⅓ to ½ cm of root left. This will have a considerable amount of possibly vital tissue (pulp) left in the root and could give rise to problems later.

If less than ⅓ to ½ cm is left, this small fragment (and the amount of bone that will be removed and the amount of "digging" that will occur in order to pursue this small root) will often lead to more damage and loss of tissue than it is worth. If one suspects the piece remaining is small, an x-ray should be taken to confirm the size of the remnant and the patient informed that it is a very small piece (less than ½ cm) and there is no infection. The likelihood of any deleterious sequelae is very small, and leaving the segment is likely the most prudent step to take. I have never in my career had a patient disagree or even intimate that they would prefer "I went after it."

The roots of an ankylosed tooth if orthodontics is to follow. Sometimes one has to remove a deciduous molar that has become ankylosed (synonym = osseointegrated), and if the space is needed for another tooth, the ankylosed root will have to be burred out—it can't be extracted. However, these roots are not very deep.

If orthodontics is to occur, then this may lead to loss of the buccal bone and subsequently a high gingival line that may be less than aesthetic, and the orthodontist may have preferred one to leave the root tip.

The reader will, I think, realize that, on reflection, I'm not advocating the leaving of many roots. If the root tip is longer than ½ cm and the operator intends to remove it, and if one knows that the root tip is loose, then a root pick can be used. The notion that these fine hard steel instruments can somehow be used to extricate small pieces of root that are not loose is fallacious. At the root tip the periodontal membrane is 0.1 mm wide, and there is no root tip elevator or pick, nor any other instrument, that is fine enough to be inserted into that space. Furthermore, if one could insert it into the space then one would be simply wedging the root tip even more firmly into position. A further point to remember is that the root tip is extremely hard and the cancellous bone is soft. If pushing with a root pick at the root tip, then the likelihood is that at some juncture the tooth fragment will be displaced either into the inferior alveolar canal, into the maxillary sinus, or through the lingual plate of the mandible into the floor of the mouth. Thus, only if the fragment is loose and there isn't an instrument available that is fine enough to extricate it, then the root tip instrument can be used. This should be insinuated into the cancellous bone alongside the loose fragment and then worked to further dislodge the root tip. If the remaining root is larger than ½ cm and is loose, then, if not the root tip, sometimes a curette or other elevator will be useful to dislodge it. If it is not loose, then one has several techniques to consider.

Fractured Maxillary Molars

In the case of a maxillary molar, if the crown has snapped off at the gingival level, then one can divide the roots by using a surgical bur (S.S. White 701/702/703) that is 5 mm long and making a fissure of 5 or 6 mm depth (the length of the bur) from the distal aspect of the tooth to the mesial aspect of the tooth between the palatal and buccal roots. Then a further cut should be made between the two buccal roots, thus one has triangulated the roots, and if they have been sectioned, then the insertion of an elevator will dislodge them one at a time. If they have not been completely cut, then the cleavage line is deep enough such that when the elevator is inserted, generally the cut will run on to completely cleave them into separate segments. If one fails to make a fissure of 5 or 6 mm in depth, then the insertion of the elevator will only lead to chipping out a small segment of root. This will therefore exacerbate the problem. The likelihood of entering the antrum with a cut of 5 or 6 mm depth is extremely small.

Once the cleavage cuts have been made and the Seldin 34S or similar elevator used to dislodge one root, then usually the palatal root can be removed with a pair of fine nosed forceps (#65), and sometimes the 190/191 elevator can be used to dislodge the distal root. If the roots are fused, then this technique cannot be used and a flap procedure will be utilized (later referenced in this chapter).

Fractured Mandibular Molars

The quickest way to address the fractured mandibular molar (provided it does not have fused roots) is to section the tooth between the mesial and distal root to a depth of about 7 or 8 mm. There is no likelihood of damage to the lingual nerve in dividing a mandibular first or second molar, because the lingual nerve is only at risk at the distal lingual aspect of the third molar.

The inferior alveolar nerve is well below the apices of the roots and thus would not be at risk in this division of the molar, and the long buccal nerve is in the cheek and not at risk. The bur should be taken from the lingual bone through the tooth to the buccal bone between the two roots. Be sure that one is at least 7 or 8 mm in depth below the gingival margin. It is important to thoroughly section the roots. Then either the mesial or distal root can be dislodged into the space created. Removal of the remaining root is usually described as fairly easy by using the 190/191 elevator and pushing the root out. Sometimes this doesn't turn out to be quite so easy, in part because of a thick segment of interceptal bone. One technique that I occasionally use is to gently retract the papilla adjacent to the root that remains, making a slot with a fine fissure bur into the remaining root and the intercrestal bone between the root and the adjacent tooth, and then insert a 190 or straight elevator in order to dislodge the root. This sometimes proves an easier way to get the root out than attempting to utilize an elevator in the socket of a dislodged root.

Maxillary and Mandibular Roots

If the root cannot be removed by these "non flap" techniques, then one should be prepared to make a flap. That is usually the most expeditious action to take, and unfortunately a lot of time and perspiration is lost in attempting to do everything but make a flap! The reader will be familiar with many flaps, but the one used in the clinic in which I was employed is fairly small and quick. It is a three-sided flap and includes the papilla on each side of the root. The base must be broader than the edge and a cut should be made around the cervical margin of the tooth. A periosteal elevator or Molt is used to lift the flap, and it is retracted with the Minnesota retractor. Once the tissue is retracted, then one can remove the bone, again with the surgical bur, and then protect the tissues before using the elevator. This means putting aside the retractors and, with the finger and thumb of the left hand on the lingual and buccal aspect of the tooth, and with the other hand use the elevator. This is a way of protecting the tissues and preventing the elevator from impaling the patient's soft tissues.

Once the roots have been removed, the bone edges should be rasped, the area flushed with saline, and then the wound sutured. Care should be taken so that the sutures are placed so that the papillae return to the position they were prior to the flap. This usually means taking the suture material and passing it through the flaps and then around an adjacent tooth in order to secure the papillae in the appropriate site.

Dry Socket

A dry socket is defined as any socket from which the patient is getting pain two or more days post extraction. Frequently, there will be an offensive odor that can be detected by inserting a small pledglett of cotton wool into the socket and smelling the deposit on the cotton roll. On other occasions, there may be a more severe reaction including a malaise, lymphadenopathy, trismus, considerable pain, halitosis, and a raised temperature.

If the patient is new to the practice, then I would advocate an x-ray of the socket be taken to be sure there is no root remnant. If there is no root remnant, then proceed to flush the socket, usually with saline or a mixture of ⅔ saline and ⅓ peroxide. There is usually a free flow of rather smelly detritus.

There are a vast number of dressings, but we find Nu-foam gauze is a reliable dressing, but it does have to be changed every other day. More often we use Whitehead's varnish. We place the Nu-foam gauze in a small amount of Whitehead varnish and then dry off the gauze, because if the varnish spills onto a blouse or shirt, it does cause a stain that is difficult to remove. The dressing can be left for as long as a week or more.

Note: The prescription for Whitehead's varnish: Benzoine 10g; Iodoform 10g; Balsam of Tolu 5g; Storax 7.5g; Ether to 100 mls.

Since using the gel foam tetracycline mix referred to earlier, our incidence of dry socket is in the region of 3% or less.

Other materials that have an oily base are not recommended, as they do not resorb and can leave areas of radiolucency in the mandible or maxilla that may provoke investigation at a subsequent date.

Certainly, if a pack is inserted then the doctor should be sure to see the patient at a later date in order to remove the pack or to confirm that the pack has been lost from the socket.

Torn Tissues

In the practice of surgery, the tearing of tissue is always a risk, but hopefully with good planning and proper flap design, it should be a rare event. A tear, particularly if long, can be a frightening event for the practitioner. The best way to approach the repair is with simple sutures. A continuous locking suture may give the best result in the hands of the expert surgeon, but the tyro is often in a panic and will find the placement of simple sutures to be easier and more effective. The place to start is at the midpoint of the tear. If the tear is ripped then one wants to suture from the continuous tissue on one side of the tear over to the continuous tissue on the other side, so locking the torn tissue in the loop.

Once the suture is placed at the halfway mark, then another suture should be placed between one end point of the tear and the halfway suture on one side, and then on the other side. This "suturing by halves" is an easy way to repair torn tissue.

It is well to remember that there are three indications for suturing:

- Torn tissue
- Loose tissue
- Bleeding tissue

Suturing

Suturing can be with absorbable or non-absorbable materials, though the former usually take two and even three weeks to resorb. Nylon and even silk are about the best non-absorbable, and the preferred width is the 3/0. The knots run easy with these materials, and the only disadvantage is that the patient has to come back to have them removed.

This is frequently not so great a disadvantage, because it allows you to see the results of your own surgery.

The absorbable materials are also 3/0 gauge, but although they make a return visit unnecessary, they are more difficult to handle and run less smoothly, and the knot is sometimes at a distance from the selected site. Pulling on the ends of the material will not advance the knot and usually leads to a break of the material. When using the absorbable materials, it is well to keep the loops as large as possible until the knot can be snugly sited.

Tissue Emphysema

When an air-driven hand piece is used to prepare a crown or in other restorative procedures, air and water are blown out onto the bur to cool it. As this mist hits the periodontal/tooth interface, it flows into the sulcus and can be removed by the suction apparatus.

If an attempt has been made to remove a tooth, then the periodontal/tooth interface, which in nature is normally an extremely close and remarkable attachment, has been disrupted and torn, with the result that if the high speed hand piece is used, then air and water are soon blown into the tissues. On occasion, this does no harm, but it can lead to air in the tissues that will make them balloon up—this is described as an emphysema. If this occurs, then the patient should be prescribed Amoxicillin, 1 gm stat and then 500 mg b.i.d. for five days. This should be done until such time as the emphysema has completely evacuated. There are many reports of where the amount of air in the tissues has been of such dimension that it has lead to either loss or impairment of vision, or necrotizing facitis in the neck.

In order to prevent this problem, the operator is urged to use a surgical hand piece in which the air is eliminated from the back of the hand piece, and although slower in speed, nevertheless, it's much safer.

There are several such devices on the market, and none of them cost more than about $400 or $500.

Oro-Antral Perforation

A perforation of the antrum can occur in the course of pursuing maxillary molar roots and occasionally the first or second bicuspid roots, though the latter is a much rarer cause for the perforation to the antrum. It is considered that perforations probably take place far more often than we are aware, but heal without incident.[6] Certainly, oral and maxillofacial surgeons know that over the last 25 to 30 years, they have done simply thousands of maxillary osteotomies, and this entails opening into the maxillary sinus, and the number of occasions in which sinusitis has followed or an intractable opening has occurred are extremely few.

Creating a fistula is not a malpractice; failing to tell the patient is a malpractice.

If the perforation occurred and the practitioner is confident that the entire root was removed, then tell the patient about the perforation and place a gel foam pack over the site. In my experience, this seems to be a very effective mode of treatment. I don't prescribe antibiotics or decongestants, because I don't feel there is any indication or need for them at this stage.

On a return visit, one can test whether the fistula is still patent by occluding the patient's nostrils and asking him/her to blow whilst at the same time holding a wisp of cotton beneath the site of the perforation. If the cotton wool moves, then this is evidence that the fistula is still patent, and if it doesn't, then this is pretty good evidence that the site has closed over.

If at the end of three to four weeks, the area is still patent and is giving rise to problems so far as liquids, etc. passing from the mouth into the nose, then the patient should be referred to an oral and maxillofacial surgeon who can proceed to close the fistula. It's my opinion that unless one is doing a closure procedure with some degree of frequency or one has had some experience on how to do it, then it's best not to try it. The problem that occurs in inexperienced hands is that an insufficiently large flap is raised and the tissue is brought from the buccal aspect of the maxilla too tightly with the result that over a few days the sutures will pull out and a gap is left. The tissue to be raised is a large segment, and then the periosteum has to be properly incised. That allows the mucosa to pass with ease, without tension, so that it can be sutured to the palatal aspect of the opening.

The sutures are then usually left in for 17 days or so, and very slowly, over a long period of time, the buccal sulcus will reestablish itself, though never as full as prior to the fistula-closing procedure.

If part of a root is pushed into the antrum, then one can say that it is virtually impossible to remove this root through the fistula. As the patient is tilted back, the root will fall into the tuberosity region and be beyond the scope of recapture.

Such a patient should be referred at once to an oral and maxillofacial surgeon, who will make arrangements for the fistula to be closed, a nasal antrostomy performed, and the root remnant removed at the same time by way of a Caldwell-Luc approach. This is an incision over the apex of the cuspid and entry into the sinuses to retrieve the roots.

In either event of closure—without a root fragment in the antrum or after a Caldwell-Luc procedure—the patient is placed on antibiotics and decongestants.

Fracture of the Tuberosity

From time to time, it will transpire that in the course of removing a maxillary third molar, one realizes that a large segment of the tuberosity has broken away from the maxilla. Older texts used to advocate that the practitioner stop the extraction and have the patient bite on a gauze and wait for six weeks until the area had healed. I don't think this is feasible. If the tuberosity broke on application of forceps, it is unlikely that a further six weeks will heal the tuberosity to the maxilla such that when the forceps are reapplied this time, only the tooth will come out. Furthermore, if the patient came in for a toothache, it doesn't seem to me to be a very acceptable treatment to ask the patient to wait for a further six weeks.

When this occurs, the only thing to do is take a scalpel blade and as carefully as possible pare away the mucosa from the bone. A periosteal elevator will not easily allow one to lift the tissues. Thus, with a pair of 150 forceps held in the left hand and placed on the tooth, and with an assistant retracting the cheek, the operator can with the right hand use the scalpel blade to pare the tissue from around the tuberosity. Gradually, the tuberosity bone and the tooth will come free, and when they do so one will be left with a large gaping wound and an opening into the tuberosity. This should be sutured with a continuous suture, but if not with simple suture,s and the area closed to the best of the ability of the operator. It may be that the area has to be revised at a later date, but it is an unfortunate complication and rarely can be predicted.

Syncope

Syncope is more common in males than females, primarily in the 18 to 35 year age group, and more often in the morning than in the afternoon. There are a host of reasons as to what may cause it,[7] but the most effective means of preventing the condition if you suspect it is about to happen or the patient indicates that he/she is feeling faint, is to tilt the chair back, remove heavy clothing such as sweaters and jackets, apply a cold towel to the neck and forehead regions, and provide the patient with a drink of glutol. Glutol is a lemon-flavored glucose drink, and since many episodes of syncope are due to hypoglycemia, it addresses the essential etiological agent directly.

Giving cups of sugared tea or candy bars is not so successful, because these contain sucrose. This has to be metabolized to glucose in the liver before it can be metabolized in the brain cells. Glucose is the only material that can be metabolized in the brain cells, and the syncopal attack is frequently due to a lowered blood glucose level.

Once the patient has been tilted back and provided with a glucose drink, heavy clothing removed, and cold towels applied around the neck and forehead, he/she usually feels much better, and the procedure can continue. The provision of odiferous agents such as ammonia is of momentary help, because as soon as the agents are removed, the patient lapses back into his/her syncopal episode. If the patient actually has a syncopal attack, then the same steps are taken and one should really endeavor to be sure that the tilting back is such that the legs are above the abdomen and the heart above the head, so there will be a downflow of blood to the brain.

If the patient is already in a syncopal episode, the same steps are taken as before, except the glucose drink cannot be given. The provision of oxygen is not a useful step, as it has to be realized that the hemoglobin (15 gm per 100 mls of blood) is fully oxygenated at the altitude of most every spot in the United States with the exception perhaps of the peaks of the Rockies. Thus, providing oxygen to a patient does not enhance the oxygenation of the hemoglobin nor does it enhance the amount of oxygen carried in the plasma, which is about 0.5 mils at normal atmospheric pressures.

The problem has occurred because of a failure of movement of blood to the brain rather than a lack of material in the blood so far as oxygen is concerned. Thus, to cool the patient off with the ice water towels does more to enhance the venous return, the cardiac output of blood, the blood pressure, and the perfusion of the brain than giving oxygen.

Hemorrhage

Episodes of hemorrhage can occur following an extraction and may be due to small vessels that have been incompletely sectioned and continue to ooze and pump. If the patient comes back with a complaint of bleeding, then one should provide him/her with a saline rinse in order to remove all the remnants of blood and then carefully examine the surgical site. If one can spot the bleeding area, then pressure will of course stop it, but the only way one can sustain the pressure is with a suture, and this should be undertaken.

Sometimes the ooze and hemorrhage are not from one particular vessel that is continuing to pump, but seems to be a general ooze. In this case, the first step is to check over the history to be sure the patient is not taking an excessive number of aspirins or alcohol (at one time brandy purchased in a drug store was called "medicinal"), and then if there is no aspect of the medical history that makes one think of a more general reason for the bleeding, then local measures such as the application of gel foam or oxycell are advocated. In my experience, though these agents have their attributes, the downside is that as soon as they are moist, they seem to be swept away in the suction. Over the past few years, we have used Colostat (Vitaphore Corporation, Plainsboro, NJ 08536), which is a microfibular material. We found the application of the small cone is very effective, and as an alternative we use Avatine (Davol Inc., Woburn, MA 01801), which is more expensive, but also a very efficacious material.

In addition, there is a material called Instat by Johnson and Johnson, and it is provided in small sheets. This can be applied in the socket and sutured.

It was the usual practice to reduce anticoagulant therapy, such as Coumadin, in patients prior to their extraction.

Wahl recommended, after a large study of patients on anticoagulant therapy, that this procedure not be followed and that the extractions proceed as normal, but extra measures be taken to provoke hematosis.[8]

Infection

It's a good practice, and one that will pay off handsomely in terms of patient appreciation, to call patients the day of a surgery and probably three or four days later to check on their progress.

If a patient has any concerns about swelling or continued pain, then the prudent practitioner will invite the patient back to the office to see for him/herself the amount of swelling or sequelae of the procedure.

One can summarize a patient's progress in one of three possibilities.

The patient is improving. A certain amount of swelling and discomfort is expected after any surgical procedure, but if there is no rise in the pulse, no rise in the temperature, no evidence of malaise (the patient having been off his/her food or feeling unwell, etc.), no throbbing in the area, and the tissue itself looks pink and healing, and it is not malodorous, then it can be concluded that this patient is healing in a normal fashion and, within a few more days, whatever swelling present will have resolved and the pain abated completely.

There is evidence of a worsening. The patient may have more pain than you would expect, there may be a temperature of 100° F or more, there may be considerable swelling and the swelling itself feels warm, there is trismus or inability to open his/her mouth, and there may be inability to take a normal diet. This patient is one whom you can strongly suspect, if not treated with antibiotics, will go on to an infection. The ideal antibiotic for oral infections is, without doubt, penicillin. No oral organisms have become resistant to it in the 55 years since its introduction, and it has very few side effects and a very low incidence of allergy. It does not interfere with the pill in women who are on a contraceptive technique, nor does it interfere or cause any abnormalities in the fetus of a pregnant individual. Apart from that, its other great attributes are that it can be given to patients without worrying about whether they have any cardiac, respiratory, hepatic, or other disease, and one can be sure that it won't interfere with any medications that they happen to be on. It's also very cheap.

One downside of penicillin is that, nowadays, the 500 mg tablet, 2 stat and 1 qid for 5 days, is the normal prescription, but some people do get an esophogitis on taking a 500 mg tablet. In addition, a lot of patients do not fill their prescriptions; thus, in the clinic, we give it intramuscularly in the buttock (1 million units of Crystalline penicillin and 1-2 million units of Benzalthine penicillin), which will provide a three-day course of antibiotic.

As an alternative to penicillin, Amoxicillin is sometimes used (500 mg x 2 and one tablet bid for five days). This, too, is effective against oral flora.

If the patient is allergic to penicillin, then Clindomycin, 600 mg stat and then 150 mg twice a day for five days, can be substituted.

If at the end of this time, the patient has not made any improvement, and there is evidence of pus formation (pus is liquefied necrotic material and an antibiotic will not remove it—it will only render it sterile), then the pus has to be relieved. In an infected tooth, one does this by opening the tooth and proceeding to endodontic therapy. In the mouth, it may be necessary to do an incision and drainage, but if it's a very large swelling and it's in a dependent area, then this patient should be referred to an oral surgeon for him/her to either institute incision and drainage under a general anesthetic or, in addition, to provide intravenous antibiotics.

If, on the patient's return, you feel that there is a distinct possibility of an infective process in addition to the trismus, difficulty in swallowing, and an inability to imbibe fluids, then it's best to refer this patient to a colleague who specializes in oral and maxillofacial surgery rather than trying to handle the condition with oral antibiotics.

The patient is not really improving. At the same time the patient is not improving, he/she certainly is not showing evident signs of an infective process.

The best thing with these patients is simply to see them in another day or two, and just continue to monitor them. I don't think there is any particular reason to institute antibiotics, but this is going to be a judgment call that the practitioner is going to have to make with the patient at hand.

Notes

[1] Leonard, M.S. The Efficacy of an Intraosseous Injection System of Delivering Local Anesthetic, *JADA*, 1995, 126:81-86

[2] Leonard, M.S. Stabident System of Intraosseous Anesthesia, *Dental Economics*, 1997, 87:51-60

[3] Leonard, M.S. Anatomy of the Intraosseous Injection, *Dentistry Today*, 1998, 17:86-89

[4] McLean, C., Reader, A., Beck, M., and Meyers, W.J. An Evaluation of 4% Privocaine and 3% Mepivacaine Compared with 2% Lidocaine for Inferior Alveolar Nerve Block, *J.Endod*, 1998, 19:146-50

[5] Leonard, M.S. Overcoming the Challenge of Alveoplasty, *Dentistry Today*, 1994, 13:92-94

[6] Laskin, D.M. Management of Oral Antral Fistular and Other Sinus Related Complications, *Oral and Maxillofacial Clinics of North America*, Philadelphia: W.B. Saunders, 1999, 11:155-164

[7] Leonard, M.S. Syncope, *Dentistry Today*, 1996, 15:72-73

[8] Wahl, M.J. Myths of Dental Surgery in Patients Receiving Anticoagulant Therapy, *JADA*, 2000, 131:77-82

Chapter 11

Crown and Bridge

By Larry Lopez, D.D.S.

Introduction

The restoration of the devastated dentition has challenged man from the beginning of his existence. There are numerous references in historical accounts of artificial teeth being carved from wood or ivory and cast with various metals. In ancient times, the loss of teeth usually was a death sentence. Advances in medicine and sanitation have made it possible for man to reasonably expect to live to 90 years or more. This fact makes it even more advantageous for an individual to desire to retain his/her teeth and to repair teeth as they become defective. Additionally, the smile is now regarded by most societies to be a major element in the overall beauty of an individual. Developments in the art and science of indirect restorative dentistry has made meeting the demands of function and esthetics more possible than has ever been enjoyed in the history of the human species.

Materials

In the past two decades, there has been a plethora of new materials come available as restorative options. And though that has caused great confusion to dentists in choosing materials, it has afforded the restorative dentist with unprecedented opportunities to create restorations that are both esthetic and biologically appropriate. The following discussion will attempt to sort through the many choices in contemporary materials.

In essence, there are three categories of materials for indirect restorations:

- Metal
- Esthetic material bonded to metal
- Non-metal restoratives

In the class of metals, there are three basic types:

- Non-precious or base metals
- Semi-precious metals, including milled titanium
- Gold

Non-precious or base metals oftentimes contain nickel for strength and corrosion resistance. Fifteen percent of American women and 1% of American men are allergic to nickel. It is extremely important that the restoring dentist using these materials takes the time to seriously quiz their patients to ascertain whether they are allergic to nickel. Responses may vary from chronic inflammation to massive bone loss and loss of teeth. It is this author's opinion that these metals should only be used in rare occasions where exceptional strength is needed. Cast gold is still an excellent restorative material that possesses great strength and requires the least amount of occlusal reduction, and therefore is particularly suited to the restoration of second molar teeth. The use of CAD-CAM machines in the fabrication of prosthesis has now allowed the milling of titanium substructures for dental fixed prosthesis. Titanium with its light-weight, remarkable strength and high biocompatibility holds great promise for a substrate for long span restorations.

Esthetic materials bonded to metal are ceramics, acrylic, and composites. Acrylic is rarely used now, because of its high wear rate and propensity to stain. Since the 1960's, when the first successful porcelain fused to metal system was introduced, there has been an increasing demand for ceramic materials. Because of its low tensile strength and brittleness, it has usually been fused to metal to increase its resistance to fracture. The metal substrate, however, can affect the esthetics of the porcelain by inhibiting light transmission through the glass matrix and can cause metal ion discoloration.

An exception to this limitation is the Captek system. This system creates copings of platinum and palladium that are completely covered inside and out with rich 22-carat gold. This rich color has the advantage of allowing the technician to use less opaquer and to create highly esthetic restorations that are much thinner in the cervical areas than previously possible. Additionally, these restorations are particularly suited for subgingival extensions of indirect restorations because of their unique properties of inhibiting plaque growth.[1] Because these restorations are not cast, they produce exceptional fits and have less stress at the porcelain-metal interface.

The drawbacks of the cast oxide metals as copings and the relatively complex procedures necessary to produce them have led to the creation of metal-free systems. These new systems are two principal types:

- All ceramic
- Composites

The all-ceramic restorative materials are typically bonded to the underlying tooth, adding strength to the restoration. The most important factor in the predictable longevity of porcelain restorations is the thickness of the occlusal surface material. With a recommended 2 mm of occlusal material, the restoration is strong enough to give good statistical results.

The all-ceramic restorative systems are the following types:

Powder slurry ceramics. This class of ceramics is supplied as a powder to the ceramist and is mixed with water to be built up in layers to form the restoration. Various translucencies, stains, and shades are available. Examples are: Duceram LFC and Optec HSP.

Pressable ceramics. These ceramics are supplied as ingots that are melted and pressed into molds that were created using the lost wax technique. The resulting restoration may be made to full form or used as a substrate for feldspathic porcelains. Examples are: OPC, OPC 3G, and Empress.

Cast ceramics. Supplied as ingots, these ceramics are melted and cast centrifugally with a lost wax technique much like metal. Usually, the ingots are one shade and other porcelains are added to create final form and shades. An example is Dicor.

CAD/CAM ceramics. These ingots of porcelain are machined using computer-aided design/computer-aided manufacturing (CAD/CAM). The resulting crowns are then stained for characterization, or a CAD/CAM coping is built up with feldspathic porcelains. Examples are: Cerec and Procera.

Infiltrated ceramics. This system is composed of a powder (aluminum oxide or spinnel) that is fabricated into a porous substrate, and a glass that is infiltrated into the substrate. This is then veneered using conventional feldspathic porcelains. Examples are: In-Ceram and In-Ceram Spinnel.

The lab-processed composite materials have been introduced to address the problems of porcelain's poor flexural strength and its tendency to wear antagonistic teeth. Studies by Suzuki[2] have shown high fusing porcelains to be some 30 times as abrasive as enamel. His studies have also shown the supposed "softer" porcelains to be approximately 10 times as abrasive as enamel. These properties of porcelain can have disastrous effects on the opposing dentition when they are used in areas tracking anterior guidance.

Both nocturnal bruxism and diurnal bruxism are parafunctional movements of the mandible that pose a danger to the longevity of indirect restorations. These phenomena must be considered in the selection of anterior materials when there is cuspid-guided disclusion, and also considered in the selection of posterior materials when lateral excursive movements are in group function. Active bruxism may be assumed if wear facets are shiny and may be considered dormant when wear facets appear dull. Studies by Rugh, et al, indicate that only 10% of adults and 5% of children are aware that they brux.[3] However, their studies have found that 80-90% of people show signs and symptoms of bruxism.[4] Sleep lab studies performed at the University of Texas Health Science Center at San Antonio have indicated that people may brux four times more strenuously when they sleep than when trying to brux while they are awake. The study postulates there is some defense mechanism existing in the conscious mind that prevents diurnal highly detrimental bruxism that shuts off when we sleep. It is apparent, therefore, the benefit of using an occlusal splint of some sort when bruxism is suspected. It is also apparent that there is potential for tremendous damage to opposing dentitions when highly abrasive porcelains oppose natural teeth in the bruxxer in the areas of anterior guidance. Figure 11-1 shows the severe wear to the opposing dentition in a male patient after wearing maxillary anterior restorations on the central incisors comprised of a high fusing and abrasive porcelain.

Optimally-cured composite systems such as Sculpture/fibrekor (Jeneric/Pentron), BelleGlass, Cristobal (Dentsply/Caulk), and ArtGlass (Heraeus Kulzer) have produced restorations that have much greater flexural strength than porcelain and will not wear the opposing dentition. These materials are at least equally as beautiful as porcelain and may be actually more esthetic than the ceramic materials in some shades and opacities. Additionally, these materials are easy to repair intraorally with any visible-light-cured composite. These materials have successfully been veneered to metal frames for posterior bridgework and may be veneered to fiber-reinforced composite frames for anterior bridges. These materials are particularly suited for inlay-onlay restorations in that they will not

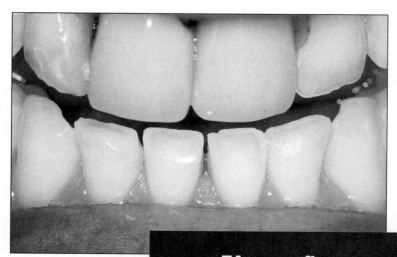

Fig. 11-1 Severe wear resulting from oppositional porcelain restorations

Fig. 11-2 The Alamo crown

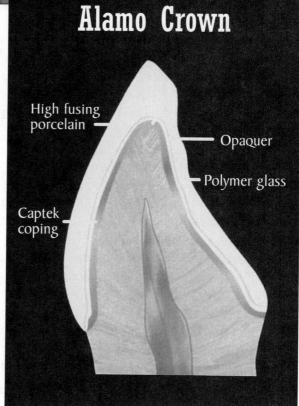

Alamo Crown

High fusing porcelain

Opaquer

Polymer glass

Captek coping

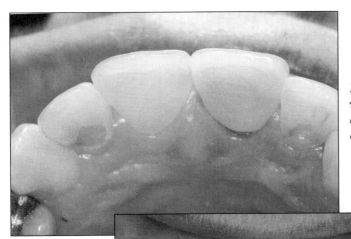

Fig. 11-3 Lingual
view of Alamo
crown showing
composite surface

Fig. 11-4
Post-op view of
Alamo Crown

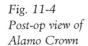

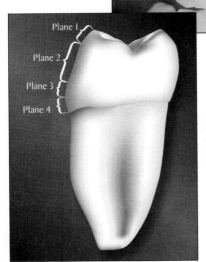

Fig. 11-5 Lateral
view of tooth to
be prepared

break as easily as porcelain inlays in the pre-luting handling. High fusing porcelains have been perfected to be highly resistant to stain, and ceramists have mastered the beauty of this material. The composites also possess the characteristics of being kind to the opposing dentition. Is it possible to have the best of both worlds?

Figure 11-2 demonstrates an attempt to incorporate both materials in a single restoration. This restoration utilizes a Captek metal coping that provides the substrate for a high fusing porcelain face and a softer composite lingual surface. The lingual composite surface provides a more compatible material for the anterior teeth to work against while tracking anterior guidance. The crown was fabricated by first making the coping and applying all the porcelain including all stains and glazes. Next the lingual surface of the porcelain was sandblasted and etched with hydroflouric acid and silanated. The lab-processed composite material was then applied to this prepared surface and light cured in place in a chamber of nitrogen under 40 psi of pressure.

Figures 11-3 and 11-4 illustrate the resultant restoration on tooth #8.

Preparations

Regardless of the material chosen by the restorative dentist, the predictably successful restoration begins with a good preparation. A proper preparation will allow sufficient room for the restorative material to be both strong and esthetically pleasing—if a tooth-colored material is chosen. In addition, the preparation will be biologically compatible with the supporting tissues. The following technique is simple and will in most cases satisfy the desired criteria. Figure 11-5 shows a lateral view of a bicuspid tooth indicating the planes that exist on the buccal and lingual surfaces. It is essential to reduce equally each plane to a depth indicated for the restorative material of choice. (Figs 11-6 through 11-9) This concept extends on to the occlusal surface, allowing an equal stripping of tooth material. This technique allows the laboratory technician sufficient

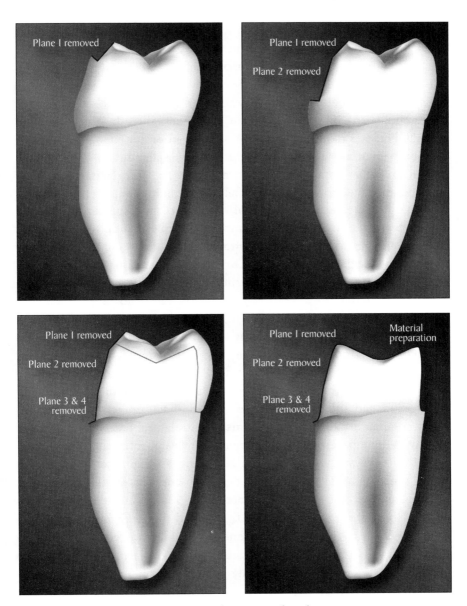

Fig. 11-6/11-9 Equal stripping of tooth structure for correct form and material strength

space to recreate the natural tooth forms, providing enough material for strength and beauty and proper emergence profiles.

It is essential to use a gauge to measure adequate occlusal reduction (Fig. 11-10). This point cannot be over-emphasized. When the author began using an occlusal clearance gauge, he was stunned to find how much he was under-preparing the occlusal surfaces of molar teeth. Porcelain fused to metal crowns requires 2 mm occlusal reduction for adequate strength. Composite crowns require a minimum occlusal reduction of 1.5 mm. When preparations are under-reduced, anatomy and strength are jeopardized and the opportunities for failure are multiplied.

Margin placement is of critical importance in respecting the health of the periodontal structures. A simple technique is simply to follow the gingival margin. Allowing the gingival margin to be your guide, you will notice that the greatest amount of interproximal cresting is in the anterior teeth and gradually becomes flatter as you move distally in the arch. Figure 11-11 demonstrates the preparation bur following the gingival margin. In almost all cases, this will keep you out of the biologic width and prevent the seqeulae of chronic inflammation. These two techniques will allow for strong, well-contoured crowns that respect the periodontal health. Studies by Orkin, Reddy, and Bradshaw[5] indicate that it is far healthier to leave the margin supragingivally. They examined 423 crowns where 355 had subgingival margins and 68 had supragingival margins. They compared them to the untreated contralateral teeth for incidences of bleeding on probing and for the occurrences of recession. They found that the teeth with crowns having subgingival margins tended to bleed upon probing 2.42 times more often than the contralateral untreated teeth, and that they were associated with recession 2.65 times more often. Contrasting those findings, they found the teeth with supragingival margins to have no more incidence of bleeding or recession than the contralateral untreated teeth. Contemporary materials have afforded our profession the opportunity to create esthetic restorations with supragingival margins (Fig. 11-12).

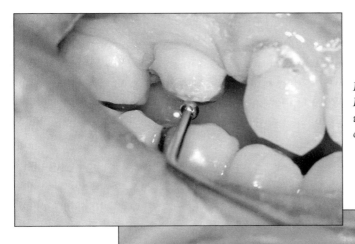

*Fig. 11-10
Reduction gauge
used to measure
occlusal clearance*

*Fig. 11-11
Diamond bur
following gingival
margin*

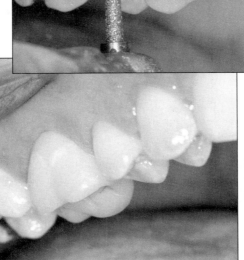

*Fig. 11-12
Crown with esthetic
supragingival margins*

Impressions

An accurate impression is also an essential element in the successful fabrication of a well-fitting prosthesis, and tissue management may be the most challenging component of the impressioning procedure. We have many medicaments and instruments available to us for the control of hemorrhage. These include ferric sulfate, aluminum sulfate, epinephrine, vinyl polysiloxanes impregnated with one of the above medicaments, electro-surgery, radio-surgery, and laser cauterization. A relatively new material, Expasyl (Kerr), is a clay-impregnated with aluminum sulfate and injected into the sulcus. Though this material has its applications, it is not the panacea we have hoped for. Cords with medicaments, lasers, and radio-surgery remain the most effective and reliable methods of handling tissue retraction and hemorrhage. It should be noted that new esthetic materials have offered the routine placement of supragingival esthetic margins, which are healthier, and in the majority of cases do not need retraction for the impression. If the impression is not perfect, it is far more profitable and clinically prudent for the operator to throw it out and take another than to accept something less than perfect, or to attempt to "fix" a defective impression.

Laboratory Communication

With a well-reduced preparation and a clear impression, the case is ready to be sent to the dental laboratory. It is essential that the technician have enough information to correctly construct a prosthesis that will fit well, look good, and last a long time. Several tools are available for communicating essential information to the lab—bite registrations, face bow transfer, preoperative models, diagnostic wax-ups and incisal edge matrices, photographs, and shade maps.

The bite registration can either be recorded in the triple-tray impression technique or taken separately in the case of full-arch impressions. When recorded separately, it is easier and neater to do so utilizing a triple-tray and a very fast setting polyvinylsiloxane bite registration material with a high shore hardness. The bite should be trimmed interproximally by the dental office before sending to the lab and labeled as a "bite" to prevent inadvertent pouring by a busy laboratory (Fig.11-13). Face bows should be used whenever there is a reconstruction of anterior guidance or where significant posterior reconstruction is considered. It is most convenient to utilize a system where the dentist's articulator and the laboratory's articulator are equilibrated to be the same, precluding shipping an entire articulator to the lab. The system illustrated in Figure 11-14 requires only the small stand and bite fork to be shipped with the case, allowing the face bow and articulator to remain in the dentist's office. Preoperative models will give the technician an idea of what the patient was functioning with before the preparations and may help set boundaries for reconstruction. The diagnostic wax-up (Fig. 11-15) and incisal edge matrix will guide the technician in the placement of incisal edges and the reestablishment of landmarks, such as the curves of Spee and Wilson and relate those planes spatially to the TMJs.

Shade taking is both a learned technique and a learned art. We need to communicate to the ceramist color shades of the teeth and texture and morphology of the surface. The language of color is hue, value, and chroma. Hue is the color itself, such as blue. Chroma is the intensity of the hue, such as light blue or dark blue. Hence, more chroma would be a more intense color. Value may be described as a black and white photograph of the object, in this case a tooth. The higher the value, the whiter the tooth, and the lower the value, the darker the tooth. When one squints and looks across a room, he will notice that colors largely disappear, and values in the form of light and dark areas become apparent. The value is probably the most important consideration in the choosing of shades for the matching of teeth. If the value is too high, *i.e.*, too light, the patient will reject the shade choice.

When one views a pickle under full spectrum light, it appears green. However, if the same pickle is viewed in light devoid of the green wavelength, it will no longer appear green. Therefore, what shade is that front tooth you are trying to match? The answer depends on the wavelength of

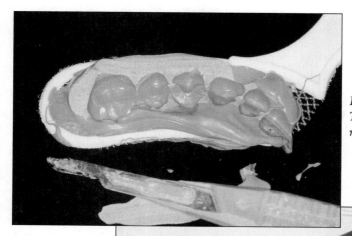

Fig. 11-13
Trimmed bite
relationship

Fig. 11-14 Artex
articulator system

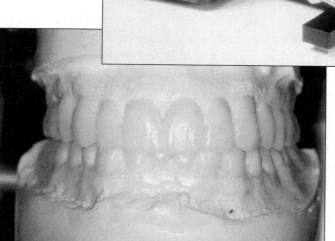

Fig. 11-15
Diagnostic
wax-up for lab
communication

light under which you are viewing it. Therefore, it is essential to view teeth for shade taking under ideal lighting situations. The most ideal light source will have a color temperature of 5,500 degrees Kelvin, and have a color-rendering index, which is the balance of the spectrum, above 90. It is both more efficacious and more affordable to have hand-held light rather than putting balanced lights in the ceiling. Ceiling lights will bounce off of your clothes, those of your patient and assistant, and any other colored objects in the operatory to deliver a light of unknown temperature to the viewing area. The shade-taking light should be held about 12 inches from the patient's mouth so as not to cause a blinding glare, and the patient napkin should ideally be light blue, the complement to orange on the color wheel. There is a phenomenon in our eyes known as "hue adaptation", which is a depletion of photo pigments in the cones, causing the hues to begin to look the same after 20 seconds or so. To prevent this from happening, the correct procedure for choosing a shade requires that we look at the teeth with the shade tab for 5 seconds and then look away at something that is light blue or light gray for 20 seconds to allow our eyes time to recover photo pigments. Then we may look back at the shades for another 5 seconds and then back at the light blue objects, repeating this procedure until the correct shade is chosen. A light blue patient napkin serves this purpose well. It should be noted that, despite our best efforts to match shades (an apparent success in our offices), the shades might be slightly off when viewed under different temperature lights. This is due to the fact that porcelain, composite, and enamel all have different spectral curves and hence, through a phenomenon known as metamerism, will reflect and absorb light slightly differently. Therefore, it may be helpful to also check the chosen shades under the cool fluorescents in ceiling lights and the warmer operatory lights.

Photographs, whether silver halide or digital, can be a valuable tool to communicate shade, texture, and morphology of anterior teeth to the laboratory. Figure 11-16 demonstrates how shade and texture were relayed to the ceramist in an attempt to match a challenging anterior tooth. Figure 11-17 shows the resulting restoration and how effective this form of communication can be in this process. Photos should be taken of

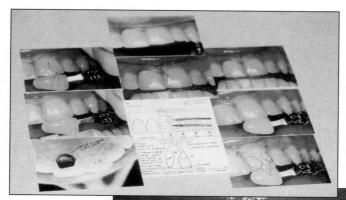

Fig. 11-16 Photos
used for lab
communication

Fig. 11-17
Definitive
restoration from
Figure 11-16

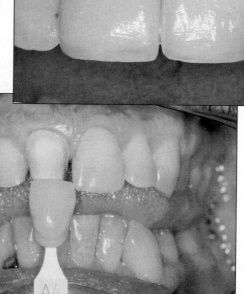

Fig. 11-18
Photo with shade
tab in place

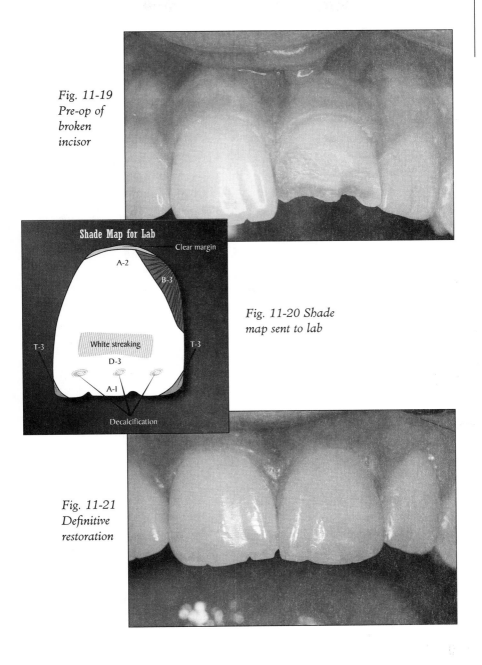

Fig. 11-19
Pre-op of
broken
incisor

Shade Map for Lab

Clear margin

A-2

B-3

White streaking

T-3

T-3

D-3

A-1

Decalcification

Fig. 11-20 Shade
map sent to lab

Fig. 11-21
Definitive
restoration

the preoperative situation, the prepped tooth, and the tooth you are trying to match from several different angles with the shade tabs in the same
plane as the tooth to be matched. (Fig. 11-18)

If photographs cannot be taken, a shade map may also be utilized to
communicate shade and texture. Figures 11-19, 20, and 21 illustrate a
shade map done for a broken tooth on a 11-year-old patient and the
results of that mapping. The goal is always to get it right the first time,
but if there is some variation that needs changing, then there is no more
effective way than to seat the tooth and photograph it in place before
sending it back to the laboratory.

To communicate nuances in the characteristics of posterior teeth,
there is the "Mosaic" shade guide as shown in Figure 11-22. With the
ability to illustrate amounts of groove staining, and the amount of decalcification as well as the degree of occlusal enamel translucency, this system can help the operator to match perfectly the posterior teeth. Figure
11-23 exhibits the results possible with this system.

Posts and Cores

Recent developments in polymer chemistry have produced resin fiber
posts that have reduced dramatically the threat of vertical root fracture
posed by metal posts. A unique new system, Fibrefill (The Pentron
Group, Wallingford, CT) allows the placement of the resin fiber post and
the obturation of the canal at the same time. It has been proposed by
Leonard et al. that endodontic failures are possibly due more to coronal
leakage than to apical leakage.[6] Other studies have proven that bonded
resin sealers seal best in both the apical and coronal directions.
Gutmann's studies suggest that the coronal opening be sealed with bonded resin immediately at the time of obturation. Studies by M. Trope and
others have proved that bonded resin/fiber posts in roots strengthen roots
against the possibility of catastrophic fracture.[7] This Fiberfill system seals
the apex and coronal opening with bonded resin and bonds in a rein-
forcing resin fiber post in a quick and simple manner. This gives optimal

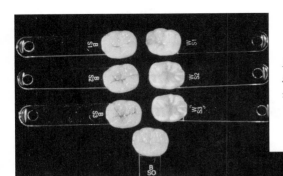

Fig. 11-22 Mosaic
shade guide for
molar shades

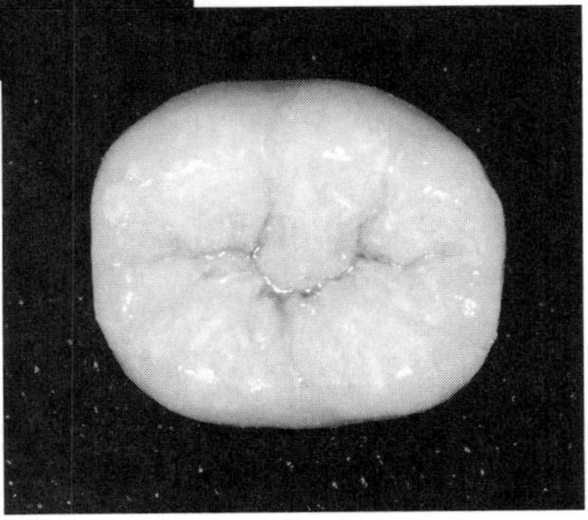

Fig. 11-23 Molar restored
using mosaic shade guide

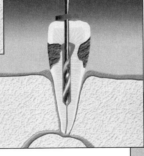

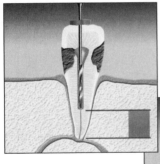

Fig. 11-24 Creating the post space length

Fig. 11-25 Creating the post space width

Fig. 11-26 Cleaning and shaping the apical third

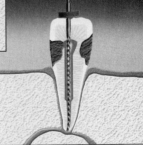

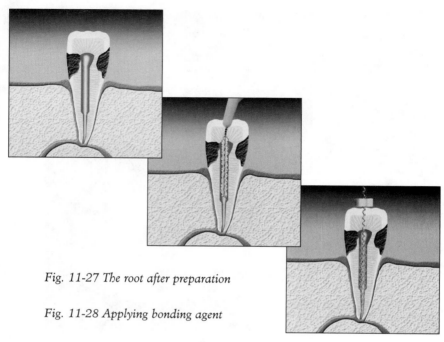

Fig. 11-27 *The root after preparation*

Fig. 11-28 *Applying bonding agent*

Fig. 11-29 *Filling the root with resin sealer*

Fig. 11-30 *The Fibrefill Obturator/post fully seated*

Fig. 11-31 *Obturator, post, and core in monobloc*

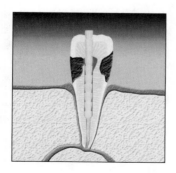

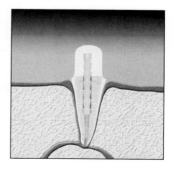

seal to the apex and the coronal end, a strengthened root, and a post for the support of build-up core material. The resulting restoration is bio-compatible, strong, esthetic, and easy to accomplish. Figures 11-24 to 11-31 illustrate the procedure.

Temporaries

A good temporary restoration is esthetic, strong, able to stabilize the prepped tooth, and easy and fast to make. Temporary restorations can be fabricated in the mouth, may be custom fabricated in a commercial laboratory, or may be made in the dental office laboratory. The custom intra-oral temporary is fabricated from a preoperative impression. This is most easily accomplished with a plastic triple tray and a fast-setting inexpensive polyvinylsiloxane material (Fig. 11-32). Once the preparation is completed and the impression is taken, the preop impression is loaded with temporary material in the area of the prepared tooth and it is placed back into the mouth. After it sets for the manufacturer's suggested amount of time, it is removed in a rubbery state and allowed to cure completely in the impression. The temporary restoration is trimmed, polished, sealed, and cemented with a suitable temporary cement.

The commercial laboratory-fabricated temporary restoration is usually reserved for large cases where long-term provisionalization is anticipated (Fig. 11-33). This may apply in cases where other procedures, such as periodontal therapies, must be completed before definitive restorations can be made. Another case where long-term provisionalization is desirous is in cases where occlusal schemes are altered, such as in full mouth reconstruction therapies. The diagnostic wax-up is invaluable as a guide for the technician in the fabrication of the long-term provisional. These restorations are usually stronger and more resistant to staining than the temporary restorations fabricated intra-orally.

A third method of temporary fabrication is the method of taking an impression of the prepared teeth and pouring that with quick setting stone, and while the patient waits, the temporary is fabricated on that stone model. The technique from that point is very similar to the intra-oral method.

Long span provisional bridges present challenges because of their propensity to fracture, particularly when utilized for long periods of time. To solve the problem of adding strength to long span bridges, they may be reinforced with glass fibers such as Ribbond or Splint-it (Pentron Clinical Technologies, Wallingford, CT). These fibers may be laid over the temporary material when it is initially placed in the matrix, and then seated over the prepared teeth or a model of prepared teeth. The fibers then become incorporated into the resinous material and may enhance the flexural strength up to 400%. The author has enjoyed great success with this technique. Occasionally, the fibers will become so displaced when the matrix is seated that the resulting restoration is unusable, but to remake it is a quick and simple procedure.

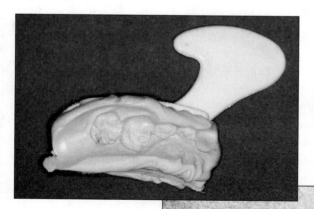

Fig. 11-32 Pre-op PVS impression for a temporary stent

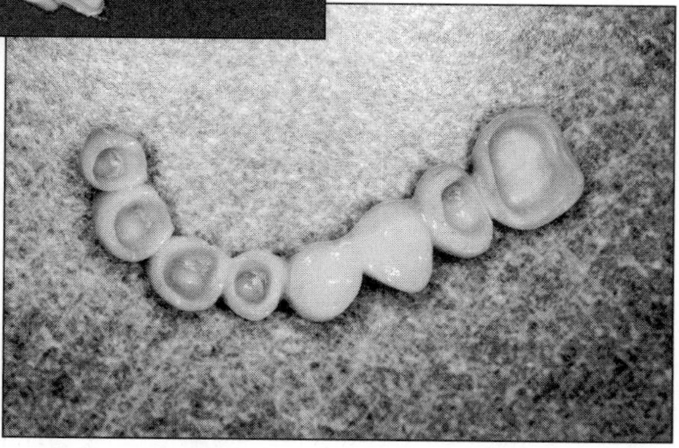

Fig. 11-33 Lab-fabricated temporary restoration

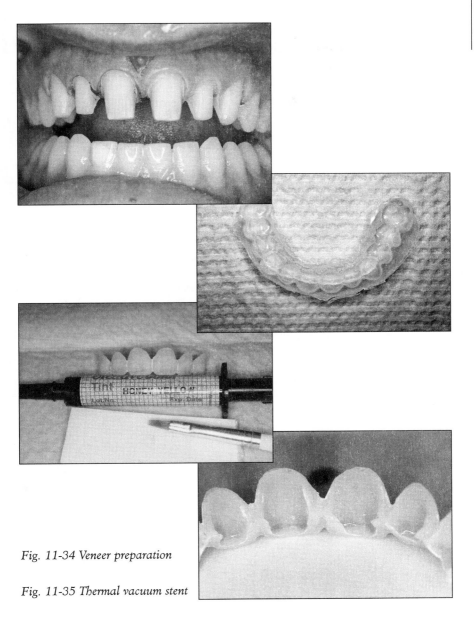

Fig. 11-34 Veneer preparation

Fig. 11-35 Thermal vacuum stent

Fig. 11-36 Application of neck stains

Fig. 11-37 Application of incisal stains

363

When esthetics of the provisional is critical, customization may be accomplished quickly and simply. Figure 11-34 shows veneer preparations on a young photographic model who was extremely sensitive about the look of the temporary restorations. He was unable to take off from work the two weeks necessary to fabricate the definitive restorations. In this case, a thermal vacuum splint was fabricated on an optimally altered model (Fig. 11-35). The challenge of making the temporaries look life-like was accomplished by applying a honey yellow stain over the necks of the provisionals (Fig. 11-36) and by applying a violet stain in the incisal areas to mimic the translucency of the incisal enamel (Fig. 11-37). Figure 11-38 demonstrates the results that allowed this young man to return to work.

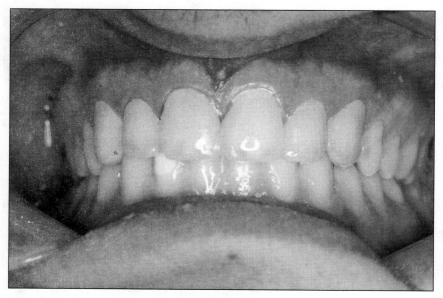

Fig. 11-38 Temporary veneers

Bonding

When the definitive restorations return from the laboratory, they have to be x-rayed in place to check for complete seating. The advent of digital radiography with its almost instantaneous images facilitates this procedure. When it is ascertained that the restoration is fully seated and the margins are closed, the restoration is appraised for its shade texture and morphology match to the rest of the teeth. If any of these don't match on anterior teeth, take a photograph of the restoration in place and send both to the laboratory for alteration. If the match is good, then the restorative dentist should proceed with the cementation process. The following is the protocol utilized by the author in luting restorations using resin cement:

1. Rinse the restoration with water and dry
2. If porcelain, then silanate and allow the silane to remain for 3 minutes
3. Air-dry the volatiles of the silane
4. Acid-etch the tooth's enamel and dentin for 15 seconds with 17% phosphoric acid
5. Rinse well and dry
6. Re-wet with Gluma desensitizer (Heraeus/Kulzer, Armonk, NY)—This is a mixture of 5% glutaraldehyde and 35% HEMA
7. Apply three coats of a primer/adhesive
8. Gently air dry
9. Light-cure the primer adhesive for 20 seconds
10. Place the resin cement of choice in the restoration and seat fully. (Use dual-cured cement for thick restoration and only a light-cured material for thin restorations)
11. Light-cure the material for 5-10 seconds until the cement has a consistency of soft calculus (The time will vary from one manufacturer's material to another)

12. Carve away excess semi-solid cement with a sharp scalpel blade or periodontal instrument and immediately use floss to clean the interproximal areas while the assistant steadies the prosthesis

13. If the contact area is impassable, then completely cure the material and saw through the contact area with a serrated saw (*e.g.*, Cerisaw, Denmat Corp.)

14. Adjust the occlusion

Metal crowns essentially follow the same protocol with the exception that a dual-cured cement is always used, and silane and hydroflouric acid are not applied to the metal surface, but rather, the metal in the crown is sandblasted to increase bonding surface area.

Conclusion

This chapter has sought to give you guidelines in accomplishing the difficult task of creating restorations that will look good, fit good, feel good, and last a long time. We have looked at the proper selection of materials and how to prepare the teeth to receive those materials. We have considered the impact those materials have on the opposing dentition and the pericoronal structures. Impressioning was discussed as well as the challenges of tissue retraction and hemostasis. Laboratory records and communication were elaborated, as were the protocols for bonding and desensitization. In spite of our diligence with each of these subjects, it is a fact that we will still experience an occasional failure. When this happens, remember that we are attempting to replace something that God made and the patient destroyed. Realize that, all in all, we do a great service to mankind.

Notes

[1] Weiss, ?, and Metzger, Z. *Bacterial Attachment to Metal Composite—a preliminary report.* Tel-Aviv University School of Dental Medicine, Feb. 1995

[2] Suzuki, S. *Antagonistic Enamel Wear of SoftSpar and Finesse Porcelains,* IADR Abstract #2454, 1997

[3] Rugh, J.D., and Ohrbach, R. Occlusal parafunction. In Mohl, N., et al., eds. *A Textbook of Occlusion.* Chicago: Quintessence, 1988

[4] *Ibid.*

[5] Orkin, D.A., Reddy, J., and Bradshaw, D. The relationship of the position of crown margins to gingival health. *J Prosthet Dent* 1987; 57: 421-424

[6] Leonard, J.E., Gutmann, J.L., and Guo, I.Y. Apical and coronal seal roots obturated with a dentin bonding agent and resin. Inter Endod J 1996; 29, 76-83

[7] Tripe, M., et al.

[8] Rugh, J.D., and Harlan, J. Nocturnal Bruxism and Temporomandibular Disorder. In Jankovic, J., and Tolosa, Ed., eds. *Advances in Neurology 49: Facial Diskinesias.* New York, Raven Press, 1988

Chapter 12

The Impact of Digital Imaging Technology on the Dental Practice

By Dale A. Miles, B.A., D.D.S., F.R.C.D.

Introduction

In the modern dental practice, nothing is making more of an impact on the way we assess and manage the patient's dental problems than "digital imaging." From clinical photography, intraoral video camera examination, and digital x-ray acquisition to fabrication of dental copings, digital imaging technology (DIT) has now touched part of almost everything we do in our dental practices. Recently, I wrote a brief opinion piece on my web site (www.learndigital.net) that describes how most of the recognized specialties have adopted DIT.[1] Even prosthodontists have adopted digital technology using solid-state imaging. Table 12-1 lists the specialty and the technology/technologies used by each discipline.

Specialty	Technology Used
Endodontics	digital intraoral x-ray, surgical video
Oral and Maxillofacial Radiology	CT, MR, intraoral and panoramic x-ray
Oral and Maxillofacial Surgery	as above
Oral and Maxillofacial Pathology	confocal microscopy, photomicrography
Orthodontics	digital intraoral and cephalometric x-ray digital clinical photography Invisalign aligner fabrication*
Pediatrics	digital intraoral x-ray
Periodontics	digital subtraction radiography, digital clinical photography
Prosthodontics	digital scanning for CAD CAM† restorations

*Invisalign—a set of clear, plastic appliances for minor adult tooth movement
† CAD CAM—computer assisted design, computer assisted manufacture as with a CEREC 2 system (Figure 1)

Table 12-1 Imaging by the "specialities"

Solid-state imaging detectors and DIT

The reason DIT has begun to impact so ubiquitously is due to the emergence of three technologies:

- The computer
- The digital detector
- Image processing software

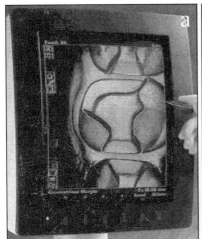 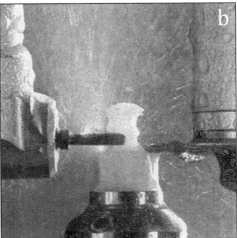

Fig. 12-1 CEREC 2 CAD-CAM system. These images of the CEREC 2 CAD CAM system depict the video image (a) of an inlay/onlay preparation on the monitor. The scanned image data will be used by the computer to mill (robotically) the temporary or final restoration (b). (Photo courtesy of Sirona USA, Charlotte, NC.)

The computer

Nothing digital in the dental office can be done without the computer. Dentists first adopted computers to help perform patient management functions more precisely and quickly. It soon became clear to dentists using computers that they could add peripheral devices for doing image acquisition and many other tasks, because the language to handle the text, images, voice, and video information was a common one; *i.e.*, the binary language of computers. The computer simply uses 0s and 1s, called a binary language, to translate every bit of information generated in the office into a common language in order to process that information. Thus, even the scanned image of a restorative preparation could be interpreted by the computer to tell a milling machine to fabricate the final restoration (Fig. 12-1).

Because of this ability to image patients, access the Internet for managing their care, and integrate text, voice, video, x-ray, and clinical still images, in addition to patient management tasks like appointment scheduling and billing, computers are now being used in the operatory as well as at the "front desk" for total patient management. This migration of the computer into the treatment area will only continue to grow.

In fact, dentists are now taking this "computerization" of their practice to the next level, by using wireless technology like a PDA (personal digital assistant) like a PalmPilot to wirelessly bring the patient information home with them or to their dental meeting so that they can always be "in touch" and "in contact" with important patient data. For example, if a patient is having post-operative pain and needs medication, the dentist can review his/her record at home, and prescribe the necessary drug more appropriately and safely, since he/she can also review on the PDA a drug database to help avoid any interactions that may occur with what they're about to prescribe and avoid a potential problem. Dental supply companies are creating dental programs for these wireless devices. Figure 12-2 shows a PDA device with a screen from the dental chart.

The digital detectors

The device behind much of the success of DIT and the first of the digital detectors to be introduced to dentists was the CCD or charge-coupled device. This is a solid-state imaging device made up of silicon (just like in the computer) and circuitry. More recently, the solid-state silicon chip that runs the operations in your computer, the CMOS chip, has had an imaging region integrated into (or more appropriately onto) the chip itself to act as an image receptor. CMOS stands for complementary metal oxide semiconductor. The term adopted by the imaging industry has been a "camera-on-a-chip." The CMOS chip is the device behind the vast majority of digital cameras now flooding the consumer and health professional market. One company, Schick Technologies, has opted to make this type of solid-state device its primary detector or sensor. Most other companies still use the CCD chip. For more detail about these devices, the reader can go to my web site or read several articles I've cited

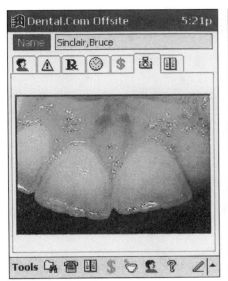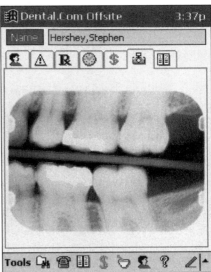

Fig. 12-2 PDA screen images. Screens for clinical photographs and radiographs of the dentist's patient. (Courtesy of Thompson Dental Company, product is Dental.com Offsite.)

in the references.[2-5] One company even marketed a hybrid CCD/CMOS detector for image capture. In addition to these solid-state detectors, there are reusable plastic plates with phosphor material imbedded in them called PSPs (photostimulable phosphors) that can be used to make digital images. They acquire the image much like a dental x-ray film, by storing the image latently until scanned by a laser light or beam. When scanned, they release the stored energy contained in the phosphor, and an image is created from the electric signal detected as the light transmission. Figure 12-3 shows images from all three types of detectors.

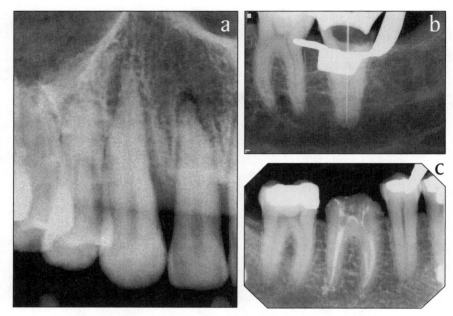

Fig. 12-3 Typical digital images. Left, CCD/CMOS image from DMD MPDx sensor (DMD, Inc. is no longer in business. This sensor will be sold through another dental company soon.) Top (b), CCD image (Schick Technologies, Inc., Long Island, NY). Lower (c), PSP image from Gendex (Denstply/Gendex, Des Plaines, IL).

How digital detectors work

The solid-state detectors are silicon chips with embedded electronic circuits that are usually fiber-optically-coupled to a computer. These detectors have various coatings on them called scintillators (phosphor materials) that the remnant x-rays leaving the patient bombard. The more efficient the phosphor material or scintillator is at gathering the x-rays, the better will be the image. When an x-ray strikes the scintillator material, the x-ray energy is converted to light that, in turn, strikes a layer of pure, amorphous silicon and breaks a covalent bond; one bond is broken for every light photon that strikes the silicon. Each bond broken results in an electron being released that is attracted to yet another layer in the silicon chip, called the "electron well." The electrons are stored in the well until a circuit embedded in the middle layer of the silicon chip (called the gate) is opened, and the electronic signal is sent to the computer. This electric, analog signal is converted to a digital image by assigning a gray shade to a certain signal strength. All of the grays of the image are displayed on the computer monitor as a "radiographic image" in small squares called pixels (picture elements). In a typical pixel array, there are from 307,200 pixels (640 x 480) to as many as 786,432 pixels (1,024 x 768). Some newer digital still cameras actually capture images (in color) that have as many as 3 megapixels or 3 million pixels or more. Some newer x-ray sensors also have a megapixel (1 million pixels) display. Figure 12-4 is a generic diagram of a solid-state detector capture system.

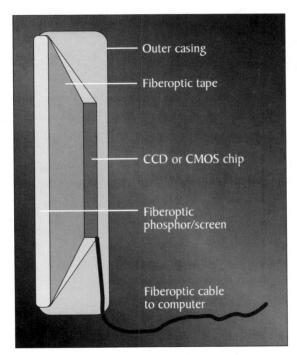

Fig. 12-4 A schematic diagram of the solid-sate image capture device

How x-rays and light are detected by the solid-state imager is important to understand. Figure 12-5 is a diagram of a CCD-type detector with legend to explain this process.

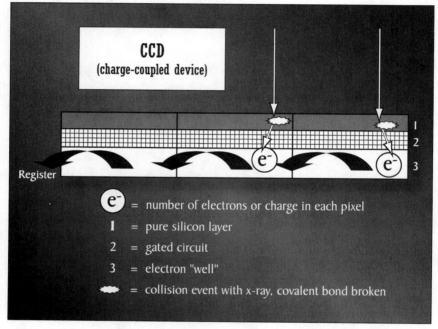

Fig. 12-5 A cross section through several pixels. There are three layers of silicon. X-rays exit the patient and strike the first layer of silicon (1). Each x-ray photon breaks a covalent bond (see collision event) in the amorphous silicon layer, releasing an electron. The electrons are drawn to a positively charged "well" (3), where they are held until the layer of silicon containing the embedded circuit or "gate" (2) is opened to allow the electronic analog signal to be detected by the computer and converted to a digital image. The signal or "charge" is read out at the far left side by a register in a "bucket brigade" fashion (black arrows), with the charge from the far right passing through each pixel until it reaches the read out register.

The CMOS-type detector uses a different method of interpreting the electronic charge that is said to be "non-destructive." The number of electrons in each pixel is read out independently, unlike the "bucket brigade" approach of the CCD. This means that each pixel can be "addressed" individually and read, without destroying the signal at each pixel. Computer operations can also be performed independently at each pixel site, which has advantages in "image processing." Figure 12-6 details the CMOS read-out process.

These detectors can be CCD-based, CMOS-based, or a combination of CCD/CMOS functions. More information can be found about the operation and characteristics of these devices elsewhere.[1-6]

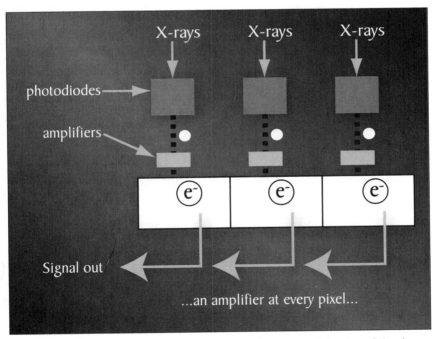

Fig. 12-6 Diagram of a CMOS-type detector showing amplification of the electronic signal at each of three pixels and the individualized "read-out" of the charge

Photostimulable phosphors (reusable phosphor plates, storage phosphors)

Solid-state detectors are not the only way to directly capture a digital x-ray image. More recently, several manufacturers have introduced another type of "digital" receptor called a PSP or photostimulable phosphor. All of these plates consist of a plastic substrate coated with a phosphor of differing types that can "store" a latent image in the phosphor until it is excited by laser light in a scanner to release the light as an electronic signal for conversion to a digital image on a computer monitor. Phosphors are found in your panoramic or cephalometric x-ray cassettes. But, unlike the storage phosphors, the ones in your panoramic cassettes immediately release light photons when struck by x-rays to expose a film. This amplification of the incoming x-rays to light photons means that we can use much less exposure time with our patient. This x-ray exposure reduction is the reason we employ screen/film combinations for conventional head and neck radiography.

The PSPs are a different story. They require longer exposures to saturate the phosphor for processing to a digital image, but still they are faster than some dental x-ray films. They are not as fast as CCD or CMOS detectors. In addition, the PSPs must be discharged after processing to eliminate any residual image in the phosphor before reuse. This entails waiting longer for an ultraviolet (UV) light source to "discharge" the plate in some phosphor systems, and in others, it means placing the plates on your x-ray view box for several minutes before re-exposure. This takes more time than the solid-state systems. In addition, the plates must be handled like x-ray film for infection control purposes. This means wrapping and unwrapping the plates and using new gloves to handle them while placing the plates in the laser scanner or in a template holder for placement into a drum-type laser scanner. Figures 12-7a and 12-7b show two commercially available scanners: the Gendex DenOptix system (Gendex Dental X-ray Division, Dentsply International, Inc., Des Plaines, IL) and the Soredex Digora system (Soredex, Inc., Marietta, GA).

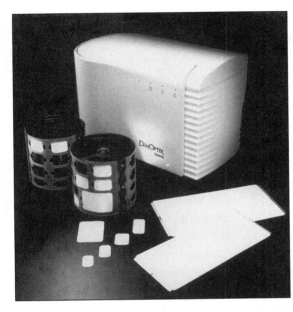

Fig. 12-7a The Gendex
DenOptix PSP system

Fig. 12-7b The Soredex
Digora PSP system

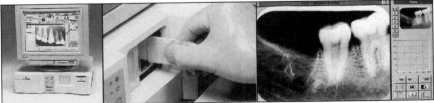

The phosphor material in the plates has one advantage over the solid-state type detectors. The PSPs can be exposed at a wider range of exposure times and still capture the image information. This means they have a wider "exposure latitude." You can give them a little exposure and you'll still have an image. Or, you can expose them for a much longer time than conventional x-ray film, CCD, or CMOS receptors, and they will still be able to display the image when processed. This may or may not be an advantage over the solid-state detectors. The CCD or CMOS detectors need only to be "sleeved" once for infection control. The image appears immediately on the computer monitor for interpretation. If you need to

379

"re-take" an image, you will know right away with solid-state systems, whereas you must wait for the laser scanning cycle to complete and for the complete discharge process also before you can re-use the PSP for a "re-take." More information is available from other authors.[6]

Digital image processing (electronic image processing—EIP)

Regardless of how you acquire the image digitally, you can perform electronic image processing on the digital image on your computer. There are a number of useful image processing "tools" or programs usually displayed on the top of the menu bar in the vendor's software program on your computer. Many of these "tools" have been borrowed from the "desktop publishing industry." The operator can alter things like the overall image contrast or density. In addition, some "tools" allow you to reverse the image contrast or use various computer algorithms called "filters" to change some feature in the image. Some even allow you to colorize the image, although at this time, there is little utility in coloring the information. One recent study used colorization to study how well clinicians could perceive bone defects at the bone/implant interface compared to gray scale images. The examiners did better with interpreting the change for this particular task. Dentists will have to use the software programs and researchers will have to continue to examine image processing "tools" in order to see what tasks in dentistry will be helped by which "tools."

What we are really doing is using electronic image processing to improve the feature detection of the disease process we are searching for. Medical radiologists have done this for more than 25 years. They alter the raw images of a patient to perform "feature extraction" to look for subtle nodules in a chest film or very small calcifications in the breast tissue that signal breast cancer. Radiologists, including oral and maxillofacial radiologists perform EIP (electronic image processing) on TMJ images acquired in CT and MR studies and for implant site assessment. Everything "digital" in radiology and now in dentistry should be altered by EIP to get the most out of the image in order to make better treatment decisions about our patients! It is *not* image "manipulation." It is electronic image *processing*, a necessary and desirable method of improving image and lesion features.

Figures 12-8 and 12-9 are examples of what can be done with image processing.

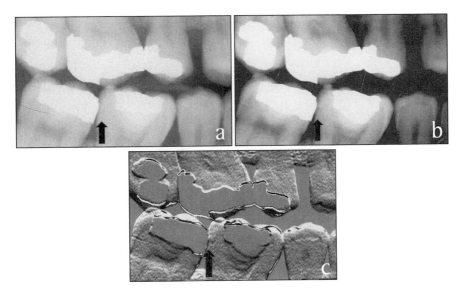

Fig. 12-8 Image processing applied to caries detection. In "A," try to see the interproximal carious lesion on tooth number 30. In "B," see how altering the image contrast improves the lesion appearance. Although the image is quite different from what we as dentists are used to looking at, see how the lesion appearance in "C" appears almost three dimensional, including a break at the interface of the DEJ.

In Figure 12-9, the processed image called "Clearview" represents one manufacturer's (Provision Dental Systems, Inc., Palo Alto, CA) proprietary algorithm using a "high-pass" filter technique. Although the image is grainier (has more noise or quantum mottle), the image is quite good for helping the clinician visualize the interproximal carious lesions present. Read the legend to see how we processed the image even further to optimize it for clinical evaluation. Image optimization for different dental imaging tasks is the goal for several image management/processing companies. Someday, we'll only have to "worry" about three buttons on our computer menu for image processing: a "caries" button, a "periodontal bone" button, and a "periapical change" button. Clicking one of these on your digital image will optimize the image for you to make it the best possible for you to evaluate.

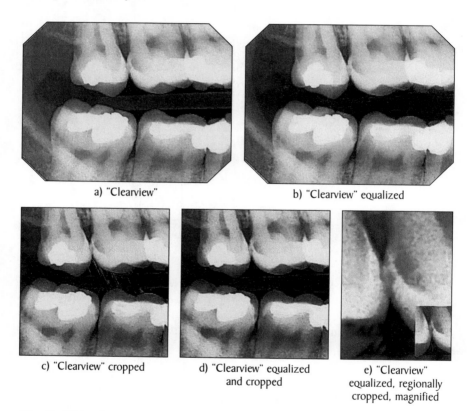

a) "Clearview"

b) "Clearview" equalized

c) "Clearview" cropped

d) "Clearview" equalized and cropped

e) "Clearview" equalized, regionally cropped, magnified

Fig. 12-9 "Equalization" procedures applied to a bitewing image. The "Clearview" equalized image (b) has slightly better overall image density for caries detection. The "Clearview" cropped image (c) eliminated the manufacturer's white corners. This improved the image once again, because the bright white "gray scale" values or numbers were not used in the mathematical algorithm to compute the gray scale changes. You can detect a slight improvement in the overall image quality between this image and the "Clearview" equalized one (d). Image (e) shows a smaller segment of the original image cropped and magnified. Note the increase in image noise when it was magnified, but also see the inserted image in the corner. It was an excellent view of the carious lesions until it was "exploded."

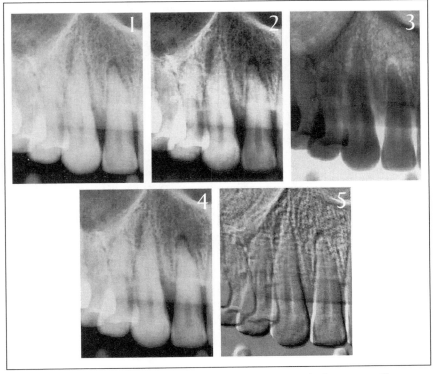

Fig. 12-10a Various image processing procedures applied to a maxillary cuspid view. 1. Raw image 2. Equalized image 3. Inverted contrast image 4. Reduced brightness, increased contrast image 5. Embossed image

Finally, we will show a palette of images that have been processed from the original to demonstrate what the images look like when subjected to various image processing "tools" (Fig. 12-10a). The original image was taken on a prototype portable x-ray generator weighing only 3.5 lbs using 60 kV and 3 mA. Other characteristics of this x-ray generator have been designed to take advantage of the faster image receptors like solid-state detectors, PSPs, and even the new faster F-speed dental x-ray films like Kodak's Insight (Eastman Kodak Company, Rochester, NY). Figure 12-10b shows an image acquired with two different x-ray generators, a conventional AC x-ray device (image on right) and a new prototype DC x-ray generator (image on left) with the image-processing menu opened for performing EIP on the images for carious lesion detection.

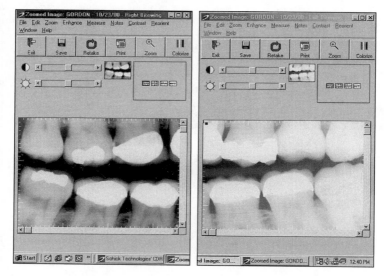

Fig. 12-10b Digital images taken with two different x-ray machines. Bitewing image on left screen taken with new x-ray machine designed to match the new, faster receptors. Image on right screen taken with a conventional x-ray generator. (Image courtesy of Dr. Claudio Levato, Bloomingdale, IL.)

Summary

Digital imaging and digital technology are here to stay. Every day, more and more dentists are adopting digital clinical cameras, computers, intraoral video cameras, image management systems, and digital x-ray systems. The advantages are many and obvious and have been demonstrated by researchers and clinicians alike. The only real change is in handling the information by computer and learning to perform EIP. It's not only making dentistry more fun, it's helping dentists make better clinical decisions and improve patient care.

Notes

[1] Miles, D.A. *Digital Imaging in the Specialties*, www.learndigital.net, May, 2001

[2] Miles, D.A., Langlais, R.P., and Parks, E.T. *Digital X-rays Are Here; Why Aren't You Using Them?* CDA Journal 27, (12):926-934, 1999

[3] Miles, D.A., and Razzano, M.R: *The Future of Digital Imaging In Dentistry*, DCNA, 44 (2): 427-438, 2000

[4] Miles, D.A. *Making Sense of Sensors*, Dental Practice Report 2001 Technology Guide, January, 2001, pp. 10-11

[5] Miles, D.A. *Understanding Digital Radiography*, Dental Practice Report 2001 Technology Guide, January, 2001, pp. 8-12

[6] Hildebolt, C.F., Couture, R.A., and Whiting, B.R. Dental Photostimulable Phosphor Radiography, DCNA, 44 (2): 273-297, 2000

Chapter 13

Orthodontics in the Progressive Dental Practice

By Elliott M. Moskowitz, D.D.S., M.Sd.

Introduction

Modern dental practice is both rewarding and challenging. Never have we seen such a consequential integration of yesterday's "separate disciplines" into what has now been termed interdisciplinary dental care delivery. The incorporation of surgical, prosthodontic, periodontic, orthodontic, and restorative concepts into the treatment of a single patient challenges all of us to learn more about techniques and materials that might not have been taught to us on the predoctoral or even postgraduate level. Orthodontics is no exception. The demand for orthodontic services is extraordinary. These services range from adjunctive orthodontic procedures as part of an overall management of a complex oral rehabilitation to comprehensive orthodontic treatment, requiring considerable knowledge of facial and dental growth and development as well as the use of significantly sophisticated diagnostic equipment and applied force mechanotherapy. It is not the purpose of this chapter to include every aspect of the wide range of orthodontic services provided to patients, but rather to selectively present practical information to aid the clinician in the management of some of the more commonly encountered clinical situations. As such, the chapter is appliance or "gadget" oriented. Much of the chapter is devoted to removable appliances. Some of these appliances will be familiar and have been used in orthodontics for many years. Others, such as Invisalign, are relatively new to both the orthodontic specialty and dental profession at large.

Fixed appliances are generally more complicated mechanical devices and not as easily presented or quickly learned as removable appliances. Consequently, sectional or partial fixed appliances have been used to demonstrate some of the advantages of utilizing fixed orthodontic appliances in selected clinical situations.

It is hoped that the clinician will find many of the techniques and materials presented in this chapter useful to his/her own dental practice. Incorporating orthodontic techniques and materials into a modern dental practice will provide patients with more treatment options as well as continue to stimulate the clinician in his/her daily practice. A selected bibliography has been included for those who might wish to explore some of these concepts in greater depth.

Removable Appliances

Removable appliances can be useful devices when employed in appropriate situations. Removable orthodontic appliances can be used to:

- Move teeth
- Retain teeth after active tooth movement has been completed
- Help in the elimination of noxious habits (thumbsucking)
- Serve as intermediate esthetic appliances as in the case of missing anterior teeth
- Maintain space in the posterior and anterior segments when primary teeth are lost prematurely

- Serve as functional appliances as part of comprehensive orthodontic treatment involving disharmonious relationships between the maxillary and mandibular dental arches

This chapter will deal mainly with appliances that either actively move teeth with relatively simple tipping movements or retain teeth that have already been moved.

Conventional removable appliances have a stabilizing element as well as an active portion. The Hawley type of appliance in Figure 13-1 has "C" clasps that will fit around the maxillary molars to help retain the appliance, a labial bow that will aid to both stabilize the appliance in the labial segment and move incisor teeth if desired, and a palatal acrylic section that will provide much of the "anchorage" during any active tooth movement.

Numerous designs of removable appliances have been developed. Many of these developments have focused upon the need to improve the esthetics of these appliances while tooth movement or retention efforts are effected. Figure 13-2 illustrates an attempt to decrease the visibility of a removable appliance by substituting a clear plastic strip to replace the conventional stainless steel wire labial bow. The plastic strip is supplying the needed force to retract and align the maxillary incisors.

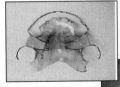

Fig. 13-1 Conventional Hawley retainer

Fig. 13-2 A more esthetic removable retainer with a clear plastic strip replacing a more visible labial bow

389

The Spring Aligner

The Spring Aligner is a removable orthodontic appliance specifically designed to correct labial and lingual malpositions and rotations of mandibular and/or maxillary incisor teeth. Following the successful alignment of the incisor teeth, the Spring Aligner can also serve as an effective removable retention device. Various designs of this appliance range from a relatively small "canine to canine" design to a more conventional type of retainer that extends to the posterior segments (Figs. 13-3, 13-4, and 13-5).

In general, severe crowding of mandibular anterior teeth can only be eliminated by the removal of teeth (usually an incisor or two premolars) to provide sufficient space to align the remaining teeth in functional,

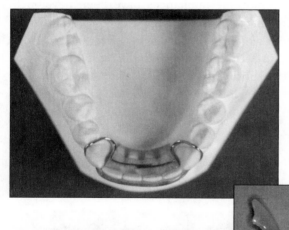

Fig. 13-3 Basic canine to canine Spring Aligner

Fig. 13-4 Additional clasping can be added to the Spring Aligner for greater retention

Fig. 13-5 The addition of a posteriorly extended acrylic section adds Spring Aligner capabilities to a conventional removable appliance

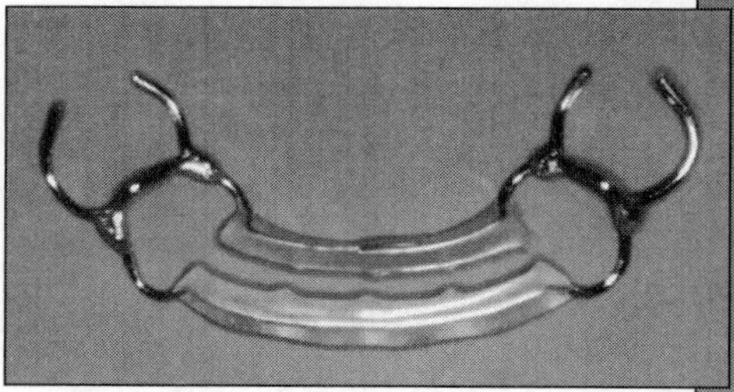

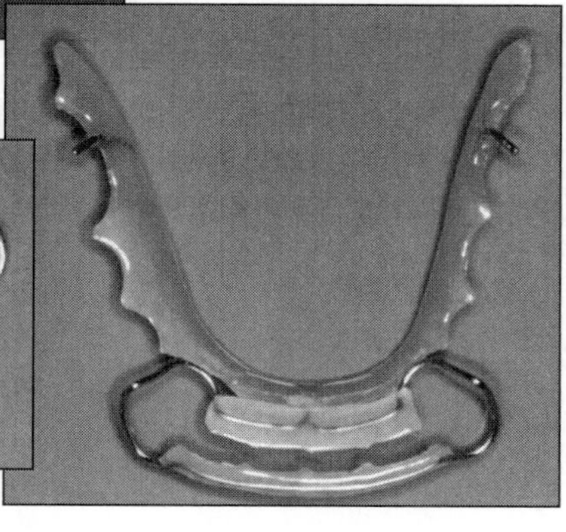

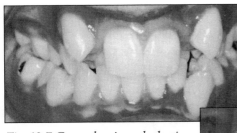

Fig. 13-6 Severe malocclusion with a significant arch length insufficiency resulting in gross crowding and other inter-arch disharmonies

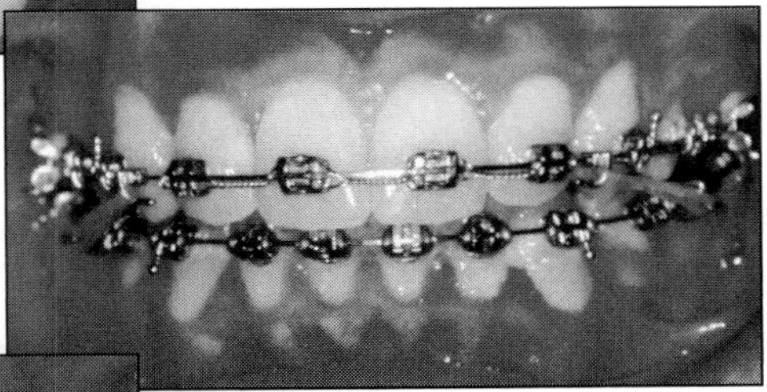

Fig. 13-7 Comprehensive orthodontic treatment with fixed multibonded orthodontic appliances. Extractions of first premolars were required as part of the overall treatment effort

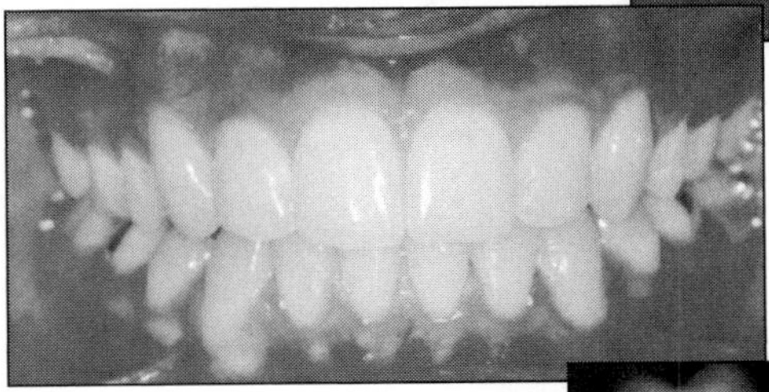

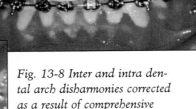

Fig. 13-8 Inter and intra dental arch disharmonies corrected as a result of comprehensive orthodontic treatment

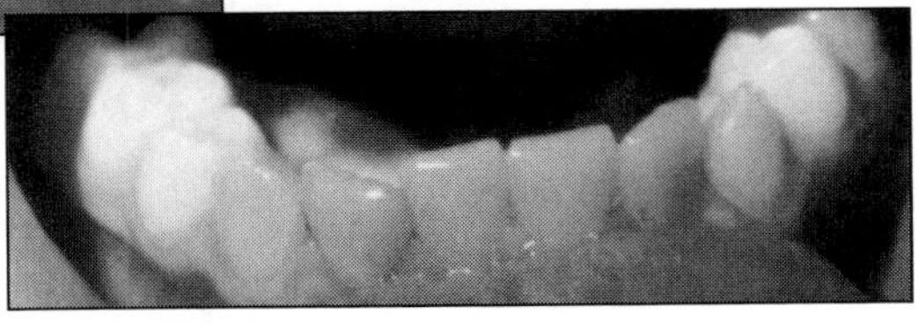

Fig. 13-9 An example of localized and relatively mild mandibular incisor malpositions. The degree of crowding is less than 3 mm

esthetic, and stable positions. This type of treatment is part of an overall comprehensive treatment effort requiring fixed, multi-bonded orthodontic appliances. An example of such a severe arch length insufficiency and its successful resolution utilizing fixed orthodontic appliances is shown in Figures 13-6, 13-7, and 13-8.

Differentiating between these types of cases and more localized situations is critical. Localized crowding of perhaps 3 mm or less might be appropriate cases for the Spring Aligner appliance (Fig. 13-9).

The additional dental arch length in these localized crowding situations can often be resolved with judicious interproximal reduction. Therefore, cases that have a predictable degree of success with the Spring Aligner appliance should have the following characteristics:

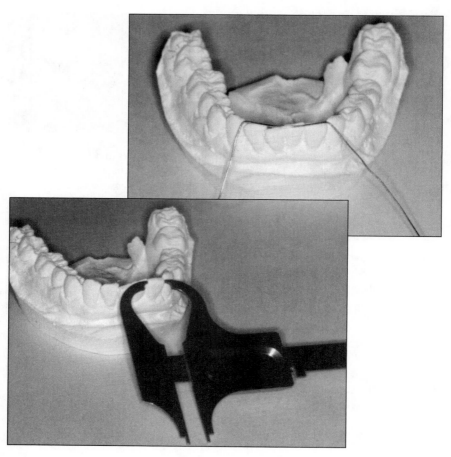

Fig. 13-10 Measuring the available space using brass separating wire along the mean arc of the incisal edges

Fig. 13-11 Measuring the required space by totaling the mesio-distal widths of the mandibular incisors

- Mild to moderate localized crowding of the maxillary and/or mandibular incisors not exceeding 2.5-3 mm
- Canines in acceptable positions
- Rotations and/or labio-lingual incisor malpositions
- Adequate periodontal support
- Axial inclinations of incisors are acceptable (the Spring Aligner is not effective in correcting mesio-distal tipping or axial inclination problems)

Treatment of crowded incisors that appear to be clinically manageable with the Spring Aligner should proceed as follows:

- Radiographs (panoramic or periapical) of the periodontium are examined to ascertain that orthodontic tooth movement is feasible (at least ⅔ of the root length in healthy bone)
- A study cast is examined to measure the incisor crowding in order to determine whether or not the Spring Aligner is an appropriate modality of treatment for the problem (3 mm or less of crowding, acceptable canine positions, and no objectionable mesial or distal tipping of incisors). First, measure the space *available* by measuring the distance from mesial of canine to mesial of canine along the mean arc of the incisal edges (Fig. 13-10). Secondly, the mesio-distal diameter (width) of each incisor is measured. Total the four incisor widths to obtain the space *required* (Fig. 13-11). Subtract the space *available* from the space *required* measurement. The difference is the arch length discrepancy that must be accounted for in the uncrowding and alignment procedure of the incisor teeth. Again, keep in mind the 3 mm or less rule, accepting the canine positions "as is," and avoiding cases that might require uprighting of tipped teeth

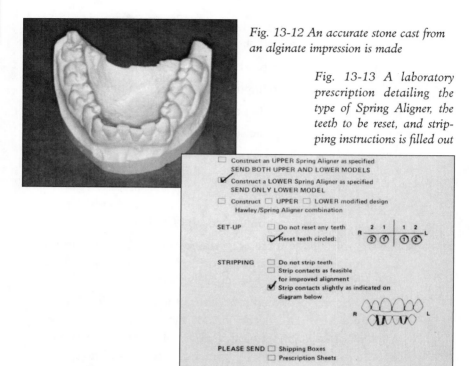

Fig. 13-12 An accurate stone cast from an alginate impression is made

Fig. 13-13 A laboratory prescription detailing the type of Spring Aligner, the teeth to be reset, and stripping instructions is filled out

- A laboratory cast (from an alginate impression) and a laboratory prescription for indicating the amount and location of desired interproximal reduction are prepared (Figs. 13-12 and 13-13)

- These procedures will greatly impact upon the actual clinical management of the Spring Aligner procedure. Alginate impressions should be poured as soon as possible and be free from artifacts (bubbles) and distortion

- The orthodontic laboratory, following your prescription, will remove (by saw cuts) the indicated incisors from the cast, strip the cast teeth, and replace the incisors on the cast in ideal positions with set-up wax. A spring wire framework (0.028 or 0.030 inch diameter stainless steel wire) is made on the set-up casts, and clear acrylic is "sprinkled" to the labial and lingual sections of the wire framework. The acrylic is pressure-cured, trimmed, polished, and returned to you on the set-up cast. See Figures 13-14 through 13-21.

Clinical Procedures

1. Fit the Spring Aligner and check its retention
2. Perform interproximal reduction (stripping) no more than ⅓ of the total amount of planned stripping amount
3. The patient is instructed in the placement and care of the appliance. The patient is given an appliance case, told to expect soreness of the incisor teeth for two or three days, and instructed to wear the appliance on a 24 hour basis (ideally only removing the appliance to brush the teeth and to eat). Reappointment time is two or three weeks
4. At observation visits, progress is noted, teeth are stripped additionally as is necessary, and the appliance is activated or modified with a Howe plier as required (Fig. 13-22)

Patient F.G. is a 39-year-old female patient who had received orthodontic treatment as a youngster. Her chief concern focused upon the malaligned mandibular incisor teeth. A Spring Aligner appliance was constructed to resolve the crowding. Figures 13-23 and 13-24 show the pre-treatment malalignment of the mandibular incisors.

Figure 13-25 shows the Spring Aligner in place after about six months. During treatment it became desirable to place a little extra rotational force on the mandibular right central incisor (Fig. 13-26). "Dimples" were placed on a new in-treatment cast with a round bur and when the second appliance was made, it had the effect of "supercharging" the appliance by placing more force (more acrylic) in that area (Fig. 13-27).

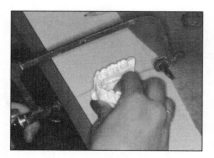

Fig. 13-14 The mandibular central and lateral incisors are removed from the cast with saw cuts

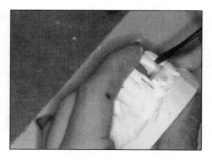

Fig. 13-15 The teeth are appropriately reduced in size (simulating the stripping that will be performed clinically) and reset

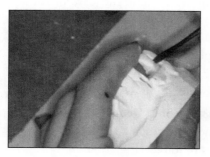

Fig. 13-16 The teeth have now been reset to simulate the final desired clinical result

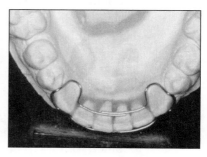

Fig. 13-17 A spring wire framework (either .028 or .030 inch diameter stainless steel wire) is constructed on the completed set-up cast

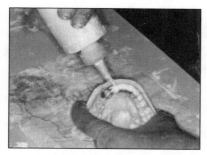

Fig. 13-18 The acrylic framework portion is fabricated on the labial and lingual aspects of the wire framework

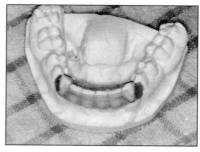

Fig. 13-19 The cured framework ready to be separated from the cast

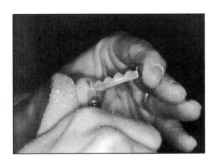

Fig. 13-20 The completed acrylic framework is trimmed and polished

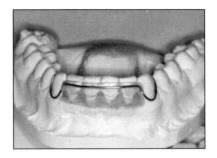

Fig. 13-21 The finished Spring Aligner is placed on the cast and is ready to be delivered to the patient

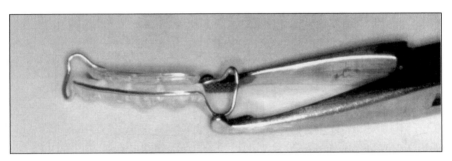

Fig. 13-22 At observation visits, the Spring Aligner is adjusted with a Howe Plier by gently squeezing the clasps

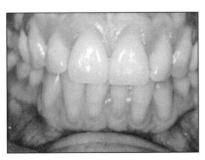

Fig. 13-23 Pre-treatment frontal intraoral view

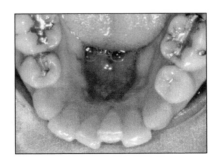

Fig. 13-24 Pre-treatment occlusal view showing the malalignment of the mandibular incisors

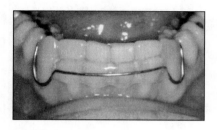

Fig. 13-25 The Spring Aligner in place

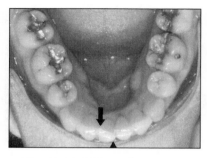

Fig. 13-26 Additional rotation is needed to correct the mandibular right central incisor

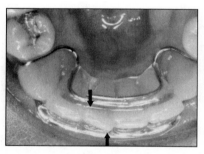

13-27 After a new in-treatment cast was made and "dimples" were placed in the area of needed rotation, the "extra" acrylic in this area serves to "supercharge" the rotational movement

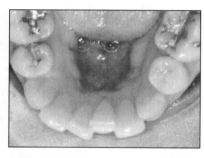

Fig. 13-28 Pre-treatment occlusal view of patient F.G.

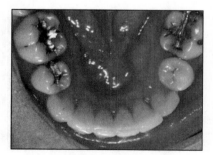

Fig. 13-29 Post-treatment occlusal view of patient F.G. after 10 months of treatment

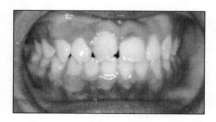

Fig. 13-30 Frontal intra-oral view of a patient with a severely rotated maxillary right central incisor

The patient was seen approximately once every 3-4 weeks. The pre-treatment (Fig. 13-28) and post-treatment result (Fig. 13-29) shows a dramatic correction.

The second case depicts a patient who had a severe rotation of the maxillary right central incisor. The Spring Aligner was effective in correcting the rotation of the maxillary right central incisor in approximately four months (Figs. 13-30 through 13-33).

Severe rotations of incisor teeth require special attention in retention due to the high tendency for relapse. A bonded lingual wire was placed in this particular case to prevent relapse (Fig. 13-34).

The Spring Aligner is a useful mechanical device for managing localized incisor malpositions. As always, case selection is an important aspect in the overall successful use of this appliance. Following active tooth movement, the Spring Aligner can serve as a nighttime-worn retention appliance.

Anterior Crossbites

Anterior crossbites in young patients are commonly encountered. Etiological factors in the development of anterior crossbites of permanent teeth may include delayed exfoliation or removal of a primary tooth (Fig. 13-35), insufficient arch length for the permanent tooth in crossbite, and skeletal disharmonies between the maxilla and mandible. Crossbites of permanent anterior teeth should be corrected to prevent further arch length loss, eliminate developing periodontal involvement (Fig. 13-36), correct jaw deflections due to prematurities, prevent damage to enamel surfaces, and improve esthetics.

Removable appliances can often be utilized to correct anterior crossbites in the mixed dentition as well as the permanent dentition. A young patient (age nine) presented with a crossbite of the maxillary right permanent central incisor that was due to an over-retained maxillary right

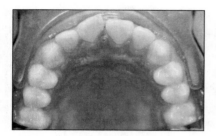

Fig. 13-31 Occlusal view of the rotated maxillary right central incisor

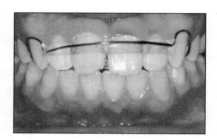

Fig. 13-32 The Spring Aligner in place

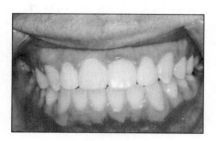

Fig. 13-33 The rotation corrected

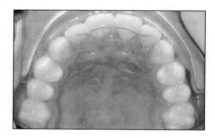

Fig. 13-34 A bonded lingual wire was placed to prevent relapse of the maxillary right central incisor

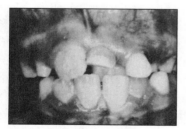

Fig. 13-35 Delayed exfoliation of a primary maxillary incisor can cause the erupting permanent tooth to assume a lingual crossbite position

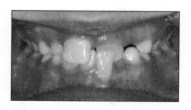

Fig. 13-36 Early adverse gingival response of the mandibular incisor in a patient with an anterior crossbite

central incisor (Fig.13-37). A removable appliance (Figs. 13-38 and 13-39) with an auxiliary spring placed lingual to the maxillary right central incisor applied a light tipping force. The crossbite was successfully "jumped" in less than three months (Fig. 13-40).

Frequently, the depth of bite and resulting lack of clearance will require some modification of the removable appliance to "raise the bite" and remove potentially traumatic forces while the tooth in crossbite is being corrected. Figures 13-41 and 13-42 demonstrate the use of occlusally built acrylic over the posterior portion of the removable appliance to remove mechanical interferences while a maxillary left central incisor is being moved labially by a lingual finger spring.

Removable appliances can also be used in adult patients to selectively tip teeth. Figures 13-43a, b, and c show an adult patient with a maxillary right lateral incisor in crossbite.

Auxiliary springs are placed to move the maxillary central incisors to the left to gain additional space while the maxillary right lateral incisor is moved labially. Occlusal acrylic to remove mechanical interferences while these movements are taking place is an important appliance modification for adult patients (Figs. 13-44a, b, and c).

Figures 13-45a and b show the completed case with the crossbite corrected and the position of the maxillary incisors improved. Treatment extended approximately nine months.

Anterior crossbites that may be corrected by moving one or several teeth should be differentiated from cases that might appear to be similar, but indeed are reflective of a more serious underlying skeletal disharmony between the maxillary and mandibular skeletal bases. These skeletally based malocclusions almost always require more sophisticated treatment protocols that could include dentofacial orthopedics and/or orthognathic surgery. Differential diagnosis and treatment planning of such cases demand a thorough knowledge of cephalometric radiography and analysis, growth, and development, as well as skills in the use of more complicated orthodontic appliances.

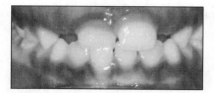

Fig. 13-37 An anterior crossbite of the maxillary right central incisor in the mixed dentition

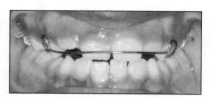

Fig. 13-38 A conventional removable appliance used to correct the crossbite

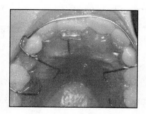

Fig. 13-39 Auxiliary spring lingual to the maxillary right central incisor applies force in a labial direction

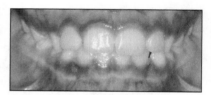

Fig. 13-40 The crossbite of the maxillary right central incisor successfully corrected

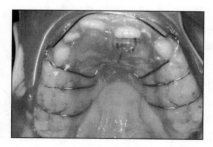

Fig. 13-41 Maxillary removable appliance with occlusal coverage used to remove occlusal interferences

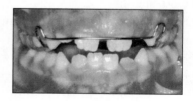

Fig. 13-42 The resultant effect of the occlusal coverage in providing the necessary "clearance" to resolve the anterior crossbite

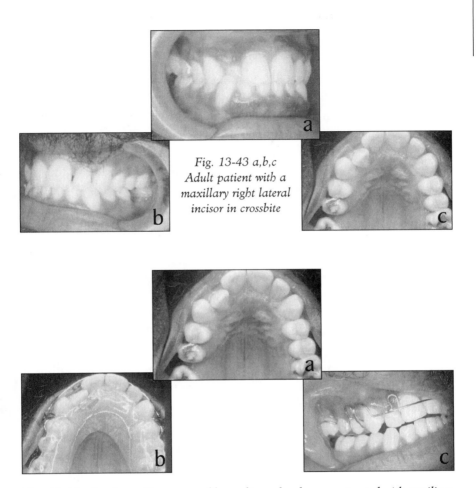

Fig. 13-43 a,b,c
Adult patient with a
maxillary right lateral
incisor in crossbite

Fig. 13-44 a,b,c A maxillary removable appliance has been constructed with auxiliary
springs and occlusal acrylic to remove mechanical interferences

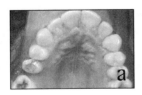

Fig. 13-45 a,b The maxillary right lateral incisor
crossbite corrected

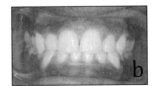

Functional Crossbites

Crossbite relationships of opposing teeth may occur in the posterior segments. Posterior crossbite relationships may be due to dental, functional, or skeletal mal-relationships between the maxillary and mandibular dentition and/or the maxillary and mandibular skeletal bases. Differentiating between dental, functional, and skeletal components of a clinically encountered crossbite(s) is an important element in the successful resolution of such problems.

Dental crossbites

Dental crossbites (illustrated in Fig. 13-46) have definite occlusal stops and have normal bucco-lingual inclinations of the opposing molars on the right side. The dental midlines coincide, and it is the left side that displays a lingually-positioned maxillary molar and a somewhat buccally-inclined mandibular molar. These situations may be treated with either removable or limited fixed appliances. Figure 13-47 shows a dental crossbite treated with a traditional intermaxillary "cross" elastic. Dental crossbites are most commonly encountered in which the maxillary tooth is in lingual position to the mandibular counterpart, however, buccal crossbites can occur as well (Fig. 13-48).

Functional crossbites

Posterior functional crossbites generally have a distinctive pattern in which, when the teeth are in maximum intercuspation, a unilateral crossbite is seen. The opposite side appears to occlude normally. The mandibular midline is shifted toward the crossbite side (Fig. 13-49).

This may be accompanied by a mandibular frontal asymmetry, as functional crossbites frequently cause a shift of the mandible to the centric occlusion-observed, crossbite-affected side. With the mandible in the rest position (Fig. 13-50), the dental midlines now coincide. The posterior teeth appear to be positioned with the buccal cusps of the maxillary teeth over the buccal cusps of the mandibular teeth. Now, it becomes apparent that what is needed is bilateral movement of the maxillary pos-

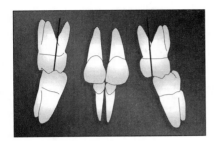

Fig. 13-46 Dental crossbite - definite occlusal stops and normal bucco-lingual inclinations of the opposing molars on the right side. The dental midlines coincide, and the left side displays a lingually positioned maxillary molar and a buccally inclined mandibular molar

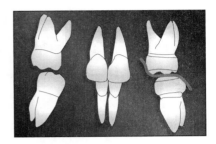

Fig. 13-47 "Cross" elastics used to correct dental crossbites

Fig. 13-48 Dental crossbites include buccal crossbites

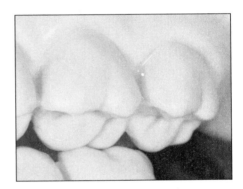

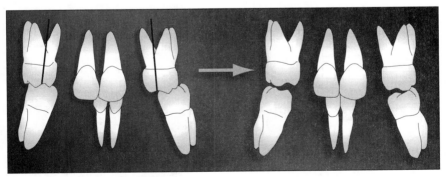

Fig. 13-49 Functional crossbite—the maxillary and mandibular dental midlines do not coincide

Fig. 13-50 When the mandible is positioned to its normal transverse rest position (midlines coinciding), it becomes apparent that bilateral expansion is required

terior segments and not merely expanding one side, as might be suggested by only observing the static crossbite relationship in centric occlusion. Accurately assessing maxillary and mandibular dental midlines is an important clinical examination step that will greatly aid the clinician in differentiating dental crossbites from functional crossbites.

Long-standing functional shifts in growing patients can contribute to facial asymmetries, and it has been suggested that transverse disharmonies involving mandibular asymmetries

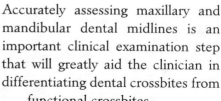

Fig. 13-51 Functional crossbite in the mixed dentition. Note the dental midline shift towards the side that displays a crossbite relationship reflecting the mandibular displacement upon closure

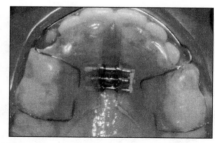

Fig. 13-52 A removable expansion device with occlusal acrylic and expansion screw

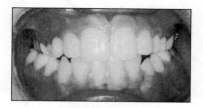

Fig. 13-53a Pre-treatment frontal intraoral view illustrating the initial dental midline relationship

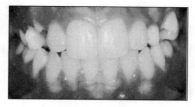

Fig. 13-53b Post-treatment frontal intraoral view with the midlines coinciding, functional crossbite corrected, and normal transverse mandibular position

might be a predisposing factor in certain adult temporomandibular disorder (TMD) patients. Functional crossbites should be treated earlier rather than later in growing patients, and the feasibility of beginning orthodontic corrective procedures in these cases will be largely dictated by favorable or unfavorable patient management conditions.

Expansion of the maxillary dentition and/or the maxillary base can be accomplished with a number of different appliances. The Quad Helix, cross elastics with arch wires, rapid maxillary expansion, slow maxillary expansion, removable appliances, and in certain cases surgery or a combination of surgery and orthodontics (surgically assisted rapid palatal expansion) are devices or techniques that can be used to effect an increase in either the maxillary dentition or actual maxillary skeletal base.

Figure 13-51 show frontal and lateral views of a functional crossbite (unilateral posterior crossbite of the right side observed in the centric occlusion position) seen in the in the mixed dentition treated with a removable expansion device (Fig. 13-52) that is activated by turning the midpalatal expansion screw by the patient's parent one turn per day. Occlusal acrylic is used to remove mechanical interferences. This acrylic is extended well up on the buccal surfaces to minimize the amount of dental tipping that might occur.

The mandible is allowed to assume its normal transverse position after "functional prematurities" are removed by the maxillary dental arch expansion. Note the initial dental midline relationship before (Fig. 13-53a) and after treatment (Fig. 13-53b)

Skeletal Posterior Crossbites

Certain observed posterior crossbites are indicators of severe skeletal disharmonies requiring comprehensive and often multidisciplinary treatment. Figure 13-54 displays a characteristic finding of skeletal crossbites. Note that the axial inclinations of the posterior teeth are normal despite the significant crossbite relationship. Dental midlines may or may not coincide in these instances. Figures 13-55 and 13-56 show a

Fig. 13-54 Skeletal crossbite with normal bucco-lingual positions of the maxillary and mandible molars

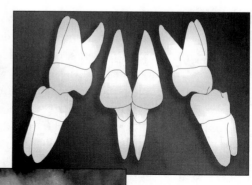

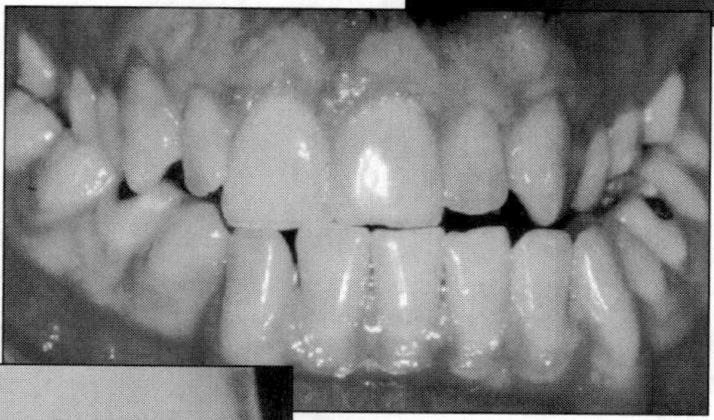

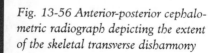

Fig. 13-55 Clinical photograph of a skeletal crossbite requiring comprehensive orthodontic treatment and orthognathic surgery

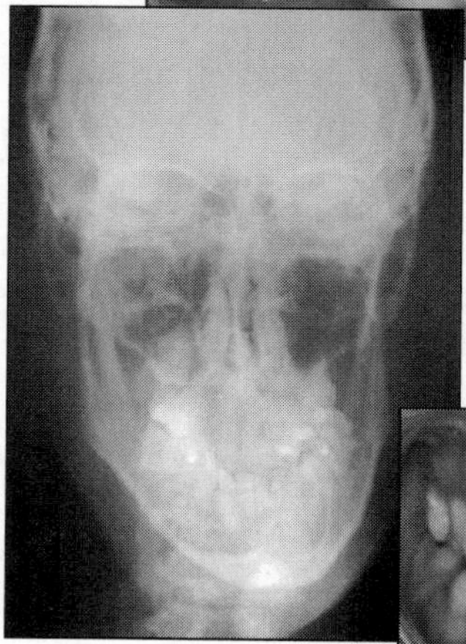

Fig. 13-56 Anterior-posterior cephalometric radiograph depicting the extent of the skeletal transverse disharmony

Fig. 13-57 Maxillary "canine-to-canine" ESSIX retainer

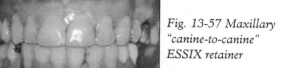

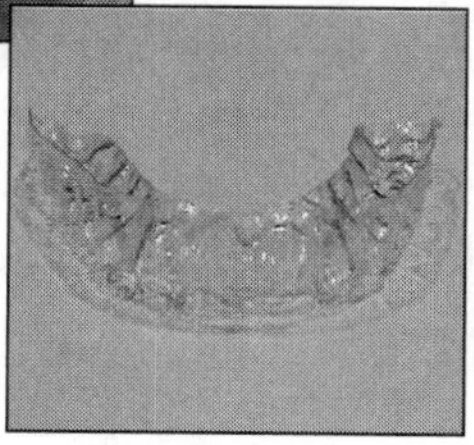

Fig. 13-58 Full arch ESSIX retainer covering all the teeth in the maxillary dental arch

patient with a severe mandibular asymmetry and a significant narrow maxillary dental arch that required both comprehensive orthodontic treatment and orthognathic surgery to resolve functional and esthetic skeletal and dental issues.

ESSIX Removable Appliances

ESSIX appliances are clear, virtually invisible, removable appliances that can retain incisor teeth, perform minor tooth movements, and serve as a useful and extremely esthetic provisional anterior prosthesis for pre- and/or post-implant patients. They are constructed from thermoformed plastic material and are most commonly constructed as "canine to canine" appliances (Fig. 13-57), although they can be fabricated to extend the entire dental arch (Fig. 13-58).

Steps in making an ESSIX retainer

1. Obtain an accurate working cast (Fig. 13-59)

   a. Use a polyvinylsilox-
      ane material or
      high grade
      alginate impression

   b. Pour the
      impression in a
      "crown and bridge"
      quality stone

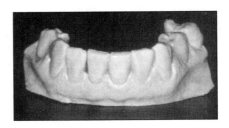

Fig. 13-59 An accurate working cast is fabricated in a "crown and bridge" quality stone

2. Thermoform a clear sheet of 0.030" thickness thermoplastic material

   a. Remove appliance from cast

   b. Trim appliance with scissors and smooth with a nail file

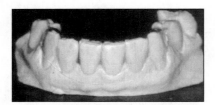

Fig. 13-60 The clear plastic ESSIX
retainer is constructed on the working cast

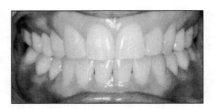

Fig. 13-61 The canine to canine
ESSIX mandibular retainer is
virtually invisible

Figures 13-60 and 13-61 show a constructed canine-to-canine mandibular ESSIX retainer on a working cast and in the mouth. Numerous retainers can be constructed from the same cast and kept as "spares" if an ESSIX retainer is lost or becomes worn.

Patients who require a single tooth implant have a special requirement of wearing an esthetic provisional appliance that does not "load" the implant during the process of osseous integration. The patient in Figure 13-62 is congenitally missing maxillary lateral incisors and has just completed orthodontic treatment.

The patient is several years away from having her implant fixtures placed and wanted an alternative to the "flipper" or Hawley type appliances with pontic replacements (Fig. 13-63). These conventional removable appliances are bulky, can cause palatal irritations due to "settling" with prolonged use, and, in the case of a modified Hawley appliance, can be notably unesthetic.

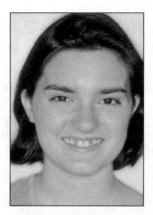

Fig. 13-62 Patient requiring implants in need of a transitional esthetic appliance before the implants are placed

Appropriately sized, shaped, and color-matched pontics were included in the thermoforming process during the construction of a modified ESSIX™ retainer (Figs. 13-64 and 13-65). Retention of the pontics are provided by undercut "trenches" that have been placed in the lingual surfaces of the pontics prior to being encased by the thermoplastic material during the vacuum form procedure (Fig. 13-66). The final esthetic result is shown in Figure 13-67.

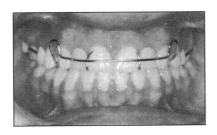

Fig. 13-63 A traditional Hawley type of removable appliance with pontics replacing the maxillary lateral incisors

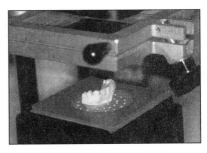

Fig. 13-64 Thermoforming process of an ESSIX retainer with a pontic secured to the working cast

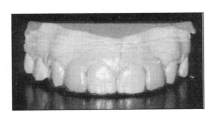

Fig. 13-65 The completed canine to canine ESSIX retainer with pontics in place

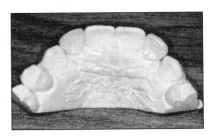

Fig. 13-66 Undercut "trenches" have been created on the lingual surfaces of the maxillary lateral incisor pontics to aid retention of the thermoplastic material

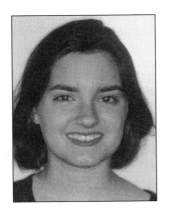

Fig. 13-67 The esthetic modified ESSIX retainer serves as an excellent transitional appliance until implants and subsequent implant supported restorations can be fabricated

Invisalign

No doubt, the single most significant factor that deters adult patients in seeking orthodontic treatment is the visibility of orthodontic appliances. Fixed orthodontic appliances have undergone considerable design modifications in an effort to reduce the visibility of the orthodontic hardware. Ceramic porcelain orthodontic brackets, tooth-colored wires, and lingual fixed orthodontic appliances are examples of this effort to make fixed orthodontic appliances more attractive to adult patients. A relatively new technology introduced by Align Technology, Inc. is the Invisalign system. Invisalign uses a unique 3-D computer graphics technology to produce multiple virtually invisible full arch removable appliances (Figs. 13-68 and 13-69) that, when worn as prescribed, are capable of moving teeth into their desired positions.

How the Invisalign system works

1. The clinician selects an appropriate case for Invisalign. Guidelines for cases that are appropriate for Invisalign have been established by Align Technology, Inc. Accurate impressions utilizing polyvinylsiloxane impression materials are made and, along with other important diagnostic data/records, are sent to Align Technology, Inc.

2. At Align Technology, Inc., a mold is poured of the patient's teeth and digitized. A proprietary computer software program is used to generate a start-to-finish 3-D movie that shows the series of movements of the patient's teeth from the current position to the desired final position

3. The clinician can then review the 3-D movie on Align Technology Inc.'s website (www.invisalign.com) and, from these images, a series of clear, plastic aligners are fabricated

4. The patient wears each stage of aligners (for approximately two weeks) before switching to the next in the series. Week by week, the patient's teeth are aligned in small increments until they are moved to their final positions

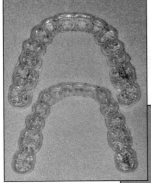

Fig. 13-68 Full arch Invisalign appliances

Fig. 13-69 Invisalign appliances on a typodont display their near invisibility quality

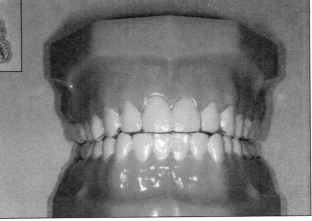

An example of Invisalign's capabilities can be seen in the case of an adult patient who exhibited a significant degree of mandibular incisor crowding (Figure 13-70). The esthetic and practically invisible mandibular Invisalign appliance is illustrated in Figure 13-71. Subsequent photographs taken at approximately 2 month intervals from the use of the very first Invisalign appliance show a marked improvement in the position of the malaligned mandibular incisors as orthodontic treatment progressed (Figures 13-72, 13-73, 13-74,13-75, and 13-76).

Successful results with the Invisalign system are dependent upon a number of factors that include initial case selection and meticulous attention to the detailed steps outlined by Align Technology, Inc. Align Technology, Inc. offers training to prospective clinicians who are contemplating utilizing the Invisalign system.

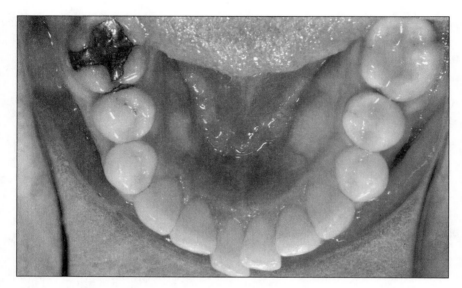

Fig. 13-70 *Adult patient exhibited a significant degree of mandibular incisor crowding*

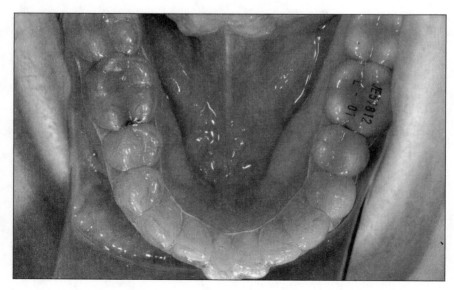

Fig. 13-71 *The mandibular Invisalign appliance is virtually invisible when worn*

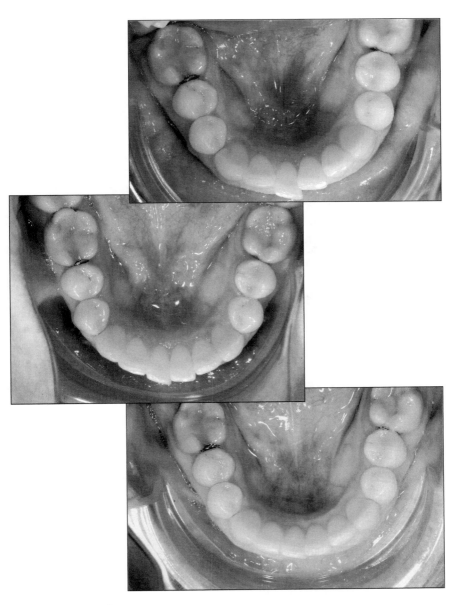

Fig. 13-72 2 month progress

Fig. 13-73 4 month progress

Fig. 13-74 6 month progress

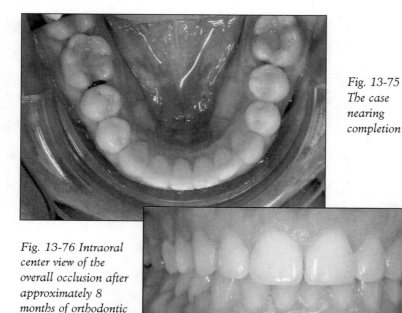

Fig. 13-75
The case
nearing
completion

Fig. 13-76 Intraoral
center view of the
overall occlusion after
approximately 8
months of orthodontic
treatment

Fixed Orthodontic Appliances

Fixed orthodontic appliances are capable of delivering a much wider range of different types of tooth movement than removable appliances. They can be used as relatively simple sectional appliances to effect minor or localized tooth malpositions or can be highly complex in design and action in more comprehensive clinical situations. The discussion of biomechanics, comprehensive use of fixed orthodontic appliances, and the more recent advances in bracket design (pre-adjusted prescription brackets, "friction-free" ligationless brackets, etc.) are well out of the scope of this chapter. Numerous texts have been devoted to the use of fixed orthodontic appliances as the mechanical device of choice in the overall treatment of complex malocclusions. Some of these references are included at the end of this chapter.

A practical approach to the use of limited fixed appliances involves some basic knowledge of the placement of orthodontic attachments and orthodontic wires as well as the different ways to activate these appliances. These orthodontic attachments (bands and brackets) can be considered "handles" that are cemented or bonded to the teeth themselves. Forces are actually delivered to these "handles" and, in turn, to the teeth themselves, resulting in tooth movement. The point of force application, amount of force, and the duration of force will greatly influence how an individual tooth will actually move. Tipping, intrusion, extrusion, and "torquing" movements can be achieved depending upon how the force is delivered to the teeth. In some instances, such as in the use of extra-oral force (*e.g.*, headgear), an orthopedic effect can be achieved over a long period of time as the entire maxillary growth is restrained and the mandible appears to "catch-up" in an anterior-posterior direction, thereby resolving skeletal disharmonies in Class II types of cases.

The placement of orthodontic attachments

Separation. Although more and more clinicians are bonding orthodontic attachments to posterior teeth, the placement of bands is still preferred by practitioners in many cases, especially when auxiliary devices such as extra-oral force, lingual arches, and palatal bars are utilized. Adequate separation must be present before a band can be properly seated. Separation is generally achieved by the placement of an elastomeric module or a brass separator wire if elastomerics cannot be used because of unusually tight contact points (*e.g.*, adult dentition with restorations, etc.). A special plier is used to both stretch and place the separator until it is well positioned interproximally (Fig. 13-77).

In cases in which the contact points are very tight, dental floss may be used to place the separator from the gingival aspect occlusally (Fig. 13-78). The goal is to have the elastomeric separator wedged between the contact points (Fig. 13-79). Adequate separation is usually accomplished in four to seven days. The brass wire separation method entails cutting a

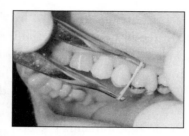

Fig. 13-77 A special plier is used to place the elastomeric
separator. The separator is situated interproximally

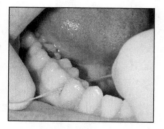

Fig. 13-78 Dental floss can be
used to carry the separator to
place in tight contacts. The floss is
worked from the
gingival to occlusal

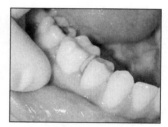

Fig. 13-79 The elastomeric
separator in place

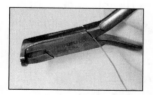

Fig. 13-80 A piece of
brass separating wire is
flattened at one end
using a plier

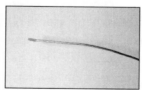

Fig. 13-81 The flattened
end of the separator
is shown

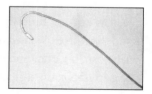

Fig. 13-82 The flattened
end is curved prior to
intraoral insertion

piece of brass separating wire, flattening one end with the heel of a plier, curving the segment to be placed in the embrasure, twisting the wire, and then cutting it off and placing the sharp end interproximally for patient comfort. Adequate space is usually accomplished in about one week (Figs. 13-80 through 13-86).

Both methods of separation (elastomerics and brass separating wire) consistently cause some initial discomfort to the patient. Patients should be cautioned about the possibility of discomfort after a separation visit and an appropriate analgesic prescribed if necessary. Recent evidence suggests that premedicating patients with a patient-appropriate dose of Ibuprofen may reduce the level of discomfort following separation.

Molar banding. The accurate placement of orthodontic bands is an important step in fixed orthodontic appliance use and can be considered a "capital investment" in the overall management of a patient who has fixed orthodontic appliances. Since the "handles" or tubes attached to the band will be transmitting forces to the teeth, their accurate placement is important. Bands are supplied by numerous orthodontic suppliers in cases with a range of sizes to accommodate most teeth. Figure 13-87 shows such a band case and some of the essential instruments used in band placement. These instruments from left to right include a band pusher, band seater, and a band-removing plier.

Bands may be "prefitted" to a tooth on a cast (Fig. 13-88) so that an approximate size may be obtained prior to fitting bands in the mouth. The procedure involves placing the band on the tooth, using the band pusher to initially seat the band and having the patient bite on the band seater stick (Figs. 13-89a through e). The band pusher is then used to burnish the band into grooves and other anatomy of the tooth. The band is removed, an appropriate cementing medium is applied to the interior of the band, and finally cemented to the tooth. Glass Ionomer cement with fluoride-releasing capability is recommended. Excess cement can be removed before final set with a cotton roll and/or toothbrush. After setting, any excess or "flash" is removed with a scaling instrument.

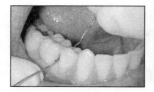

Fig. 13-83 The separating wire is placed between the embrassures. The wire is brought to the lingual surface and extended.

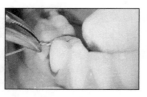

Fig. 13-84 Using a Howe plier or hemostat, the wire is twisted upon itself

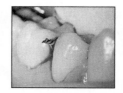

Fig. 13-85 The wire is then cut with a ligature cutter

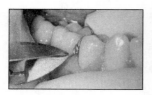

Fig. 13-86 The excess wire is then pushed interproximally so as not to irritate the soft tissues

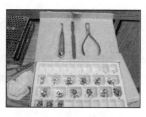

Fig. 13-87 Typical band case with numbered sizes of bands. The instruments needed from left to right are a band pusher, band seating bite stick, and band removing plier

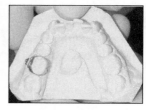

Fig. 13-88 Bands may be "prefitted" on a study cast before actually placing them intraorally.

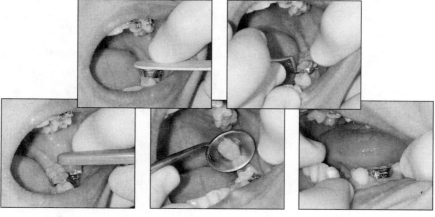

13-89 a-e The fitting, contouring, and cementation steps in the placement of a mandibular molar band

Direct bonding of orthodontic attachments

The bonding of orthodontic attachments is based upon the mechanical locking of an adhesive to irregularities in the enamel surface of the tooth and to mechanical (in most cases) locks formed in the base of the orthodontic attachments. The advantages of bonded attachments when compared to banding (specifically in the anterior and premolar area) are numerous and include:

1. No need for separation
2. Faster and simpler
3. More accurate placement of attachment
4. Less discomfort caused to the patient
5. More esthetic (especially when some of the more esthetic ceramic brackets are used)
6. Partially erupted (or impacted teeth following surgery) can receive attachments
7. No increase in arch length due to thickness of band material
8. Interproximal enamel reduction is possible during orthodontic treatment
9. Interproximal caries formed during treatment may be treated
10. Better access for cleaning and oral hygiene
11. No interproximal spaces to close after orthodontic treatment.

Some of the disadvantages or current limitations of the use of bonded attachments include the difficulty of removal with possible injury to the teeth and questionable use of bonded attachments to molar teeth when extraoral force or other adjunctive appliances must be used. On balance, however, the advantages of bonded attachments greatly outweigh the routine use of traditional orthodontic bands on incisors, and at least in the anterior segment, have all but replaced the use of bands on maxillary or mandibular anterior teeth. Modern bonding resins have been shown to be predictable and clinically invaluable to orthodontic attachment bonding efforts. There are so many techniques and excellent materials to choose from today that suggesting one bonding method over another would be foolish. However, what should be stressed is the meticulous attention to detail in any bonding technique to assure long-term success with bonded orthodontic attachments.

Ten important steps in the direct bonding technique (Fig. 13-90)

1. Inspection of tooth and documentation of defects
2. Thorough prophylaxis with pumice
   (steps 2 and 3 can be interchanged)
3. Appropriate isolation for individual patient
4. Acid etch (gel or liquid etchant?)
5. Thorough removal of etchant material
6. Application of drying agent (optional)
7. Application of sealant
8. Mixing of bonding material and placement to brackets
9. Meticulous placement of bracket to tooth
10. Removal of excess bonding material around bracket

Indirect bonding of orthodontic attachments

Arguably, most orthodontic clinicians prefer to use a direct bonding technique, however, there are distinct advantages to using an indirect bonding technique. Although much more technique-sensitive and laboratory-intensive, the indirect bonding method can be much less stressful to the clinician chairside and offer other advantages as well. There are numerous indirect bonding techniques available both "in-house" and as offered by commercial laboratories. Essentially, the technique entails placement of the orthodontic brackets on a stone cast in the laboratory, creating a suitable template that will accurately carry the brackets to the patient's dentition, and placement of the entire template "en masse" so that all of the brackets are bonded simultaneously. The various steps of one such indirect method are summarized in Figures 13-91, 13-92, and 13-93. Proponents of indirect bonding methods purport that the indirect technique offers greater accuracy in bracket placement than can be routinely achieved by direct bonding techniques.

Fixed appliances demand accurate placement of orthodontic attachments, and whether one uses the direct or indirect method, chemical or light-cured bonding resins, the criteria for bracket placement (and consequences for poor bracket placement) remain the same. Imprecise bracket placement in the vertical plane causes inciso-gingival tooth position discrepancies. Poor mesio-distal positioning causes rotational disharmonies, and axial mispositioning causes axial inclination, vertical, and rotational problems.

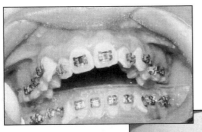

Fig. 13-90 Orthodontic attachments that have been directly bonded to the facial surfaces of the maxillary mandibular teeth

Fig. 13-91 Orthodontic brackets have been directly bonded to an accurate cast with an intervening bonding material

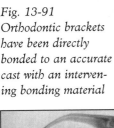

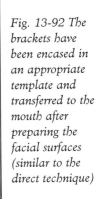

Fig. 13-92 The brackets have been encased in an appropriate template and transferred to the mouth after preparing the facial surfaces (similar to the direct technique)

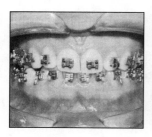

Fig. 13-93 After removing the templates, the brackets are in place and ready to receive arch wires

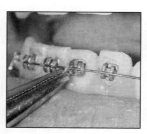

Fig. 13-94 Elastomeric modules securing the wire to the orthodontic attachment

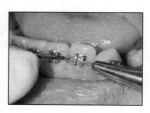

Fig. 13-95 Stainless steel ligature securing the arch wire to the bracket

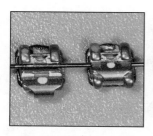

Fig. 13-96 The use of the In-ovation bracket (GAC, Corporation) offers a new dimension in bracket/arch-wire relationship which significantly reduces friction between the arch wire and bracket

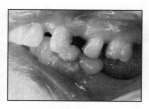

Fig. 13-97 Multiple missing teeth and resultant tipping of teeth adjacent to the missing teeth

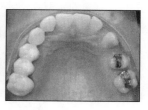

Fig. 13-98 An occlusal view further illustrating a prosthetic dilemma with respect to the present difficulty in tooth replacement

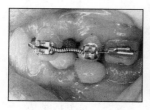

Fig. 13-99 An open coil spring that has been compressed supplies reciprocal force to reposition the teeth

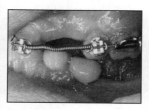

Fig. 13-100 Significant tooth movement has occurred using the reciprocal force of the open coil spring

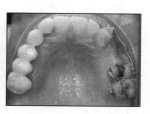

Fig. 13-101 An occlusal view of the completed tooth movement and resulting simplified prosthetic clinical situation

Orthodontic wire placement

Orthodontic wires secured to the brackets can serve as an important "track" for teeth to precisely move into desired positions. They can also be used to actually supply the needed force to cause tooth displacement. Orthodontic wires are secured to brackets with either elastomeric rings or steel ligature wire. Recently, "self-ligation" brackets, or brackets that require neither elastomeric rings nor steel ligatures to engage the orthodontic arch wire have been introduced to orthodontics. Ease of placement and removal of arch wires, significantly reduced friction between the arch wire, and bracket, and other associated advantages (less force needed to produce tooth movement) are attributes claimed by the manufacturers and developers of these brackets. The use of elastomeric modules to secure arch wires to brackets is illustrated in Figure 13-94. Stainless steel ligation is shown in Figure 13-95. The most recently developed "self-ligating" or "ligationless" bracket is illustrated in Figure 13-96.

The use of fixed sectional appliances

Sectional or partial fixed appliances can be useful in the resolution of localized or isolated areas of tooth malpositions. In addition, the forces applied are usually "reciprocal" in intent (in fact, every force has a reciprocal element), and this reciprocal force and response are generally desired. This may be in contrast to the use of more complex orthodontic mechanisms in which the reciprocal response to force application might be undesirable and only through great lengths and other collateral force systems may be prevented or at least minimized. An example of the latter situation is when we retract maxillary incisors and attempt to hold the posterior segments as close to their original positions as possible. Lingual arches, palatal buttons, extra-oral force, and intra-oral elastics might be some examples of additional and important adjuncts or mechanisms involved in comprehensive orthodontic systems.

Tooth movement prior to implant and/or prosthodontic procedures

Individual tooth malpositions can pose substantial obstacles to successful esthetic and functional prosthodontic procedures. The consequences of missing teeth often result in tipping of adjacent teeth, thereby compromising what otherwise might be a routine prosthetic replacement procedure.

The patient in Figure 13-97 and Figure 13-98 had multiple missing teeth on the maxillary left side. The missing maxillary left first premolar and teeth posterior have caused considerable tipping of adjacent teeth. The objective was to simply tip the canine mesially and posterior teeth distally, thereby creating a more routine prosthetic solution to what might appear to be difficult prosthetic challenge without adjunctive orthodontic treatment. A stainless steel sectional wire was placed in the orthodontic attachments, and an open coil spring was compressed (Fig. 13-99). The force generated by the open coil spring (60-90 grams) was enough to tip the teeth into their final positions (Figs. 13-100 and 13-101).

Sectional appliances are useful in providing a precise track for the teeth to move along. Figures 13-102, 13-103, and 13-104 show the closure of a diastema within two months. A tooth-colored wire was used.

Forced eruption

Forced eruption utilizing fixed appliances can be a useful technique in providing biologically sound "crown lengthening." The maxillary right second premolar in Figure 13-105 has fractured below the alveolar crestal bone. Erupting this tooth allowed the fabrication of a restoration on sound tooth structure (Figs. 13-106 and 13-107).

Uprighting molars

Sectional appliances can sometimes be used to upright mesially tipped molars. Figure 13-108 illustrates the classic example of uprighting a mandibular second molar with a sectional appliance in anticipation of an implant/restorative procedure.

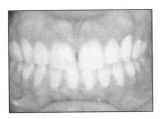

Fig. 13-102 Pretreatment maxillary midline diastema

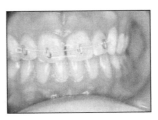

Fig. 13-103 A sectional appliance with a clear elastomeric thread supplies the force to move the maxillary incisors along a "track" to effect the desired tooth movement

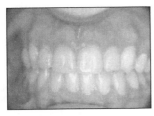

Fig. 13-104 Post-treatment result of the maxillary midline diastema closure

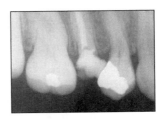

Fig. 13-105 The maxillary right second premolar has been fractured below the alveolar crest, making a predictable restoration difficult

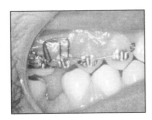

Fig. 13-106 A sectional appliance is used with a "box loop" to forcibly erupt the maxillary right second premolar

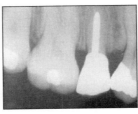

Fig. 13-107 The maxillary right second premolar and surrounding alveolar bone have been repositioned to facilitate the fabrication of a full crown on sound tooth structure

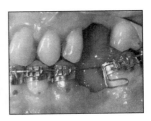

Fig. 13-108 The uprighting of tipped posterior teeth to facilitate either an implant supported restoration or conventional fixed bridge

Summary

Incorporating orthodontic techniques and materials into a progressive dental practice can be very rewarding. Patients are provided with additional options and can often benefit from limited or localized tooth movement procedures. The author has attempted to present a number of commonly encountered clinical situations that have been resolved with either a sole orthodontic procedure or adjunctive orthodontic treatment in combination with other dental treatment procedures. It is hoped that one or more of the techniques and/or appliances presented will be of some interest to the clinician. Every effort was made to keep the focus practical and appropriate to clinical practice. Covering every aspect of orthodontic treatment was not the author's intent. Complex craniofacial and/or comprehensive long-term treatment of significant malocclusions were intentionally omitted from this chapter. The clinician, as he/she has done in the past, must distinguish those orthodontic problems appropriate for limited orthodontic treatment (such as the problems presented in this chapter) from those that might require a more detailed and comprehensive approach that invariably requires additional and advanced training in orthodontics and/or dentofacial orthopedics.

Notes

1 Proffit, W.R., and Fields, H.W., *Contemporary Orthodontics*, 3rd ed., St. Louis, MO: Mosby, 2000

2 Proffit, W.R., and White, R.P., *Surgical Orthodontic Treatment*, St. Louis, MO: Mosby, 1991

3 McNamara, Jr., J.A., and Brudon, W.L., *Orthodontic and Orthopedic Treatment in the Mixed Dentition*, Ann Arbor, MI: Neeham Press, 1993

4 Thurow, R.C., *Edgewise Orthodontics*, St. Louis, MO: C.V. Mosby Company, 1982

5 Graber, T.M., and Vanardsdall, Robert, *Orthodontics, Current Principles and Techniques*, 2nd ed., C.V. Mosby, 1994

6 Nanda, R., and Burstone, C.J., *Retention and Stability in Orthodontics*, Philadelphia: W.B. Saunders Company, 1993

7 Bennett, J.C., and McLaughlin, R. P., *Orthodontic Treatment Mechanics and the Preadjusted Appliance*, London, England: Wolfe Publishing, 1993

8 Brantley, W., and Eliades, T., *Orthodontic Materials- Scientific and Clinical Aspects*, Stuttgart, New York: Thieme, 2001

9 Moskowitz, E., *The Spring Aligner*, Teaching Monograph, NYU College of Dentistry, Department of Orthodontics, New York, NY, 1995

[10] Moskowitz, E., Sheridan, J., et al. *Provisional Anterior Prosthesis for Pre and Post Implant Patients*, New York State Dental Journal, April, 1997, pp. 32-35

[11] Moskowitz, E., Sheridan, J., et al. *A New Look at Indirect Bonding*, *Journal of Clinical Orthodontics*, Vol. XXX, No. 5, May, 1996, pp. 277-281

[12] Sheridan, J., LeDoux, W., and McMinn, R. *ESSIX Retainers: Fabrication and Supervision for Permanent Retention*, JCO, January, 1993

Chapter 14

Removable Prosthodontics

By M. Nader Sharifi, D.D.S., M.S.

To be successful, a removable prosthesis must exhibit certain factors. It must have retention to keep the prosthesis seated in its proper position and stability to limit its side-to-side movement. The prosthesis must receive support from the anatomical structures that can provide it without compromising those structures that cannot. A removable prosthesis must replace the missing teeth, fulfilling the patient's esthetic and phonetic requirements. Lastly, it must restore the function of mastication for the missing teeth without allowing these artificial teeth to compromise any of the previous tenets. This is true of a partial or full arch prosthesis.

To achieve this, we must understand five factors that will define our success. We need to know the anatomical structures that will be relied upon to provide stability, support, and retention to the final prosthesis. In addition, we will need a clear understanding of how we can best utilize these anatomical structures to better serve and protect our needs.

It is required that we record this information intra-orally and transfer it accurately to the laboratory for prosthesis fabrication. We should have knowledge regarding the various materials used to fabricate our prostheses and when to prescribe the appropriate material or method. Finally, we need to understand how to deliver the prosthesis and maintain it at its highest operable level. These five factors are: patient evaluation; framework design and tooth preparation; impression making and record collecting; tooth selection and occlusal design; and prosthesis delivery.

Patient Evaluation

Patients who are missing one, some, or all of their teeth must rely upon alternative structures of the mouth to aid in replacing those that are missing. The two goals of patient evaluation are to determine (1) what alternative structures are available to provide stability, support, and retention to the new prosthesis, and (2) what anatomic limitations may exist to those structures. The anatomic limitations must be weighed against the complaints and concerns of each patient in order to determine realistic options.

The existing prostheses must be critically evaluated as a part of this procedure. Patients often present numerous complaints about their current conditions. However, those complaints need to be weighed against the critical evaluation of the existing prostheses. In addition, patients should be asked about what is working well for them and describe how they felt when restorations were initially placed. All three of these factors: complaints, positive comments, and initial reactions, will influence the recommended treatments.

While a patient could have significant complaints about a wonderful prosthesis that would be difficult to be improve, another patient might have mild complaints about a very poor prosthesis. What must be clear is that the complaints mean very little until the anatomic limitations of each patient are evaluated in combination with their comments.

When evaluating the anatomic form of a patient, we are drawn to observe edentulous and non-edentulous areas.[1-3] In addition, we are attempting to determine if these areas will be beneficial, hurtful, or neutral to placing a removable prosthesis. Obviously, some anatomic areas are of greater influence to the final prosthesis than others. When a patient is partially edentulous, little can help the stability, support, and retention better than the remaining teeth. In the edentulous patient, we have to rely entirely upon the hard and soft tissues of the remaining arch.

The remaining teeth should be evaluated for any existing restorations and any existing conditions that require treatment. This should also include plane of occlusion discrepancies and vertical dimension of occlusion discrepancies as well as the periodontal health. A tooth that can support itself adequately may not be able to support others as a RPD abutment. Individual teeth should be evaluated for contours that would support the use of clasps, guide planes, and rest seats.

Any area that is missing teeth can provide stability and support to the final prosthesis. The arch form can be U-shaped or square and offer excellent stability, although a square-shaped arch may have undercuts at the "corners." A V-shaped arch may provide lateral stability, but tends to result in anterior cantilevers when the replacement teeth are placed in an arch form. That can compromise vertical stability. An O-shaped arch will provide the least amount of support, since the prosthesis can rotate on the arch form like a steering wheel.

Dr. Atwood has classified the ridge shape.[4] The ridge shape creates stability as well as offering a little support. A high, well-rounded ridge offers the greatest stability due to the height of the ridges. A low, well-rounded ridge can still offer excellent stability even though it has a shorter ridge height. A knife-edged ridge can often be found in the mandibular posterior quadrants. This shape will not compromise a removable partial denture (RPD), since support is not expected from the ridge. The knife-edged ridge does provide good stability to a removable prosthesis. The ridge of only basal bone will not provide adequate stability for a removable prosthesis.

Tuberocities can provide excellent support and stability. By engaging all walls of a tuberocity, prosthesis gains stability. Support is derived from the crest of the ridge in this area. This is the only area of the ridge that offers primary support in either arch. All other areas of the ridge should be considered supportive in a secondary manner only. Larger tuberocities offer greater stability and support than smaller ones.

The hard palate is the area of the maxillary arch where removable prostheses will get the most support (Figure 14-1). Stability can also be gained along the lateral walls of the hard palate. Typically, the larger the hard palate, the greater the support and stability; however, a hard palate that is deep can complicate matters. The deep, hard palate is difficult to accurately record with impression techniques. Further, the ability to fabricate a well-adapted prosthesis is also compromised by the laboratory phase of RPDs. Planning on delivering a prosthesis with a reline and using materials in the deep hard palate that can be relined will offer a solution for this anatomic limitation.

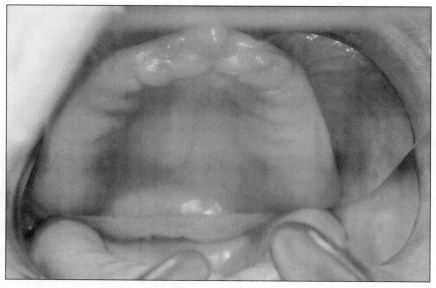

Figure 14-1 An edentulous maxilla with characteristics that will provide excellent stability for a complete denture. The ridges are high and well rounded, the arch form is U-shaped, there are large tuberocities, and the hard palate is of medium depth

In the mandibular arch, the greatest degree of support comes from the buccal shelf. This is the area lateral to the mandibular molars. This support area is the one that provides the most horizontal support for the mandibular prosthesis. The larger this area is, the better support the prosthesis will have.

On the lingual side of the mandibular molars, the lateral throat form offers stability to the prosthesis by allowing the lingual flange to adapt to the vertical wall of the mandible. The deeper the lateral throat form, the more stability is available (Figure 14-2). This can be evaluated using an intra-oral mirror. If the mirror is held in the lingual flange area and the patient swallows, the mirror will be moved by the floor of the mouth. If the entire mirror head is still below the crest of the ridge, the patient has a large lateral throat form and it is considered class I. A class II lateral throat form is one where the mirror moves up to a point where the top of the mirror head is visible, but the handle is still below the crest of the ridge. In a class III situation, the handle is visible, due to the extremely short lateral throat form.

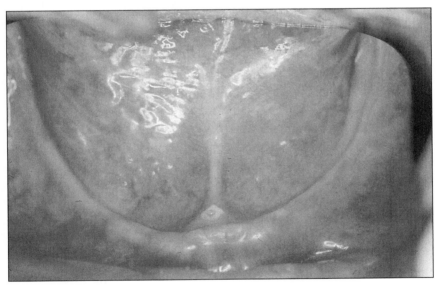

Figure 14-2: An edentulous mandible with characteristics that do not provide good stability for a complete denture. The ridges are resorbed to basal bone, the arch form is O-shaped, the buccal shelves are small, and there does not appear to be a deep lateral throat form

A torus can be present to alter the stability or support of an RPD. The lateral throat form in the mandibular arch can be compromised by the existence of torus. In the maxillary arch, a torus on the hard palate might be large enough to create a problem. In either case, surgical removal may be indicated to eliminate the anatomic limitation.

The soft tissue is evaluated for patient comfort and movement. In the upper arch, the hard palate is entirely made up of attached mucosa. To ensure patient comfort, more than 70% attached mucosa should be visualized. In the mandibular arch, at least 30% is desirable for patient comfort. The soft tissue also needs to be firmly attached to the hard tissue below. Movable mucosa can create movement in the prosthesis and could compromise the stability and retention.

Evaluating the frenum can also be of importance. The anterior frenum should not be visible during the biggest smile. In an immediate denture patient, a visible anterior frenum will result in a visible frenum notch in the denture. The notch will create an esthetic compromise. In addition, the peripheral seal can be lost when the notch is exposed during a smile. Lateral frenums may alter clasp selection for RPDs. An infra-bulge clasp should not be used in any area where a lateral frenum maintains an attachment near the free-marginal tissue. The movement of the cheek will cause the frenum to rub against this clasp. This complication typically is only solved by surgery or by exchanging the infra-bulge clasp for a supra-bulge clasp. Neither of these are easy solutions for a new RPD.

An additional benefit can be derived from the patient evaluation if the existing prostheses are evaluated. Once an understanding is reached regarding the anatomic limitations of the patient, then the existing prostheses can be critically checked. A critical evaluation of the existing prostheses helps the practitioner determine if the patient's complaints are founded or not.

The prosthesis is evaluated for stability, support, retention, esthetics, phonetics, and occlusion. Stability, support, and retention are evaluated by the practitioner's perspective only. Both the practitioner and the patient question esthetics, phonetics, and occlusion. Since the anatomic limitations have been evaluated, we should have a relatively good understanding of what could be expected with a removable prosthesis in this patient's mouth. The prosthesis is rated against the anatomic limitations as good, adequate, or poor for all these factors.

Retention should not be checked by pressing on the prosthesis and then pulling it away from the tissues. This is a false evaluation, since there is not a natural function to provide pressure in this fashion. Instead, have the patient take a drink of water. During a swallow, the teeth touch and will set the prosthesis against the tissue in its usual functional manner. Now, an attempt can be made to pull the prosthesis away from the tissue and check retention. To evaluate stability, a prosthesis is checked for side-to-side movement. Support is checked by pressing it into the soft and hard tissues to look for any rocking.

Esthetics are evaluated by the patient by asking if the teeth look like they are similar to what they had prior to wearing removable prostheses. Phonetics can be evaluated by asking the patient if he is often asked to repeat himself when speaking on the telephone.[5] For occlusion, is the patient able to eat salad, are they slow eaters, do they often prefer fish or pasta to chicken or beef?

For the practitioner, there are other questions to answer.[6-8] For esthetics, is the pleasure curve fulfilled? Do the shape and the amount of teeth that show at rest and while smiling match the patient's age and gender? Phonetically, is a lisp noticeable or does the patient whistle? From an occlusion perspective, it is critical to know if the prosthesis offers contralateral contact when making a working-side movement. This balancing side contact is much more important than cusp form or the existence of tertiary anatomy.

The patient evaluation provides an opportunity to envision what appearance a final prosthesis may have. The final prosthesis will be confined by the anatomic limitations with which the patient presents. Evaluation of the existing prosthesis helps identify complaints and unrealistic expectations. Understanding those limitations and their consequences offers a practitioner a chance to set an appropriate treatment plan with realistic expectations for the final prosthesis.

Tooth Preparation

Our goal in RPD design is to use the teeth that remain to give us stability, support, and retention without compromising their own long-term success. Different design factors will provide different results in each consideration. We must weigh the need for retention, stability, and support against the compromise that these needs cause. In framework design, stability will come from guide planes, support from occlusal rests, and retention from clasps.

Guide planes will provide stability. They will connect the partial denture to the remaining teeth and their roots. By creating a flat plane on the proximal surface of an abutment tooth, the framework can have a mating surface that engages the help of the adjacent tooth in providing resistance to side-to-side movement. When that adjacent tooth has interproximal contact to an additional tooth, then the additional tooth is also engaged in this stabilizing support.

We can design the guide plane to provide this stability and not overly tax the abutment tooth that provides it. This can be done by ensuring an open area apical the guide plane into which it would have an opportunity to move during load. When the partial denture is under load, the hard and soft tissues that support the saddle areas will allow some displacement of the saddle. The open area provides an opportunity for the guide plane to move into that will reduce the strain on the abutment tooth itself.

The optimal design for a guide plane is one that is two to three millimeters tall and three to four millimeters wide. Its most coronal aspect will be at the occlusal table. Apical to the guide plane will be an undercut before reaching the gingival crest. Guide planes should be parallel to each other throughout the entire arch.

In the posterior region, the guide planes tend to be perpendicular to the plane of occlusion, but will be influenced by the undercuts on the remaining teeth. In the anterior region, the guide planes tend to be angular and not perpendicular to the plane of occlusion. When we are restoring an anterior edentulous area, we will use the angular guide planes.

When we are restoring an edentulous posterior area, we will use the perpendicular guide planes.

When we have a mixed case, with edentulous areas in the anterior and the posterior, then we will face difficulties. If we choose the angular guide plane of the anterior area and attempt to apply that to the posterior region, we will require significant modifications of the posterior proximal surfaces to create parallelism to the anterior guide planes. If we choose the posterior guide plane, the tooth modification is minimal in the anterior region; however, other complications arise (Figure 14-3).

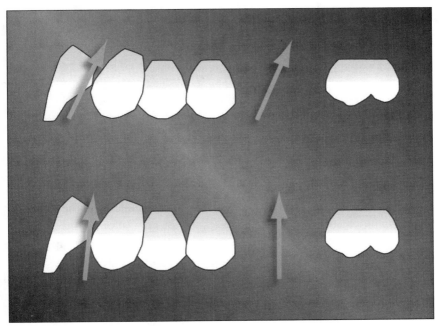

Figure 14-3: With edentulous areas in the anterior and posterior, the path of insertion is best selected from the posterior teeth

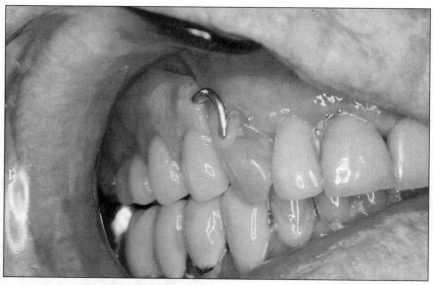

Figure 14-4: The narrow cervical area in the neck of the artificial tooth #7 is due to passing through the interproximal contacts to seat with the posterior path of insertion. The esthetics are improved here with the use of a subgingival pontic

Since the guide planes dictate the path of insertion, the posterior guide plane path will require that the anterior edentulous saddle be seated from a palatal approach. This tends to result in a narrowing of the proximal surfaces of the partial denture base in the cervical third area in order to provide passage between the guide planes. Clinically, this will result in an open area that could cause some complications (Figure 14-4). It could be esthetically displeasing if visible in the smile. It could cause some phonetic compromise if air were able to pass through the area. In addition, it could become a hygienic complication, attracting food and plaque in the area. It is best recommended to separate anterior and posterior edentulous areas by restoring one of them with a fixed partial denture and the remaining with the removable partial prosthesis.

The vertical support is provided in RPD frameworks through the use of occlusal rests. The occlusal rest transfers some of the forces of occlusion from the missing teeth to those teeth with rests. While it might seem appropriate to place rests on all remaining teeth and gain vertical support whereever available, this is not necessarily prudent. The philosophy of placing the minimum required rests, without excess, is recommended.

For an occlusal rest to truly provide support to a RPD, it must transfer those forces down the long axis of the tooth. A simple rule of thumb will help achieve this tenet; the angle of the occlusal rest to the long axis of the tooth should always be less than 90° (Figure 14-5). This acute angle will ensure that the supporting tooth is not loaded angularly.

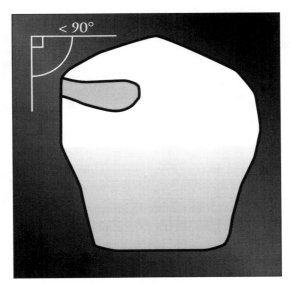

Figure 14-5: All occlusal rests should create acute angles

The shape of an occlusal rest is similar to that of a spoon. It has smooth and rounded contours. It is prepared into the tooth structure sufficiently to ensure at least 1 mm clearance to the opposing occlusion. In the area where the occlusal rest attaches to guide planes and clasps, the rest should be rounded to prevent fractures (Figure 14-6).

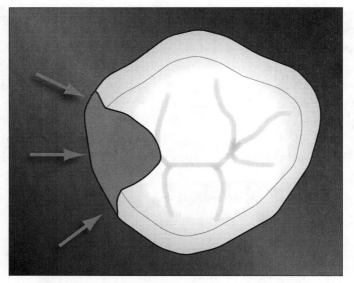

Figure 14-6: Fracture risk areas are identified. The rest should be rounded to all minor connectors and clasp arms

The size of the rest should be adequate for strength without compromising the abutment tooth itself. The mesial or distal pit of molars and premolars offers excellent contours for preparing these occlusal rests. In the premolar region, the length should be approximately one-half the mesial-distal length of the tooth. In the molar region, the size of the tooth is greater, so the length should be approximately one-third the length of the tooth. The width of the occlusal rest should be approximately one-half the occlusal table width of either a molar or a premolar.

An occlusal rest can be prepared into an existing restoration. Should a perforation of the restoration occur, consideration should be given to replace the restoration before completing the framework. When the existing restoration is an occlusal filling, the occlusal rest should be prepared beyond the outline of that restoration. Should replacement of the occlusal filling be necessary in the future, the outline of the occlusal rest will be apparent when shaping the new restoration.

In the anterior region, greater challenges exist to create acute angles between the rest seat and the long axis of the tooth. When a strong cingulum is present, its contours can be enhanced with a parallel-sided bur to provide this acute angle. Should a sufficient cingulum not be available, then an incisal rest is the only non-restorative option that remains. An incisal rest is prepared with a round bur and should create a 180° preparation into the incisal edge. When neither option is available or desirable, a crown or a pin-ledge inlay can be fabricated with the appropriately-shaped rest. Using a button of composite cannot be recommended, because it does not provide adequate load-bearing properties and it is difficult to retrofit a replacement after failure.

Rests are placed according to clasp design and the need for indirect retention. When attachments are used, rests are still required and must be planned for in the framework design.

Once the lateral support has been created with guide planes and the vertical support planned with rest preps, then the retention can be designed with clasps or attachments.

Clasp Design

There are basically three types of clasp retention. Infra-bulge clasps and supra-bulge clasps are two types of clasps, and the third, attachments, although clasp-free, are a form of clasps since they are used to provide retention.

A complete understanding of the clasp design for a bilateral distal extension framework is vital to success with partial dentures.[9] Dentists will often encounter the distal extension patient in both the unilateral and bilateral situations. The knowledge of these situations can also be applied to the Kennedy Class IV, anterior edentulous scenario.

The Kennedy Class IV case should not be looked at as a tooth-born partial denture.[10] Instead, it is really two free-end extensions. One is on the left and the other on the right, they just happen to be meet in the middle. The fact that this scenario occurs in the anterior rather than the posterior is irrelevant. The simple bilateral distal extension RPD can be turned around and applied to the anterior edentulous patient with simplicity and success.

The only clinical situation that remains is the tooth-born situation. One option with this scenario is to create a design that can work well today and is adaptable for the future. To do this, the partial denture should be designed as if the posterior abutment or abutments creating the tooth-born edentulous area were not present. That would create a free-end saddle. The framework would be designed as an ideal distal extension and then a clasp added for the posterior abutment tooth.

The distal extension design is applicable, but not required for the anterior abutments. In the future, should the distal abutment be lost, the RPD can be easily modified. Even if the distal abutment tooth were not lost, the RPD may act like a distal extension if the clasp loosens on that tooth. For a tooth-born situation, the RPD may act like a free-end saddle or may become a free-end saddle. Designing the framework with this in mind is an ideal option for these clinical situations.

The other option for a tooth-born partial denture would be to treat the patient for success today, but eliminate flexibility for the future. This would be with a rotational path design. The rotational path partial denture is not feasible as a distal extension. Therefore, this design only works as long as all the existing teeth remain.

In partial denture framework design, it is important to understand the distal extension. Kennedy Class I and Class II RPDs are distal extensions. Kennedy Class III RPDs may act like or even become distal extensions, and Kennedy Class IV RPDs are really bilateral distal extensions turned around to the anterior. With an understanding of the options for clasp design in the distal extension, one can apply it throughout dentistry.

Standard clasps are separated into two categories: supra-bulge and infra-bulge (Figure 14-7). Supra-bulge clasps begin along the occlusal table, typically from a rest seat. They have clasp arms that lay above the height of contour until the tip of the clasp arm reaches into an undercut for retention.

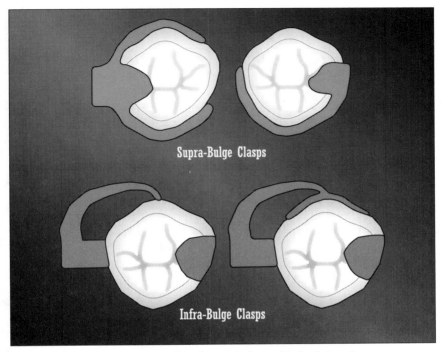

Figure 14-7: Examples of supra-bulge and infra-bulge clasps

An infra-bulge clasp arm is typically connected to the framework in the saddle area. This clasp arm travels through the acrylic of the saddle and exits in the buccal vestibule. The clasp arm lays in space until the retentive tip comes in contact with the abutment tooth. The entire clasp assembly is below the height of contour. The infra-bulge clasp arm only has contact with the abutment tooth at the retentive tip.

The use of a supra-bulge clasp has been debated versus the infra-bulge clasp. Using the Kennedy class I bilateral distal extension free-end saddle as an example (Figure 14-8), both options will be discussed. The two will be compared with regard to retention, clasp longevity, saddle load, and esthetics. This knowledge can then be carried to the other Kennedy classifications as necessary.

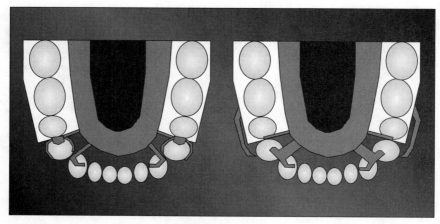

Figure 14-8: A bilateral distal extension partial denture designed with
a supra-bulge clasp system and an infra-bulge clasp system

The typical supra-bulge clasp arm for a free-end saddle is an Akers clasp.[11] The use of this clasp arm is typically paired with a distal guide plane and distal occlusal rest. The typical design of an infra-bulge clasp arm is the rest plate I-bar (RPI) complex.[12] This system includes a distal guide plane, a mesial rest, and an I-Bar with the tip of the clasp arm in the center of the tooth mesial-distally.

The supra-bulge clasp has a pulling action of retention. The clasp arm is above the height of contour and pulls the retentive tip from the under-cut. The infra-bulge clasp arm is below the height of contour and has a pushing action of retention. It is a universal truth in physics; if one wants to overcome an obstruction, such as an undercut, then it would be easi-er to pull over the obstruction than it is to push. Therefore, with equal undercut, an infra-bulge clasp arm with its pushing action of retention will be more retentive.

Clasp longevity deals with the need for adjustment. The Akers clasp has tight, intimate contact against the tooth and should be well main-tained. On the other hand, the typical infra-bulge clasp only contacts the tooth at the retentive tip. The Akers clasp assembly typically requires more adjustment than the I-Bar clasp. This is not a result of the clasps themselves, but the position of the rest seats.

The rest seat is the fulcrum point through which rotation will occur. If the saddle is well adapted to the edentulous ridge, then little rotation can occur. When the ridges have resorbed and the saddle has not been relined, then increased rotation can occur. Regardless of the amount of rotation, the movement is occurring through the rest seat associated with the free-end saddle clasp.

Because this fulcrum point acts as a class I lever arm—like a teeter-totter—it is simple to evaluate. Everything that is on one side of the fulcrum point will move the same direction. Anything that is on the other side of the fulcrum point will move in the opposite direction. When a load is applied to the saddle, everything on the saddle side of the fulcrum point will move downward. All the components on the opposite side of the rest seat will move in the opposite direction.

When we use a distal rest, everything associated with the RPD framework is on the other side of the fulcrum point except the distal guide plane. When we use a mesial rest, there is an opportunity to have more than just the distal guide plan on the same side of the fulcrum point as the load.[13] When using the mesial rest, it is imperative to maintain the tip of the clasp arm on the same side of the fulcrum as the load.

Under load, the saddles of an RPD framework with a distal rest will move downward. During this load, the other side of the framework will move upward. Since the Akers clasp arm is on the other side, it will move upward. This upward movement causes the retentive tip to engage the tooth and flexes the clasp arm. The I-Bar, with its mesial rest, can move downward under load as long as the retentive tip is placed distal to the mesial rest (Figure 14-9). Under load, the I-Bar will move downward and disengage from the tooth.

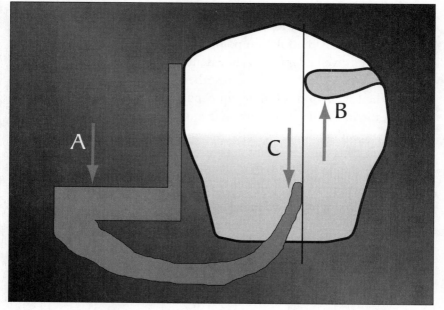

Figure 14-9: With the tip of the I-Bar distal to the rest seat (B), the clasp arm (C) moves downward with the saddle (A) every time a load is applied

The increased movement associated with a distal rest Akers assembly will change the physical properties of the metal clasp arm. The increased movement will lead to a work hardening of the metal that will make the metal more brittle.

The load that the saddle applies to the residual ridge will also be different. It is different with the two different clasp arms because of the location of the rest seat. The rest seat is the fulcrum point. The further a load is from the fulcrum point, the more vertical that load will travel. The closer to the fulcrum point, then the movement will be more rotational.

Because the supra-bulge system incorporates a distal rest, the fulcrum point is as close to the saddle as possible. In the infra-bulge system, the fulcrum point is a mesial rest. The distance is not great from the distal of a tooth to the mesial. Any change in position in the rest will make a difference.[14-16] The degree of difference has not been found to be substantial; however, a difference does occur.

The esthetics of the two options are also different. The amount of metal that shows when a patient smiles with these options will depend upon the location of the RPD and the patient's smile line. In the lower arch, mesial rests will be more visible than distal rests since they are closer to the front of the mouth. The smile line rarely presents a problem in the lower arch. The exposed metal on the buccal surface usually will be hidden by the cheek and lips in the lower arch. Typically, each option will be esthetic for most patients in the lower arch.

In the upper arch, the smile line can expose more of the buccal surfaces of posterior teeth than are visible at rest. To minimize the show of metal, it is desirable to keep the clasps as close to the cervical one-third as possible. While both the supra-bulge and infra-bulge clasps can be maintained in the cervical one-third, the infra-bulge typically will show less metal due to less metal in contact with the tooth.

Considering the potential benefits of the two different clasp systems, it becomes evident that the factor responsible for most issues is the mesial rest. It follows then to fabricate an RPD with mesial rests and Akers clasps wrapping from the mesial to the distal.[17] This will change the direction of movement of the clasp arm during load. The subsequent downward movement under load will eliminate most of the flexure of the Akers clasp arm that is evident with the distal rest design.

Further, the load to the residual ridge will also mimic that of the infra-bulge design. The esthetics will result in a major difference. The Akers clasp arm will be more visible with this orientation than in any other orientation. Maintaining an esthetic design with the Akers clasp arm and a mesial rest may not be possible. The RPI system with a mesial rest distal guide plane and I-Bar clasp with the retentive tip in an undercut on the mesial-distal height of contour appears to be a preferred clasp design for a free-end saddle.

Attachments are readily available and significantly varied.[18-19] Each different attachment requires a different body of knowledge as to its use, effectiveness, and concerns. Space does not allow a thorough discussion of individual attachments. What should be fully understood, however, that attachments are replacements for clasps. Attachments provide retention, not stability or support. Attachments do not generally replace the need for rest seats or guide planes. Guide planes should be planned first for lateral stability, rest seats second for vertical support, then your choice of attachments for retention.

Multiple options exist when considering clasp design for RPD frameworks. Simplifying the myriad of potential patient scenarios is possible when a thorough understanding of the free-end saddle clasp system is achieved. The RPI clasp system can be applied to most clinical situations with success.

Impression Techniques

An impression of the mouth is made to accurately transfer the size and shape of structures in the oral cavity to the laboratory for prosthesis fabrication. Numerous impressions can be made; however, an initial and a final impression should be adequate for nearly all cases. Initial impressions offer information such as diagnosis and case design, but more is available than just those issues. Since each impression is more accurate than the previous one, the initial impression is really a trial run at the final impression.[20]

Initial impressions should be simple, quick, and inexpensive. An irreversible hydrocolloid material in a stock tray fulfills these requirements and offers excellent results within reasonable parameters. The greatest drawback to using alginate is the short period of time before deformation of the impression begins. It has been shown that accuracy begins to diminish after 12 minutes. These impressions should be poured as quickly as infection control procedures allow.

While it may be enticing to have a staff member make initial impressions as a time saver, this eliminates the opportunity to make a trial run at the final impression. Much is learned about the anatomic form of the patient with each impression. Each subsequent impression then sifts out finer detail. Experience with the initial impression may alter the technique for the final impression.

Final impressions should be the most accurate representation of the tissues of the mouth that are required to support the removable prosthesis.[21] Different materials hold certain advantages and disadvantages over others. When making a final impression for a cast RPD framework, we may choose one material versus a different material for a complete upper denture final impression. Therefore, many materials and their properties should be understood.

Irreversible Hydrocolloid

Alginate material's greatest attribute is that it is hydrophilic. This material is not negatively affected by saliva, blood, or any moisture. That makes it a wonderful option to use in the mouth where those issues exist. The greatest challenge is its accuracy. As previously mentioned, the impression must be poured within 12 minutes to maintain the accuracy necessary for any final impression step.

Alginate is a mucostatic material that often results in an overextended impression. In addition, a mucostatic material records the tissue at rest rather than when subjected to a load. The overextension must be compensated for in the laboratory by fabricating the prosthesis short of the final impression borders. And, if desired, functional load may be recorded in the saddle areas.

Although alginate is an excellent material to use in the oral environment, its challenges will limit its usefulness. The mucostatic result and overextended borders will limit its effectiveness for any saddle area or complete denture.[22] Alginate is an excellent choice for final impressions of RPD frameworks (Figure 14-10). Excess material should be pressed into occlusal rests and along guide planes to ensure complete registration of these key areas. Care should be taken to pour these models as quickly as infection control procedures will allow.

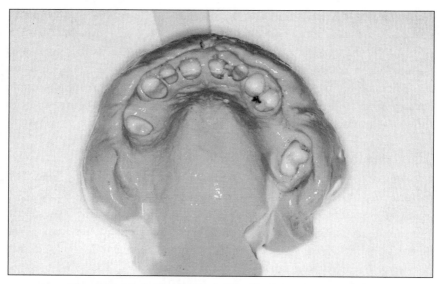

Figure 14-10: An irreversible hydrocolloid impression made by syringing blue material into the vestibules and pressing it into the occlusal form, then using a green material in the tray

Polysulfide Rubber Base

If this material came in a gun delivery system, it would be a favorite of many practitioners. The most negative issue related to rubber base impression material is the delivery system. This material does not mix easily; it has a bad aroma and an unusual taste. Rubber base impression materials do have excellent characteristics that make it an excellent choice for use in removable prosthodontics.

Rubber base material exhibits very good memory, so it will bounce back after being removed from an undercut area. This material also registers soft tissue very well (Figure 14-11). Rubber base is available in packages of heavy, medium, and light body material. Using the heavy and light body materials, the consistency of the material can be altered to create varying amounts of load on the tissue. This allows for customizing the load to the tissue based upon the depressability and movement of that tissue.

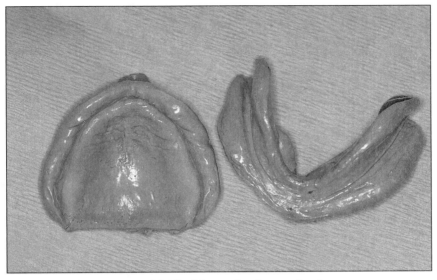

Figure 14-11: Final impression for complete lower denture made with polysulfide rubber base.

Rubber base impressions require the use of a border-molded custom tray. The custom tray fabricated from the initial impressions is one more step in sifting out the detail of the final impression. The custom tray is then "customized" in the mouth through border molding. This step essentially sifts out greater detail than the initial impression could. The border-molded custom tray is a customized custom tray, ready for the most accurate final impression. Prior to making the final impression, any wax spacer should be removed from the custom tray and the border molding should be trimmed approximately 1 mm. Each of these steps ensures that there will be adequate room for the final impression material.

Using the patient's existing prosthesis as a final impression tray cannot be recommended. If this is an appealing impression technique, it is recommended to duplicate the existing prosthesis for use as an impression tray. This will preserve the integrity of the patient's original prosthesis. However, the existing prosthesis should exhibit the necessary extensions that a custom tray would have. It is not advisable to significantly border-mold the duplicated denture. If more border molding than usual is necessary, then a custom tray would be a better option for the final impression.

The memory and soft tissue registration make rubber base an excellent material for final impressions. Complete upper and lower dentures can both be fabricated from these models. In addition, RPD frameworks can be accurately fabricated when there is a large discrepancy between the remaining teeth and saddle areas. Rubber base is also an excellent material choice for laboratory reline procedures on complete or partial dentures.

Polyether

Polyether's greatest attribute over all other materials is its rigidity. It is because of this rigidity that we obtain excellent accuracy with impressions on implants with square impression copings. Tapered impression copings require memory and vinyl polysiloxane (VPS) tends to be a better material with that technique. However, this rigidity also can cause some problems.

When making an impression for a RPD framework, a lone-standing tooth is often encountered. The rigidity of polyether can cause these teeth to fracture from the cast when separating the cast from the impression. A repaired cast is not going to be an accurate representation of the oral environment.

Similar to a fracture occurring on a lone-standing tooth, an area with deep undercuts can also create a fracture problem. Further, polyether impression material will not demonstrate as much accuracy as some alternative materials when making impressions of areas with strong undercuts, since memory of polyether is not its greatest attribute.

Polyether is a fine choice for completely edentulous impressions. The technique used for final impressions for complete dentures would be the same as described for polysulfide rubber base. The most ideal use for polyether in removable prosthodontics is as a final impression material with square impression copings for implant-supported overdentures.

Vinyl polysiloxane

Vinyl polysiloxane (VPS) is one of the most commonly used impression materials in dentistry today. The ease of use with the gun delivery systems and positive attributes such as tear strength and memory offer a winning combination (Figure 14-12). The material is available in a number of different bodies as well as bite registration and die material. The biggest problem with VPS is dealing with the hydrophobic nature of the material.

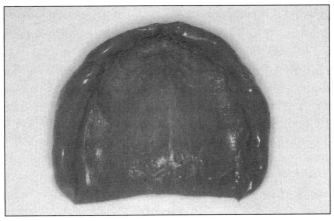

Figure 14-12: Medium-body VPS impression made for an upper complete denture

The VPS material will bond to itself very well. This allows one variation of the material to be used for the border molding and another for the final wash impression. Using a custom-fabricated impression tray and fast-setting VPS bite registration material, a border-molded tray can be fabricated in minutes. A material can be selected between medium-, heavy-, and light-body options to vary the functional load applied to the tissues during the impression procedure.

The tear strength and memory associated with VPS provide practitioners with the option of this material for any impression step in removable prosthodontics. Partial denture frameworks, complete den-

455

ture impressions, and laboratory relines can all be completed with equal success. However, due to the hydrophobic nature of these materials, care must be taken to control the moisture in the oral environment for greatest accuracy.

Border Molding

Border molding a custom tray is "customizing" the custom tray. This step is not associated with the final impression. This step does help to sift out finer detail than the initial impression provided. Border molding is recommended for all impression techniques, regardless of final impression material. However, the final impression material may influence the material and technique used for border molding.

Border molding is most commonly completed with compound. Stick compound provides ideal characteristics and simplicity of use. Compound remains shiny when it has failed to come in contact with tissue. This characteristic provides excellent guidance to the practitioner regarding deficient areas. Compound also exhibits good heat retention, which maintains its moldable characteristics while entering the mouth. The material will not be easily displaced if it comes in contact with the lips or cheeks while being seated. These are all favorable characteristics of compound.

In the upper arch, there are four areas to mold (Figure 14-13), while the lower has five different areas. The areas are the left and right buccal sides, and the anterior and the posterior palate in the upper arch. The lower arch includes the left and right lingual sides in lieu of the palatal.

A piece of compound, one-half to two-thirds the length of the stick, is broken off and tempered in a water bath. The tempered compound is pressed onto the tray in the area to be registered. For the buccal vestibules, this would be the area from the distal of the second molar to the cuspid region. The tray can then be taken directly to the mouth or held in the water bath to improve the temperature of the compound. Since compound will develop a chalky appearance if cooling in air, it is easily determined if returning to the water bath is necessary.

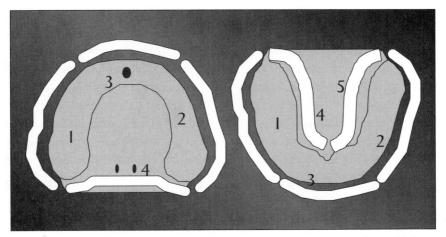

Figure 14-13: Four maxillary and five mandibular areas to be border molded

When border molding any of the buccal vestibules, the corner of the mouth is held and gently pulled away from the arch being molded and posteriorly. This motion is repeated twice. This will shorten the buccal vestibule and create an area for movement of the buccal frenum. The buccal frenum will often create a V-shaped notch in the compound. Once the right and left buccal vestibules are competed, the anterior can be molded.

Again, tempered compound is pressed onto the tray in this region. An alcohol torch is used to flow the new, tempered compound into the previously molded and set compound at both right and left junctions. The anterior part of the tray is placed back into the water bath to temper these areas before seating intra-orally. Both the upper and lower areas are border molded by having the patient create a big smile and by blowing a kiss. Both of these actions should be repeated twice. The big smile will tighten the obicularis oris muscle and thin the compound in the anterior area. Blowing a kiss will shorten the vestibule.

In the upper arch, the posterior region is completed last. Again, the torch is used to flow the new, tempered compound into the set compound on the right and left junctions. The junction is the area lateral to the tuberocities. Once the material is tempered, it can be seated in the mouth and the patient can border mold.

The posterior region is molded by having the patient open his/her mouth as wide as possible. The patient is then instructed to close part way and move the jaw from side-to-side. The motions are then repeated. Opening wide will accentuate the hamular notch regions. Moving the jaw from side-to-side causes the coronoid process of the mandible to move close to the tuberocity of the maxilla. The side-to-side movement tends to create a thinly molded area of compound immediately next to a wide area of the buccal vestibule. The tray should exhibit strong suction upon removal. Should the tray not exhibit strong suction, the posterior area should be rechecked.

In the lower arch, the lingual vestibules are completed independent of each other, but identically. It is very easy to border mold this area too aggressively. When the patient is asked to protrude her tongue – or worse, to press it into each cheek – the floor of the mouth moves much more than is necessary to adequately border mold. The result is a short lingual vestibule that will compromise the stability and retention of the final prosthesis.

The tempered compound is pressed onto the tray and seated. Very slight pressure is applied with the practitioner's fingers onto the top of the tongue (Figure 14-11). The patient is asked to resist this very slight pressure. That resistance will stimulate a contraction of the muscles of the floor of the mouth. This procedure is completed for both sides of the floor of the mouth.

If the tray is evaluated with the tongue maintaining the peripheral seal, suction should also be evident in the lower arch. However, if the tongue is retracted, then the peripheral seal will be lost and no suction will exist. While this technique is meant to create an ideal length to the lingual vestibule, if an error is to be made, let it be made such that the flange of the denture is too long. An adjustment to remove excess flange length in a final prosthesis is much simpler to complete than adding length to a completed prosthesis.

A sharp scalpel is used to scrape and trim approximately 1 mm of compound from the internal and external surface of the border mold. The length of the vestibule is shortened when the surface of the compound is scraped. This will allow for final impression material to record the tissue rather than the compound. The wax spacer should be removed and adhesive placed over the entire internal surface of the impression tray as well as on the compound overlapping onto its exterior surface.

The described technique can also be completed using VPS fast-setting bite registration material in lieu of compound. The characteristics of this material do require some alterations in the technique. Those alterations make this material easy to use in the maxilla, although more of a challenge in the mandible.

Since fast-setting bite registration material tends to have an airy characteristic, it displaces easily. If contact is made between unset material and any anatomic structures such as the cheek or lips, then the material can be pulled from the tray and an inaccurate mold will be made. Therefore, in regions where contact will be made between the unset material and anatomic structures before the tray is seated, an alteration in the technique is necessary. The only area that does not require a change in technique is the maxillary posterior area.

Adhesive is necessary on the custom tray's entire border. Using a hand-held mixing gun, the fast-setting bite registration material is injected directly into the vestibule to be border molded (Figure 14-14). The tray is seated and the area border molded as previously described. Fast-setting material will set within 60 seconds, and then the next area can be molded. Using this technique, the maxilla is completed in three different sections: the upper right from tuberocity to the midline, the upper left from tuberocity to the midline, and the posterior between the tuberocities.

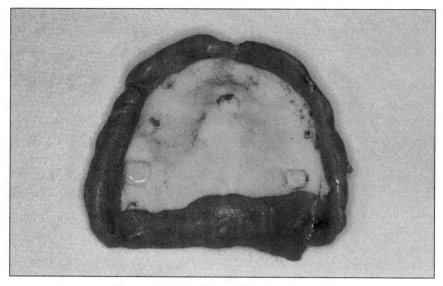

Figure 14-14: Border molding completed with
fast-setting VPS bite registration material

As with all border-molding techniques, this still is a customization of the custom tray. Therefore, the border mold should be trimmed approximately 1 mm. A sharp scalpel works well to trim this material. The wax spacer should also be removed at this time. Regardless of border-molding material or final-impression material, an adhesive should be used on the entire tray as well as the buccal surface of the border molding itself. Now the custom tray has been customized, and we have sifted out finer detail for the final impression.

Wax Records

A wax records appointment is completed so that the upper and lower models can be related to each other and the temporal-mandibular joints in space. We can also estimate other aspects of the final removable prosthesis with a wax record that offers the opportunity to make quick and easy modifications.

The wax record baseplate should be rigid, well adapted to the model, and comfortable for the patient. Many options are available for baseplate material. Acrylic is the most common baseplate material, but must be made at least 24 hours in advance to account for distortion. Composite works well when that period of time is unavailable, but is a more expensive material. Vacuum form plastics and other materials are also available for consideration. As long as the requirements of rigidity, comfort, and adaptation are met, any of these options will do just fine.

The wax should estimate the size and shape of the horizontal and vertical height of the missing teeth. Hard baseplate waxes are more difficult to remove, but hold up better in the mouth. Soft waxes allow for easy adjustments, but may show distortion in warm environments. Of course, the records have been collected; the same wax will be used to hold the denture teeth for a wax trial appointment. Soft baseplate waxes will allow for more tooth migration once set. Hard waxes will hold a tooth position better than the soft alternative.

The size of the wax rim can be manufactured with an estimate of the final shape, or with more specific methods. Generalized measurements have been made of the edentulous patient. These measurements have deduced averages that can be used as a starting point for wax rim fabrication. An Alma Gauge is an instrument used for such a procedure indicating the protrusion of the incisal edge from the middle of the incisive foramen (Figure 14-15). The facial height of the

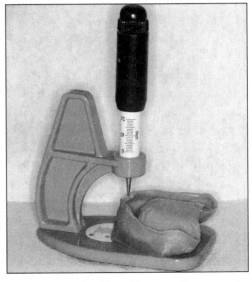

Figure 14-15: An Alma Gauge used to create the starting point for size and shape of a wax rim

wax rim has been estimated. These two measurements can make up the anterior segment of the wax rim. A spatula is also available to estimate the posterior occlusal plane to the length of the anterior segment.

Intra-orally, the first evaluation of the wax rim is for esthetics. Contours of the face are evaluated from the facial as well as from profile. Palpation is used to verify that adequate thickness exists to support the corners of the nose. Insufficient support for the corners of the nose will result in an increased aged appearance. Between the canine eminences, it is uncommon to require thick buccal vestibules for esthetics.

The length of the maxillary wax rim is determined by esthetics and phonetics.[6] Varying the amount of wax that shows at rest and while speaking will alter the esthetics of the patient. A younger patient will show more of their upper anterior teeth than an older patient will. This is true at rest as well as while speaking. A female patient has been found to show more length than a male.

Due to esthetic variability, the use of phonetics can aid in the final determination of maxillary incisor length. Fricative sounds are made when the lower lip comes in contact with the incisal edge of the maxillary incisors. Fricative sounds are "F" and "V". Asking patients to repeat their name, address, and phone number will typically require the use of a few words with fricatives.

Since the human body is adaptable, it is not advisable to have the patient count up from 40. The continual fricative sounds will offer that patient an opportunity to hear her own deficiencies and self-correct them. This would create confusion for the practitioner trying to determine if strong fricatives existed. Wax should be added or removed as necessary to fulfill the requirements of esthetics and phonetics.

Once the maxillary wax rim has been finalized for anterior length, that length must be carried throughout the entire wax rim. Using a paralleling device, such as a Fox Plane (Figure 14-16), viewed from the anterior, the wax rim is contoured to have a length parallel to the pupils of the eyes. Then the wax rim is paralleled to the ala-tragus line on the right and left side. The ala is the lower corner of the nose and the tragus is the piece of skin that protects the auditory canal. The imaginary line between these two creates an ideal anterior-posterior horizontal occlusal plane. This completes the upper wax rim for facial support, esthetics, and phonetics.

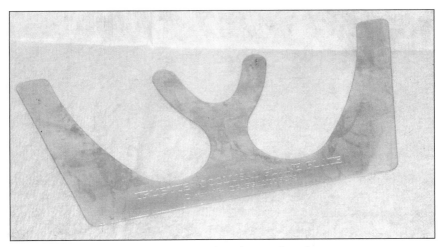

Figure 14-16: A Fox Plane from Trubyte for creating a horizontal plane with an upper wax rim

The lower wax rim is used to complete the record taking. Using a lower wax rim with the posterior wax built up short of the vertical height will allow the anterior portion of the wax rim to be used for phonetic evaluation. Sibilant sounds are sharply made when the lower anterior incisal edge protrudes and just misses the upper anterior incisal edges. Most patients will create this sound in an edge-to-edge incisal relationship. Some true skeletal class III patients can actually protrude to a negative overjet position. Alternatively, some skeletal class II patients will still maintain an overjet and overbite while making sharp sibilant sounds.

The height of the lower anterior wax rim is adjusted until a sharp sibilant sound is located.[6,23] There should be no whistling or signs of a lisp and no contact between the upper and lower wax rims. What must be clear is that this is not the vertical dimension of occlusion. It is more than the vertical dimension of occlusion, but it is less than the vertical dimension of occlusion and the freeway space (Figure 14-17). The closest speaking space is made between the incisors when the lower jaw opens and protrudes (Figure 14-18).

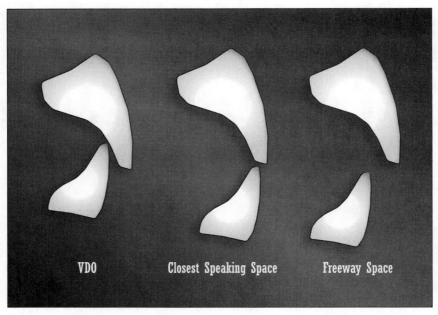

Figure 14-17: When the lower wax record creates the closest speaking space, the incisors are creating the vertical dimension of occlusion and some of the freeway space

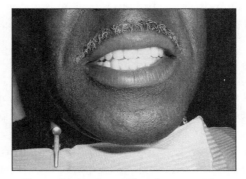

Figure 14-18: A complete denture patient demonstrating the closest speaking space

The difference between the vertical dimension of occlusion and the closest speaking space will be corrected on the articulator during the wax up of the denture teeth. Prior to completing the centric record, the overbite can be measured. The wax rims are adjusted to allow the mandibular rim fit inside the maxillary rim in centric relation. The patient is asked to close into centric. In a skeletal class I relationship, there will be 2-3 mm of overbite. Calipers can be used to measure a distance between an indentation made in the maxillary wax rim and one made in the mandibular wax rim. In the lab, the upper and lower denture teeth will be waxed up. After all the upper denture teeth and the lower anteriors have been waxed up, then the incisal pin will be closed to create the desired overbite. The lower posterior teeth are set at this position – vertical dimension of occlusion.

Class III patients may have zero overbite, and they will require an average of 3 mm of freeway space. Class II patients may have as much as 8 mm of overbite in centric. That overbite must be evaluated against the overbite during sibilant sounds for closest speaking space determination.

The height of the posterior wax rim is now adjusted to be at the same level as the anterior wax rim. This is done intra-orally with warm wax. Baseplate wax is added to the posterior segment of the lower wax rim. This wax should still be warm and moldable without flowing.

The wax rim is seated and supported with finger pressure on the flanges. The patient is instructed to gently bite into the wax rim. When the anterior area is just coming into contact, the patient is instructed to open quickly. The lower rim is cooled and rechecked for even contact all around. We are now ready to obtain a centric record.

For the partially edentulous patient, intra-occlusal records should be made at maximum intercuspation. Should insufficient teeth remain to provide a clearly reproducible maximum intercuspation, then a record will be made as if the patient were completely edentulous. These records are made at centric relation.

Many patients who lack sufficient teeth for maximum intercuspation or who have lost all their teeth tend to function in centric relation. Obtaining centric relation records for these patients is relatively easy.

Midline marks can be made on the maxillary and mandibular wax rims. The patient can be guided into centric relation using bilateral manipulation to seat the condyles in a superior position of the fossae.

When the patient is guided into this position, a mark can be made on the occlusal table of the maxillary wax rim as it relates to the midline of the mandibular wax rim. This is, in a sense, a mark of the overjet.

The patient is released and asked to state his name and address. He is then asked to close together. Most often, edentulous and near edentulous patients can reproduce this centric without manipulation. The overjet mark is used as the confirmation. Two centric relation records can be made with fast-setting bite registration material. Ensure that the material completes the arch lingually in the anterior so as to not block the overjet mark being used for confirmation.

When this method is insufficient, an intra-oral tracing device should be used. An intra-oral tracing device will have a single point of contact against a flat plate (Figure 14-19). They are attached to the upper and lower wax rims following the determination of the vertical dimension of occlusion and closest speaking space. A gothic arch is traced to aid the patient into centric relation. An open bite registration is made, and a second can be obtained for confirmation.

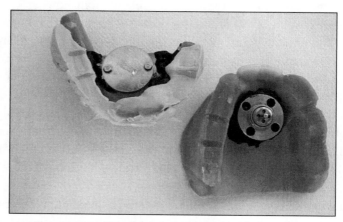

Figure 14-19: An open bite registration of centric relation obtained with the Coble Balancer intra-oral tracing device for a completely edentulous patient

To obtain the most from an articulator, a protrusive record and a facebow transfer are made.[24] The facebow transfer allows the maxillary model to be related appropriately to the condyles on the articulator. Further, the protrusive record can then be used to program the condylar inclination (Figure 14-20). Right and left working records to program the progressive side shift are not generally recommended.

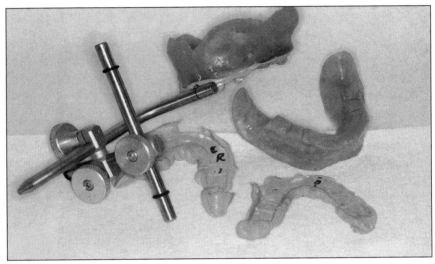

Figure 14-20: Records to be returned to the laboratory for an esthetic wax trial

The final step in the wax records appointment is tooth selection. Teeth are selected based upon the age and gender of the patient as well as the patient's size and shape.[7,9] The shade of the teeth is selected by the age and gender of the patient and their esthetic desires.[8] Tooth selection is an opportunity for patients to express their desire for prosthodontic privacy by selecting age- and gender-appropriate shade and shape. Often, patients desire a younger looking smile than prosthodontic privacy can provide.

The shape of the central incisor mimics the shape of the patient's face. The height and width of the face have been shown to be related to the height and width of the central incisor by a factor of 16. Both of these factors will influence the mold selection in addition to the age and gender of the patient.

Posterior teeth are selected based upon the desires and needs of the patient. A cusp form tooth will provide greater chewing efficiency and better esthetics.[25] However, the cusp form tooth requires good muscle control and adequate supporting bone. When little bone remains or muscle control is inadequate, then flat plane teeth are recommended regardless of the lack of esthetics.[26]

A good compromise is lingualized occlusion.[27] In lingualized occlusion, the esthetics and chewing function of the cusp form tooth is combined with the reduced stress related to the flat plane tooth. The maxillary posterior cusp form teeth are combined with a lower cusp angle tooth form in the mandible. The teeth are set with working side and balancing side contacts – both in-group function. Unlike a typical bilateral balanced occlusion, the teeth on the working side have no buccal contacts in centric or eccentric movements.

The wax records appointment has provided the opportunity to estimate the final removable prosthesis with a wax record enabling quick and easy modifications. The size, shape, and shade of the denture teeth have been selected, and the posterior tooth mold and occlusal designs have been decided. The laboratory now has a clear understanding as to how the upper and lower models can be related to each other and can return an appropriate set-up.

Prosthesis Trial

The trial seating of a prosthesis offers the practitioner and the patient an opportunity to see what the final result may be like while still being able to make any changes that may be desirable. A cast framework should be tried-in prior to adding baseplates, wax rims, or denture teeth. A trial with denture teeth should be completed with complete and partial denture cases.

The framework try-in will be completed to evaluate the complete seating of the framework, the movement of the framework so that the soft and hard tissues of the edentulous areas can support the occlusal load, and the occlusion with the opposing arch. Seating of the framework is confirmed with the use of disclosing mediums. A coat of disclosing medium is placed on the guide planes and rest seats, and the framework is seated in the mouth. Any area of contact that may be a high point restricting the complete seating of the prosthesis is evident as a shiny area of metal that shows through the disclosing medium. Magnification is a benefit for this technique. These areas are adjusted until the prosthesis seats completely.

Again, using disclosing medium on the most distal minor connectors, guide planes, and rest seats, the framework is seated. Transferring the load from the rest seats to the saddle areas should create movement as the framework rotates and moves along the abutment teeth. This movement is necessary to limit the support required by the abutment teeth by gaining support from the hard and soft tissues under load.[21] Typically, the minor connector requires some adjustment apical to the most distal guide plane to provide adequate movement for this support.

The last adjustment is to check the occlusion with articulating paper and shim-stock. Polished frameworks do not mark well with articulating paper. Using air abrasion or a white stone on the rest seats prior to checking the occlusion is beneficial. Adjustments should be made until the shim-stock is maintained equally and similarly with the framework in the mouth as well as with the framework out of the mouth.

Another evaluation that should be completed is a wax trial of the final denture teeth in the final arrangement. The patient should invite a person whose opinion they respect to accompany him/her on this appointment. The patient and the colleague will be asked to evaluate the size, shape, shade, and position of the denture teeth once the practitioner has completed the evaluation.

The practitioner's evaluation actually begins in the laboratory. The denture tooth set-up is evaluated on the articulator. Most manufacturers of denture teeth provide guidelines for setting up their teeth in dentures. Using these guidelines, a practitioner can critically evaluate the work of the technician.

Typically, the denture teeth should be set in a class I occlusal arrangement as evaluated in the cuspid and molar region (Figure 14-21). The teeth should appear to be tight mesial-distally and from maxillary to mandibular arch. The plane of occlusion should not exhibit any disruptions outside of the appropriate curve of Spee and curve of Wilson. Evaluating the balancing side contacts from the buccal and from the lingual should determine that strong contra-lateral contact exists on the articulator.

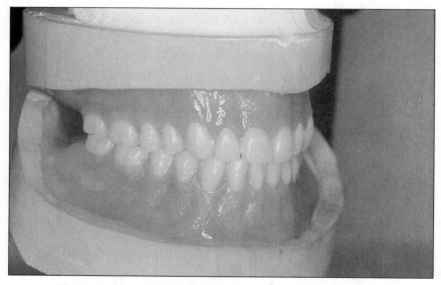

Figure 14-21: An articulator with a complete denture set up for a wax trial. The denture teeth are set in a Class I relationship

In the mouth, the plane of occlusion is evaluated with a Fox Plane. This is done from the facial using the intra-pupil line as well as from both lateral positions using the ala-tragus line exactly as done during the wax records appointment. Centric relation is confirmed and centric contacts checked with shim-stock. Again, balancing side contacts are evaluated to confirm contra-lateral contact.

The phonetics are evaluated using fricative sounds to confirm the appropriate length of the maxillary anterior teeth. Sibilant sounds are used to confirm that the vertical dimension of occlusion is accurate. If the closest speaking space is insufficient, then the lower teeth should be brought closer to the uppers. If contact occurs during sibilant sounds, then the vertical needs to be closed. That would result in an increase in the anterior overbite.

Once the practitioner has been satisfied with the occlusion and phonetics, the patient and their colleague can evaluate the esthetics. They are asked to consider the size, shape, shade, and position of the teeth. In addition, they are asked to evaluate the amount of wax that shows while speaking and when smiling. The fit of the prosthesis is not a consideration during this appointment although a lack of comfort could indicate an occlusal problem and should be investigated.

With any aspect of the wax trial appointment, small changes can be easily be made at this time. This is why we completed the procedure. Major changes such as vertical dimension of occlusion or shade selection will need a laboratory correction and may require the repetition of the records appointment.

When everything has been evaluated and is considered acceptable, the prosthesis is ready to be processed. Having the patient sign an informed consent form will not absolve a practitioner from litigation. However, there are patients who require an informed consent form to understand that this is their last chance to make changes.

Prosthesis Delivery

Now that the prosthesis is fabricated, the esthetics, phonetics, occlusion, as well as the fit to the tissue all need to be evaluated. In the fabrication process, significant appointment time has been spent fitting the fine details of the fit of the prosthesis to the tissue. For that reason, we should spend little time on the fit and concentrate on other pertinent issues. The esthetics and phonetics could be evaluated at the time of delivery; however, they will be more accurately criticized in one week.

Therefore, it is best to concentrate time on the occlusion on the day the prosthesis is delivered.

Prior to evaluating the occlusion, the prosthesis must be seated in the patient's mouth. Since the impression techniques discussed could record undercuts, the prosthesis should also engage these undercuts. Rather than eliminate them, an attempt should be made to maintain them (Figure 14-22). The engagement of an undercut will help the stability and retention of the final prosthesis. However, it is common that undercuts cause sore areas when seating and removing a prosthesis.

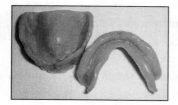

Figure 14-22: A set of processed upper and lower dentures with undercut areas on the flanges

The seating surface area of the prosthesis is covered with a material that will indicate areas of contact. Pressure-indicating paste is an ideal material for this procedure. With brush marks of the pressure indicating paste on the denture, the patient is given the denture. The patient is instructed to try and seat the denture. They are told to "rock" the denture back and forth so as to slip around any undercuts. If the undercut is too great, the patient will feel pressure in this area and will remove the prosthesis. Any area of contact will show in the pressure-indicating paste and can be adjusted.

Once the prosthesis has been seated, the patient is instructed to bite on cotton rolls for five minutes. This helps to "de-program" the muscles from the previous denture's occlusion and seat the condyles in the fossae, both of which will improve the evaluation of the new occlusion. It will also mold the denture-bearing tissue to the prosthesis, which will increase the retention and the patient's confidence.

Prior to evaluating the eccentric occlusion, the centric contacts should be idealized. Even centric contacts are achieved when no premature contacts exist. Articulating paper is not an appropriate material for this evaluation. The premature contact will act as a fulcrum point and still allows other contacts to be created. In fact, with articulating paper, an alternative contact may mark as the heaviest point of occlusion, while the actual prematurity appears as a donut contact point.

Occlusal indicator wax (Figure 14-23) is a material that will hold light contacts from touching while a prematurity is making contact. The wax will be penetrated by the opposing arch cusps at varying depths, allowing a premature contact to break through. The premature cusp will contact the opposing arch, while cusps with light contacts do not break through.

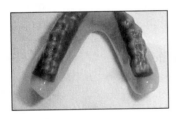

Figure 14-23: Occlusal indicator wax being used on a denture to mark centric occlusion prematurities

These premature contacts can be marked and adjusted by having the patient bite into the wax while in centric. If the patient is allowed to squeeze together as strong as he/she can, then the wax will work just like articulating paper. Therefore, the patient is instructed to "tap-tap-tap and squeeze with 75% power." Each time an adjustment is made, the patient will add 5% until reaching full power. The patient should then have even contact on the right and left sides as well as the anterior and posterior.

The prosthesis should also exhibit excellent retention following a swallow at this time. Should any difficulty arise in achieving centric contacts, a clinical remount should be completed. In completing a clinical remount, an open bite registration is obtained.

An open bite registration is completed by placing four small pieces of metal-impregnated wax on one arch. These pieces are placed in the second molar and first premolar areas. The patient will bite into these four pieces of wax without penetrating them. The metal-impregnated wax is cooled. When the prosthesis is returned to the mouth, the patient is instructed to close gently into the wax and hold, while fast-setting bite registration material is injected between the dentures.

If a remount index was not fabricated in the lab prior to processing, then a new facebow will be necessary. Once the prosthesis is mounted, the centric can be evaluated and adjusted with articulating paper. Even centric contacts are desired from a clinical remount. Gross eccentric discrepancies, if they exist, can be eliminated, but fine eccentric adjustments are made in the mouth.

Eccentric adjustments are made intra-orally with articulating paper. Marking one working movement at a time simplifies the adjustment. The patient should complete one working movement with a light-colored articulating paper such as red. Then the centric is marked with a darker color, such as black or blue.

The prosthesis is evaluated visually to determine what eccentric adjustment is necessary to improve the group function on the working side as well as the balancing side. If lingualized occlusion is being developed, then all buccal contacts are removed on the working side while the palatal – or lingual – contacts are developed in-group function. In a balanced occlusion, the maxillary arch buccal and palatal cusps are maintained in-group function.

In addition to finalizing the occlusion, the patient must be instructed in home care procedures at the delivery appointment. Patients need to understand the need to remove dentures at night. The oral mucosa requires time and oxygen to aid in the recovery of bearing the load of function. Removing the dentures at night should be recognized as similar to taking off shoes before going to bed.

Brushing the dentures after every meal is ideal. At times, it is not easy to brush them, but effort should be made to remove and rinse them as well as the mouth following meals. A denture toothbrush has longer bristles that can reach into the intaglio of the denture base and help keep it free of plaque and calculus.

When time is available to brush the dentures, an appropriate paste should be used. Denture toothpastes have gentle cleansing actions and are preferred to regular toothpaste. For partially edentulous patients, the toothpaste they use for their remaining teeth will suffice. The simplicity of this option will result in greater compliance.

Following brushing, the denture should be rinsed and dried. When dried, any remaining plaque or calculus will be evident as chalky white material. This material can be cleaned off with additional brushing or a toothpick. The dentures should be kept moist overnight. A glass of tap water is preferred to any over the counter cleaners. The patient should be welcomed to bring their dentures in at any time for a "professional" cleaning in the ultra-sonic cleaner in the office. Often, this is the only opportunity available to complete a periodic exam and oral cancer screening.

Using occlusal indicator wax, even centric contacts can be created on the right and left sides as well as from the anterior to the posterior. Once even centric has been created, then disclusive contacts are eliminated, and a group function is created on the working side and balancing side. The patient is instructed on oral hygiene and released to return in one week for a post delivery adjustment.

Post-Delivery Adjustment

The post-delivery adjustment can be set up for any interval of time. To instill confidence, it is recommended to schedule this visit one week after delivery of any removable prosthesis. The patient should be told, however, that he/she is welcome to call and come in sooner if there is a problem. In addition, the previous dentures should be kept in the dental office during the first adjustment period. The patients are told that this is done to complete a professional ultrasonic cleaning and ready them for emergency use in the future.

When a patient returns for the first post delivery adjustment, there are three typical problems that may occur: a lack of comfort due to sore areas, a lack of retention, and an inability to chew. There are also patients who return and are doing well and desire no particular change whatsoever. These patients should be evaluated as if they were coming in for a periodic exam. The occlusion is rechecked, the denture-bearing areas are evaluated, an oral cancer screening is completed, and home care is reviewed. Periodic exams should be scheduled annually and usually require little time.

If a patient has a lack of comfort due to a sore area, then it must be determined what is causing the soreness. If the sore area is related to the termination of the flanges, then typically the adjustment will need to be made to the pink acrylic. If the soreness is related to the area around the ridges, then typically the adjustment will need to be on the denture teeth.

Adjustments to the flanges can be additions or subtractions. Obviously, subtractions are much easier to complete. A pressure-indicating paste is brushed onto the intaglio of the denture as well as over the flanges themselves. The denture is carefully seated to not mark the paste. Once seated, the patient is asked to repeat the movements that make or accentuate the soreness. Often, this includes chewing and can be replicated with cotton rolls.

The denture is then carefully removed and the paste can be read for areas that burn through (Figure 14-24). On a flange, the areas of burn-through are indicators of overextension. These areas should be adjusted lightly and polished, remembering that the flanges tend to be well rounded and never knife-edged. The evaluation with pressure-indicating paste is repeated. When a patient reports that it feels a little bit better, then the adjustment is probably perfect. If the report is that it feels perfect, then the adjustment may have been too much.

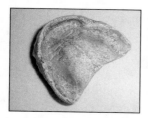

Figure 14-24: Pressure-indicating paste brushed onto a complete upper denture to identify sore areas

If the flange is cutting into the tissue, it may be due to a knife-edged finish line, when a well-rounded finish is required. Adding to an existing denture is never easy, and care should be taken to avoid such adjustments before they are necessary. However, when necessary, a flange can be extended and rounded with hard chairside reline acrylic.

The flange to be improved is lightly adjusted with an acrylic bur to create a slightly roughened surface. A round bur is used to create a butt joint end to the area that will be extended. This should be done on the intaglio as well as the external surface. Chairside reline acrylic is mixed and rolled into ropes of necessary thickness following the appropriate bench setting. It is adapted to the flange and seated in the mouth. In addition to the border molding reviewed previously, the patient should read aloud while the material is still in the working phase. Any flash is removed to the butt joint and the improved flange is polished.

Any sore spots on or near the crest of the ridge are probably related to the occlusion. It is easiest to check for a centric prematurity. That is completed first with occlusal indicator wax. These sore areas tend to be located nearest the crest of the ridge, but can also be found on the buccal inclines.

Articulating paper is used to identify what occlusal adjustment is necessary. Most often, these adjustments are made to the occlusion only. No adjustment is necessary on the acrylic.

If the patient has had a dramatic adjustment, then an additional one-week post delivery adjustment is made. When little was required, the patient is scheduled for the appropriate periodic examination. As always, if at any time patients have needs related to anything intra-orally, encourage them to contact the office for an appointment.

Conclusion

The five factors that define our success (Figure 14-25) in removable prosthodontics have been reviewed. The anatomical structures that are relied upon to provide stability, support, and retention for the final prosthesis have been identified. A clear understanding of how to best utilize these anatomical structures to serve and protect the patient's needs has been achieved.

The recording of the intra-oral information and transfer of that information to the laboratory has been outlined as well as a review of some of the materials available for completing these records. The delivery and maintenance of the final prosthesis have been clearly defined. These five factors for critical patient success with removable prosthodontics are: patient evaluation; framework design and tooth preparation; impression making and record collecting; tooth selection and occlusal design; and prosthesis delivery.

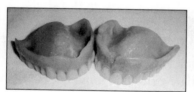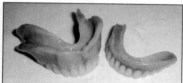

Figure 14-25: The evaluation of the patient's previous and new prosthesis. Areas are scrutinized with the patient to educate them regarding the benefits of a well-extended denture base with ideal occlusal contacts

Notes

1 Jacoboson, T., and Krol, A. A contemporary review of the factors involved in complete denture retention, stability and support: Part I: Retention. *J Prosthet Dent* 1983; 49:5.

2 Jacoboson, T., and Krol, A. A contemporary review of the factors involved in complete denture retention, stability and support: Part II: Stability. *J Prosthet Dent* 1983; 49:165.

3 Jacoboson, T., and Krol, A. A contemporary review of the factors involved in complete denture retention, stability and support: Part III: Support. *J Prosthet Dent* 1983; 49:306.

4 Atwood, D. Clinical, cephalometric and densitometric study of reduction of residual ridges. *J Prosthet Dent* 1971; 26:280.

5 Pound, E. Let "S" be your guide. *J Prosthet Dent* 1977; 38:482.

6 Frush, J.P., and Fisher, R.D. How dentogenic restorations interpret the sex factor. *J Prosthet Dent* 1956; 6:160-172.

7 Frush, J.P., and Fisher, R.D. How dentogenic restorations interpret the personality factor. *J Prosthet Dent* 1956; 6:441-449.

8 Frush, J.P., and Fisher, R.D. The age factor in dentogenics. *J Prosthet Dent* 1957; 7:5-13.

9 Barco, M.T. Jr., and Flinton, R.H. An overview of four removable partial denture clasps. *Int J Pros* 1988; 1:159-64.

10 Chow, T.W., Clark, R.K., and Clarke, D.A. Improved designs for removable partial dentures in Kennedy Class IV cases. *Quintessence Int.* 1988; 19:797-800.

[11] Stewart, K.L., Rudd, K.D., and Kuebker, W.A. *Clinical Removable Partial Prosthodontics.* C.V. Mosby, St. Louis, MO 1983.

[12] Krol, A.H., Jacobson, T.E., and Finzen, F.C. *Removable Partial Denture Design - Outline Syllabus.* University of the Pacific School of Dentistry, 1990.

[13] Browning, J.D., Meadors, L.W., and Eick, J.X. Movement of three removable partial denture clasp assemblies under occlusal loading. *J Prosthet Dent* 1986; 13:549-557.

[14] Myers, R.E., et al. A photoelastic study of rests on solitary abutments for distal-extension removable partial dentures. *J Prosthet Dent* 1986; 56:702-707.

[15] Ko, S.H., McDowell, G.C., and Kotowicz, W.E. Photoelastic stress analysis of mandibular removable partial dentures with mesial and distal occlusal rests. *J Prosthet Dent* 1986; 56:454-460.

[16] Feingold, G.M., Grant, A.A., and Johnson, W. The effect of partial denture design on abutment tooth and saddle movement. *Journal of Oral Rehabilitation* 1986; 13:549-557.

[17] Eliason, C. RPA clasp design for distal extension removable partial dentures. *J Prosthet Dent* 1983; 49:25.

[18] Burns, D.R., and Ward, J.E. A review of attachments for removable partial denture design: Part 2 - Treatment Planning and attachment selection. *Int J Pros* 1990; 3:169-170.

[19] Burns, D.R., and Ward, J.E. A review of attachments for removable partial denture design: Part 1 - Classification. *Int J Pros* 1990; 3:98-102.

[20] Brudvick, J.S. *Advanced Removable Partial Dentures*. Quintessence Publishing Co., Inc. Chicago, IL 1999.

[21] Levin, B. *Complete Denture Impressions*. Quintessence Publishing Co., Inc. Chicago, IL 1984.

[22] Leupold, R.J., Flinton, R.J., and Pfeifer, D.I. Comparison of vertical movement occurring during loading of distal extension removable partial denture bases made by three impressions techniques. *J Prosthet Dent* 1992; 68:290-293.

[23] Pound, E. Controlling anomalies of vertical dimension and speech. *J Prosthet Dent* 1976; 36:124.

[24] Pound, E. Accurate protrusive registration for patients edentulous in one or both jaws. *J Prosthet Dent* 1983; 50:584.

[25] Shannan, J. A bilaterally balanced occlusal scheme for patients with arch width and curvature discrepancies. *J Prosthet Dent* 1980; 44:101.

[26] Clough, H., Knodle, J., Pudwill, S., Myron, L., and Taylor, D. A comparison of lingualized occlusion and monoplane occlusion in complete dentures. *J Prosthet Dent* 1983; 50:176.

[27] Becker, C.M., Swoope, C.C., and Guckes, A.D. Lingualized occlusion for removable prosthodontics. *J Prosthet Dent* 1977; 38:601.

Chapter 15

Oral Mucosal Disorders Commonly Encountered in Oral Medicine

by Michael A. Siegel, D.D.S., M.S.

Dentists are frequently asked by their patients to diagnose and treat oral mucosal disorders, which are often painful and/or disfiguring. These lesions may represent an oral manifestation of a systemic disease, a reactive or neoplastic process, or may be a component of a dermatologic disorder. The diagnosis of these conditions is usually based on case-specific historical findings, clinical appearance, and the results of diagnostic procedures. This chapter will discuss the diagnosis and management of commonly encountered oral mucosal conditions such as herpes virus infection, recurrent aphthous ulceration, lichen planus, and candidosis.

Dentists are frequently called upon to evaluate and manage oral mucosal conditions. This chapter will present four of the most frequently encountered oral conditions:

- Herpes virus infection
- Recurrent aphthous ulceration
- Lichen planus
- Candidosis

Diagnosis of these lesions as well as therapeutic and palliative modalities for management of these lesions will be presented.

Herpes Simplex Virus Infection

Herpes simplex virus (HSV) is responsible for the most commonly occurring viral infections of the oral cavity and perioral soft tissues. The HSV has two distinct types:

- HSV-I—primarily associated with oral and labial lesions
- HSV-II—usually associated with genital lesions

Studies have shown that the predilection of a specific viral serotype to an anatomic site is changing, possibly due to varying sexual practices. In a review of 336 cases of primary genital herpes, 10.7% were associated with HSV-I.[1] A similar study of 160 cases of primary herpetic gingivostomatitis indicated that 2.5% of these infections were associated with HSV-II.[1]

Exposure to HSV-I is widespread in the United States. HSV-I serum antibodies can be found in up to 90% of the Americans who have been tested. Primary herpetic infections occur in individuals who have not been previously exposed to the virus. They are seen most often in children and adolescents. Primary herpetic infections do occur in adults, but are often misdiagnosed by health care practitioners. Most often, exposure to the HSV virus in children results in a subclinical infection. The child may complain of a mild flu-like condition that is commonly overlooked by the parents. Only a small percentage of patients will develop clinical manifestations of primary herpetic gingivostomatitis, pharyngitis, or both.

Primary herpetic gingivostomatitis has systemic manifestations and accompanying oral lesions. This primary viral disorder is recognized by a rapid onset of generalized prodromal symptoms and signs, such as malaise, headache, irritability, fever, and head and neck lymphadenopathy. These systemic symptoms are followed by the development of vesicular mucosal and gingival lesions. The initial oral manifestation is usually severe generalized gingival inflammation. Within several days, development of oral vesicles can occur on any of the oral mucous membranes (Fig. 15-1). The blisters rupture very rapidly, forming shallow, extremely painful erosions with a yellowish center and erythematous, irregular borders. These discrete erosions then merge, forming larger jagged lesions. Labial erosions will often appear crusted. Oral mucosal lesions are usually accompanied by severe pain, fetid odor, and sialorrhea.

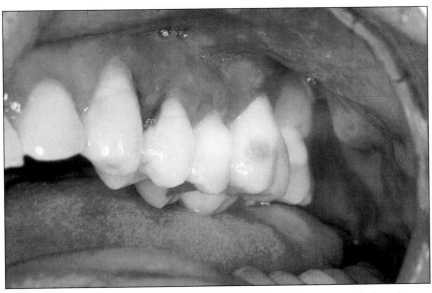

Fig. 15-1 Primary herpetic gingivostomatitis in a 67-year-old grandfather who was exposed to HSV by his grandchildren. Note the bleeding and erosion of the gingival tissues as well as the involvement of the buccal mucosal

Acute primary herpetic infections may also present as pharyngitis without any other oral lesions. This occurs most often in adolescents and is characterized by a sore throat, fever and headache, dysphagia, and cervical lymphadenitis.

The diagnosis of primary herpetic gingivostomatitis is based on the presence of both prodromal systemic signs and symptoms and the characteristic clinical appearance of generalized irregularly-shaped, shallow oral erosions. Diagnostic tests such as viral isolation in tissue culture and direct immunofluorescent antibody testing are available to confirm the diagnosis, but they are not routinely used in an otherwise healthy patient.

In a healthy individual, primary herpetic oral infection is self limiting, lasts approximately 10-14 days, and the lesions heal without scarring. Since this is an acute viral infection, the usual supportive measures such as the maintenance of adequate fluid intake and nutrition should be encouraged to prevent dehydration and electrolyte imbalance. Patients often present with severe pain. Systemic analgesics such as acetaminophen with or without codeine are useful for the pain control. Aspirin and non-steroidal anti-inflammatory medications should be avoided in acute viral infections, especially in children because of the risk of Reye's syndrome.[2]

Systemic anti-viral agents such as acyclovir are not routinely indicated for primary herpetic gingivostomatitis except in severely immunocompromised patients or when ophthalmologic involvement exists. However, if the use of a systemic antiviral medication is considered, it will be most effective if prescribed very early in the clinical course of the infection. The usual dosage of acyclovir is 200 mg, five times daily for 7-10 days[3] (Table 15-1). The current Food and Drug Administration recommendation is that this regimen be used to treat oral herpes only in immunocompromised patients.

Recurrent Herpetic Infections

Approximately 30-40% of patients who have been exposed to HSV will develop recurrent infections. Recurrent HSV infections can occur as either recurrent herpes labialis (RHL) or recurrent intraoral herpes (RIH). These recurrent infections represent reactivation and not reinfection of the HSV, which persists in a latent state in the trigeminal (semi-

MEDICATION	FORMS	DISPENSE	INSTRUCTIONS	ADVANTAGES/DISADVANTAGES/COST
penciclovir	1% cream	2 gm tube	Apply every two hours during waking hours for a period of four days. Treatment should be started during the prodromal symptoms, if possible.	High compliance Decreased duration and pain of episode Primary indication is RHL Safe Expensive
docosanol	OTC cream	2 gm tube	Apply five times per day during waking hours for a period of four days. Treatment should be started during the prodromal symptoms, if possible.	High compliance Decreased duration and pain of episode Only indication is RHL Safe Moderately expensive
acyclovir[†]	200 mg capsules	50	Take one capsule five times daily until gone.	Safe Must be initiated during prodrome to be effective Inexpensive
acyclovir[‡]	400 mg capsules	14	Take two capsules daily starting one day prior to anticipated sun exposure until gone.	Safe Inexpensive

[†] Recommended regimen for primary herpetic gingivostomatitis. The current Food and Drug Administration recommendation is that this regimen be used to treat oral herpes only in immunocompromised patients.

[‡] Recommended prophylactic regimen for severe episodes of recurrent herpes labialis in a patient at-risk for sun exposure. The current Food and Drug Administration recommendation is that this regimen be used to treat oral herpes only in immunocompromised patients.

Table 15-1 Medications used to treat herpetic infections. (Modified from Siegel, M.A. Strategies for management of commonly encountered oral mucosal disorders, J Cal Dent Assoc, 27(3):210-27, 1999)

lunar) ganglion. Recurrent infections are characterized by a mild clinical course. Recurrent HSV infections have been associated with exposure to sunlight, stress, fatigue, stress, menstruation, and oral trauma.

RHL (cold sore, fever blister) is preceded by prodromal signs or symptoms such as burning, tingling, soreness, or swelling in the site where the lesions will develop. Within hours, small vesicles develop in clusters along the vermilion border of the lips (Figs. 15-2a and 15-2b). The vesicles quickly rupture resulting in erosions that can coalesce to

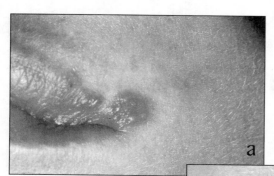

Fig. 15-2a Recurrent herpes labialis: early vesicle

Fig. 15-2b Recurrent herpes labialis: crusted lesions

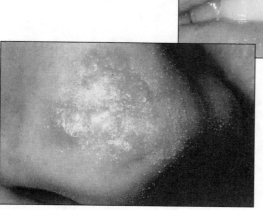

Fig. 15-3 Vesicles on the tip of the nose caused by shedding of recurrent HSV along the second division of the trigeminal nerve

form larger irregular lesions with a crusted surface. In an otherwise healthy individual, the lesions heal in 7-14 days without scarring. Lesions of recurrent extraoral herpetic infections can occur at sites other than the lips that are served by the trigeminal nerve (Fig. 15-3).

The diagnosis of RHL is based on its characteristic clinical appearance. The treatment for RHL is still primarily symptomatic. Ice, ether, chloroform, and rubbing alcohol have been used as topical agents with mixed results. Historically, topical antiviral agents such as acyclovir ointment have also been used with limited success, primarily because of poor cutaneous absorption. Penciclovir 1% topical cream is available by prescription for the treatment of RHL[4] (Table 15-1). Penciclovir 1% cream has been shown to reduce the severity and duration of the viral outbreak by inhibiting viral replication. Recently, docosanol has become available as an over-the-counter therapy for the treatment of RHL.[5] The mechanism of action of docosanol is via alteration of healthy cell membranes to prevent viral entry.

Lysine tablets have also been used with varying degrees of success. Some investigators reported that lysine resulted in milder episodes of RHL if taken in high doses (2-3 gm) at the first prodromal signs.[6] In some individuals, it was also found to be effective in preventing recurrences if the patient continued to take 1,000 mg per day. Systemic antiviral agents, such as acyclovir, are primarily used in severe cases of mucocutaneous or ophthalmologic herpes simplex infections in immunocompromised patients. However, in patients known to have RHL induced by exposure to sunlight, a prophylactic regimen of acyclovir, 400 mg twice daily, may be employed if prolonged actinic exposure is anticipated.[7] (Table 15-1) In otherwise healthy patients, RIH occurs less frequently than RHL. Lesions of RIH may be triggered by dental therapy; local, thermal, or chemical injury; or trauma from mastication. Lesions of RIH begin as clusters of tiny vesicles that rupture very rapidly, leaving small discrete erosions of the keratinized oral tissues (Fig. 15-4). These erosions can coalesce, forming larger irregular lesions. RIH occurs primarily on oral tissues that are firmly bound down to the underlying bone, *i.e.*, the hard palate, attached gingiva, and alveolar ridges.

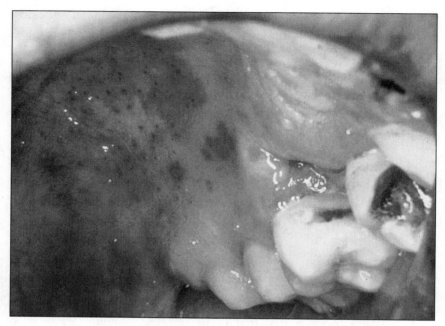

Fig. 15-4 Localized erosions of the keratinized palatal soft tissues resulting from ruptured vesicles of recurrent intraoral herpes following extraction of a maxillary premolar tooth

The diagnosis of RIH is based on the clinical appearance of the lesions and their location. The amount of discomfort associated with these lesions varies, and they heal without scarring in 7-14 days. The management of pain in RIH would involve the same topical palliative agents as were recommended for the painful lesions of primary herpetic gingivostomatitis.

Patients must be informed of the infectious nature of both acute and recurrent oral herpetic conditions. The vesicles of oral herpetic infections are extremely contagious, so care must be exercised to avoid autoinoculation of other mucosal sites as well as transmission to others. All stages of these viral lesions are potentially infectious until complete re-epithelialization has occurred.

Recurrent Aphthous Ulceration

Recurrent aphthous ulcerations (RAU, canker sores) are the most commonly occurring non-traumatic ulcerations of the oral cavity. The incidence rate varies from 20% to 60% of the population.[8-9] The etiology of RAUs is still unknown. Current investigations suggest an immunologic reaction in which there is a focal immune dysfunction involving the lymphocytes.[10] A number of factors play a triggering or modifying role in the development of RAUs. These include hormonal changes, trauma, stress, and/or food allergies.[11-12] Foods associated as triggering agents of RAUs include cinnamon, spices and preservatives, bovine milk protein, chocolate, glutens, and nuts.[13] Medications are also known to cause RAUs. One of the most commonly used medication classes reported to cause intraoral aphthous-like lesions are the non-steroidal anti-inflammatory drugs.[14] Deficiencies of ferritin and vitamin B12 have also been associated with RAUs.[15] RAUs have long been associated with inflammatory bowel diseases (IBD). IBD may have extra-abdominal intraoral signs such as aphthous-like ulcers that may appear one year prior to radiographic abdominal changes.[16] However, controversy exists as to whether the RAUs represent a primary manifestation of granulomatous bowel diseases or a result of the medical management of these conditions.[17]

RAUs have a characteristic clinical appearance. They appear as a shallow round or ovoid ulceration with a whitish center and an erythematous border. Clinically, RAUs present as single or multiple shallow ulcerations that occur on freely movable mucous membranes such as the lips, tongue, buccal mucosa, soft palate, floor of the mouth, and oropharynx. RAUs are categorized as minor, major, or herpetiform depending on their size and duration (Figs. 15-5a, 15-5b and 15-6a, 15-6b). Minor RAUs heal within a two week period and are less than or equal to 0.5 cm in diameter. Major RAUs are larger than 0.5 cm in diameter, take six weeks to three months to resolve, and may heal with residual scarring.

Herpetiform RAUs are very small (0.1-0.2 cm) and occur in clusters; therefore, this clinical appearance is very suggestive of a viral infection.

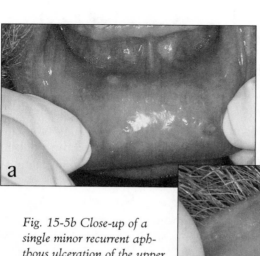

Fig. 15-5a Minor recurrent aphthous ulcerations of the lower lip in a 47-year-old male

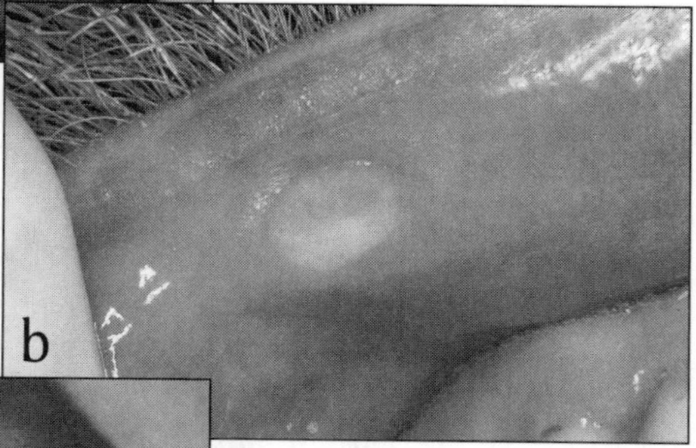

Fig. 15-5b Close-up of a single minor recurrent aphthous ulceration of the upper lip in the same patient

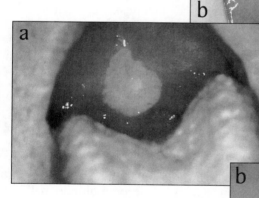

Fig. 15-6a Major aphthous ulceration of the soft palate in a 66-year-old male caused by a non-steroidal anti-inflammatory drug

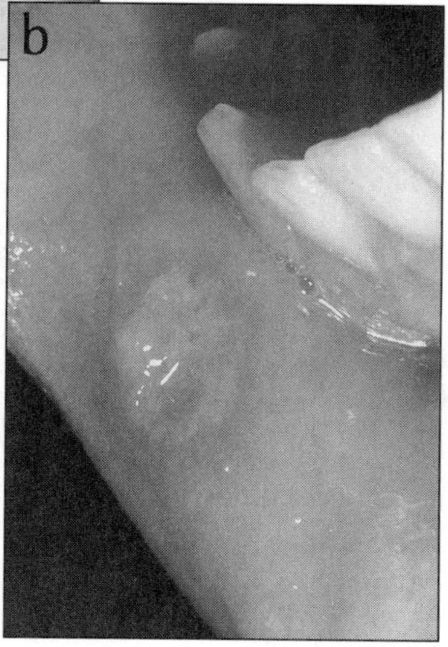

Fig. 15-6b Major aphthous ulceration of the lower lip in a 27-year-old male. Note the size and depth of the lesion

However, these lesions are not viral in etiology, as "herpetiform" inappropriately suggests. The distribution of herpetiform RAUs are on movable mucosa. The lesions do not begin as vesicles or blisters. Viral culture is usually negative, suggesting against HSV as a primary etiologic agent.

The diagnosis of RAUs is based on the presence of characteristic historical, clinical and, if necessary, laboratory findings. A previous history of similar lesions, the classic round-to-ovoid clinical appearance of the lesions, and the location of these lesions on freely movable mucous membranes will often establish the diagnosis. The patient's daily medication regimen, including prescribed, over-the-counter and homeopathic medications, must be carefully scrutinized to ensure that the lesions are not drug-related. Care should be taken to ensure that an adequate allergy and gastrointestinal history is obtained from the patient. A family history of IBD may also be significant. A complete blood count with a differential as well as serum ferritin and B12 levels may be necessary for some patients, especially those with refractory lesions.

To date, the treatment of RAUs is primarily palliative and symptomatic. Every effort should be made to eliminate predisposing allergens from the patient's diet. It is often helpful to have the patient maintain a food diary for a period of two weeks in order to identify dietary triggers of RAU. Once identified, the recurrence rate will decrease commensurate with the allergen's role in predisposing the patient to RAU. Therapeutic agents such as topical steroids and amlexanox 5% oral paste have been effective in decreasing the symptoms and healing time, but nothing has been found effective in decreasing the recurrence rate unless a trigger or serum deficiency can be identified and corrected. Recently, a sealant containing 2-octyl-cyanoacrylate has become available for the management of RAUs. This over-the-counter product provides immediate pain relief and provides a thin, flexible seal for RAUs that can last for up to six hours.[18]

Topical steroids are frequently used for the treatment of minor RAUs (Table 15-2). These drugs seem to be effective by decreasing the inflammatory response, which results in minimizing both the symptoms and the healing time. One of the most effective topical steroid preparations is

493

MEDICATION	FORMS	DISPENSE	INSTRUCTIONS	ADVANTAGES/DISADVANTAGES/COST
fluocinonide	0.05% cream ointment	30 gm tube	Apply thin coat to ulcer after meals and at bedtime. Do not eat or drink for 30 minutes following application. DO NOT USE FOR MORE THAN TWO WEEKS.	Shortens the duration and severity of lesions Prompt relief of pain Patient must carefully follow directions Risk of mucosal atrophy and absorption with prolonged use
amlexanox	5% oral paste	5 gm tube	Apply thin coat to ulcer after meals and at bedtime. Do not eat or drink for 30 minutes following application.	Primary indication for use is aphthous ulcers Very safe Minimal side effects Moderately expensive
dexamethasone	elixir	0.5 mg/ 5 ml 100 ml	Rinse with one teaspoonful for 3 minutes four times daily and expectorate until lesions resolve. DO NOT SWALLOW.	Shortens the duration and severity of lesions Prompt relief of pain Patient must carefully follow directions Risk of mucosal atrophy and absorption with prolonged use Risk of secondary candidosis
2-octyl cyanoacrylate	drops and applicator	OTC	Apply thin barrier directly to ulcer as per the instructions on the package. May be used every six hours.	No side effects Immediate pain relief May be difficult to use on multiple lesions and in the posterior pharynx. Moderately expensive

0.05% fluocinonide, which is available in a cream, ointment, or gel vehicle. Patients must be warned that chronic use of topical steroids will likely result in mucosal atrophy as well as systemic absorption of the steroid. Patients must be instructed not to use topical steroid medications on virally-induced lesions. Topical steroid therapy should not exceed two weeks for any occurrence of aphthous ulcers. Patients must discontinue topical steroid applications for a period of at least two weeks before reinstituting therapy for a recurrence of lesions. Cases of disseminated RAUs can be treated with a steroid rinse such as dexamethasone elixir 0.5 mg/5 ml. The same information regarding steroid use should be given to the patient. The extensive mucosal contact of steroid rinses may predispose the patient to secondary candidosis.

In severe cases of RAUs that are not responsive to topical steroids, systemic steroids such as prednisone may become necessary. When prescribing systemic steroids or steroid rinses for severe oral ulcerations, concurrent therapy with antifungal agents should be considered.

Amlexanox 5% oral paste is a new medication specifically indicated for the management of RAUs.[19-20] This medication has antihistamine properties and has been shown clinically to reduce both the symptoms and duration of the lesions.

Other types of treatment options include topical anesthetics, caustic agents, and laser ablation. Topical anesthetics such as 2% viscous lidocaine hydrochloride will provide temporary relief of pain. Caustic agents such as silver nitrate or sulfuric acid have been used to cauterize the central portion of the ulcer, thus providing relief of pain. Cautery may result in mucosal scarring. Laser ablation has been used to manage RAUs in some individuals, but is limited by both the availability of the laser and the cost to the patient for repeated treatments.

Table 15-2 (left) Topical medications used to treat recurrent aphthous ulcers. (Modified from Siegel MA. Strategies for management of commonly encountered oral mucosal disorders, J Cal Dent Assoc, 27(3):210-27, 1999)

Lichen Planus

Lichen planus is a disorder of unknown etiology and represents the most common cutaneous disorder with oral manifestations. The skin lesions occur as violaceous papules with a fine scale on the flexor surface of the arms and legs. The oral lesions vary greatly in appearance and frequently represent the only clinical sign of disease. Lichen planus is usually found in patients over the age of 40 and has been associated with stress and anxiety. Numerous medications have been reported to cause oral lichenoid drug reactions.[21-22] Commonly encountered medications may include thiazide diuretics and tetracyclines. Dental amalgam restorations with direct mucosal contact have also been implicated in lichenoid reactions.[23-25] The patient may be unaware of the intraoral form of the disease, because it is often asymptomatic. Therefore, the oral soft tissues of patients with signs and symptoms of dermal lichen planus must be examined.

Oral lichen planus is often identified by the presence of fine, reticular white lines (striae of Wickham) on the lateral borders of the tongue, buccal mucosa, and gingiva (Figs. 15-7a, 15-7b and 15-8a, 15-8b, 15-8c). However, striae are not always present, especially in the atrophic or ulcerative forms of the disease (Fig. 15-9). Biopsy may be necessary in order to establish a definitive diagnosis. Although prospective studies have failed to demonstrate that lichen planus is a premalignant disorder, it is recommended that all patients exhibiting this condition intraorally, particularly those who have had the ulcerative form, receive long-term follow-up.[26-28] Fluocinonide cream, ointment, or gel is quite effective in treating mucosal lesions and has not been shown to cause adrenal suppression (Table 15-3).[29] Ultrapotent topical steroids such as clobetasol propionate ointment may also be used intraorally and appear to be both safe and effective.[30] However, because of potential systemic adverse reactions from long-term use of ultrapotency topical steroids on the skin, patients must be monitored regularly.[31] Occlusive steroid therapy using custom-made flexible mouthguards to localize fluocinonide gel is extremely effective in controlling the gingi-

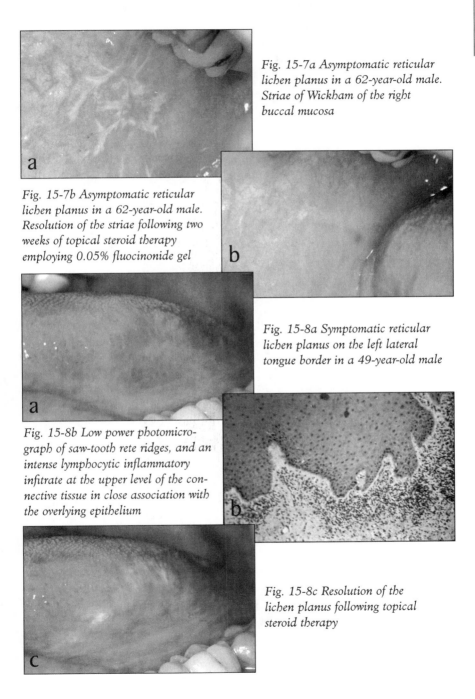

Fig. 15-7a Asymptomatic reticular lichen planus in a 62-year-old male. Striae of Wickham of the right buccal mucosa

Fig. 15-7b Asymptomatic reticular lichen planus in a 62-year-old male. Resolution of the striae following two weeks of topical steroid therapy employing 0.05% fluocinonide gel

Fig. 15-8a Symptomatic reticular lichen planus on the left lateral tongue border in a 49-year-old male

Fig. 15-8b Low power photomicrograph of saw-tooth rete ridges, and an intense lymphocytic inflammatory infiltrate at the upper level of the connective tissue in close association with the overlying epithelium

Fig. 15-8c Resolution of the lichen planus following topical steroid therapy

MEDICATION	FORMS	DISPENSE	INSTRUCTIONS	ADVANTAGES/DISADVANTAGES/COST
fluocinonide	0.05% cream ointment gel	30 gm tube	Apply thin coat to ulcer after meals and at bedtime. Do not eat or drink for 30 minutes following application. DO NOT USE FOR MORE THAN TWO WEEKS.	Shortens the duration and severity of lesions Relief of pain Patient must carefully follow directions Risk of mucosal atrophy and absorption with prolonged use Gel form should be used with custom carrier(s)
clobetasol propionate	0.05% ointment	30 gm tube	Apply thin coat to ulcer after meals and at bedtime. Do not eat or drink for 30 minutes following application. DO NOT USE FOR MORE THAN TWO WEEKS.	Shortens the duration and severity of lesions Relief of pain Patient must carefully follow directions Risk of mucosal atrophy and absorption with prolonged use Risk of systemic absorption
dexamethasone elixir	0.5 mg/ 5 ml	100 ml	Rinse with one teaspoonful for 3 minutes four times daily and expectorate until lesions resolve. DO NOT SWALLOW.	Shortens the duration and severity of lesions Relief of pain Patient must carefully follow directions Risk of mucosal atrophy and absorption with prolonged use Risk of secondary candidosis

Table 15-3 Topical medications used to treat lichen planus. (Modified from Siegel, MA. Strategies for management of commonly encountered oral mucosal disorders, J Cal Dent Assoc, *27(3):210-27, 1999)*

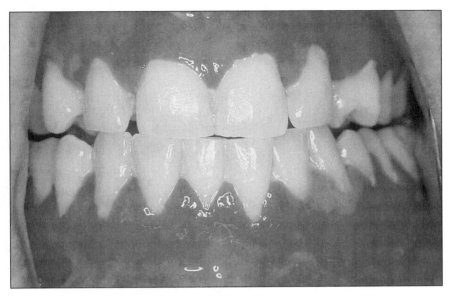

Fig. 15-9 Atrophic gingival lichen planus in a 40-year-old female with biopsy-proven cutaneous lichen planus. Note the intense erythema in the presence of good plaque control

val lesions of lichen planus.[32-33] Fluocinonide 0.5% gel is applied to the mouthguards; patients are instructed to wear the mouthguards for 30 minutes per application. Therapy can be instituted with a regimen of four applications daily, preferably after meals and at bedtime. The frequency of daily use depends on the response of the lesions. Long-term control of persistent lesions can often be achieved with a 30-minute application every other evening.

Disseminated lesions can be controlled with dexamethasone rinses. Refractory, persistent, localized lesions respond very favorably to intralesional injection of triamcinalone (10 mg/ml) in lidocaine. Secondary candidosis should be considered when ulcerated lesions remain refractory to conventional therapy or when an unexplained relapse occurs in a patient using topical steroids.[22] Systemic corticosteroids will resolve oral lesions that occur coincidently with skin lesions of lichen planus, but recurrence of oral lichen planus is likely. Use of systemic steroids for periods of time greater than two weeks given at doses greater than 40 mg daily are likely to result in side effects that may not resolve once the steroids are discontinued. These side effects include but are not limited to oral candidosis, hypertension, fluid retention, gastrointestinal discomfort, insomnia, fat deposition, and/or skin rash.[31] Intraoral mucosal conditions that are refractory to therapeutic trial or remain present for a period of greater than two to four weeks should be biopsied in order to establish a definitive diagnosis. Routine removal of amalgam restorations for the management of lichen planus is contraindicated. If a refractory lesion is in direct contact with an amalgam restoration, polishing of the restoration under a rubber dam and application of a copal varnish to the surface to establish the metallic restoration as the causative agent of the lesion is prudent. If a number of restorations are planned for removal, patch testing for oxides of silver, tin, and mercury may provide the dentist with a rationale for restoration removal. Referral to an allergist in these cases is suggested.

Oral Candidosis

Candidosis, the most commonly occurring oral fungal infection in the non-immunocompromised patient, is caused by *candida albicans*. Up to 60% of healthy individuals may harbor this fungal organism as host flora in the oral cavity.[34] In individuals who have candida albicans as a normal component of their oral microflora, their own immune system and the competing bacteria keep the fungal organisms from overgrowing.[35] This opportunistic infection may occur due to a variety of systemic factors or as a result of local changes in the oral environment.

Systemic conditions associated with the development of candidosis include endocrine disturbances such as diabetes, pregnancy, and hypoparathyroidism or systemic steroid therapy. Other systemic factors that may favor the development of candidosis include immunosuppression such as seen in AIDS patients, malabsorption and malnutrition,

Sjogren's syndrome, and cancer chemotherapy.[36-37] Local factors that favor the development of candidosis include changes in the oral flora resulting from decreased tissue resistance due to xerostomia or chronic local irritants (dentures, orthodontic appliances, smoking) and/or antibiotic therapy.

The clinical appearance of the oral lesions can vary greatly. Pindborg reported four clinical varieties of oral candidosis found in HIV-infected individuals—pseudomembranous, erythematous, hyperplastic, and angular cheilosis.[38] These clinical fungal subtypes are also useful in diagnosing and managing these lesions in non-HIV infected individuals. The two most common oral presentations are pseudomembranous candidosis and erythematous candidosis (denture sore mouth).

Pseudomembranous candidosis is characterized by the presence of white curd-like lesions that can be easily removed with a tongue blade or gauze, exposing an erythematous, erosive surface underneath (Figs. 15-10a, 15-10b, and 15-10c). The term thrush should be reserved for use in a pediatric patient population. The white curds consist of fungal organisms, bacteria, inflammatory cells, fibrin, and desquamated epithelial cells. The lesions occur most commonly on the buccal mucosa and mucobuccal folds, the dorsal surface of the tongue, and the oropharynx. If the white lesions have not been rubbed off, the patients are usually asymptomatic. Patients with extensive erosive areas may complain of a burning dysesthesia, tenderness, or dysphagia.

Erythematous candidosis is frequently noted in patients who wear maxillary complete or partial dentures, especially in cases when the prosthesis is not removed prior to bedtime (Figs. 15-11a and 15-11b). This form of candidosis seems to occur as a result of decreased tissue resistance from the prosthetic appliance. The lesions have a distinct predilection for the palatal mucosa, but may also occur under mandibular dentures. Clinically, erythematous candidosis appears as red, atrophic lesions. The erythema may diffuse, involving the entire denture-bearing area or it may present as patchy areas of erythema that resemble petechiae.

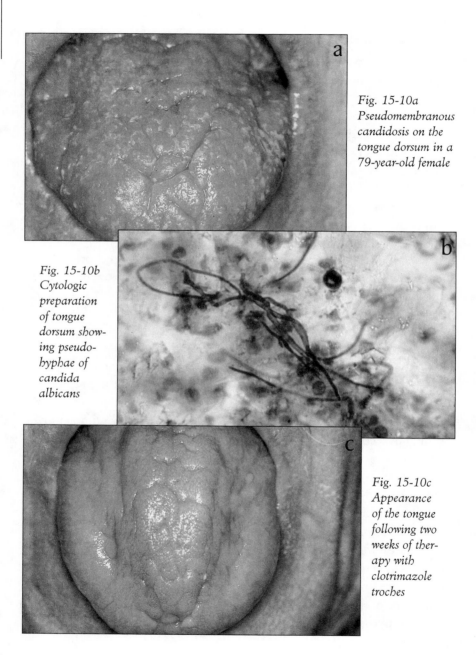

Fig. 15-10a
Pseudomembranous
candidosis on the
tongue dorsum in a
79-year-old female

Fig. 15-10b
Cytologic
preparation
of tongue
dorsum show-
ing pseudo-
hyphae of
candida
albicans

Fig. 15-10c
Appearance
of the tongue
following two
weeks of ther-
apy with
clotrimazole
troches

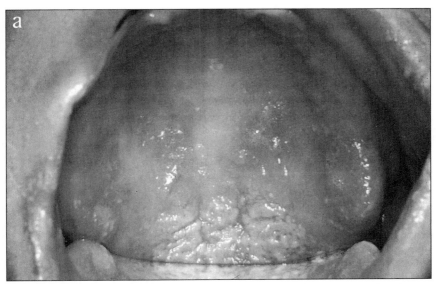

Fig. 15-11a *Erythematous candidosis of the palate in a 44-year-old female under an ill-fitting maxillary complete denture. Note the pseudomembranous candidosis along the posterior border of the hard palate*

Fig. 15-11b *Appearance of the palate following temporary reline of the denture and two weeks of therapy with nystatin ointment*

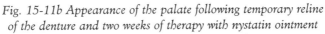

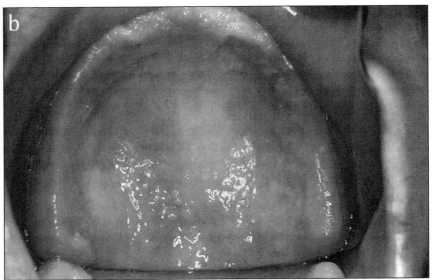

Hyperplastic candidosis is unlike the pseudomembranous and erythematous forms in that it cannot be wiped off of the mucosa. It is seen as elevated white plaques that resemble clinical leukoplakia. Hyperplastic candidosis most often involves the dorsal surface of the tongue or the hard palate. It must be differentiated from other keratoses by cytologic smear, culture, biopsy, or therapeutic trial with antifungal medication. Lesions that do not respond to a trial of antifungal medication must be biopsied to establish a diagnosis.

Angular cheilosis is due to candidal infection of the labial commissures. Angular cheilosis may occur with or without concurrent oral candidal lesions. It is characterized by redness and/or fissures radiating from one or both corners of the mouth and is often associated with small white plaques (Figs. 15-12a, 15-12b, and 15-12c,d). Angular cheilosis has long been associated with vitamin B deficiency and decreased occluding vertical dimension. While these conditions may serve as predisposing factors for the development of angular cheilosis, the management of the lesions must be directed at their fungal etiology.

The diagnosis of candidosis can often be made from the patient history and the clinical appearance and distribution of the mucosal lesions. When necessary, especially in an immunocompromised individual, identification of the organisms is made from a cytology smear stained with periodic-acid Schiff (PAS) reagent, or on a wet smear macerated with 10% potassium hydroxide.

If is becomes necessary to speciate the fungal organisms from a lesion, they can be grown in a culture on a selective medium available from a hospital medical laboratory or commercial service. Oral candidosis is most often treated with topical antifungal agents such as clotrimazole troches or nystatin ointment (Table 15-4). Oral preparations in the form of troches provide the advantage of prolonged contact of the medication with the lesions. They are safe to use because of their poor systemic absorption. Oral hygiene must be reinforced when prescribing oral antifungal troches because of their sugar content. The sugar content of these medications can also present a problem when prescribed for diabetic patients who are on a strict carbohydrate diet. While nystatin sus-

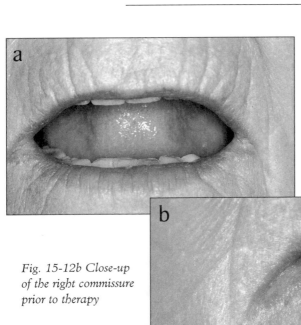

Fig. 15-12a Severe bilateral angular cheilosis in a 71-year-old female patient

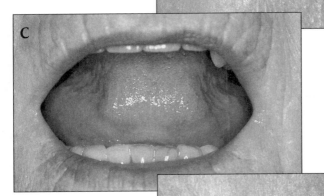

Fig. 15-12b Close-up of the right commissure prior to therapy

Fig. 15-12c,d Resolution of the labial commissures following 4 weeks of therapy using nystatin with triamcinalone acetonide ointment

MEDICATION	FORMS	DISPENSE	INSTRUCTIONS	ADVANTAGES/ DISADVANTAGES/COST
nystatin	ointment	30 gm tube	Apply thin coat to inner aspect of denture(s) after each meal. Do not eat or drink for 30 minutes following application.	Safe High compliance Inexpensive
clotrimazole	troches	70	Dissolve slowly five times/day until gone. DO NOT CHEW.	Safe High compliance Pleasant tasting High sugar content Expensive
nystatin- triamcinalone acetonide	ointment	15 gm tube	Apply to corners of mouth after meals and at bedtime for two weeks. DO NOT LICK.	Safe High compliance Inexpensive

Table 15-4 Topical medications used to treat candidosis. (Modified from Siegel MA. Strategies for management of commonly encountered oral mucosal disorders, J Cal Dent Assoc, 27(3):210-27, 1999)

pension is frequently prescribed, in general, rinses are less effective than other forms of topical antifungal therapy because the duration of tissue contact is insufficient.[39] Patients who wear dentures must remove the dentures prior to using an antifungal rinse or troche.

When treating cases of erythematous candidosis under a denture, the prosthetic appliance must be addressed as well as the oral lesions. After each meal, nystatin ointment or clotrimazole cream should be applied to the tissue side of the denture before replacement in the mouth. Patients should be reminded to remove their dentures at bedtime and soak them overnight in an antifungal solution. Most commercially available denture soaking tablets are fungicidal; it should not be necessary to prescribe nystatin suspension specifically for this purpose.

Angular cheilosis is a mixed infection of candida albicans and salivary species of streptococci. These lesions respond very well to combination therapy containing an antifungal and a topical steroid in a cream or ointment vehicle. Nystatin with triamcinalone acetonide or clotrimazole with betamethasone dipropionate preparations are quite useful for this purpose. Patients should be encouraged not to "lick" the lesion,s as this will serve to superinfect the cheilosis with salivary bacteria.

In cases of refractory candidosis, mucocutaneous candidosis, patients in whom compliance is a problem, or in women who have a concurrent candida vaginitis, a systemic antifungal therapy with ketaconazole or fluconazole is recommended (Table 15-5). If either of these medications is used for longer than two weeks, liver function tests should be performed to ensure against hepatotoxicity.

Discussion

Management of painful oral mucosal conditions may be either topical or systemic. Oral therapy should address patient nutrition and hydration, oral discomfort, oral hygiene, management of secondary infection, as well as local control of the disease process. Depending on the extent, severity, and location of oral lesions, consideration should be given to obtaining a consultation from a dentist who specializes in oral medicine, oral pathology, oral surgery, or periodontics.[40] If the oral lesions are painful enough to limit normal dietary intake, nutritional supplementation and adequate hydration must be stressed to the patient. Commercially available weight-control beverages serve this purpose in a cost-effective manner. Cold beverages or the use of ice chips may provide temporary relief of oral pain. Citrus fruits, carbonated beverages, and other acid-containing or spicy foods will exacerbate oral discomfort, so they should be avoided. Symptomatic relief can be provided with topical preparations such as 2% viscous lidocaine hydrochloride applied

MEDICATION	FORMS	DISPENSE	INSTRUCTIONS	ADVANTAGES/ DISADVANTAGES/COST
ketaconazole	200 mg tabs	14	Take one tablet daily with a meal until gone.	High compliance Potential for hepatotoxicity Must take with meal Poor absorption Inexpensive
fluconazole	100 mg tabs	15	Take two tablets the first day, then one tablet daily until gone.	High compliance Good absorption Potential for hepatotoxicity Expensive

Table 15-5 Systemic medications used to treat candidosis. (Modified from Siegel MA. Strategies for management of commonly encountered oral mucosal disorders, J Cal Dent Assoc, 27(3):210-27, 1999)

prior to meals to facilitate eating (Table 15-6). Topical anesthetics can be used as a rinse in adults, but should be applied with a cotton swab in a child so that the child does not swallow the medication. Swallowing these anesthetics is contraindicated, in part, because they may interfere with the patient's gag-reflex. Symptomatic relief can also be obtained by mixing equal parts of diphenhydramine hydrochloride elixir and magnesium hydroxide/aluminum hydroxide. Children's formula diphenhydramine hydrochloride elixir does not contain alcohol. Sucralfate suspension may also be used prior to meals. The diphenhydramine mixture and the sucralfate coat the ulcerated lesions and allow the patient to eat more comfortably.

Mouth rinses containing a hydro-alcoholic vehicle should be avoided because of the oral discomfort that will result from their use. The amount of oral discomfort experienced by patients with oral mucosal lesions varies and can often be controlled without the use of narcotic analgesics.

Meticulous oral hygiene is absolutely mandatory for these patients. Mucosal lesions contacting bacterial plaque present on the dentition are more likely to become secondarily infected. Patients should be seen by the dentist or hygienist for scaling and root planing, under local anesthesia when necessary, in all cases where oral hygiene is sub-optimal. Patients must be encouraged to brush and floss their teeth after meals in a gentle, yet efficient manner. This may be enhanced by placing a soft toothbrush under hot water to further soften the bristles. Tartar-control toothpastes containing calcium pyrophosphate should be avoided because of their caustic nature and reported involvement in circumoral dermatitis.[41] Secondary infection of ulcerative oral mucosal lesions is most commonly fungal in etiology. While long standing oral ulceration alone may predispose some patients to secondary candidosis, therapeutic regimens of antibiotics or steroids will increase the frequency of mycotic infection in susceptible individuals.[22] Bacterial infection is less common. Unless the lesions become indurated, purulent, or are associated with an acute tender lymphadenopathy, antibiotic coverage should be unnecessary.

MEDICATION	FORMS	DISPENSE	INSTRUCTIONS	ADVANTAGES/DISADVANTAGES/COST
lidocaine HCl	2% viscous	100 ml bottle	Apply with cotton swab or rinse for two minutes prior to meals and expectorate. DO NOT GARGLE OR SWALLOW.	Safe Fast acting pain relief Short duration May compromise gag reflex Inexpensive
diphenhydramine HCl and magnesium hydroxide/ aluminum hydroxide	children's elixir suspension	OTC Mix equal parts (50% mixture of each)	Rinse with two teaspoonfuls for two minutes as necessary for pain and expectorate.	Safe Fast acting pain relief Provides coating over ulceration Short duration Children's elixir contains no alcohol Inexpensive
sucralfate	suspension	14 oz bottle	Rinse with two teaspoonfuls for two minutes prior to meals and at bedtime and expectorate.	Safe Fast acting pain relief Provides coating over ulceration Moderate duration Expensive

Table 15-6 Medications used to palliate oral mucosal ulcerations. (Modified from Siegel MA. Strategies for management of Assoc, 27(3):210-27, 1999)

Notes

1 Nahmias, A.J., and Starr, S.E. Infections caused by herpes simplex viruses. In *Infectious diseases: a modern treatise of infectious processes*. 2nd ed., edited by P.D. Hoeprich. Hagerstown, MD: Harper and Row, 726-35, 1977

2 Ward, M.R. Reye's syndrome: an update. *Nurse Practitioner*, 1997, 22(12):45-53

3 *Physicians Desk Reference*, 55th ed. Montvale: Medical Economics, 2001

4 Wynn, R.L. New drugs approvals in 1996. *Gen Dent*, 1997, 45:224-7

5 Pope, L., Marcelletti, J., Katz, L., et al. The anti-herpes simplex virus activity of n-docosanol includes inhibition of the viral entry process. *Antiviral Res*, 1998, 40:85-94

6 Griffith, R.S., Norins, A.L., and Kagan, C. A multicentered study of lysine therapy in herpes simplex infection. *Dermatologica*, 1978, 156:257-67

7 Scully, C. Orofacial herpes simplex virus infections: current concepts in the epidemiology, pathogenesis, and treatment, and disorders in which the virus may be implicated. *Oral Surg Oral Med Oral Pathol*, 1989, 68:701-10

8 Shapiro, S., Olson, D.L., and Chellemi, S.J. The association between smoking and aphthous ulcers. *Oral Surg Oral Med Oral Pathol*, 1970, 30:624-30

[9] Ship II. Epidemiologic aspects of recurrent aphthous ulcerations. *Oral Surg Oral Med Oral Pathol*, 1972, 33:400-6

[10] Regezi J.A., and Sciubba, J.J. Ulcerative conditions. In *Oral Pathology Clinical Pathologic Correlations*. 2nd ed., Philadelphia, PA: W.B. Saunders Company, 52-60, 1993

[11] Balciunas, B.A., Kelly, M.A., and Siegel, M.A. Clinical management of common oral lesions. *Cutis*, 1991, 47:31-6

[12] Ship, J.A. Recurrent aphthous stomatitis. *Oral Surg Oral Med Oral Pathol Oral Radiol Endod*, 1996, 81:141-7

[13] Woo, S.B., and Sonis, S.T. Recurrent aphthous ulcers: a review of diagnosis and treatment. *JADA*, 1996, 127:1202-13

[14] Siegel, M.A., and Balciunas, B.A. Medication can cause severe ulcerations. *JADA*, 1991, 122:75-7

[15] Porter, S.R., Kingsmill, V., and Scully, C. Audit of diagnosis and investigations in patients with recurrent aphthous stomatitis. *Oral Surg Oral Med Oral Pathol*, 1993, 76:449-52

[16] Siegel, M.A. Oral manifestations of gastrointestinal disease: diagnosis and treatment. In *Current therapy in gastroenterology and liver disease*. 3rd ed, edited by T.M. Bayless. Burlington, Ontario: BC Decker, 1989, pp. 1-7

[17] Siegel, M.A. Gastrodontology: a clinical perspective worth consideration. *Am J Gastroenterol*, 1996, 91:1-2

[18] Kutcher, M.J., Ludlow, J.B., Samuelson, A.D., Campbell, T., and Pusek, S.N. Evaluation of a bioadhesive device for the management of aphthous ulcers. *JADA*, 2001, 132(3):368-76

[19] Khandwala, A., Van Inwegen, R.G., and Alfano, M.C. 5% amlexanox oral paste, a new treatment for recurrent minor aphthous ulcers. II. pharmacokinetics and demonstration of clinical safety. *Oral Surg Oral Med Oral Pathol Oral Radiol Endod*, 1997, 83:231-8

[20] Khandwala, A., Van Inwegen, R.G., and Alfano, M.C. 5% amlexanox oral paste, a new treatment for recurrent minor aphthous ulcers. I. clinical demonstration of acceleration of healing and resolution of pain. *Oral Surg Oral Med Oral Pathol Oral Radiol Endod*, 1997, 83:222-30

[21] Van Dis, M.L., and Parks, E.T. Prevalence of oral lichen planus in patients with diabetes mellitus. *Oral Surg Oral Med Oral Pathol Oral Radiol Endod*, 1995, 79:696-700

[22] Vincent, S.D., Fotos, P.G., Baker, K.A., and Williams, T.P. Oral lichen planus: The clinical, historical, and therapeutic features of 100 cases. *Oral Surg Oral Med Oral Pathol*, 1990, 70:165-71

[23] Ostman, P., Anneroth, G., and Skoglund, A. Amalgam-associated oral lichenoid reactions. *Oral Surg Oral Med Oral Pathol Oral Radiol Endod*, 1996, 81:459-465

[24] Bratel, J., Hakeberg, M., and Jontell, M. Effect of replacement of dental amalgam on oral lichenoid reactions. *J Dent*, 1996, 24:41-5

[25] Pang, B.K., and Freeman, S. Oral lichenoid lesions caused by allergy to mercury in amalgam fillings. *Contact Dermatitis*, 1995, 33:423-7

[26] Silverman, Jr., S., Gorsky, M., and Lozada-Nur, F. A prospective follow-up study of 570 patients with oral lichen planus: persistence remission and malignant association. *Oral Surg Oral Med Oral Pathol*, 1985, 60:30-4

[27] Silverman, S., Gorsky, M., Lozada-Nur, F., et al. A prospective study of findings and management in 214 patients with oral lichen planus. *Oral Surg Oral Med Oral Pathol*, 1991, 72:665-70

[28] Silverman, Jr., S., and Bahl, S. Oral lichen planus update, clinical characteristics, treatment responses, and malignant transformation. *Am J. Dent*, 1997, 10:259-63

[29] Plemons, J.M., Rees, T.D., and Zachariah, N.Y. Absorption of a topical steroid and evaluation of adrenal suppression in patients with erosive lichen planus. *Oral Surg Oral Med Oral Pathol*, 1990, 69:688-93

[30] Lozada-Nur, F., Huang, M.Z., and Zhou, G. Open preliminary clinical trial of clobetasol propionate ointment in adhesive paste for treatment of chronic oral vesiculoerosive diseases. *Oral Surg Oral Med Oral Pathol*, 1991, 71:283-7

[31] Lozada, F., Silverman, Jr., S., and Migliorati, C. Adverse side effects associated with prednisone in the treatment of patients with oral inflammatory ulcerative diseases. *JADA*, 1984, 109:269-70

[32] Aufdemorte, T.B., Villez, R.L., and Parel, S.M. Modified topical steroid therapy for the treatment of oral mucous membrane pemphigoid. *Oral Surg Oral Med Oral Path*, 1985, 59:256-60

[33] Wray, D., and McCord, J.F. Labial veneers in the management of desquamative gingivitis. *Oral Surg Oral Med Oral Pathol*, 1987, 64:41-2

[34] Fotos, P.G., Vincent, S.D., and Hellstein, J.W. Oral Candidosis. Oral Surg Oral Med Oral Pathol, 1992; 74:41-9.Allen CM. Diagnosing and managing oral candidiasis. *JADA*, 1992, 123:77-82

[35] Allen, C.M. Diagnosing and managing oral candidiasis. *JADA*, 1992, 123:77-82

[36] Muzyka, B.C., and Glick, M. A review of oral fungal infections and appropriate therapy. *JADA*, 1995, 126:63-72

[37] Patton, L.L., and Shugars, D.C. Immunologic and viral markers of HIV-1 disease progression: implications for dentistry. *JADA*, 1999, 130(9):1313-22

[38] Pindborg, J.J. Classification of oral lesions associated with HIV infection. *Oral Surg Oral Med Oral Pathol*, 1989, 67:292-5

[39] Epstein, J.B. Antifungal therapy in oropharyngeal mycotic infections. *Oral Surg Oral Med Oral Pathol*, 1990, 69:32-41

[40] Siegel, M.A. Strategies for management of commonly encountered oral mucosal disorders. *J Cal Dent Assoc*, 1999, 27(3):210-27

[41] Beacham, B.E., Kurgansky, D., and Gould, M. Circumoral dermatitis and cheilitis caused by tartar control dentifrices. *J Am Acad Dermatol*, 1990, 22:1029-32

Chapter 16

Periodontics

By Michael Sonick, D.M.D

Periodontics has undergone a significant metamorphosis in the last three decades. The goal of periodontal treatment has always been to arrest the progression of bone loss, which frequently led to the demise of the dentition. In the past, periodontal treatment frequently left patients with less than optimum esthetics. Teeth were saved but at the expense of cosmetics. Figure 16-1 shows a patient who had undergone periodontal surgery 25 years previously. The pockets have been eliminated and the teeth saved. However, each time the patient speaks, air and saliva are forced through the open embrasures of his teeth labially. Food gets caught between them and he is esthetically compromised. This type of periodontal result should be avoided at all costs. (See section on papilla retention procedure.) What was previously thought of as clinical success is now deemed a failure. For whom do we perform treatment, the patient or the clinician? Pocket elimination alone is not clinical success if the patient is not happy. To paraphrase the Hippocratic Oath—*above all do no harm*.

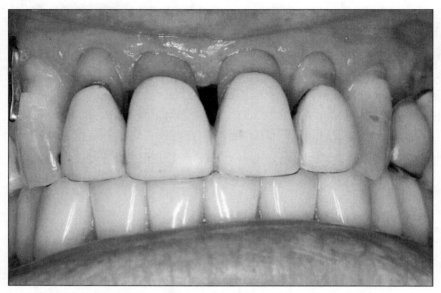

Fig. 16-1 This patient had resective periodontal surgery 30 years ago. He was treated with a full thickness apically repositioned flap. Note the loss of interdental papillae. Periodontal pockets have been eliminated, however the patient is esthetically compromised

Periodontal treatment today still includes the prevention, control, and elimination of periodontal disease. However, with advances in research and technology, periodontal therapy provides clinicians with the ability to regenerate lost alveolar bone, replace lost gingival tissues with root coverage techniques, augment ridges in preparation for restorative dentistry and implants, and to perform esthetic crown-lengthening procedures in preparation for smile design. Periodontal therapy today includes:

- Preventative therapy
- Control of disease
- Elimination of disease
- Regeneration of hard tissue
- Regeneration of soft tissue

- Periodontal plastic surgery
  ◊ mucogingival therapy
  ◊ root coverage procedures
  ◊ soft tissue ridge augmentation
  ◊ esthetic crown lengthening
- Pre-implant regenerative therapy (site therapy)
- Implant therapy

Periodontics is considered the foundation of dental health. In the absence of healthy bone and gingiva, teeth are unstable, restorations are not placed on solid foundations, and the patient is not dentally stable. Periodontics is the therapeutic pillar on which solid clinical dentistry rests.

Etiology of Inflammatory Periodontal Diseases

The healthy periodontium

Before entering a discussion of periodontal disease, periodontal health must first be defined. Supporting tissues of the teeth are known collectively as the *periodontium* (from the Greek *peri*, around, and *odontos*, a tooth). The periodontium is made up of four structures—the gingiva, periodontal ligament, cementum, and alveolar bone.

Macroscopic anatomy. Figure 16-2 shows the teeth and gingiva of a periodontally healthy individual. The color of the gingiva is uniform and pale pink. Variation occurs due to differences in keratinazation, pigmentation, thickness, and vascularity.[1-3] The gingival margin thins as it moves coronally, and the marginal gingiva is scalloped. The embrasure spaces are filled with interdental gingiva. The interdental gingiva has a labial and a vestibular peak, which is connected beneath the contact point of the teeth by a col.[4] Healthy gingiva is firm and non-mobile. It does not detach from the teeth when blown with air from a syringe (Fig. 16-3a). The gingival sulcus is healthy and can be probed to approxi-

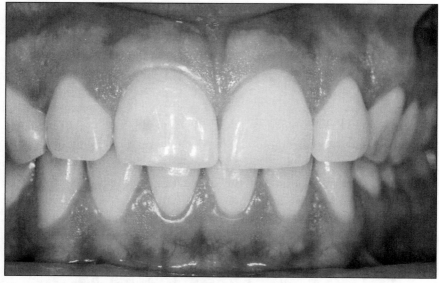

Fig. 16-2 Teeth and gingiva of a periodontally healthy individual. Gingival color is uniform and pale pink. Variation occurs due to differences in keratinazation, pigmentation, thickness, and vascularity. The gingival margin thins as it moves coronally, and the marginal gingiva is scalloped. The embrasure spaces are filled with interdental gingiva

mately 1 mm or more in depth (Fig. 16-3b). Two parts of the gingiva can be differentiated:

- Free gingiva
- Attached gingiva

The free gingiva extends from the coronal aspect of the gingival margin (the free gingival margin) to the base of the sulcus circumferentially. The attached gingival extends apically from the free gingival until it meets the alveolar mucosa. The junction between the attached gingival and the alveolar mucosa is called the mucogingival junction. The alveolar mucosa is darker red in color than the free and attached gingiva, and is loosely bound to the underlying bone. In contrast to attached gingiva, the alveolar mucosa is mobile in relation to the underlying tissue.

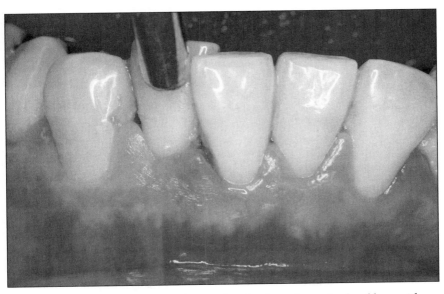

Fig. 16-3a Edematous inflamed tissue detaches from the tooth when blown with air from a syringe. Sub-gingival calculus is evident in the periodontal pocket

Fig. 16-3b Gingival health was attained after patient in Figure 16-3a was treated with oral hygiene instructions and scaling and root planning. Tissue is firm, pink, fibrotic, and no longer is detachable. Pocket depth is 1 mm

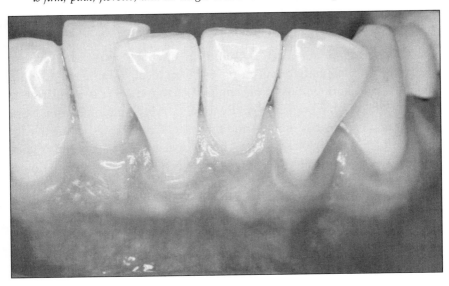

Microscopic anatomy. The free gingiva is the most frequently visited dental tissue by the clinician. It is where all the action takes place. Periodontal disease begins here. Dentists spend much time taking impressions and hiding margins of restorations here. Yet little time is spent in discussion of this important area in relation to its importance in the performance of ideal dentistry.

The free gingiva comprises all three structures coronal to the alveolar bone:

- Gingival sulcus
- Junctional epithelial attachment
- Connective tissue attachment

The epithelial attachment and the connective tissue attachment have been described as the biologic width (Fig. 16-4a). The gingival sulcus is approximately 1 mm in length and in line with the oral sulcular epithelium, which faces the tooth without being in contact with the tooth surface.[5] The junctional epithelial attachment is the epithelium, which forms a hemidesmosonal attachment from the gingiva to the tooth. It is usually 1 mm in length. The boundary between the epithelial attachment and the apically-positioned bone and periodontal ligament is taken up by the connective tissue attachment. This tissue is usually 1 mm in length and connects the gingival to the cementum of the tooth by horizontal fibers.

Clinical tip! Sound (Fig. 16-4b) (locate the bone's position relative to the free gingival margin by probing under local anesthesia) to bone before taking impressions to determine where the bone is in relation to the margin of the preparation. Be sure a minimum of 3 mm exists between the restoration margin and the bone. Crown lengthening may be necessary to avoid violating this "sacred space." Recession and inflammation will be avoided, and a predictable result will ensue. Violation of this tissue by the placement of subgingival restorations frequently results in recession or chronic inflammation (Fig. 16-5a, b). These two tissues, the epithelial attachment and the connective tissue attachment, average 2 mm in length. They have been dubbed the dental gingival complex.[5]

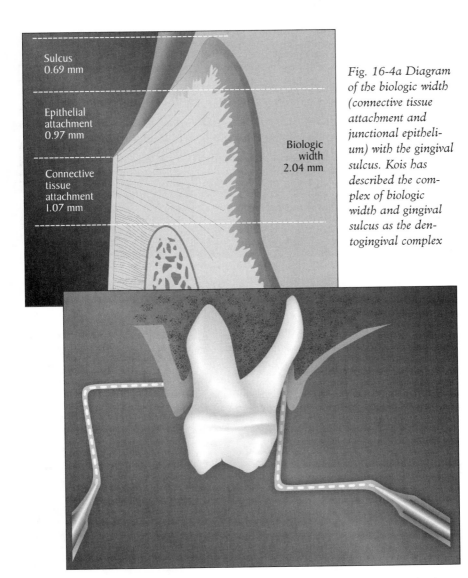

Sulcus
0.69 mm

Epithelial
attachment
0.97 mm

Connective
tissue
attachment
1.07 mm

Biologic
width
2.04 mm

Fig. 16-4a Diagram of the biologic width (connective tissue attachment and junctional epithelium) with the gingival sulcus. Kois has described the complex of biologic width and gingival sulcus as the dentogingival complex

Fig. 16-4b Sounding the bone is a technique to determine the position of the alveolar bone in relation to the free gingival margin. Under local anesthesia, a periodontal probe is placed into the sulcus and pushed apically until contact with the bone is made. Thus, the clinician can determine the amount of space that exists apical to the potential restoration margin so that the biologic width is not invaded

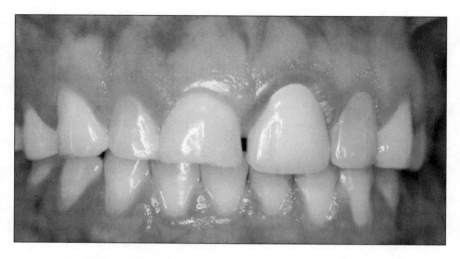

*Fig. 16-5a Inflammation around crown with a violated biologic width.
The inflamed cyanotic reddish margin will remain until the problem is corrected*

*Fig. 16-5b Recession present around teeth # 8, #9, #10, and #11, for the biologic width
was invaded at the time of cementation. Recession was not present at the time of cementation. Note crown recently placed on tooth #7 has early recession and inflammation. In
time, additional recession will most likely occur. When biologic width is violated by the
presence of a crown margin or restoration, inflammation or recession is usually the result*

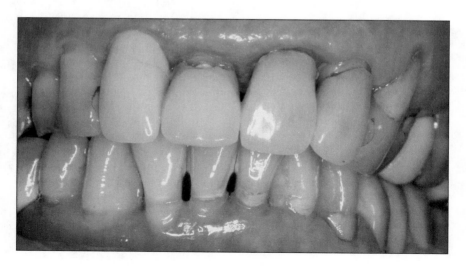

The body has a tendency to protect itself from the outside world. Gingiva, like skin, has a primary purpose to protect the underlying tissues. It is the body's first line of defense. Orally, 2 mm is the minimal amount of tissue needed from bone to outside world to achieve a lack of gingival inflammation.

Diagnosis and Classification of Periodontal Diseases

Periodontal disease was previously classified as either gingivitis or periodontitis. It was also previously believed that gingivitis progressed inevitably to periodontitis. It has been currently shown that there are a number of different manifestations of gingivitis and periodontitis.[6] Differences exist in microbiology, progression, host-parasite interactions, and clinical manifestations. Moreover, gingivitis does not invariably lead to periodontitis.[7]

Periodontal diseases have evolved as new information has emerged relating to pathogenesis, etiology, and host factors. In light of this, a new classification was established at the 1989 World Workshop in Clinical Periodontics. While this classification is not perfect, it has served as a template from which to work for the past decade. Changes will be made, as our knowledge of the etiology, pathogenesis, and parasite host interaction becomes clearer.

The 1989 classification of periodontal diseases is seen in Table 16-1. [8-9]

However, in 1999, at the International Workshop for a classification of periodontal diseases, a new classification was developed. This classification provided for eight major disease categories. The classification is quite voluminous and detailed. A summary of the classification follows in Table 16-2.[10]

Gingivitis

1. Experimental gingivitis
2. Acute necrotizing ulcerative gingivitis (ANUG)
3. Steroid hormone-influenced gingivitis
4. Medication-influenced gingival overgrowth gingivitis
5. Desquamative gingivitis

Periodontitis

1. Adult periodontitis
2. Early onset periodontitis
3. Prepubertal periodontitis
   ◊ generalized
   ◊ localized
4. Juvenile periodontitis
   ◊ generalized
   ◊ localized
5. Rapidly progressive periodontitis
6. Periodontitis associated with systemic disease
7. Necrotizing ulcerative periodontitis
8. Refractory periodontitis

Table 16-1 Previous classification of periodontal diseases (From Proceedings of the World Workshop in Clinical Periodontics, *American Academy of Periodontology, Chicago, 1989 and* Annals of Periodontology, *1996 World Workshop in Periodontics, American Academy of Periodontology, Chicago, 1996)*

Gingival Diseases

This new category defines gingival diseases as being both dental plaque-induced and non-plaque induced. Gingival diseases have been described for almost 3,500 years.[11] The notions of the various forms and manifestations of gingival diseases are constantly evolving and will continue to evolve as our knowledge increases. A review of the current concepts of the most *prevalent* of gingival disease follows. A more detailed follow-up of gingival and periodontal conditions not discussed can be found in the 1999 International Workshop for a classification of periodontal diseases and conditions.[12]

Dental plaque-induced gingival diseases

These diseases are seen in patients without attachment loss (Figs. 16-6a and 16-6b). They are further subdivided into gingival diseases that are modified by systemic factors, predominantly hormonal conditions, diabetes, taking of medications, and malnutrition.

Gingivitis associated with dental plaque only. Plaque-associated gingivitis is the most common of dental periodontal diseases. No one is immune to the development of gingivitis if dental hygiene is suspended completely. Dr. Harold Loe's classic study in 1965 was the first to prove that bacteria were necessary for gingival inflammation to occur.[13] He took perfectly healthy dental students who had no gingivitis and were clinically plaque free. He required them to stop brushing for three weeks. Every one of the students developed gingivitis and an increase in bacteria in their mouths within three weeks. No one was immune. Within three weeks, all students enrolled in the study had gingivitis. Plaque associated with gingivitis includes *actinomyces* and *streptococcus* in the supragingival plaque and *F. Nucleatum, V. parvula,* and the *treponema* species in the subgingival gram-negative flora. The patient in (Fig. 16-7a) exhibits much plaque on her teeth and inflammation of the gingiva. She has no bone loss, only gingival inflammation. After the institution of oral hygiene instructions and scaling and root planing, a resolution in inflammation is

Gingival diseases

A. Dental plaque-induced gingival diseases
   1. Gingivitis associated with dental plaque only
   2. Gingival diseases that are modified by systemic factors
      a) Associated with the endocrine system
         1) Puberty associated gingivitis
         2) Menstrual associated gingivitis
         3) Pregnancy associate
            • gingivitis
            • pyogenic granuloma
         4) Diabetes mellitus associated gingivitis
      b) Associated with blood dyscrasias
   3. Gingival diseases modified by medications
   4. Gingival diseases modified by malnutrition
B. Non-plaque-induced gingival lesions
   1. Gingival diseases of specific bacterial origin
   2. Gingival disease of viral origin
   3. Gingival diseases of fungal origin
   4. Gingival lesions of genetic origin
   5. Gingival manifestations of systemic conditions
      a) Mucocutaneous disorders
         1) lichen planus
         2) pemphigoid
         3) pemphigus vulgaris
         4) erythema multiforme
         5) lupus erythematosus
         6) drug induced
      b) Allergic reactions
   6. Traumatic lesions
   7. Foreign body reactions

Chronic periodontitis

A. Localized
B. Generalized

Aggressive periodontitis

A. Localized
B. Generalized

   1. Periodontitis as a manifestation of systemic diseases

   2. Acquired with hematological disorders

   3. Associated with genetic disorders

   4. Necrotizing periodontal diseases

     a) Necrotizing ulcerative gingivitis (NUG)

     a) Necrotizing ulcerative periodontitis (NUP)

   5. Abscesses of the periodontium

   6. Periodontitis associated with endodontic lesions

   7. Developmental or acquired deformities and conditions

     a) Localized tooth-related factors that modify or predispose to plaque-induced gingival diseases/periodontitis

     a) Mucogingival deformities and conditions around teeth

     a) Mucogingival deformities and conditions on edentulous ridges

     a) Occlusal trauma

Table 16-2 Current classification of periodontal diseases and conditions. (From Armitage, G.C. Development of a classification system for periodontal diseases and conditions. An Periodontol, 4:1-6, 1999)

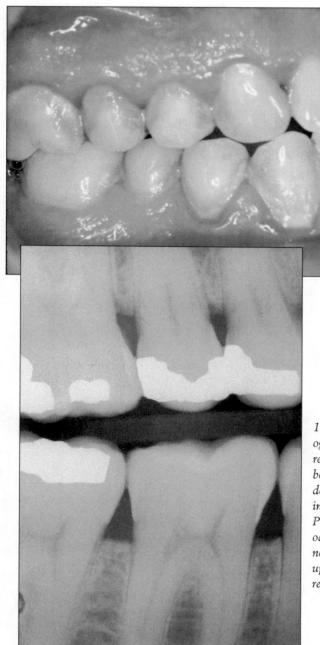

16-6a Gingival inflammation is seen in the presence of significant accumulations of plaque. Note the rolled reddened marginal gingiva

16-6b Bitewing radiograph of this patient reveals no alveolar bone loss. Patient has dental-plaque-induced gingivitis. Progression to periodontitis may or may not occur depending upon the patient's resistance to disease

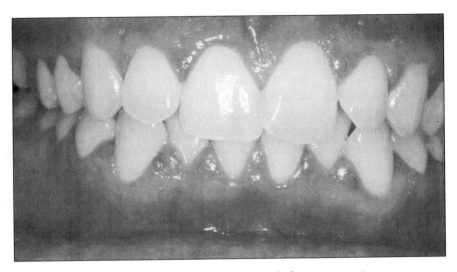

16-7a Gingivitis in a 27-year-old woman before treatment is commenced. Note the reddened edematous tissue and plaque on the teeth. Patient avoids the dentist because "cleanings'" hurt too much

16-7b The same patient 10 years following root planing and scaling under local anesthesia and instruction in oral hygiene. She has been on a 4-month recall program for 10 years. Periodontal surgery was never needed. Inflammation has been controlled, no attachment loss has occurred, and teeth cleanings no longer hurt

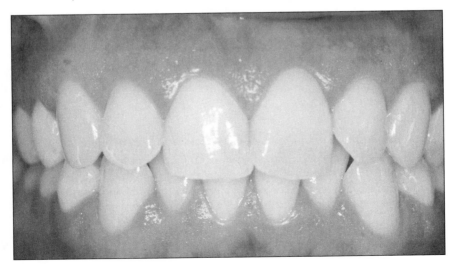

noted (Fig. 16-7b). It has been shown that gingivitis is prevalent at all ages of the dentate population and that this disease is considered to be the most common form of periodontal disease.[14]

Endocrine-influenced gingivitis. Puberty, pregnancy, birth control medications, and other alterations in the female hormonal cycle can lead to an increase in the tendency toward developing gingivitis.[15-18] The level of bacteroides found subgingivally is increased when steroid hormones are elevated.[19] It has also been shown that progesterone serves as a growth factor for bacteroides.[19] Thus, the gingival tissues serve as an incubator for the growth of bacteria, which are associated with gingivitis and periodontitis. Severe cases can lead to the formation of pyogenic granuloma, also known as the pregnancy tumor (Fig. 16-8).

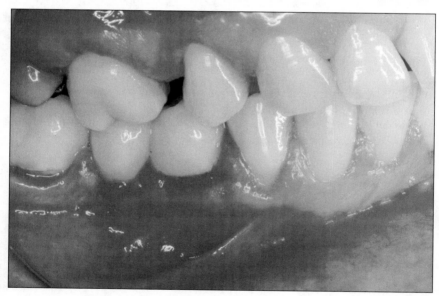

Fig. 16-8 Pregnancy gingivitis is present in this woman, now in her second trimester of pregnancy. Note the presence of the pyogenic granuloma (pregnancy tumor) associated with the mandibular second bicuspid and an early pyogenic granuloma forming interproximally between the canine and first bicuspid

Treatment. It is not advisable to give local anesthetic to pregnant women, unless absolutely necessary. The best treatment is prevention. Ideal recommendations are to maintain excellent oral hygiene and frequent recall during pregnancy, *e.g.*, routine prophylaxis every two to three months. However, if the patient has active gingival inflammation, as the patient in Figure 16-8, four visits of root planing and scaling are recommended with liberal applications of topical anesthetic. Following this, the patient should be placed on a two-month recall until end of term. Following pregnancy, a thorough examination and treatment plan should be established to control any remaining periodontal disease.

Gingival disease associated with diabetes mellitus. *Diabetes mellitus* is a chronic systemic disease characterized by a disorder in the production and metabolism of insulin. It affects the metabolism of fat, carbohydrate, and protein and has a significant effect on the blood vessels and the body's ability to handle infection. Type I diabetes—insulin-dependent diabetes mellitus or juvenile diabetes—is the more severe form. In children with this disease, gingivitis is a very common finding, especially in the poorly controlled individual.[20] Gingival and periodontal disease features in the diabetic individual are similar to the non-diabetic individual. However, plaque control in the severity of inflammation is much more important in controlling the disease.[20] In short, these patients are at a greater risk for developing periodontal disease.

Gingival disease modified by medications. Three classes of medications are known to stimulate gingival overgrowth—phenytoin (Dilantin), which is used to treat epileptic seizures,[21] cyclosporins, used for immunosuppressive therapy in transplant patients;[22] and calcium channel blockers (nifedipine, calan, verapimil, etc.), used in the management of hypertension.[23] It is unclear how much of a role plaque plays in the amount of gingival overgrowth. Some suggest it is not only plaque related, but drug dose related as well. The gingival overgrowth usually begins in the papillary regions and grows outward, leading to bacterial cul-de-sacs where oral hygiene becomes more difficult. Psuedopockets form as the papillary growths unite (Fig. 16-9a). Treatment for the severe hyperplasia is surgical removal. Gingivectomy or a periodontal flap (Fig. 16-9b) are the two surgical procedures of choice.

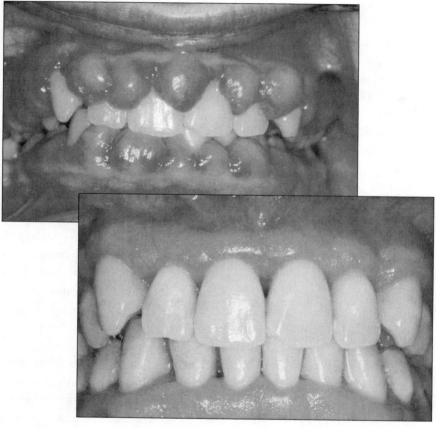

Fig. 16-9a Dilantin-induced gingival overgrowth present in a young man. Eating has become difficult due to the significant amount of gingiva present over the teeth. Note the existence of severe outpocketing of gingiva beginning in the papillary areas. The papillae are coalescing and forming "pseudo pockets"

Fig. 16-9b Patient six weeks following periodontal flap surgery to remove hyperplastic gingival tissues. Note the amount of crown that is now visible. Patient is much more comfortable. However, if excellent hygiene is not maintained, the hyperplasia will return. Note the immature granulation tissue forming mesial to the mandibular right canine

Non-plaque-induced gingival lesions

A number of types of gingival inflammation are different from that of routine plaque-associated gingivitis. These non-plaque-associated types of gingivitis often present specific clinical features. Bacterial infections such as neisseria gonorrhea and treponema present as isolated angry red edematous ulcerations. They also may be associated by non-painful cancres and associated with lesions on other parts of the body.[24-25]

Gingival diseases of viral origin. A number of gingival diseases are known to be caused by viral infections. Herpes simplex virus Types 1 and 2 and varicella zoster virus causes the most common of these infections. The herpes virus usually enters the body at childhood and lays dormant in the nerve cell. Factors that may trigger the onset of the viral infection include trauma (*e.g.*, oral surgery), sunburn, fever, or stress.[26] The clinical manifestation is usually vesicles at the area innervated by the nerve harboring the latent virus (Fig. 16-10).

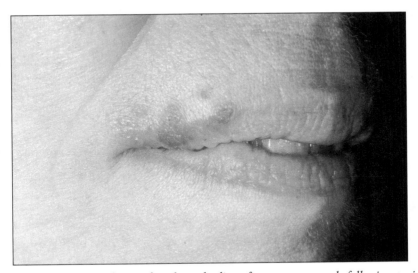

Fig. 16-10 Herpetic lesions found on the lips of woman one week following periodontal surgery. Oral surgery can trigger the activation of the virus, which lives quiesently in the nerve. Herpes virus usually manifests itself as a cluster of small ulcers

Primary herpetic gingivostomatitis is the initial manifestation of herpes simplex virus, Type I. It is mainly contacted by small children and is usually asymtomatic. However, when contacted initially by an adult it is usually characterized by painful severe gingivitis with ulcerations, edema, fever, and lymphadenopathy and extreme malaise.[27]

Gingival disease of fungal origin. A number of fungal infections may also cause gingival diseases. The most common is candida albicans.[27] This is usually an opportunistic infection and may occur as a consequence of an immunocompromised host. Erythematous lesions can be found anywhere in the oral mucosa. These lesions are particularly prominent in human immunodeficiency virus (HIV) patients.[28]

Gingival manifestations of systemic disorders

Mucocutaneous disorders. This classification of diseases used to be called *desquamative gingivitis*. They included lichen planus, pemphigoid, pemphigus vulgaris, erythema multiforme, and lupus erythematosus. These lesions are characterized by sloughing of the epithelium, frequently a sign of an underlying systemic condition[29] (Figs. 16-11a and 16-11b). Of the before-mentioned diseases, erosive lichen planis is the most common. It is frequently seen secondary to stress. Geographic tongue and Wickham's striae, delicate white lines on the buccal mucosa, are often associated with the gingival lesions. The disease is usually self-limiting. Treatment is usually of a palliative nature. However, steroid rinses are helpful in limiting the course of the disease.[30] Desquamative lesions can also be caused by allergic reactions to drugs or to overzealous toothbrushing (Fig 16-12).

Allergic reactions. Mechanical reactions in the oral mucosa are relatively uncommon. However, a number of materials have been associated with contact dermatitis. These include restorative materials, mercury, nickel, gold, zinc, chromium, palladium, and acrylics. Although rare, reactions to toothpastes and mouthwashes have also been reported. Certain foods have also been associated with Type I and Type IV allergic

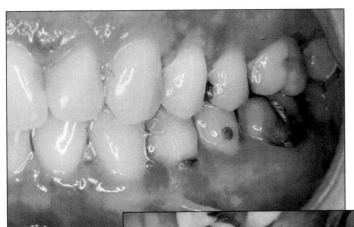

Fig. 16-11a Gingival sloughing and ulceration seen in a patient with ulcerative lichen planis

Fig. 16-11b The patient also demonstrates Wickman's striae on the buccal mucosa, a frequent finding in patients with lichen planis. It presents as a delicate lacy white pattern on the buccal mucosa

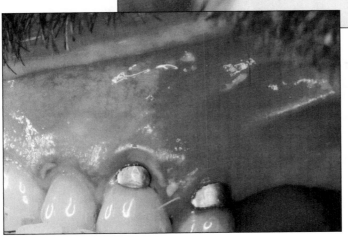

Fig. 16-12 Gingival redness and desquamation associated with an allergic reaction to chewing gum, contact dermatitis. Note the newly ulcerated marginal gingiva.

reactions. Those reported include peanuts, pumpkin seeds, kiwis, apples, chestnuts, and salami.

Traumatic lesions. Epithelial ulceration may be due to any type of trauma to the gingival tissues. This can happen through overzealous oral hygiene (Fig. 16-13). Self-inflicted injuries may also occur—termed gingivitis artefacta. They may be found in small children or in adults. Picking or scratching the gingiva with a finger or fingernail usually produces them. Sometimes musical instruments, as is shown in this flute player, may cause the lesions (Figs. 16-14a and 16-14b).

Chronic periodontitis

The previous category of *adult periodontitis* has been replaced with the category chronic periodontitis. Chronic periodontitis usually does not occur until the late 20s.[31] However, it can also be seen in adolescents. Its clinical significance does not usually manifest itself until the late 30s (Fig. 16-15). The severity of the disease is usually related to the amount of plaque and calculus present. This is directly related to the diligence of the patient in performing oral hygiene and the frequency and quality of his/her professional hygiene visits. This disease is slowly progressive and bilaterally symmetrical. There is no sex predilection, and immunologic function is usually normal.[32] The bacteria associated with adult periodontitis vary with the severity of the infection and the host response. The subgingival bacteria associated with adult periodontitis are usually gram negative anaerobic rods and spirochetes. Frequent bacterial isolates include prevotella intermedia, porphyromonous gingivalis, bacteroides forsythus, treponema denticola, peptostreptoccus micros, and campylbacter rectus.[33] Chronic periodontitis is recognized as the most frequently occurring form of periodontitis.[34]

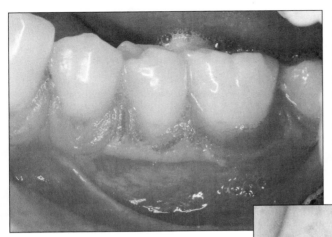

Fig. 16-13 Gingival sloughing in a patient one week after being instructed in oral hygiene. This self-induced lesion is a result of over-zealous toothbrushing in an attempt to eliminate periodontal disease in one week

Fig. 16-14a Profile of a young female flutist. She has a Class II occlusion and anterior flaring of the maxillary anterior teeth. This situation has created an open bite in which to place her flute

Fig. 16-14b Gingival recession and mucogingival defect are associated with mandibular central incisor. The trauma from the flute resting against her labial gingiva has resulted in recession

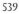

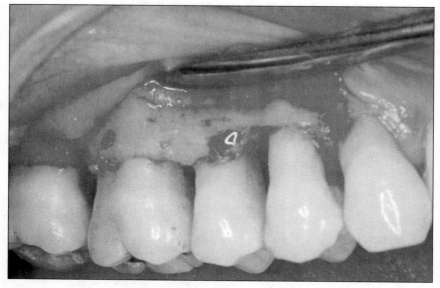

Fig. 16-15 Adult periodontitis present in a patient in her late thirties. Attachment loss and alveolar cratering are present throughout her dentition

Aggressive periodontitis

Aggressive periodontitis was previously known as early-onset periodontitis. The previous term was found to be too restrictive, for it was based solely on age and not the clinical, radiographic, historical, and laboratory findings of the disease. Under this newer classification, patients who previously met the criteria for localized juvenile periodontitis, general juvenile periodontitis, and rapidly progressive periodontitis are included as having aggressive periodontitis. The terms "localized aggressive periodontitis" or "generalized aggressive periodontitis" relate to the extent of the disease. The previous category of prepubertal periodontitis is now included under the category of "periodontitis as a manifestation of systemic diseases," for there is always a systemic component that underlies the manifestation of prepubertal periodontitis.

Hence, aggressive periodontitis can be divided into localized aggressive periodontitis, which essentially replaces the older term "localized juvenile periodontitis." The new designation "generalized aggressive periodontitis" replaces the older term "generalized juvenile periodontitis." The most common features of aggressive periodontitis are:[35]

- Except for periodontitis, the patients are otherwise clinically healthy
- Rapid attachment loss and bone destruction
- Familial aggregation. There is a genetic basis of the disease inherited as an X-linked dominant trait or an autosomal recessive trait[36]

Secondary features that are frequent, but not always found, include the following:

- There is usually minimal amount of evident plaque, low caries, and minimal clinical inflammation[37]
- The amount of alveolar bone loss appears to be much greater than the amount of microbial debris present
- Depressed neutrophil chemotaxis is a frequent finding[38]
- There are hyper-responsive macrophage phenotype, including elevated levels of PGE2 and IL-1B
- The progressive attachment loss may be self-arresting

Frequently found subgingival mircroflora include actininobacillus actinomycetemcomitans, and in some populations porphyromonas gingivalis.[39]

Localized aggressive periodontitis frequently starts out about the time of puberty. Frequently, high antibody response to infecting agents is present. It is often characterized by angular bony defects around the first permanent molars and central incisors[35] (Figs. 16-16a and 16-16b). Early treatment has been effective in eliminating and even reversing the disease. Treatment consists of systemic tetracycline for three weeks, scaling and root planing, and surgery. Significant regeneration of alveolar defects is often possible (Figs. 16-17a and 16-17b).

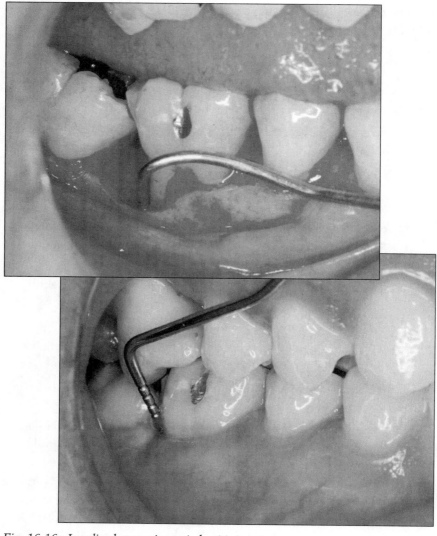

Fig. 16-16a Localized aggressive periodontitis in a teenage female. Note the bony defect distal to the first molar

Fig. 16-16b Some bone regeneration was achieved following periodontal surgical regenerative (osseous grafting) treatment

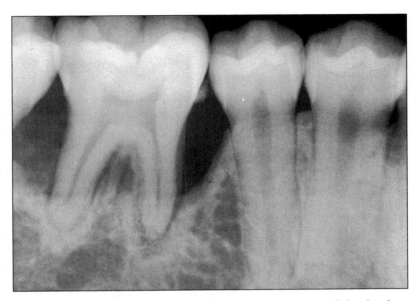

Fig. 16-17a Preoperative radiograph of a teenage patient with localized aggressive periodontitis. Angular molar defects are present

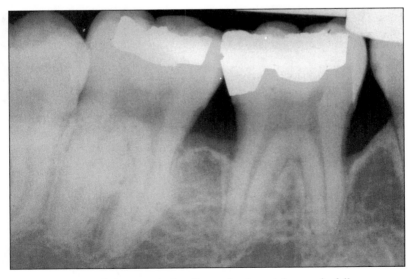

Fig. 16-17b Post-surgical radiograph taken eight months following caries control and active periodontal treatment, which included bone-grafting surgery. The amount of healing is dramatic

Generalized aggressive periodontitis generally affects persons under 30 years of age, but patients may be older. The serum antibody response is not significant to the infecting agents. The amount of bony destruction is episodic and sporadic. The areas of bone loss are not confined to the first molars and incisors. Multiple teeth are usually involved.[35] The amount of bone destruction can be quite significant and dramatic, especially at a young age (Fig. 16-18).

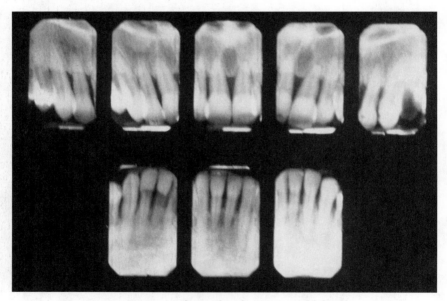

Fig. 16-18a Anterior radiographs of a 24-year-old female patient with generalized aggressive periodontitis. More than 50% alveolar bone loss is present throughout all of her dentition

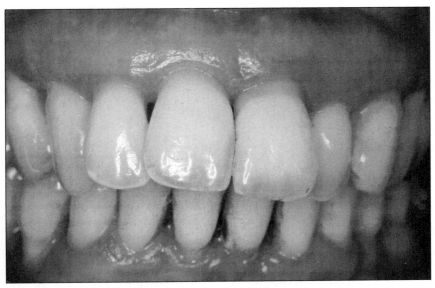

Fig. 16-18b Photograph of same 24-year patient with generalized aggressive periodontitis. Loss of papillae, recession, and some anterior flaring are evident

Periodontitis as a Manifestation of Systemic Diseases

Systemic disease can obviously alter the progression of periodontal diseases. Systemic diseases in which periodontitis are a common manifestation include hematologic diseases—acquired neutropenia, leukemias, and others. Genetic disorders such as cyclic neutropenia, Down syndrome, Papillon-Lefevre syndrome, Chediak-Higashi syndrome, Ehlers-Danlos syndrome, hypophosphataia and others can all lead to periodontal diseases.[40]

Diabetes, previously discussed, can also modify the progression of periodontal disease, as can smoking.

Necrotizing ulcerative periodontal diseases

Necrotizing ulcerative gingivitis (NUG). This was previously called acute necrotizing ulcerative gingivitis (ANUG). *NUG* is an acute, recurring, gingival infection characterized by much gingival pain and necrosis of the tips of the papilla, a fetid odor, and a metallic taste. Bleeding of the gingiva at its onset is swift and usually associated with the following— poor oral hygiene, significant stress, and smoking. HIV infection has also been shown to be associated with NUG. The etiology is bacterial. Fusiform bacteria, prevotella intermedia and spirochetes have been found to be associated with the lesions.[41]

Treatment. The patient in Figure 16-19 demonstrates the symptoms of NUG. She is a single 19-year-old mother, one pack a day smoker, on social assistance, who was recently hospitalized for hypotension following an asthmatic attack. She presented with a fetid odor, loss of gingival papilla, significant oral pain, and exquisitely painful gingiva. Following examination and diagnosis, initial treatment consisted of a 60-second debridement following the application of topical anesthetics. Total time for the debridement was 1-2 minutes. The purpose was to disturb the flora and get some irrigation of the periodontal pockets, therefore disturbing the bacteria. It is *extremely important* to initially debride the acute periodontal patient. If only antibiotics are prescribed, one loses the initial opportunity to get the infection under control—antibiotics will take at least 48 hours to have significant impact. In addition to initial debridement, the patient is placed on antibiotics for one week (usually Amoxicillin 250 mg qid for one week) and a chlorhexidine rinse two times a day. The patient is appointed in one week to begin the active phase of root planing. This is done over four visits and is essential to get the gingivitis under control. The patient looks much better after root planing and scaling (Fig. 16-20). However, papillae have still been lost. The most important aspect in treating a patient with NUG is timely diagnosis and immediate treatment. This immediate treatment should not only include the placement on antibiotics, but also, an initial debridement upon first presentation. Although the patient may be sensitive at his/her initial visit,

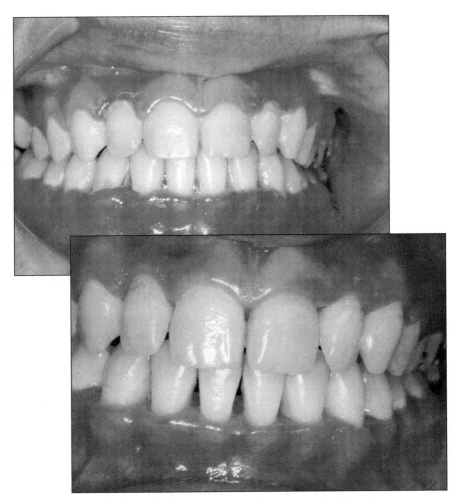

Fig. 16-19 Patient with necrotizing ulcerative periodontitis. Note the inflamed gingiva and the blunted papilla. Some of the papilla has already been lost. This 19-year-old female is a smoker, was recently hospitalized with a life-threatening asthma attack, and had not seen a dentist in a few years. Her oral hygiene is fair to poor

Fig. 16-20 Same patient as in Figure 16-19 following treatment. Therapy consisted of immediate debridement, oral hygiene instructions, and a one-week course of penicillin. This was followed up by four visits of root planing and scaling under local anesthesia with a reinforcement of oral hygiene instructions. Oral hygiene has improved, and tissues are no longer inflamed. However, the initial loss of papillae is permanent, and the embrasures are open

he/she will appreciate the fact that his/her teeth are being saved and that the cosmetic disfigurement will be minimized. Patients usually experience significant pain relief within a few hours of initial debridement.

Necrotizing ulcerative periodontitis (NUP). *NUP* is an infection characterized by the necrosis of the gingival tissues, periodontal ligament, and alveolar bone. These lesions are most frequently seen in the immunocompromised individual and/or patients with systemic conditions. These include patients with HIV, severe malnutrition, and immunosuppression.

Abscesses of the periodontium. This is a new category and was not included in the 1989 AAP classification of periodontal diseases. A *periodontal abscess* is a localized purulent infection of periodontal tissues. It may occur in a patient with untreated periodontal disease (Fig. 16-21a, b). It can also occur in a patient under regular periodontal care. Three types of abscesses have been classified. The gingival abscess is a localized collection of pus confined to the gingival tissues. Treatment of this lesion is local curretment and debridement (Fig. 16-22). Streptococcus viridian is the most common isolate in the exudate of periodontal abscesses.

Treatment of the periodontal abscess. It is of paramount importance that the periodontal abscess be treated immediately. Acute infections may lead to rapid bone loss.[42] Therefore, immediate local debridement and drainage are extremely important, similar to the treatment of NUG. Treatment should include a liberal application of topical anesthetic and a gentle curettage to establish drainage. The author also finds it advisable to irrigate the area with saline or chlorhexidine for 30 seconds to remove the suppuration and bacteria. The patient is then placed on antibiotics for one week, usually Amoxicillin 250 mg, four times a day. The patient is also instructed to rinse with chlorhexidine twice a day and warm saltwater 10 to 20 times a day for the first two days. The patient is seen one week later for a follow-up examination and to establish a periodontal treatment plan.

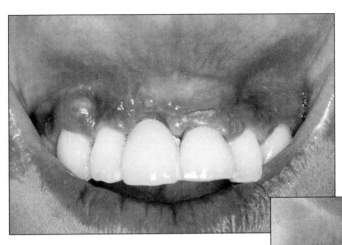

Fig. 16-21a Periodontal abscess in an untreated periodontal patient. Note the large swelling in the mucobuccal fold over right canine and central incisors. The gingival tissues between the central incisors are detachable

Fig. 16-21b Radiograph of abscessed patient reveals alveolar bone loss that approaches the apical area of the central incisor. Prompt treatment is essential

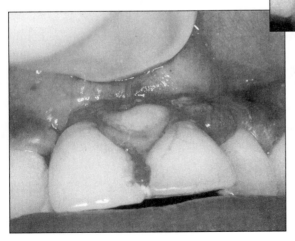

Fig. 16-22 Immediate drainage of the periodontal abscess is of paramount importance to minimize the amount of bone loss. The abscess is curreted, and the patient is place on antibiotics, warm salt-water rinses, and chlorhexidine rinses for one week. Initial therapy is commenced once the acute abscess is under control

Treatment of Periodontal Disease

Patient examination

The patient examination is one of the most important, if not the most important, parts of periodontal therapy. Without a thorough examination, a diagnosis is not possible. Without a diagnosis, an appropriate treatment plan is not possible. The adage that "diagnosis should precede treatment" is one that should not be taken lightly. All too often the dentist does not complete a thorough periodontal examination. As a practical matter for some clinicians, patients enter the dental clinic via the dental hygiene department for "teeth cleaning." This does not allow the opportunity for a complete examination. While this is a philosophical decision on the part of the practitioner, this author believes that the patient's initial visit to the dental clinic should include a comprehensive examination and treatment plan, if possible with the doctor. This chapter will explore the components of a complete examination and the philosophy of its importance. A complete dental examination should be comprehensive and include the following (see Table 16-3):

The initial visit

The initial visit should include the gathering of data about the patient's oral condition and overall general health. Rapport should be established with the patient. This is best established by taking time to perform a thorough examination and to explain to the patient the condition of his/her mouth. A menu of treatment options should then be presented to the patient. This gives the patient a sense of control over his/her treatment as well as a sense of ownership of his/her dental situation.

This chapter will take the vantage point that the initial visit is one of examination and diagnosis, rather than one of treatment. The initial visit should establish a diagnosis so that an appropriate treatment plan can be determined and presented to the patient. The *one exception* to this is the patient who presents as a dental emergency. If the patient arrives in pain or discomfort, relief of pain should be the priority (Figs. 16-21 and 16-22). If the patient presents with a periodontal abscess, pain relief and treatment of this condition should supercede a comprehensive evaluation. The initial visit should be devoted to treating the acute infection and the patient reappointed for a follow-up visit and comprehensive evaluation. Not only is this appropriate, it is effective in gaining the patient's trust. There is no more grateful patient than one that the clinician has relieved of his/her pain.

An attempt is made to have the patient fill out a comprehensive medical and dental history prior to the initial visit. It is also important to gather information during the initial telephone consultation as to why the patient is seeking care. If possible, obtain a complete series of radiographs prior to the initial patient meeting. Patient confidence is enhanced if the doctor enters the operatory with knowledge of the patient's chief complaint, dental history, medical history, and radiographic status. The tone is set for a productive hour, and rapport is readily established.

Medical history. The initial medical history is a form filled out by the patient. If possible, the form is mailed or faxed to the patient, prior to the initial visit. This accomplishes two things:

- The patient does not have the aggravation of filling out another form at the initial visit. The medical history form can be filed out at the patient's leisure and faxed or mailed back to the office prior to his/her examination. The dentist can then review the history and chief complaints prior to the patient's office visit and be better informed and prepared

- Establish rapport
- Medical history
- Dental history
- Full mouth radiographs
- Extra- and intra-oral examination
- Periodontal examination
- Occlusal examination
- Caries and teeth examination
- Photographs
- Patient education

Table 16-3 Initial examination sequence of therapy

- The patient is given a professional introduction to the dental office

A letter of introduction and informational brochure are included with the medical history.

Once seated in the operatory, the patient's blood pressure is taken and recorded. It is not unusual to find an elevated blood pressure at a patient's initial visit. If the pressure is elevated, it is retaken at the conclusion of the appointment and at the following appointment. An elevated blood pressure is a contraindication to performing dental treatment, and the patient is referred to his/her physician for evaluation.

The patient's age is another important consideration in determining the severity of periodontal disease. Periodontal disease at a young age carries more significance than attachment loss in the later decades of life. It has been shown that periodontal disease increases with each decade—for two reasons:

- The patient has had the teeth for a longer period of time in which to develop periodontal disease
- Periodontal disease and bone loss accelerate with each passing decade[43]

Other salient aspects of the patient's medical history include the presence or absence of heart disease, in particular mitral valve prolapse. The American Heart Association recommends pre-medicating patients prior to periodontal therapy if a heart murmur exists.[44] The medications the patient is taking are also important to evaluate. As discussed, a variety of medication can cause gingival changes. There are also cross-reactions to many of the medications with ones that are prescribed during periodontal therapy. The patient's allergies should also be noted.

Lastly, the history of smoking should be documented. Smokers have a greater predilection to periodontal disease.[45] Smokers also do not respond as well to regenerative therapy including implants.[46] Smokers do not heal as well from periodontal surgery. All smokers are advised to refrain from smoking one week prior to periodontal or implant therapy and for three weeks thereafter. Of course, the best advice would be for the patients to refrain from smoking forever.

Dental history. It is of paramount importance to take a thorough dental history. The amount of dental care, frequency of recall visits, patient performance of oral hygiene, and past experiences all impact upon the initial treatment plan. A patient with severe periodontal disease who has never had periodontal or significant dental care has a much better prognosis than a patient who has been under active maintenance with the same amount of attachment loss. The patient in Figures 16-23a and 16-23b is 40 years of age and has seen a dentist only twice in his life. The significant amount of calcareous deposits and poor oral hygiene bodes well for making this a successful case. The post-therapeutic result (Fig. 16-23c) reveals the remarkable improvement that is seen once oral hygiene instructions and active periodontal therapy have been instituted. The patient has undergone oral hygiene instructions, scaling and root planing, periodontal surgery, minor orthodontics, extraction of his hopeless mandibular incisors, and placement of two dental implants. The 10-year postoperative result is a testament to the benefit of excellent dental care coupled with patient cooperation.

Significant recession is seen in a patient whose dental history revealed that she had undergone full mouth gingivectomy in the 1960s (Fig. 16-24a). The patient had mobility of Class II on all of her affected teeth. The treatment plan called for mucogingival reconstruction. Free gingival grafting resulted in an increase of attached keratinized tissue and a decrease in tooth mobility (Fig. 16-24b).

The competence of a patient's oral hygiene is also important to assess. A patient with poor oral hygiene is not a good candidate for periodontal surgery.[47] Periodontal surgery in the absence of excellent plaque control is more detrimental than doing no surgery at all.[47] The patient in Figure 16-25a presented as a new patient to the dental practice. He stated that he had recently gone through full mouth root planing and scaling in the office of an excellent periodontist. The prognosis for this patient is

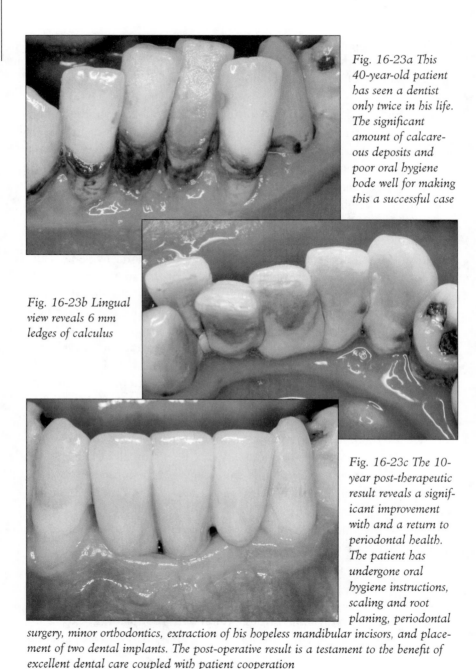

Fig. 16-23a This 40-year-old patient has seen a dentist only twice in his life. The significant amount of calcareous deposits and poor oral hygiene bode well for making this a successful case

Fig. 16-23b Lingual view reveals 6 mm ledges of calculus

Fig. 16-23c The 10-year post-therapeutic result reveals a significant improvement with and a return to periodontal health. The patient has undergone oral hygiene instructions, scaling and root planing, periodontal surgery, minor orthodontics, extraction of his hopeless mandibular incisors, and placement of two dental implants. The post-operative result is a testament to the benefit of excellent dental care coupled with patient cooperation

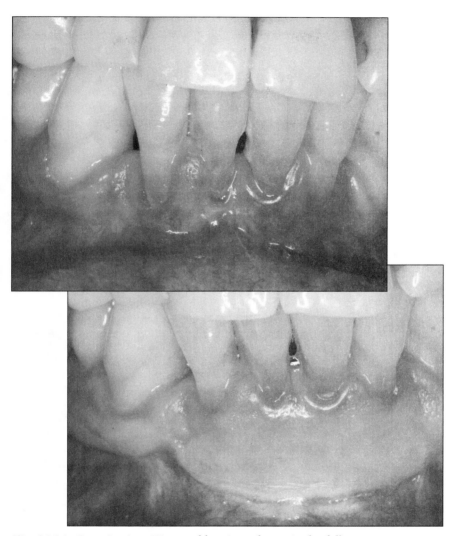

Fig. 16-24a Recession in a 55-year-old patient who received a full mouth gingivectomy in the 1960s. This therapy resulted in a loss of attached gingiva and the creation of mucogingival defects. All of her affected teeth had Class II mobility, and she found it difficult to eat

Fig. 16-24b The treatment plan called for mucogingival reconstruction with free gingival grafting. Mobility was decreased, attached gingiva and root coverage increased, and periodontal health was restored

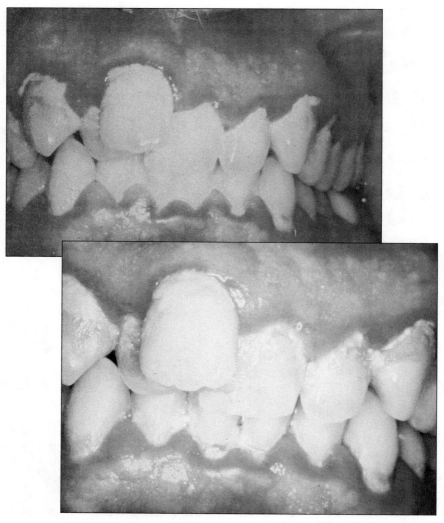

Fig. 16-25a Patient presentation at his initial visit prior to root planing and scaling and oral hygiene instructions. Oral hygiene is poor, and the gingival tissues are inflamed

Fig. 16-25b Post-initial therapy the patient is reexamined. Yellow disclosing dye reveals much plaque and little if any improvement in oral hygiene. This patient is not a good candidate for periodontal surgery and is advised to go into a three-month maintenance program

not good, unless a significant change can be made in his oral hygiene. Following a review of oral hygiene and re-scaling, little change was noted (Fig. 16-25b). The patient was not treated surgically and was placed on a three-month recall program.

Full mouth radiographs

A periodontal examination is not complete without a full mouth series of radiographs. Radiographs do have the limitation of being two-dimensional. They can not distinguish between successfully treated and untreated cases, record tooth mobility, and show hard-to-soft tissue relationships.[48] However, radiographs do record the position of septal bone on the tooth in one plan, serve as a useful adjunct to the clinical exam, record the alveolar bone and periodontal ligament on the mesial, distal, and apical aspects of the root in a single plane, document clinical crown to root ratios, allow the observation of dense calcareous deposits, demonstrate significant overhanging restorations, and demonstrate periodical pathology.[48] The author's radiographic series includes the following:

- Five maxillary anterior size one films
- Three mandibular anterior size one films
- Four vertical bitewings with size two films
- Eight posterior periapical size two films (Fig. 16-26)

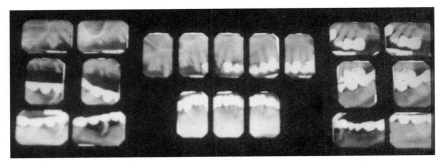

Fig. 16-26 Complete radiographic examination includes 20 films—
4 vertical bitewings, 8 anterior periapical, and 8 posterior periapical films

This complete set gives the clinician an excellent overview of the dentition, the level of alveolar bone, and the periapical regions. Panoramic radiographs are good screening tools. However, they lack the detail of periapical film.[49] Frequently distortion up to 40% is seen, and important details are missed (Figs. 16-27a, 16-27b, and 16-27c). Vertical bitewing radiographs are also preferred over horizontal bitewing radiographs. Caries is equally visible in both types of radiographs. However, the level of alveolar bone, especially in the periodontally compromised patients, is more easily seen with vertical bitewings (Figs. 16-28a and 16-28b).

Frequently, patients refuse radiographs for fear of exposure to radiation. It is this author's belief that the risk of not taking radiographs far outweighs the small level of radiation exposure that the patient will receive. The patient in Figure 16-29a refused radiographs for nine years. When she was finally convinced to have a radiograph, 10 years later, the amount of periapical pathology present was so great as to deem the tooth hopeless (Fig. 16-29b). She had let the lesion go unchecked for so long that the two adjacent teeth were also compromised.

Radiographs are a significant diagnostic tool in the diagnosis of periodontal disease. In fact, second to the periodontal probe, they are the most important diagnostic aid we have. The 25-year old male patient in Figure 16-30a has severe periodontal disease. However, the true level of bone loss is not evident until the radiographs are taken and examined (Fig. 16-30b).

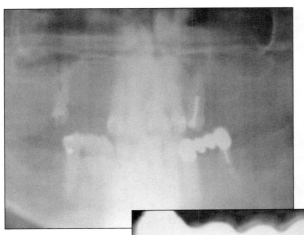

Fig. 16-27a Panoramic radiographic of the patient is a good screening tool and allows one to assess morphologic relationships. However, distortion of up to 40% can be seen, and fine details are often missed. It is not possible to visualize the defect on the distal of the lower left 2nd premolar

Fig. 16-27b The periapical radiographic is more accurate and has minimal distortion. Vertical defect on the distal of the premolar is seen, as well as root resorption at the apical extent of the post

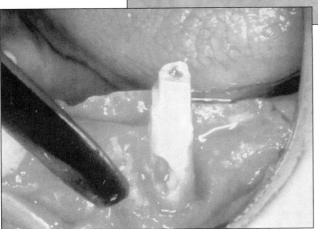

Fig. 16-27c Clinical view of the premolar at the time of surgery. If the only pre-surgical radiograph were a panoramic view, this lesion would not have been diagnosed, radiographically

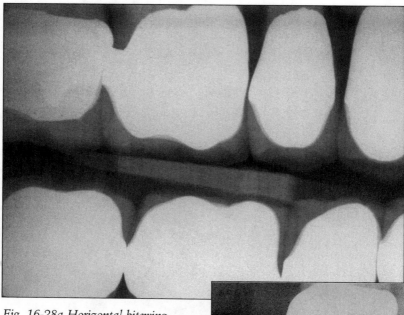

Fig. 16-28a Horizontal bitewing radiographs taken during a routine recall visit. They are not diagnostic. It is not possible to see the alveolar bone, due to bone loss, or to diagnose caries, for the crown margin is not visible in the film

Fig. 16-28b Vertical bitewing radiographs taken the same day as in 16-28a. Alveolar bone level can be evaluated and caries diagnosed. It is strongly recommended to take vertical bitewing radiographs

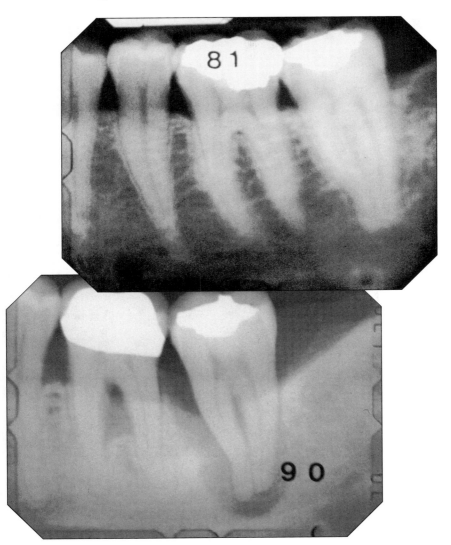

Fig. 16-29a Periapical radiograph taken in 1981. Patient felt that x-rays were detrimental to her health and refused them for nine years

Fig. 16-29b Periapical radiograph of the area in 29 A taken in 1990. It was the first x-ray taken since 1980. Severe bone loss is present in the furcation of the first molar, and a perio-endo lesion on the second molar has deemed these teeth hopeless. Not taking radiographs turned out to be tooth detrimental

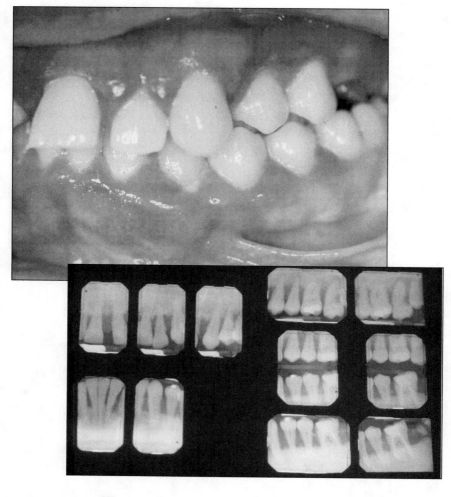

Fig. 16-30a Clinical photograph of a 25-year-old male patient at his initial visit. Clinically, severe periodontal disease is suspected. However, the level of severity is not truly comprehended until radiographs are taken

Fig. 16-30b Radiographs of the patient in 16-30a. The true level of alveolar bone loss could not be appreciated until a full mouth radiographic series was taken. The patient had 80 to 100 % loss of alveolar bone. His teeth were terminal, and they were given a hopeless prognosis

Extra and intra-oral examination

This is a very important part of the examination. All too often, this is missed, for the focus is on the dentition. However, dentists are in a unique position to diagnose many diseases and conditions that are not evaluated during routine medical examinations and "check ups." It is not only an opportunity, but also a dentist's responsibility to perform a thorough examination, including an oral cancer exam. The following table (Table 16-4) provides a checklist of the clinical areas that should be examined initially and at all recall appointments.

- Lymph nodes
- Neck and thyroid gland
- Lips
- Buccal mucosa
- Vestibule
- Hard palate
- Soft palate
- Pharynx
- Tongue
- Floor of the mouth
- Gingiva
- Oral hygiene E G F P
- Gingival index 0 1 2 3
- Teeth

Table 16-4 Extra- and intra-oral examination

Lymph nodes. The lymph nodes of the neck, including the anterior cervical, posterior cervical, and submandibular, should be palpated. Enlargement can mean infection, tumors, lymphoma, or a variety of other immunological disorders. A 40-year old male patient (Fig. 16-31a) presented following scaling and root planing. His oral hygiene was fair, as evidenced by plaque on the teeth and the root planing was performed again. During his initial examination, lymphadenopathy of his anterior cervical lymph nodes was noted. The patient had recently had a full medical examination and was told that "the neck swelling" was nothing to be concerned about. Following scaling and root planing, minimal improvement was noted in his gingival tissues. Radiographs (Fig. 16-31b)

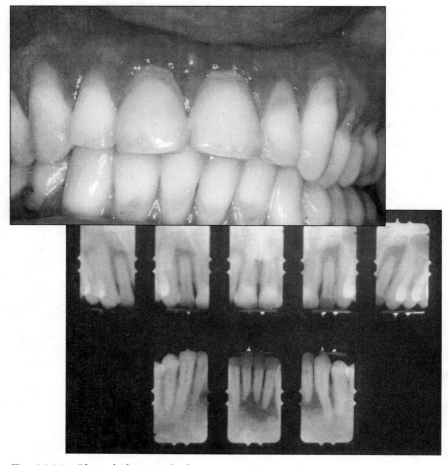

Fig. 16-31a Clinical photograph of a 40-year-old man at his initial periodontal visits. However, he has just completed root planing and scaling in the office of his restorative dentist. The gingival tissues reveal inflammation, and plaque is evident at the cervical margins. The patient was advised to redo the initial therapy. Little gingival improvement was noted following his second phase of initial therapy. This raised suspicion that a systemic problem might exist

Fig. 16-31b Radiographs of the anterior teeth. Radiolucencies are noted at the apices of the maxillary lateral incisors and the mandibular incisors. This is a reported finding in patients with sarcoidosis

revealed periapical radiolucencies on his maxillary lateral incisors and mandibular incisors. His overall gingival and dental appearance coupled with his lymphadenopathy raised suspicion. The patient was referred to an otolaryngologist for evaluation. The lymph nodes were biopsied and the patient was found to have sarcoidosis, a systemic immunological disease. Untreated, this could be fatal. The patient was treated with steroids, and today, 12 years later he is under control and leading a healthy life. The dental literature is sparse on this subject. However, a few articles do exist that discuss the association between sarcoidosis and gingival disease.

Neck and thyroid gland. The neck should be palpated to look for swellings. The thyroid gland should also be palpated to make sure it is not enlarged. This exam takes but a minute, but the value in diagnosing a patient with a thyroid problem and placing him/her into the hands of an endocrinologist is invaluable.

Lips. The external and internal aspects of the lips should be palpated and visually examined. The upper lip is more prone to skin cancer due to its proximity to sun exposure. The patient in Figure 16-32 has had this lesion present for many years. She was not advised to have it removed. Removal revealed a basal cell carcinoma. Suspicious lesions should be biopsied or removed in toto. Cancer is not something that should be watched. All patients are not compliant in returning for follow-up appointments. It is safer and wiser to remove the lesion initially than chance losing the patient to follow-up.

Herpetic lesions frequently present on the lip (Fig. 16-33). They present as a series of vesicles and are usually self-limiting, healing within 10 to 14 days.

Buccal mucosa. The buccal mucosa is frequently the sight of trauma from teeth biting. This is referred to as linea alba and follows the occlusal plane. Lichen planus is also seen on the buccal mucosa as well as other previously discussed lesions.

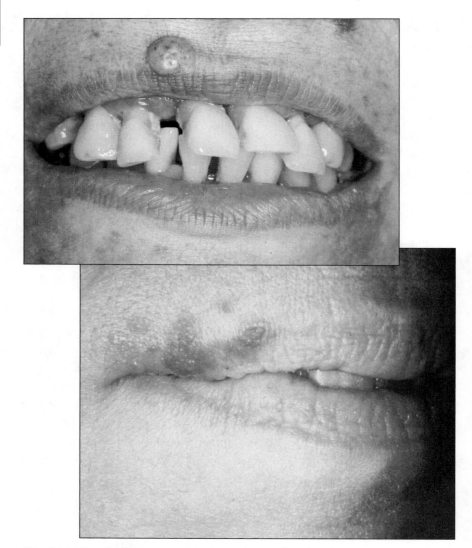

Fig. 16-32 Basal cell carcinoma present on the maxillary lip of a 50-year-old female. Despite its presence for years, she was never advised to have it removed. Undiagnosed lesions should be biopsied or removed en toto

Fig. 16-33 Herpetic lesions present on the lip of a patient one week following oral surgery. Trauma is a frequent precipitating factor

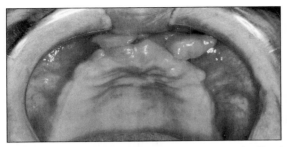

Fig. 16-34a Patients wearing complete maxillary dentures will frequently form inflammatory fibrous hyperplasia (epulis fissuratum) in the maxillary anterior region. These folds of excess tissue form in response to ill-fitting dentures and or bone resorption of the alveolar bone that leads to elongated rolls of tissue in the mucobuccal fold area into which the denture flange fits. The tissue is inflamed and serves as a nidus for plaque formation

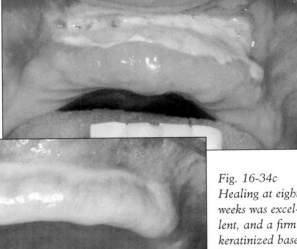

Fig. 16-34b Treatment consisted of removal and grafting with alloderm, an acellular dermal matrix processed from donated human skin

Fig. 16-34c Healing at eight weeks was excellent, and a firm keratinized base exists. The patient's denture is relined, and the occlusal is verified

Vestibule. The vestibule should be examined for lesions, especially draining fistulas. In the edentulous patient wearing prosthesis, the vestibule should be examined for epulus and denture irritation. In Figure 16-34a, the treatment is removal of the epulus, and relining or making a new prosthesis, as shown in Figures 16-34b and 16-34c.

Hard palate. The hard palate is frequently a sign of traumatic lesions. Smokers frequently present with nicotinic stomatitis, an irritation of the salivary glands from cigarette smoke (Fig. 16-35). The finding of this condition presents a unique opportunity for the dentist to warn the patient of the dangers of smoking. Patient visualization of the irritation has a profound effect in showing the patient the damage he/she is creating.

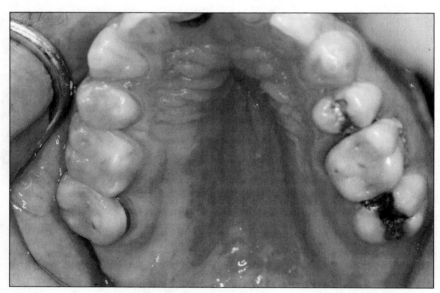

Fig. 16-35 Nicotinic stomatitis on the hard palate of a 28-year-old man with a history of smoking two packs of cigarettes a day. Thickening of the epithelium adjacent to the inflamed of the salivary glands is present. The patient is advised to quit smoking

Blunt trauma is also seen on the hard palate. It is usually painless. Nevertheless, it should be monitored and followed until the lesion resolves (Fig. 16-36). This lesion was found in a young homosexual man, secondary to penile trauma.

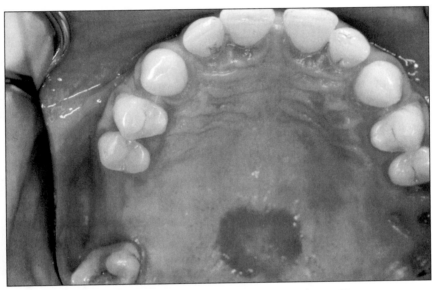

Fig. 16-36 Blunt trauma present in this 30-year-old homosexual man. He was asymtomatic except for the large ulcer present on his palate. The lesion resolved within two weeks

Soft palate and pharynx. The soft palate is a frequent site of irritation of a non-dental nature. Allergies, burns, infections, irritation due to smoking, and tonsillar infections can all lead to irritation of the soft palate. A thorough assessment and diagnosis should be made. Referral to an ear, nose, and throat (ENT) specialist or physician may be necessary.

Tongue. The tongue should be thoroughly examined. Ninety percent of all oral carcinomas are associated with the tongue and the floor of the mouth. A 2" x 2" piece of gauze should be used to retract the tongue from the mouth so that the lateral borders of the tongue can be well visualized.

Geographic tongue is also a frequent finding and is often associated with lichen planus.

Floor of the mouth. The floor of the mouth should also be meticulously examined for cancer. The patentcy of the submandibular and sublingual gland should be assessed. The present of tori should be evaluated. Frequently, they must be removed in order to place a removable partial denture or to facilitate plaque control.

Periodontal examination

The initial examination tray is the same for all patients (Fig. 16-37). It consists of a periodontal probe, single-ended explorer, mouth mirror, furcation probe (Nabers probe), 2" x 2" piece of gauge for examination of the tongue, and an 18-inch piece of dental floss for checking contact points and balancing interferences. Periodontal diagnosis is a multifactorial process and includes a thorough examination (Table 16-5).

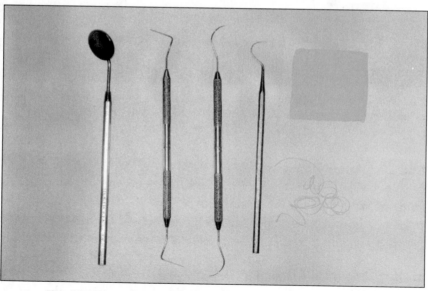

Fig. 16-37 Initial oral examination tray. It consists of mouth mirror, periodontal probe, furcation (Nabers) probe, single-ended explorer, 2 x 2 piece of gauze, and an 18-inch length of dental floss

Visual inflammation and bleeding on probing. Assessment of periodontal inflammation can be subtle. The patient shown in Figure 16-38a may or may not be seen as having gingival inflammation. This depends on the sophistication of the examining clinician. However, this 24-year female clearly has early signs of periodontal disease. Gentle probing (Fig. 16-38b) reveals that this patient has bleeding on probing—clearly an early sign of periodontal disease. It has also been stated by some that patients with bleeding on probing are more prone to further attachment loss.[50]

- Visual inflammation
- Bleeding on probing
- Suppuration
- Pocket depth and probing
- Attachment level
- Furcation involvement
- Mucogingival assessment
- Tooth mobility
- Radiographs

Table 16-5 Examination of the periodontium

Suppuration. A much more obvious form of periodontal disease is present in the patient in Figure 16-39. There is obvious suppuration, loss of attachment, papillae loss, shifting of teeth, hypereruption, and cyanosis. This is aggressive periodontitis. Some patients may exhibit flaccidity of the papillae (Figs. 16-40 and 16-3a). Gently blown air from the syringe causes the papilla to detach from the tooth. This patient was made aware of his condition and immediately opted for treatment—surgical repair of the area. Three years later, following surgery and the institution of excellent hygiene and frequent recall, a stable result is achieved (Fig. 16-3b). Absence of clinical visual inflammation is possible in the presence of periodontal pockets.[51] Therefore, it is essential to accurately probe all individuals to assess their periodontal health.

Pocket depth and probing. Probing of the periodontium is an art. Many clinicians were taught to probe along the long access of the teeth. This is often not possible if one is to probe the interproximal areas, where most

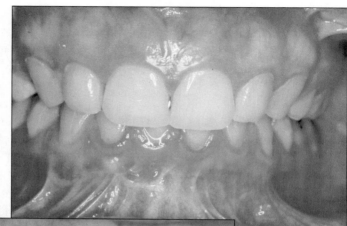

Fig. 16-38a Visual examination of this 24-year-old patient reveals minimal or no periodontal disease

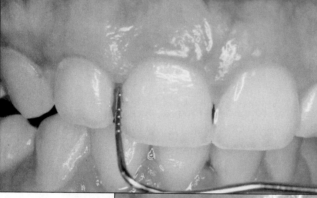

Fig. 16-38b Probing is necessary to reveal 4-mm anterior pocketing and bleeding upon probing. Patient has early gingivitis, which is easily treated at this stage

Fig. 16-39 Severe periodontitis is easily revealed upon visual examination. Loss of papillae, edema, cyanosis and suppuration, and drifting and shifting of teeth are all evident without probing or radiographs

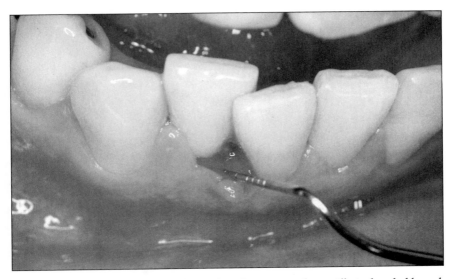

Fig. 16-40 Prior to the initiation of periodontal treatment, the papilla is detachable and calculus is present subgingivally. This is the same patient as in Figures 16-3a and 16-3b

periodontal lesions begin.[52] If the probe is inserted along the line angles strictly parallel to the long axis of the teeth, the pocket depth is a reflection of the position of the cortical plate and therefore conservative (Fig. 16-41a). Actual periodontal disease may be missed. Therefore, the probe must be angled slightly to reach the bottom of the crater (Fig. 16-41b).

The inexperienced clinician may miss significant periodontal disease if the patient is not probed accurately (Figs. 16-42a and 16-42b). Certain areas of the dentition are more prone to periodontal disease than others. These include teeth with furcation involvement, the maxillary molars, mandibular molars, and maxillary first bicuspids (Fig. 16-43). Also the mesial of the mandibular canine is prone to bone loss due to the wide buccal lingual dimension of this tooth. Plaque removal is often ineffective because of its position in the arch (Fig. 16-44).

Maxillary central and lateral incisors often present with development anomalies called palato-gingival grooves. Their frequency has been reported to be approximately 5%.[53] These areas are prone to periodontal disease due to the lack of fusion of the embryonic tooth buds (Fig. 16-45).

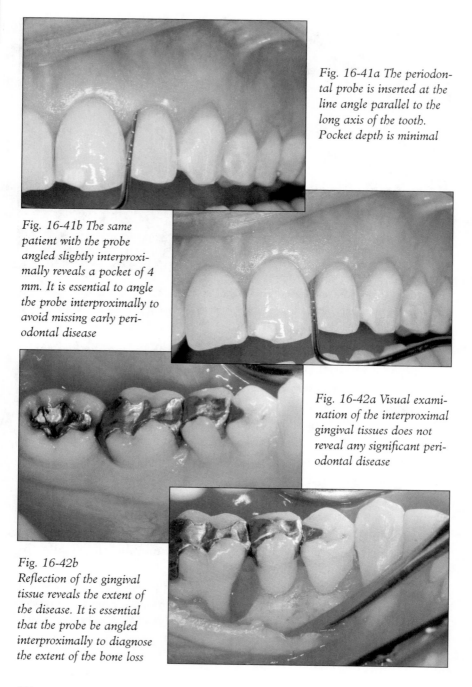

Fig. 16-41a The periodontal probe is inserted at the line angle parallel to the long axis of the tooth. Pocket depth is minimal

Fig. 16-41b The same patient with the probe angled slightly interproximally reveals a pocket of 4 mm. It is essential to angle the probe interproximally to avoid missing early periodontal disease

Fig. 16-42a Visual examination of the interproximal gingival tissues does not reveal any significant periodontal disease

Fig. 16-42b Reflection of the gingival tissue reveals the extent of the disease. It is essential that the probe be angled interproximally to diagnose the extent of the bone loss

Fig. 16-43 The mesial of the maxillary first bicuspid is predisposed to periodontal disease. Anatomically, there are two roots, which may be separate or fused. A mesial root groove or furcation is present, depending on whether the buccal and palatal roots are bifurcated or fused. Accurate probing of this interproximal area should be done on all patients. If the line angle is probed, the interproximal bony cratering may be missed

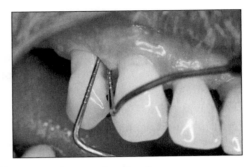

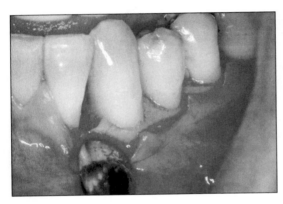

Fig. 16-44 The mesial of the mandibular canine is predisposed to plaque formation. The root is broad in a buccal lingual direction. The canine is the "cornerstone" of the arch, at the junction between the anterior and posterior teeth, and is often missed during oral hygiene. Note the absence of bone loss on the premolars and the facial of the canine

Fig. 16-45 This 78-year-old woman presents with a palatal root groove on only one of her maxillary lateral incisors. The left lateral with the root groove probes 8 mm, while the lateral incisor without the root groove probes 3 mm. The groove serves as a plaque trap. Treatment should include debridement as well as elimination of the groove with a high speed-finishing bur, if possible

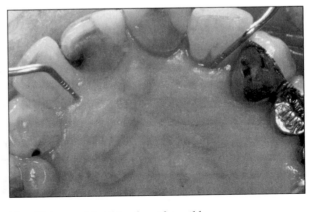

Attachment level. The position of the gingival margin must also be noted in addition to the pocket depth. The patient may have minimal pocket depth, but a gingival margin apical to the cemento-enamel junction (CEJ). A 5-mm pocket reading in which the gingival margin coincides with the CEJ is different from a 5-mm pocket in the presence of 4 mm of gingival enlargement or from a 5-mm reading where 4 mm of recession exists. These three different situations are very different and should be differentiated.

Furcation involvement. As bone is lost apically on teeth with furcations, the areas between the roots become exposed. A number of furcation classifications have been described. For the purpose of this discussion, the following furcation classification will be used (Table 16-6).

Detection of these lesions is quite important in case management

Grade I—Pocket formation into the flute of the furcation, but the interradicular bone remains intact.

Grade II—Loss of interradicular bone and pocket formation of varying depths into the furcation, but not completely through to the opposite side of the tooth.

Grade III—Through-and-through bone loss to the opposite side of the tooth.

Table 16-6 Furcation classification

and in treatment planning. A total of 34 possible furcations exist. These include three furcations in all six maxillary molars, two furcations in the six mandibular molars, and two furcations in the two maxillary first bicuspids. The possible furcation involvement could be represented as follows:

Maxilla	3	3	3	2	2	3	3	3	= 22
Mandible	2	2	2			2	2	2	= 12
Total									34

The diagnosis of furcations is best determined by using a curved furcation probe, called a Nabers probe. Buccal furcations are relatively easy to diagnose because of their accessibility (Figs. 16-46a and 16-46b). Mesial and distal maxillary molar furcations are best accessed from the palatal, for the embrasures are wider palatally than bucally on the maxilla (Figs. 16-47a and 16-47b).

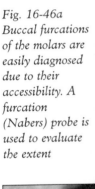

Fig. 16-46a Buccal furcations of the molars are easily diagnosed due to their accessibility. A furcation (Nabers) probe is used to evaluate the extent

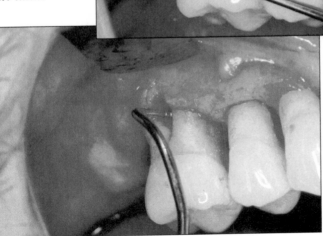

Fig. 16-46b Flap reflection reveals the horizontal extent of the furcation. The vertical extent should also be evaluated

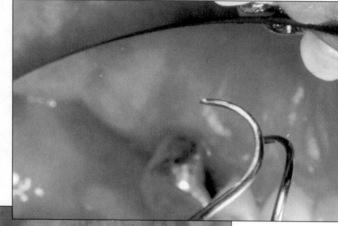

Fig. 16-47a A curved curette or furcation probe is used to access the mesial furcation of the maxillary molar

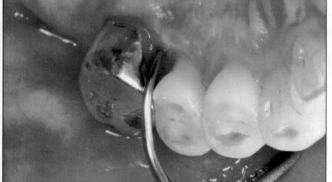

Fig. 16-47b A palatal approach used for the palatal provides better accessibility, for they are wider than the buccal embrasures of the maxillary molars

The best treatment of furcation involvement is early diagnosis. Furcation entrances are difficult to instrument. It has been reported 81% of all furcation entrance diameters measure less than 1 mm, with 58% measuring less than 0.75 mm[54] (Fig. 16-48). Another difficulty in treating furcations is the anatomy of the root morphology. The roots have significant grooves and invaginations, making complete calculus and debris removal close to impossible (Figs. 16-49a and 16-49b). Furcation therapy varies on the extent of furcation involvement. Therapy for the three classes of furcations will be reviewed.

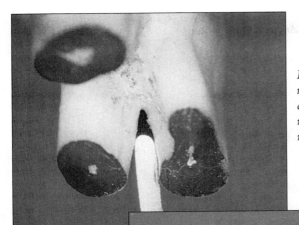

Fig. 16-48 The diameter of most cruets is too wide to enter the furcation area, making complete debridement close to impossible

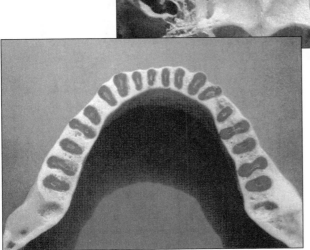

Fig. 16-49 a,b Cross sections of the maxillary and mandibular teeth reveal root grooves and concavities present on the furcal aspects of the roots of the maxillary and mandibular molars. Complete root preparation of these areas via instrumentation is not possible

Class I furcation therapy

Early furcation involvement is most easily treated with finishing burs, ultrasonic instrumentation, and curette tips. Enamel pearls on the root trunk leading to the furcation area of the root surface may manifest themselves as cervical enamel projections. The goal of therapy is to make the furcation area cleansible. Treatment may involve apically-repositioned flaps with elimination of enamel projections (Fig. 16-50). Non-surgical therapy may also be effective, if access is possible.

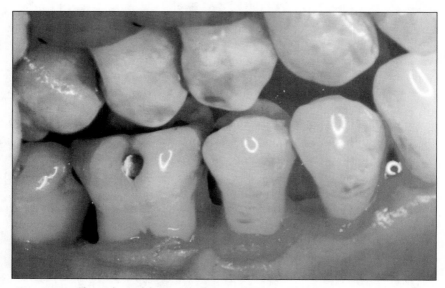

Fig. 16-50 Class I buccal furcation of a mandibular molar demonstrates early furcal bone loss and a slight enamel projection. Treatment should involve removal of the enamel projection and osseous reshaping to provide easy cleansibility of the furcation

Class II furcation therapy

Treatment of the Class II furcation is variable. Early involvement may consist of root planing and reshaping of the furcation to make it more cleansible. However, this technique provides little or no improvement.[55] Treatment of Class II furcations has been attempted with a variety of regenerative techniques, including a variety of bone grafts placed alone and in conjunction with bio-resorbale and non-bioresorbable membranes. A review of the literature by Jan Egelberg was inconclusive as to the effectiveness of regenerative treatment in eliminating Class II furcations. This author has found regenerative therapy to be effective in eliminating Class II furcations in their early stages (Figs. 16-51a, 16-51b, and 16-51c). However, Class II furcations of a more significant nature are more difficult to predictably regenerate. The most positive experience has been with early Class II furcations in mandibular molars.

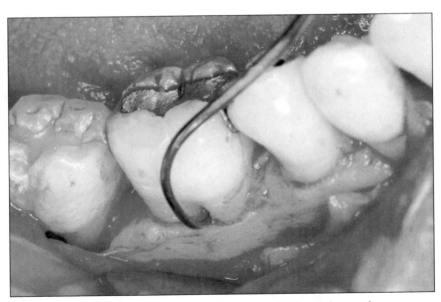

Fig. 16-51a An early Class II furcation with the Nabers probe showing its extent. It is amenable to guided bone regeneration

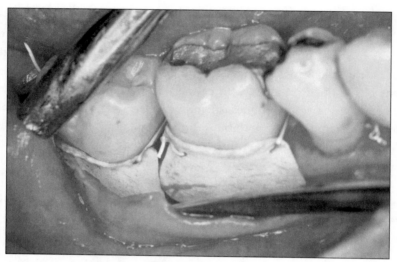

Fig. 16-51b Gore-Tex barrier membranes are placed over the furcations after the roots were debrided with finishing burs, treated with tetracycline for five minutes, and an autogenous bone was placed. The membranes are intimately adapted to prevent the ingrown of gingival connective tissue and epithelium. The buccal gingival flap was then elevated to completely cover the Gore-Tex membrane. The membrane is left for six to eight weeks before removal

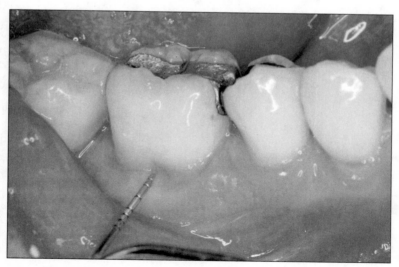

Fig. 16-51c Eight months later, the furcation is closed for bony regeneration has taken place. Probing is not possible

In maxillary molars, root amputation is frequently a viable alternative. This is dependent upon the furcation involvement including only two roots. The remaining two roots must be free of any bone loss to make this a predictable procedure. It is particularly useful when root proximity is also an issue. The treatment involves three procedures: endodontic therapy, periodontal surgery, and a crown (Figs. 16-52a through 16-52d). The published results of root resection are variable, with a failure rate ranging from 0% to 38%.[55] In this author's experience, maxillary molars fare much better than mandibular molars.

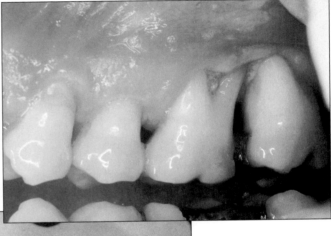

Fig. 16-52a Root proximity is present between the maxillary first and second molars. Class II furcation involvement exists on the buccal and distal furcation of the maxillary first molar

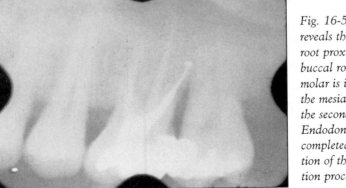

Fig. 16-52b Radiograph reveals the extent of the root proximity. The distal buccal root of the first molar is in contact with the mesial buccal root of the second molar. Endodontic therapy was completed in anticipation of the root amputation procedure

583

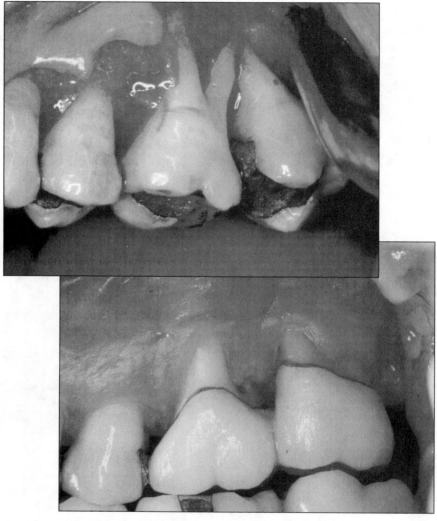

Fig. 16-52c *Flap refection reveals the buccal furcation involvement as well as the root proximity. As is, this is a non-maintainable situation*

Fig. 16-52d *Post-therapy crowns were placed on the maxillary first and second molars to establish better occlusion. Note the amount of interproximal space that exists between the molars, allowing for cleansibility. Plaque control is excellent (Restoration courtesy of Dr. Peter Ferrara, Westport, CT)*

Class III furcation therapy

Regeneration of Class III through bone grafting procedures is not predictable.[56] Hemisection of Class III furcations is possible. However, the literature is quite inconclusive. The largest problems with resected teeth are usually prosthetic in nature—caries and root fracture.[57] The case in Figures 16-53a through 16-53d lasted 10 years before caries occurred. Periodontal stability was achieved, and the patient was on a strict three-month recall. However, caries caused this case to fail. Root fracture and endodontic failure are also frequent causes of failure.

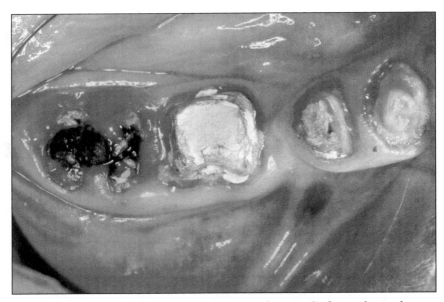

Fig. 16-53a Class III furcations are present between the first and second mandibular molars. A decision has to be made as to what roots are maintainable from both a periodontal and restorative perspective

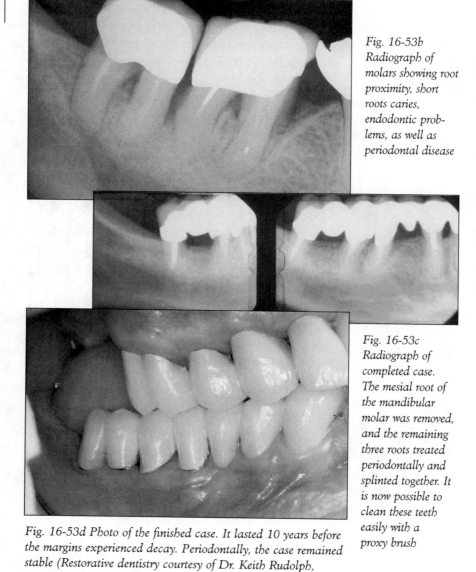

Fig. 16-53b Radiograph of molars showing root proximity, short roots caries, endodontic problems, as well as periodontal disease

Fig. 16-53c Radiograph of completed case. The mesial root of the mandibular molar was removed, and the remaining three roots treated periodontally and splinted together. It is now possible to clean these teeth easily with a proxy brush

Fig. 16-53d Photo of the finished case. It lasted 10 years before the margins experienced decay. Periodontally, the case remained stable (Restorative dentistry courtesy of Dr. Keith Rudolph, Westport, CT)

The maxillary case presented in Figures 16-54a through 16-54f was much more difficult to maintain and required excellent patient home care. This patient was extremely diligent. However, the long-term prognosis is guarded due to the amount of bone loss and difficulty in maintaining this area consistently.

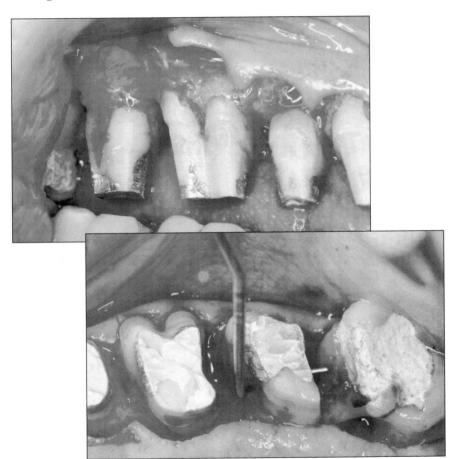

Fig. 16-54a Gingival flap reflection of trifurcated maxillary molars

Fig. 16-54b Occlusal view revealing Class III furcation of the maxillary second molar. The third molar is hopeless, and the first molar has a Class II furcation on the distal

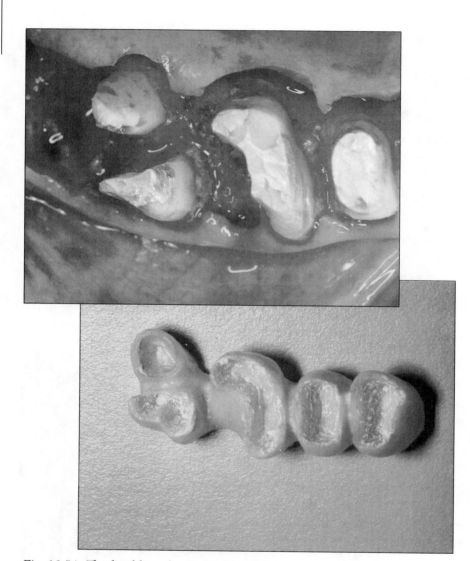

Fig. 16-54c *The distal-buccal root of the first molar was amputated, and the second molar was trisected. It was determined that the palatal and mesial-buccal roots had the best prognosis*

Fig. 16-54d *A provisional restoration was fabricated on the altered dentition. The patient is allowed to heal and is instructed in proper home care*

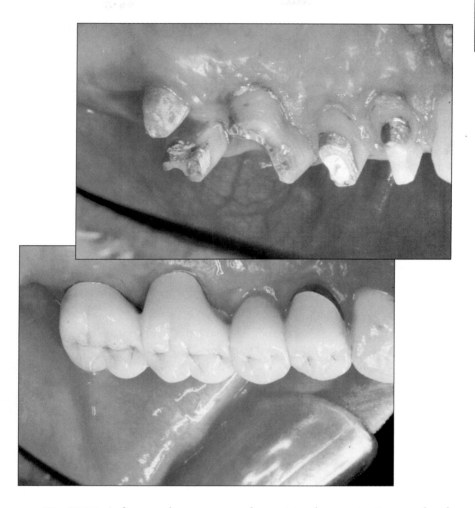

Fig. 16-54e At four months post-surgery, the provisional restoration is removed and patient compliance is assessed. At this stage, a decision is made as to whether the patient can adequately clean the remaining roots. Manual dexterity and patient commitment are essential for long-term stability. This patient demonstrated excellent hygiene, and a decision was made to proceed to the final restoration

Fig. 16-54f Palatal view of final restoration. Patient is adequately maintaining, and plaque control is excellent. Monitoring is essential for long-term success (Restorative dentistry courtesy of Dr. Robert Cieri, Wilton, CT)

Tunnel preparation of furcated teeth may be an alternative to root resection.[58] However, these teeth are prone to caries, and maintenance is difficult despite good oral hygiene and the administration of fluoride with proxybrushes (Figs. 16-55a through 16-55d).

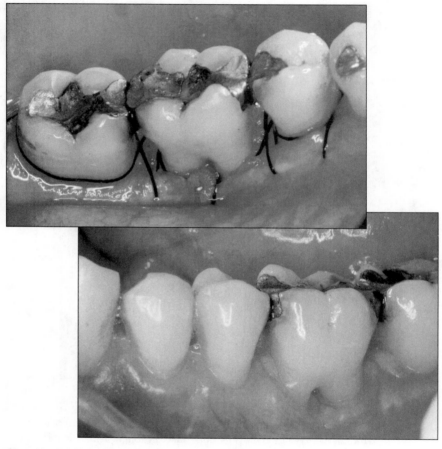

Fig. 16-55a Tunnel preparation was done at the time of surgery. A proxybrush is placed into the tunnel before suturing to maintain the patency of the Class III furcation

Fig. 16-55b Healing is uneventful, and tissue health is excellent. The opening to the Class III furcation is evident

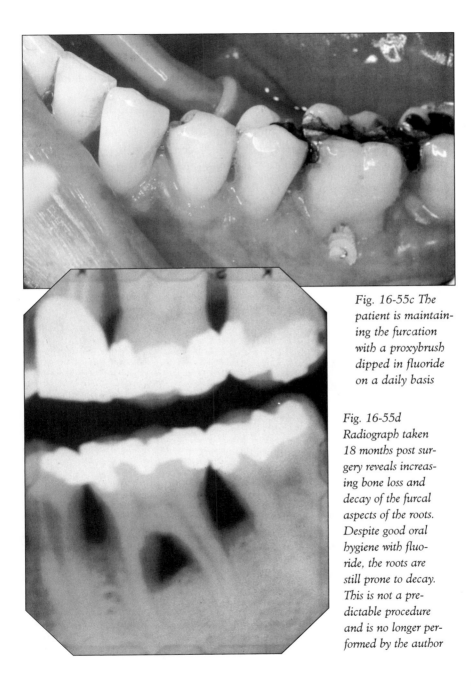

Fig. 16-55c The patient is maintaining the furcation with a proxybrush dipped in fluoride on a daily basis

Fig. 16-55d Radiograph taken 18 months post surgery reveals increasing bone loss and decay of the furcal aspects of the roots. Despite good oral hygiene with fluoride, the roots are still prone to decay. This is not a predictable procedure and is no longer performed by the author

When teeth are severely compromised by furcation involvement, watchful diligence is sometimes the best way of maintenance. Patients can be instructed to irrigate the furcations on a twice-daily basis with chlorhexidine (Figs. 16-56a and 16-56b). This disturbs the bacteria, but at best it is a compromise, and long-term studies have not substantiated any significant benefit.[55] The most predictable way of treating teeth with Class III furcations is extraction and replacement with dental implants (Figs. 16-57a, 16-57b, and 16-57c). Dental implants have a success rate upward of 90%.[59]

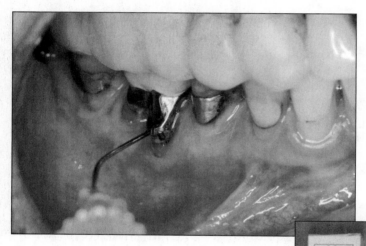

Fig. 16-56a Buccal furcation not amenable to pre-dictable treatment. Restoration is present in the furcation, making regeneration impossible. With the exception of extraction, maintenance is the only alternative. The patient was instructed to irrigate the area on a daily basis with chlorhexidine. This disturbs the bacteria and may slow down the bone loss in the furcal area. Maintaining this tooth's furcation does not impact on the adjacent teeth

Fig. 16-56b Irrigation device used by patient to deliver subgingival medications to difficult to maintain areas. Patient was instructed to fill it with chlorhexidine and irrigate two times a day

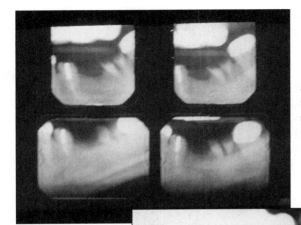

Fig. 16-57a Pretreatment radiograph of a hopeless maxillary molar with a Class III furcation

Fig. 16-57b Post-treatment radiograph of the molar replaced with two implants

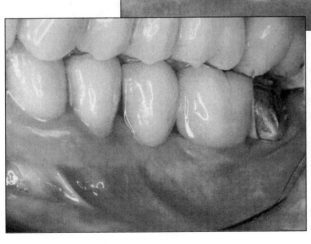

Fig. 16-57c Post-treatment photographs of mandibular molar restored with two dental implants. The predictability of this restoration is in the high 90th percentile

Mucogingival assessment is also part of the initial examination. For a thorough review, please refer to the section on mucogingival surgery.

Tooth mobility

Tooth mobility is defined as the looseness of a tooth beyond physiologic movement. The most commonly-used clinical index for tooth mobility is the Miller index.[59] Mobility is detected by using the blunt ends of instruments (Fig. 16-58). Mobility is scored as follows:

1 = first distinguishable sign of movement

2 = movement of the crown up to 1 mm in any direction

3 = movement of the crown more than 1 mm in any direction and/or vertical depression of the crown in its socket

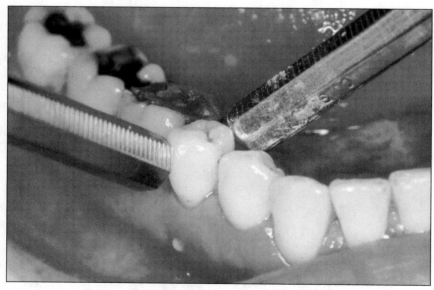

Fig. 16-58 The blunt end of the explorer and mouth mirror are used to assess tooth mobility

This scoring of mobility is very subjective. A number of instruments (microperiodontometer, Periotest, etc.) have been designed to systematize mobility scores, however, they have not gained in popularity.

Tooth mobility is caused by two factors—an increase in attachment loss and/or an increasing force acting upon a tooth. There are three situations in which tooth mobility is of concern. The first situation is when tooth mobility is increasing. This is called *progressive tooth mobility*. The periodontal ligament widens, and active bone resorption takes place. Teeth may become hypermobile.[60] Coupled with active periodontitis, an increase in alveolar bone resorption may occur. The second situation of concern is when mobility causes migration of teeth, *pathologic migration*. The third area of concern is when mobility results in patient discomfort, as in difficulty in chewing.

Lindhe[60] concluded that trauma from occlusion cannot induce periodontal tissue breakdown. Lindhe did state that trauma from occlusion does result in resorption of alveolar bone, leading to increased tooth mobility. This can be transient or permanent. Lindhe called this increased mobility a physiologic adaptation of the periodontal ligament and surrounding bone to the increased trauma. Lindhe concluded that in the presence of plaque associated periodontal disease, increased mobility can act as a co-factor in progressing alveolar bone loss.

In conclusion, it is of paramount importance to control plaque-associated periodontal disease. The control of mobility or trauma from occlusion alone, without controlling inflammation, will not arrest periodontal disease.

Radiographs, another essential part of the periodontal examination, were covered under the initial examination.

Occlusal examination

A thorough occlusal examination (Table 16-7) should also be part of the complete periodontal examination. As briefly discussed in the last section, the occlusion can be a co-factor in periodontal breakdown.

Occlusion may be a co-factor in esthetics as well as function. Untreated, bruxism can lead to severe tooth wear. Unchecked, significant amounts of tooth structure can be irreversibly lost (Figs. 16-59a and 16-59b). There is much antidotal evidence that trauma from occlusion can cause angular bony defects as well as furcation breakdown in the presence of plaque (Fig. 16-59c).

Oftentimes, lost teeth are not initially replaced. This may result in hypereruption of the opposing tooth or teeth (Fig. 16-60a). Subsequently, the plane of occlusion is altered. If not corrected before it is restored, the resulting restoration will be in an altered state. This is referred to as *conformational dentistry*.[61] The resulting restoration is built into an altered plane of occlusion.

One of the basic tenets of good restorative dentistry is to have a replacement tooth ready for a tooth that is to be extracted. All too often, teeth are extracted and not immediately temporized. This sets up the patient for hypereruption, drifting, and tipping of the teeth. Oftentimes, patients present with edentulous areas in need of restoration, where space for replacement restoration is inadequate (Figs. 16-60a and 16-60b). The patient in Figure 16-60 had two implants placed in the posterior mandible. The bone was adequate. However, there was inadequate interocclusal space for the restoration, due to hypereruption of the maxillary molars. Crown lengthening, elective endodontic therapy, crowning of the maxillary molars, and a specialized UCLA implant prosthesis were needed in order to adequately restore this patient (Figs. 16-

- Class
- Working contacts
- Balancing contacts
- Protrusive contacts
- Crossbites
- Centric prematurities
- Fremitus
- Plane of occlusion
- Bruxism
- Wear facets
- Muscles of mastication
- TMJ symptoms
- Drifting of teeth
- Tongue thrust
- Posterior bite collapse
- Radiographic findings

Table 16-7 Occlusal examination

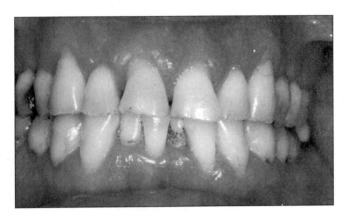

Fig. 16-59a
Significant
generalized
occlusal wear
in a 40-year-old
male bruxer

Fig. 16-59b Occlusal view of view through the
mandibular incisors. Secondary dentin is present

for the patient
has ground his
teeth through
the enamel,
into the dentin
and into the
area where the
pulp chambers
used to be

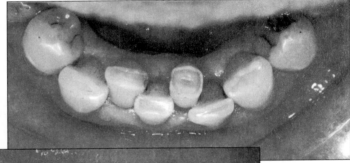

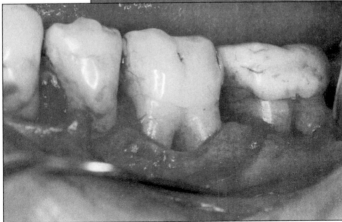

Fig. 16-59c
Class II furca-
tions present in
mandibular
molars. Some
clinicians feel
that occlusion
"may" be a
cofactor in fur-
cal bone loss

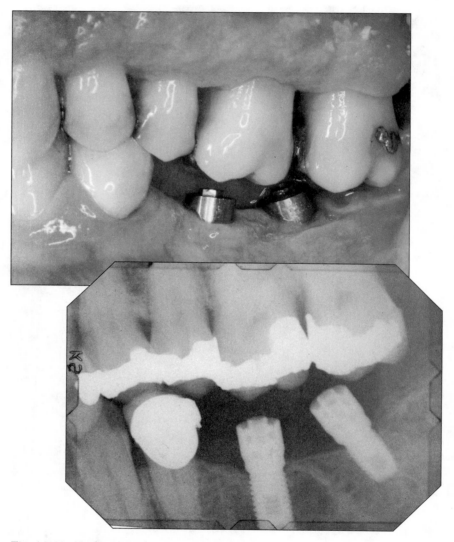

Fig. 16-60a Teeth #18 and #19 were lost and never replaced in this patient. The maxillary molars subsequently drifted into the edentulous space. Implants were eventually placed. However, there was inadequate interocclusal space

Fig. 16-60b Radiographs demonstrate the lack of room to place an adequate functional restoration

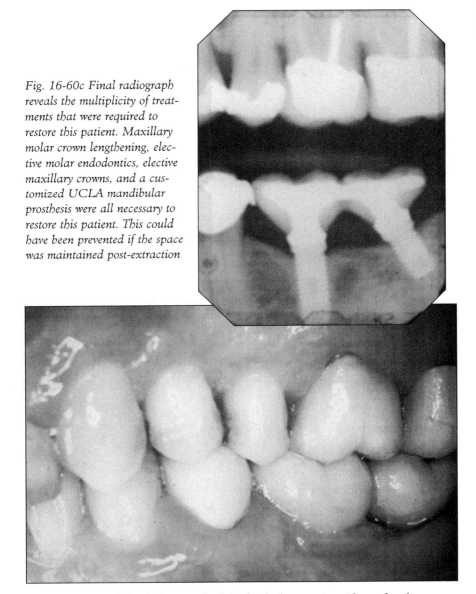

Fig. 16-60c Final radiograph
reveals the multiplicity of treatments that were required to
restore this patient. Maxillary
molar crown lengthening, elective molar endodontics, elective
maxillary crowns, and a customized UCLA mandibular
prosthesis were all necessary to
restore this patient. This could
have been prevented if the space
was maintained post-extraction

Fig. 16-60d Final photograph of the finished restoration. Plane of occlusion has been reestablished. The cost was restoration of the maxillary
molars (Restorative dentistry courtesy of Dr. Gary Horblitt, Fairfield, CT)

60c and 16-60d). Much of this dentistry could have been avoided if the maxillary arch had been stabilized following the extraction of the mandibular molars. A removable partial denture or a maxillary hard acrylic biteguard could have achieved this.

Caries and teeth examination

All missing teeth, present teeth, restorations, caries, fractured teeth, endodontically-treated teeth, and clasped teeth should be noted and charted.

Photographs

All patients have a facial photograph taken at their initial visit. The photograph is placed into the patient's chart. *A picture is worth a thousand words.* The photograph is very helpful to refamiliarize oneself with the patient. If a patient was only seen once, and calls the office a few months or years later to reschedule or discuss some aspect of care, the photograph is an excellent reminder of who the patient is.

Intraoral photographs are also very important. They serve to document procedures, educate patients, and educate dentists, and they are useful teaching tools. Photographic documentation is perhaps the best educational tool dentists have at their disposal to further their understanding and knowledge of clinical dentistry.

Patient education

At the conclusion of the initial examination, the patient is seated in the consultation room. The report of findings is discussed with the patient. The patient is given a menu of treatment options. The various options are reviewed with the patient. The costs, risks, and benefits of treatment are explained in detail. The costs, risks, and benefits of *not* performing treatment are also elucidated and reviewed with the patient. An educated, well-informed patient is best able to make the most appropriate decisions regarding his/her treatment.

Periodontal Treatment Planning

The conclusion of the patient examination is the presentation of the treatment plan. An oft-asked question is *"Who does the treatment planning?"* This is an excellent question. Who is responsible for making the treatment planning decisions? The dentist gathers information and makes the presentation to the patient. However, the decision should be mutually agreed upon. Similar to a restaurant, patients are presented with choices. Two differences exist between dental offices and restaurants. First, dentists provide services—not food. Secondly, in restaurants, patrons are usually familiar with the menu and the different choices. In a dental office, patients must be educated as to what the differences in services are. The presentation of treatment alternatives to a patient can be called a *Menu of treatment options* (Table 16-8).

The side table is merely a hypothetical example of the multiplicity of options that are available to patients. Most patients are confused by the large variety of treatment alternatives that are available today. It is the responsibility of the dentist to educate, clarify, and guide the patient to do what is in the patient's best interest. Dentist and patient become co-therapists and co-treatment planners in this process. The ideal treatment planning sequence is shown in Table 16-9. As

Non-Surgical
Root planing
Chemical
Antibiotics
Holistic
Watchful vigilance

Extract
Leave alone
Augment
Soft tissue
Bone (auto, allo, synth)
Guided bone regeneration
Combinations

Surgical
Open debridement
Osseous
Regenerative
Combination

Replace
Fixed bridge
Removable bridge
Implant

Table 16-8 Menu (treatment options)

601

previously discussed, initial therapy is the starting point, unless the patient presents in pain and is in need of emergency care.

Initial therapy

A detailed diagnosis predicated on a thorough examination should be a prerequisite for an appropriate treatment plan. Caries and periodontal disease are infections associated with bacteria. Prior to the performance of definitive therapy (Table 16-9), an attempt should be made to reduce or eliminate etiologic factors.

- Examination
- Emergency treatment
- Initial therapy
- Reevaluation
- Definitive therapy
  ◊ Periodontal surgery
  ◊ Implant surgery
  ◊ Restorative treatment
- Maintenance therapy

Table 16-9 Periodontal treatment plan

Thus, the primary goal of initial therapy is to control oral infections. The elimination and control of plaque are probably the most critical procedures in therapy.

Initial therapy is designed to set the stage for overall dental and periodontal health. In some instances, it is an end stage. However, in others it is the necessary first step in the sequence of definitive thera-

- Patient dental education
- Oral hygiene instructions
- Extraction of hopeless teeth
- Caries control
- Root planning and scaling
- Endodontics
- Temporization
- Oral hygiene instructions

Table 16-10 Initial therapy

py. Whether additional therapy is required depends on the severity of disease and the patient's response to treatment. *However, definitive therapy should not be considered or begun until the patient proceeds through the initial phase of treatment and is thoroughly evaluated.* Initial therapy may involve a multiplicity of procedures aimed at the control of infection (Table 16-10).

The objective of oral physiotherapy (oral hygiene) is the complete daily removal of dental plaque in the most efficient, efficacious manner. The patient's oral hygiene procedures will vary with the severity of disease, the soft tissue anatomy, and the patient's manual dexterity. Oral hygiene aids include toothbrushes, electric toothbrushes, dental floss, interproximal brushes, toothpicks, rubber tips, oral irrigation devices, and mouthrinses. The regimen of oral physiotherapy will vary from patient to patient. Each patient should receive a customized program specific to his or her needs, anatomy, and motivation.

It is never too early to begin good oral hygiene habits (Fig. 16-61). Lack of oral hygiene results in gingivitis in all patients.[13] No one is immune from the development of gingival inflammation (Fig. 16-62a). Subsequently, with the introduction of oral physiotherapy, and the removal of plaque, a decrease in gingival inflammation will occur (Fig. 16-62b). The dramatic changes seen in this patient following one week of oral hygiene are not unusual.

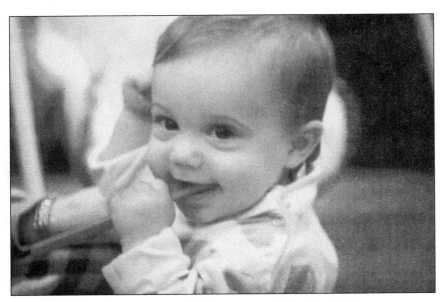

Fig. 16-61 Young child beginning tooth brushing. It is never too early to begin good oral hygiene habits

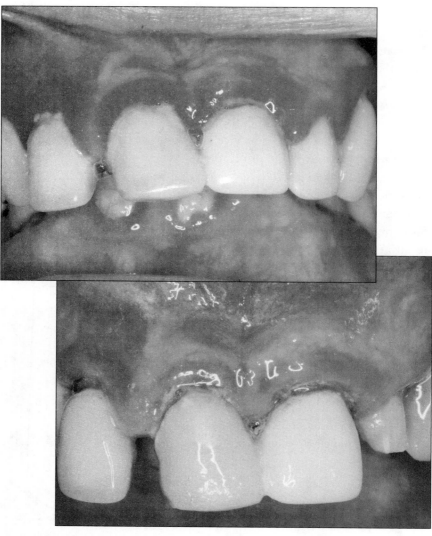

Fig. 16-62a This 38-year-old female patient has not seen the dentist in 12 years. Significant plaque accumulation with resultant angry red gingivitis is seen

Fig. 16-62b One week later, after the institution of home care in conjunction with oral hygiene instructions, some resolution of inflammation is seen

During the 1970s there was a great amount of interest in investigating the plaque-removing efficacy of different methods of toothbrushing, *e.g.*, bass, charters, circular, roll, scrub, etc. Results of the various studies were similar. Using any of the particular methods over other methods resulted in little advantage.[62] Of note was the fact that none of the toothbrushing methods were effective at removing interproximal plaque. Hence, interdental cleaning must also be done in addition to toothbrushing. Numerous devices exist with which to remove interproximal plaque (Fig. 16-63).

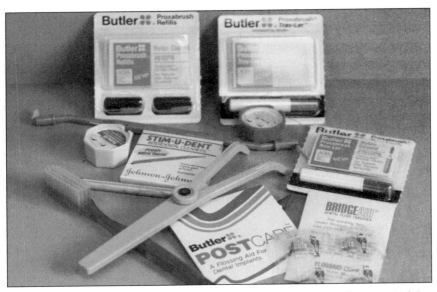

Fig. 16-63 Numerous oral hygiene aids exist to assist the patient in the control of dental plaque. They include various types of proxybrushes, dental floss, floss threaders, superfloss, stim-u-dents, floss handles, rubber tips, disclosing tablets, toothbrushes, etc.

Dental floss is the most common form of interdental cleaning. A number of different dental floss types are available, including waxed nylon, expanded polytetrafluoroethylene, and unwaxed. Little or no difference in efficacy has been found between the various floss types.[63-64]

Proper flossing technique is important to assure adequate plaque control as well as to avoid gingival injury (*e.g.*, floss cut) (Fig. 16-64). The floss should be gently inserted into the sulcus and wrapped around the tooth like a C, so as not to cause gingival clefting.

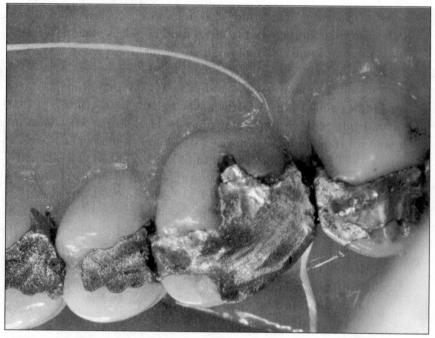

Fig. 16-64 This patient has been flossing. However, the floss has created a gingival cleft, for it was not wrapped around the tooth and placed into the sulcus. The floss should be placed into the sulcus and wrapped like a C around the tooth

Electric toothbrushes have increased in popularity after their introduction 50 years ago. Their effectiveness in comparison to manual toothbrushing is still undetermined. Many patients find the novelty of the electric toothbrush to be stimulating. However, most clinical studies are not long enough in duration to effectively assess the quality of electric toothbrushes.[65] More research in this area is needed.

The use of the rubber tip stimulator has not been greatly investigated. However, the author finds it to be a useful adjunct to toothbrushing and flossing, especially immediately after periodontal surgery (Fig. 16-65). Firm pressure directed at a right angle to the teeth results in interproximal plaque control and a firming up of the gingiva. The rubber tip is also useful in the maintenance of furcations (Fig. 16-66).

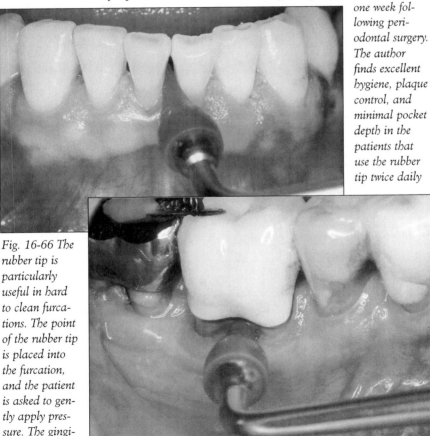

Fig. 16-65 The rubber tip is a useful adjunct in the control of plaque. Patients are instructed to begin to gently use the rubber tip one week following periodontal surgery. The author finds excellent hygiene, plaque control, and minimal pocket depth in the patients that use the rubber tip twice daily

Fig. 16-66 The rubber tip is particularly useful in hard to clean furcations. The point of the rubber tip is placed into the furcation, and the patient is asked to gently apply pressure. The gingival furcal tissue maintains firmness, and oral health is better maintained

The proxybrush is found to be an excellent interproximal cleaning device in situations where the embrasure spaces are open and allow its passage (Fig. 16-67). In one study, the use of the interdental brush in conjunction with toothbrushing was more effective than flossing and toothbrushing.[66]

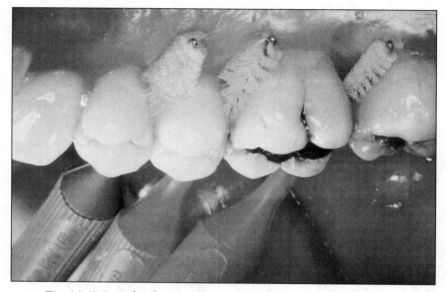

Fig. 16-67 Proxybrushes are effective at removing interproximal plaque. Embrasure space must exist to allow their passage. They are most useful after posterior periodontal surgery where there has been attachment loss

Mouthrinses have been marketed by manufacturers as being effective in reducing gingivitis. However, at the present time, none exist that replace mechanical plaque control methods. Available mouthrinses today include stannous fluoride, cetylpyridinium chloride, cetylpyridinium chloride, chlorhexidine, phonemic essential oils, sanguinarine, zinc chloride/sanguinarine, and triclosan.

With the exception of 0.12% or 0.20% chlorhexidine, mouthrinses as a supplement to mechanical plaque control appear to offer little benefit.[67] Chlorhexidine (peridex) is effective in significantly retarding the development of plaque and gingivitis.[68-69]

Chlorhexidine, while the most effective of mouthrinses in controlling plaque and gingivitis, is not without its side effects. Extrinsic tooth staining, alteration of taste, tongue staining, oral mucosal lesions, and increased accumulations of supra-gingival calculus are reported side effects of chlorhexidine use. However, chlorhexidine has its use in practice. Since it does lower the concentration of oral bacteria, chlorhexidine is useful clinically when a decrease of oral bacteria is necessary (Table 16-11). When patients find it impossible to mechanically perform oral hygiene, chlorhexidine is of great benefit. Due to its side effects, the duration of use must be kept to a minimum, two to three weeks.

Oral infections (e.g., NUG, herpes)

Compromised oral hygiene

Pre-implant surgery

Post periodontal surgery

Irrigation of extraction sites

Post exodontia rinse

Pre-treatment rinse

Office irrigation

Home irrigation

Table 16-11 Chlorhexidine indications

Root planing and scaling

Root planing and scaling coupled with plaque control is the cornerstone of non-surgical periodontal therapy. *Scaling* is defined as a procedure that removes plaque and calculus from the tooth surface. *root planing* is instrumentation of the softened "diseased" cementum of the root surface and removal of hardened calcareous deposits. The therapeutic goal of root planing is to remove the endotoxins on the root and to create a hard, smooth, glassy root surface.

Scaling and root planing are indicated at sites that manifest signs of gingival inflammation, elevated putative pathogens, and progressive loss of attachment. In some instances, root planing may represent the end point of periodontal therapy (Figs. 16-7a and 16-7b). However, in some cases, root planing serves as the initial phase of periodontal treatment, a pre-surgical therapeutic predecessor (Figs. 16-68a, 16-68b, and 16-68c). As disease progresses and pockets deepen, scaling and root planing become less effective as a therapeutic modality in eliminating periodontal disease. This is particularly true of multi-rooted teeth and teeth with surface irregularities.[70] In studies comparing the effectiveness of root planing and scaling in removing calculus versus open flap debridement, it was found that a significantly greater amount of calculus was always found in the group that was not surgically treated.[70-71]

Scaling and root planing are less predictable in pockets more than 5 mm in depth.[72] However, scaling and root planing should still be performed in order to eliminate subgingival bacteria, reduce inflammation, and allow assessment of the patient's healing response and healing potential (Fig. 16-68b).

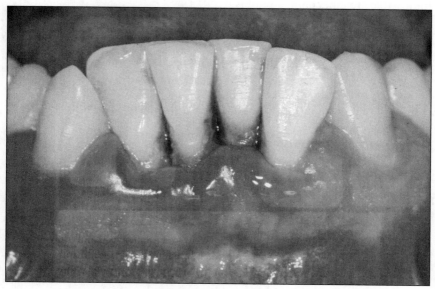

Fig. 16-68a Patient before initial therapy

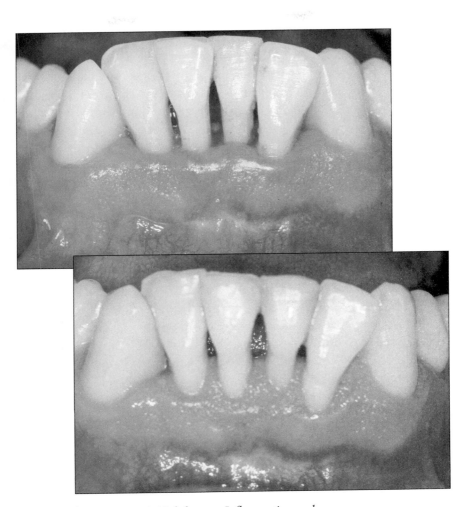

Fig. 16-68b Patient post initial therapy. Inflammation and pocket depths have decreased. However, significant pocketing still remains, and pocket elimination therapy is indicated

Fig. 16-68c Pocket elimination surgery has been performed. Gingival tissues are healthy, and pocket depth is minimal. However, more of the root has been exposed. In an esthetic area, this form of treatment is contraindicated

For scaling and root planing to be effective, an experienced operator must spend significant time. The literature is replete with confusion as to the results of scaling and root planing as a therapeutic endpoint. This confusion stems from the lack of standardization. The amount of time spent scaling and root planing each tooth varies significantly from study to study. The most effective results achieved from scaling and root planing are achieved when *significant* time per tooth was spent instrumenting under local anesthesia. In one study, teeth slated for extraction were root planed for 45 minutes by 5 different operators and then extracted and evaluated for remaining calculus.[73] Despite the amount of time and the experience of the operators, the average depth of pocket that could be instrumented to a plaque and calculus free surface, "curette efficiency," was 3.73 mm, and not deeper than 4 mm. The maximum probing depth at which evidence could be seen of instrumentation on the root surface was called the "instrument limit" and was 6.2 mm (Figs. 16-69a through 16-69f). In some studies, interdental papillae reflection is performed in order to provide better access. Thus, clarification as well as standardization is needed to accurately compare the results achievable from scaling and root planing. Regardless, the deeper the pocket, the more difficult it is to achieve a calculus-free surface.

Variations also exist in the manner in which the instrumentation is performed. Instrumentation may be accomplished by:

- Hand instruments (Fig. 16-70)
- Ultrasonic and sonic instruments (Fig. 16-71)
- High speed finishing burs (Fig. 16-72)

Several studies have evaluated the effectiveness of calculus removal using ultrasonics and hand instruments. Studies by Torfason et al. (1979), Badersten (1981), Oosterwaal et al. (1987), and Boretti et al. (1995) suggest that debridement of the contaminated root surfaces in deep pockets can be equally accomplished by ultrasonic and hand instruments.[74-77]

Loos et al. compared the effects of the Titan-S sonic instrument with the Dentsply Cavitron ultrasonic instrument.[78] Evaluation of

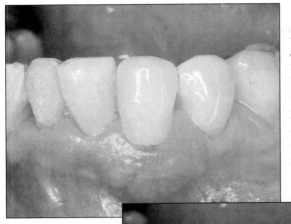

Fig. 16-69a This patient has gone through scaling and root planing one year ago. The buccal surface of tooth #22 probed 2 mm post root planing and scaling. However, she presented with a periodontal abscess one year following initial therapy

Fig. 16-69b Patient probes 6 mm the day of the abscess

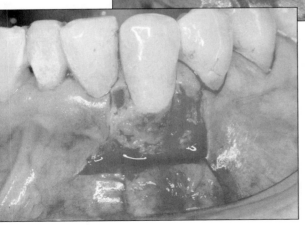

Fig. 16-69c Split thickness flap reflection reveals heavy subgingival calculus. However, the root is calculus free 3 mm apical to the CEJ. The effective area of subgingival instrumentation in this patient was 3 mm

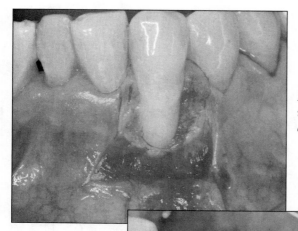

Fig. 16-69d Thorough root planing was accomplished

Fig. 16-69e The flap was repositioned with multiple sutures to assure good adaptation, similar to a free gingival graft

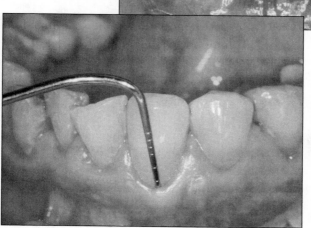

Fig. 16-69f Seven years later, the tissue is firm, and the gingival sulcus is non-probable

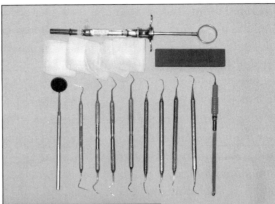

Fig. 16-70 Root planing and scaling instrument set up. A variety of curettes are used. Local anesthesia is used 95% of the time to maximize the subgingival depth that can be instrumented

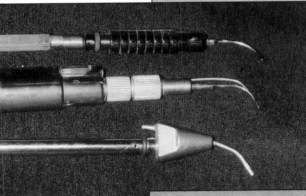

Fig. 16-71 Ultrasonic instruments are also used for scaling and root planing. In addition, a high-speed prophyjet is used to remove stains. It is more expedient than using a rubber cup and pumice

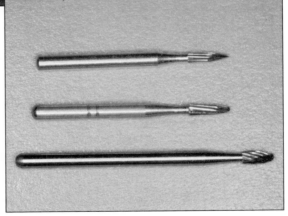

Fig. 16-72 High-speed finishing burs are also incorporated in the scaling and root planing armamentarium. The most frequently used burs are 12-fluted finishing burs and the neumeyer bur. They do not cut dentin very well and do not gouge the root surface. Patients experience less hypersensitivity than when using ultrasonics or hand instrumentation

probing depth and attachment level was recorded over one year. Similar results were obtained after the use of the ultrasonic and sonic instruments. Studies comparing hand instruments with the Titan-S sonic scaler did not disclose any differences in healing responses between the various instruments.[79]

It has been suggested that ultrasonic scalers produce an uneven root surface on a microscopic level. For this reason, some clinicians have recommended that ultrasonic scaling be supplemented with hand instrumentation to establish a smooth root surface.[80] However, many clinicians question whether a smooth root surface after treatment in subgingival areas is important for successful healing. Repeated instrumentation during the healing phase following root planing is generally not needed if adequate debridement can be accomplished during initial instrumentation. Differences between the various forms of instrumentation appear to be insignificant.

The use of high speed finishing burs for the removal of calcareous deposits has been described.[81] The author has found the use of finishing burs to be a useful adjunct in removing calculus and creating a smooth glassy root (Fig. 16-69a). A comparison of rotary diamonds and curettes in the removal of calculus from furcations found the rotary diamonds to be much more effective.[82] Finishing burs are able to access root concavities and furcation areas better than curettes, due to their smallness. Post-operative sensitivity appears to be less with rotary finishing burs than with ultrasonic and hand instrumentation. The time required for calculus removal also is significantly reduced with rotary instruments. For these reasons, they have become the author's preferred choice of root instrumentation.

The removal of caries, extraction of hopeless teeth, necessary endodontic treatment, and temporization are also important aspects of initial therapy. They can be performed concurrent with oral hygiene instructions and root planing and scaling. However, patient compliance in maintaining adequate oral hygiene is the main prerequisite for optimal healing.

Reevaluation

Reevaluation is performed at the termination of the initial phase of therapy. Initial therapy is the most important part of periodontal treatment. Therefore, a thorough examination and analysis of the dentition are essential. The reevaluation assesses the patient's healing response to periodontal therapy via a conventional periodontal examination. At present, the assessment of periodontal disease is done historically, primarily by the presence of pocket depth and inflammation. There are a number of commercially available diagnostic kits, which evaluate the presence of potentially pathogenic microorganisms and the presence of enzymes associated with tissue destruction. It would be valuable if a litmus test was available to determine the activity of periodontal disease. However, as of yet, one does not exist. Unfortunately, the predictive values of these kits have yet to be scientifically determined over an adequate length of time.[83]

In addition to an evaluation of the patient's periodontal status, of utmost importance is an evaluation of the patient's ability to adequately perform plaque control. Patients unable to perform excellent plaque control are not candidates for definitive periodontal and restorative treatment.

At the conclusion of initial therapy, data are collected and analyzed; and patients are categorized into one of the following categories:

1. The patient exhibits excellent oral hygiene, no gingival inflammation, and minimal pocket depth. No further active periodontal treatment is indicated, and the patient is placed into a maintenance program

2. The patient exhibits excellent oral hygiene and minimal gingival inflammation. However, significant pocket depth remains and some sites still continue to bleed on probing and exhibit periodontal inflammation. This patient is a candidate for corrective periodontal surgery in order to eliminate pocket depth, gain access to the roots for subgingival debridement, and possibly regenerate some of the lost attachment

617

3. The patient, despite repeated instruction in oral hygiene, exhibits poor plaque control (Fig 16-25b). Periodontal pocketing still remains, but the patient refuses or is unable to exercise proper home care. This patient is not a candidate for definitive periodontal surgery. The patient should be made aware of the problem that exists and a continued effort made to motivate the patient. This patient should be placed into a maintenance program with the goal of motivating the patient to achieve better oral hygiene so that definitive therapy can be performed and active disease eliminated. Surgical therapy in the absence of excellent plaque control is more detrimental than performing no surgery at all.[47]

Surgical Therapy

The management of plaque-induced periodontal disease is divided into phases:

- Examination
- Initial therapy
- Reevaluation
- Periodontal surgery/implant therapy/restorative therapy
- Maintenance

The goals of periodontal therapy are as follows:

- Control of disease
- Functional rehabilitation
- Regeneration
- Esthetic rehabilitation
- Maintenance of periodontal health

The goal of periodontal surgery is to restore health and function to the periodontium. Many periodontal surgical techniques exist. This chapter will explore and elucidate the procedures most useful in the practice of periodontal therapy.

Indications for surgical therapy

Four major indications for surgical therapy exist:

- Access for root debridement
- Pocket elimination
- Regeneration of soft and hard tissue
- Esthetic rehabilitation

Additional indications for periodontal surgery may also include the following:

- Removal of diseased periodontal tissues, creating a favorable environment for new attachment and/or readaptation of soft and/or osseous tissues
- Corrections of mucogingival deficiencies or defects
- Establishment of tissue contours that facilitate oral hygiene maintenance
- Creation of a favorable restorative environment
- Drainage of periodontal abscesses and biopsy and diagnosis[84]

Following initial therapy, significant pocketing and inflammation may still exist despite adequate oral hygiene. Pocket elimination therapy facilitates plaque control and allows access for further root debridement. Surgical therapy also allows for the regeneration of attachment, root coverage with soft tissue, and esthetic rehabilitation. Some of the surgical techniques available for the treatment of periodontal disease include the following:

- Gingival curettage
- Excisional new attachment procedure (ENAP)
- Gingivectomy
- Modified Widman flap
- Flap surgery
- Osseous surgery
- Osseous grafting
- Guided tissue regeneration
- Curtain procedures
- Papillary retention procedure
- Free gingival graft
- Subepithelial connective tissue graft
- Connective tissue graft for ridge augmentation
- Esthetic crown lengthening

The scope of this chapter does not permit a detailed analysis of all of the above surgical procedures. An attempt will be made to highlight the most frequently utilized and relevant of the aforementioned techniques.

Principles of Periodontal Surgery

Medical considerations

The surgical indications for periodontal surgery have been elucidated (see section on reevaluation and surgical indications). The importance of optimal-plaque control both pre-operatively and post-operatively cannot be overemphasized. Failure of a patient to comply with excellent oral hygiene is a *contraindication* to surgical treatment.[85]

Contraindications. The medical contraindications for periodontal surgery are similar to other minor outpatient surgical procedures. Hypertension should be controlled and monitored. Patients with recent myocardial infarctions should not be subjected to periodontal surgery within six months of hospitalization, and only after consultation with their physician. Patients on anticoagulant treatment have a propensity for increased bleeding. Their medications should be adjusted four to five days prior to surgery after consulting with the patient's physician. Salicylates should not be used for post-operative pain control since they further increase bleeding tendencies.

Diabetes mellitus. Uncontrolled diabetics should not be treated surgically.[86] A well-controlled diabetic may be treated providing precautions are taken so his/her insulin routine is not disturbed. It is usually recommended to treat diabetic patients early in the morning. The patient should eat breakfast and take his/her usual dose of insulin.[87] Diabetics have a lowered resistance to infection and a tendency to have a delay in wound healing. Therefore, diabetics should also be covered prophylactically with antibiotics.

Blood dyscrasias and pregnancy. Patients suffering from blood dyscrasisas, such as acute leukemia, agranulocytosis, and lymphogranulomatosis, should not be subjected to periodontal surgery. The surgical treatment of pregnant women is more controversial. Most Ob/Gyns advise against treatment during the first trimester. It is the author's opinion that periodontal surgery should be foregone until after pregnancy. The cost-risk-benefit ratio is clearly in favor of waiting six months, until the mother gives birth. From a medical/legal point of view, the benefits of waiting outweigh the risks of causing a problem with the pregnancy.

Antibiotic prophylaxis. Patients with mitral valve prolapse, congenital heart lesions, vascular implants, and prosthetic joint replacements should be premedicated with antibiotics one hour before surgery according with the recommendations of the American Heart Association, 2 grams of Amoxicillin by mouth one hour before therapy. If the patient is allergic to penicillin, clindamycin 600 mg is substituted.[44]

Smoking. Smoking is not a contraindication to performing periodontal surgery. However, smoking is a risk factor in the development of periodontal disease.[88] It negatively affects wound healing; and the healing response following bone regenerative procedures and mucogingival procedures is compromised.[89-92] Clearly, it is in the patient's best interest to not smoke. Patients should be informed of the risks smoking poses to the success of treatment. It should be noted that in implant surgery, smokers have a significantly higher failure rate than non-smokers, 28% compared to 7.5% in non-smokers.[93] Bain and Moy also found that smoking negatively impacted upon implant success.[46]

Pre-surgical instructions

Prior to surgery, all patients should have a consultation appointment with the dentist to review patient concerns, pre-operative instructions including medications, and post-operative instructions, and to obtain an informed consent. A copy of pre-surgical instructions is given to the patient during the pre-operative consultation.

Premedication. *All medications are called into the pharmacy for the patient prior to his/her appointment.* Patients appreciate the convenience of having their prescriptions ready at the pharmacy and not having to wait for them to be filled. Calling in the prescriptions also increases patient compliance. Secondly, following surgery, the patient does not have to stop at the pharmacy, for all the needed medications are at home and available for immediate use.

Analgesics. All patients are given an analgesic, to be taken one hour before their surgical appointment, usually a non-steroidal anti-inflammatory drug (NSAID). The amount of post-operative pain is diminished significantly by administering the analgesic prior to the onset of pain.[94-95] Ibuprofen, 600 mg, is the author's analgesic of choice. However, any of the other NSAIDs are acceptable. In fact, a new generation of NSAIDs has recently been introduced, called COX 2 inhibitors. Vioxx (refecoxib) 50 mg is one example. The benefit of using these medications is that there is less gastrointestinal upset, and there is increased patient compliance, for the dose is only one tablet a day.

NSAIDs not only relieve pain and reduce fever, but are anti-inflammatory as well. Some patients request acetaminophen, due to gastric sensitivity. This works well for pain, but has no anti-inflammatory properties. It has been the author's experience that patients experience minimal to no pain the day of surgery if they are premedicated and follow the postoperative protocol.

Antibiotic coverage. It is necessary to prescribe antibiotics to patients requiring prophylactic antibiotic coverage for medical reasons (see medical considerations). However, the use of antibiotics to improve surgical outcome and to prophylactically prevent postoperative infections is controversial.[96] A study of 884 operations performed without antibiotics revealed a 1% infection rate. A 2% infection rate was found in the same study on 43 operations performed with antibiotic coverage.[97] It is hard to justify antibiotic use in a healthy patient for routine periodontal surgery. However, some clinicians recommend antibiotic coverage for bone regenerative therapy, especially when a membrane is used. However, there is minimal research to support this. When an antibiotic is prescribed for regenerative therapy, Doxycycline is usually the antibiotic of choice, for it is concentrated in the gingival crevicular fluid at 5 to 7 times the concentration in the blood[98] and is effective against many of the pathogenic bacteria associated with periodontal disease.

Sedation. Pre-operative sedation for periodontal surgery is used often on several levels. Most patients experience some anxiety prior to having periodontal surgery performed. Patients like to be informed and to exercise some control over whether or not they would like to be sedated. The control of patient anxiety affects how the patient perceives the periodontal surgery as well as how much post-operative pain he/she experiences. People like to be in control. Thus, after patient education and discussion, four choices of the level of sedation are offered:

1. *Level one* is local anesthetic only. No sedation is given. The patients can drive themselves to and from the dental office. Few patients opt for this regimen, wishing rather some form of pre-operative sedation

2. *Level two* is the use of local anesthetic supplemented with nitrous oxide. This works well for many patients. However, some patients are not comfortable with nitrous oxide, for they feel they lose control. Nitrous oxide offers many benefits. It is safe, effective in the control of anxiety, potentates the effect of local anesthetic, inexpensive, and well tolerated in most patients

3. *Level three* includes the use of an oral sedative with or without the supplementation of nitrous oxide. Effective oral sedatives include diazepam (Valium), triazolam (Halcion), and zolepidem (Abien). The combination of nitrous oxide and Halcion 0.25 mg has been found to be as effective as intravenous sedation with Valium

4. *Level four* includes the use of intravenous sedation performed by a dentist/physician anesthesiologist. Intravenous conscious sedation medications may include sedatives (midazolam), narcotics (meperidine, nalbuphine), barbiturates (methohexital), and other agents, depending on each

individual patient's needs. The patient is monitored with an automatic blood pressure cuff, an electrocardiogram, pulse oximeter, and the constant presence of an anesthesiologist. It is the author's opinion that the surgeon should focus solely on the surgery, and not have the added responsibility of monitoring an IV-sedated patient. The dentist/physician anesthesiologist is responsible for monitoring the patient. This does increase the cost of the procedure, but the level of patient safety is greatly enhanced. The comfort of knowing that an anesthesiologist is monitoring the patient is immeasurable to the patient and to the operating dentist. Additional benefits include the reduction of patient anxiety, the ability to give intravenous antibiotics, analgesics, and steroids, significantly more control of the patient's level of consciousness, and the ability to reverse the level of sedation when needed.[99] It is the author's experience of more than 15 years that patients heal with less discomfort and with less pain when treated with intravenous sedation

An additional benefit is the ability to complete more patient treatment in one visit. Patients appreciate the decrease in office visits, travel time, multiple surgical events, multiple post-operative healing episodes, and the increased speed with which treatment is completed. The patient's dentists are also pleased with surgery being completed in one visit with intravenous sedation because the patient returns to their offices for restorative care much sooner than if the surgery was performed in multiple appointments.

Local anesthesia. Local anesthesia is always used during all periodontal surgical procedures, regardless of the level of sedation. The local anesthetic of choice is 2% Xylocaine (lidocaine) with 1:100,000 epinephrine. It is efficacious and controls hemostasis well in most patients. Local anesthetics with higher concentrations of epinephrine are used when additional hemostasis is needed.[100] A broad spectrum of local anesthetics is available to the dental surgeon.[101] Mepivocaine 3% (Carbocaine) without a vasoconstrictor is used when patients complain of an "allergic reaction" to local anesthetics. Some patients are hypersensitive to the presence of epinephrine in local anesthetics, and report an increase in anxiety and/or tachycardia when epinephrine is used. It is often difficult to achieve profound anesthesia in inflamed patients. The author has found that articaine (septocaine) 4% with 1:100,000 epinephrine is very effective in achieving anesthesia in these patients. This is a newer local anesthetic, recently introduced from Europe and Canada. There have been some reports of palatal sloughing, so its use on the palate should be avoided. At the conclusion of periodontal surgery, it is recommended to supplement the local anesthesia with a long-acting local anesthetic. Patients are given bupivacaine (Marcaine) with 1:200,000 epinephrine at the conclusion of periodontal surgical procedures. Bupivacine is a long-acting local anesthetic. Patients require less post-operative analgesics when bupivacaine is administered at the conclusion of surgery.[102] Soft tissue anesthesia lasts for five to eight hours. An advantage of a long-acting anesthetic is that the patient can take two to three doses of analgesic before the anesthetic has worn off. This results in significantly less post-operative pain, for the patient has achieved a significant blood level of analgesic before the onset of pain.

Surgical instrument and setup

Surgical instruments are stored in sterile, ready-to-use double-wrapped surgical packs. Various instrument sets are kept relative to the variety of surgical procedures performed—periodontal and mucogingival surgery, exodontia, autogenous block grafting and guided bone regeneration, and implant surgery. The double sterile wrapping of the instruments also serves the purpose of having two sterile drapes on which to set up the instruments during surgery. The basic periodontal surgical setup has almost all of the instruments that may be required during a periodontal surgical procedure, be it routine flap surgery, guided bone regeneration, crown lengthening, esthetic periodontal plastic surgery, gingival grafting, or ridge augmentation. The typical setup includes the following instruments (Fig. 16-73).

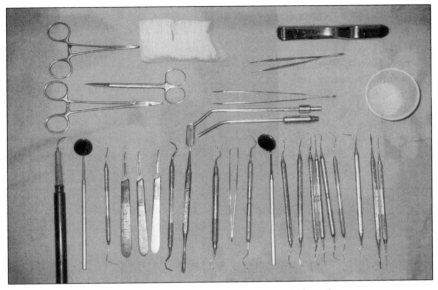

Fig. 16-73 *Typical instrument set up for periodontal surgery*

- Cavitron tip
- Two mouth mirrors
- Three scalpel handles with 15 c surgical blades
- Periodontal curettes
- Orban interproximal knife
- Prichard elevator
- Rhodes back-action chisel
- Tissue pickups
- Hirschfeld file
- Nabers furcation probe
- Explorer
- Oschenbien chisel
- Weidelstat chisel
- Interproximal file
- Tissue pliers
- Cotton pliers
- Needle holder
- Tissue scissors
- Mosquito hemostat
- Aspirator tips
- Physiologic saline
- Sterile gauze
- Cheek retractors
- Surgical burs (carbide round burs 8, 6, 4, 2; Neumeyer large and small surgical burs; 12 fluted finishing burs, 557 surgical bur, diamond burs)

Surgical procedures

There are numerous surgical procedures that exist for the treatment of periodontal disease. To further complicate matters, there are a multiplicity of periodontal diseases and periodontal situations, that present in patients who are in need of care. A thorough understanding of the multiplicity of periodontal diseases is essential if one is to perform surgical procedures. Each surgical procedure is designed to deal with a specific situation or to meet a certain objective. Surgical treatment is not cookie cutter. Surgical techniques often must be modified in order to achieve the appropriate therapeutic endpoint. An amalgamation of techniques and procedures is frequently necessary. Hence, surgery is customized and designed to meet the demands of each specific situation.

An attempt will be made to make sense out of the multiplicity of incision techniques, flap designs, regenerative, and resective procedures that are available. The scope will be limited to a discussion of the following:

- Flap surgery
- Osseous surgery
- Osseous grafting
- Guided tissue regeneration
- Papillary retention procedure
- Mucogingival surgery
- Ridge augmentation
- Esthetic crown lengthening

Flap surgery—designs and techniques

Flap surgery is all encompassing. All modalities of periodontal surgery incorporate some form of flap surgery, with the possible exception of the gingivectomy. Flap surgery is necessary when access is needed to bone or periosteum. Differences have existed in the definitions of the various forms of flap surgery. Incision design, flap thickness, and final positioning of the flap are all variable. This can be quite confusing. The indications and contraindications for each of these variables are important in the surgical decision-making process. Therefore, a classification system of flap surgical designs was developed in an attempt to clarify flap designs and techniques[103] (Table 16-12).

There are eight possible surgical flap designs based upon three different surgical criteria. The indications for each of the three criteria listed below will be elucidated:

- Sulcular versus inverse bevel incision

- Full-thickness versus partial-thickness flap

- Apically-positioned versus reposition flap

I. Sulcular
   A. Full thickness flap
      1) apically positioned
      2) repositioned
   B. Split thickness flap
      1) apically positioned
      2) repositioned
II. Inverse bevel
   A. Partial thickness flap
      1) apically positioned
      2) repositioned
   B. Split thickness flap
      1) apically positioned
      2) repositioned

Table 16-12 Surgical flap designs

Sulcular incisions

Indications for sulcular incisions include the following:

- Minimal attached gingiva

- Preservation of papillae

- Esthetic concerns

- Bone grafting

- Guided tissue regeneration

A sulcular incision is one in which the scalpel enters the sulcus and is directed along the long axis of the root until the scalpel comes in contact with the bone (Fig. 16-74a). The flap is then reflected and the surgery is performed. The flap may be full or partial thickness, depending upon the individual situation. Patients presenting with a very thin peri-

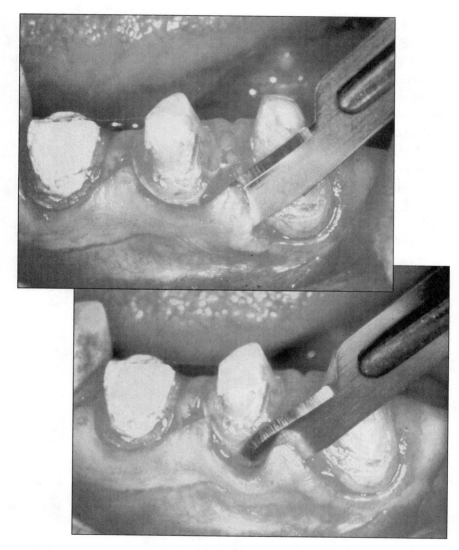

Fig. 16-74a Sulcular incision. The scalpel is placed into the sulcus and directed along the long axis of the tooth in order to preserve all of the attached gingiva

Fig. 16-74b Care is taken to preserve the entire papilla as well as all of the keratinized gingiva. The scalpel is used to incise as well as to reflect the tissue

odontium with minimal thickness of bone and minimal attached keratinized gingiva are candidates for sulcular incisions. Care is taken to preserve all of the keratinized gingiva. Note how the scalpel is directed so the keratinized gingiva, as well as the papillae, are preserved (Fig. 16-74b). It is easier to preserve tissue than to remove it and have to graft in the future.

Crown lengthening in the maxillary anterior region, the esthetic zone, is not a desirable procedure from the standpoint of esthetics. The soft tissue usually follows the underlying bony architecture,[104] thus removing bone to allow more of the root to be exposed can cause recession and an esthetic deformity. The patient in Figure 16-75a presented with a fractured lateral incisor. Treatment options included extraction and replacement with an implant, orthodontic extrusion following by crown lengthening and a new crown, or conservative esthetic crown lengthening followed by the fabrication of a new crown. The patient opted for the last option. Sulcular incisions were made to preserve the papilla, and the papillae were reflected from the palate to minimize recession (Figs. 16-75b, 16-75c, 16-75d). The larger the volume of tissue, the better the blood supply, and one is less likely to get necrosis and recession. Although care was taken to preserve papillae, minimal recession still occurred. It was necessary to remove some interproximal bone in order to expose enough tooth structure to fabricate a new crown. Papilla reformation was achieved a few years later when the adjacent crown was redone and the contact point was moved closer to the bone (Figs. 16-75e and 16-75f). The distance from the contact point to the bone was decreased. Thus, the formation of a new papilla was enhanced.[105]

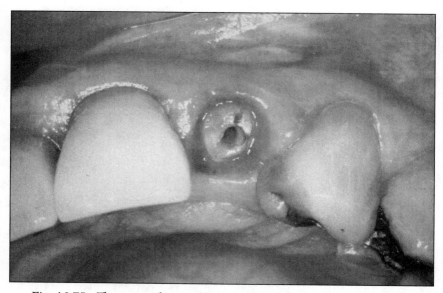

Fig. 16-75a *The patient fractured her maxillary lateral incisor subgingivally to the osseous crest. Crown lengthening was indicated in order to avoid invading the biologic width and to expose enough root to achieve crown retention*

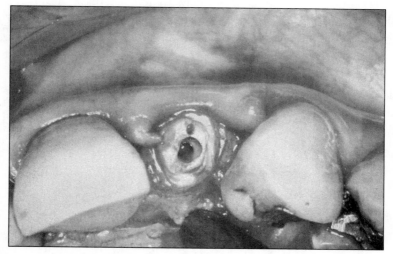

Fig. 16-75b *Sulcular incisions were made to preserve all of the keratinized tissue as well as the papillae. A palatal approach was used to preserve the entire papilla*

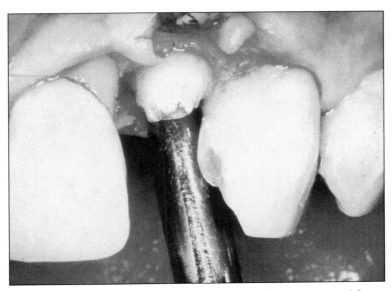

Fig. 16-75c Post-osseous surgery. Note that some bone was removed from the mesial of the central incisor. Some papillary loss will occur

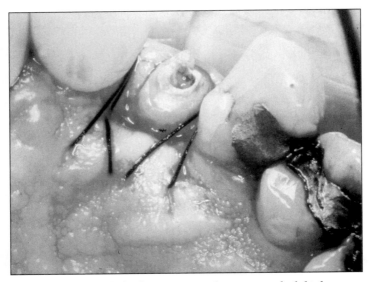

Fig. 16-75d The flap was sutured to preserve the labial papilla and eliminate pockets from the palatal

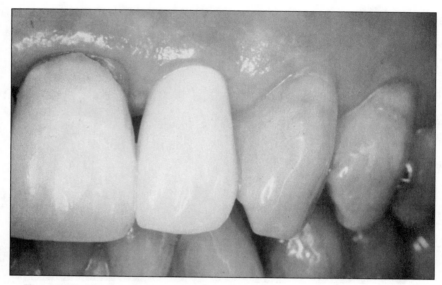

Fig. 16-75e Final restoration. Esthetics is good with the exception of the papilla between the lateral and central, which was lost due to the interproximal bone removal. Some recession is also seen on the labial of the central incisor

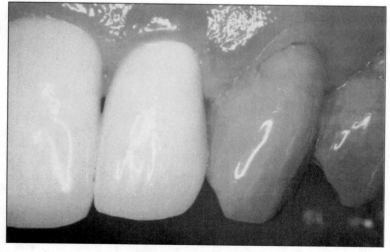

Fig. 16-75f Six years later, the central incisor crown was redone. This facilitated the growth of the papilla between the central and lateral. Ideal esthetics has now been achieved (Restorative dentistry courtesy of Dr. Keith Rudolph, Westport, CT)

Preservation of soft tissue is also desirable when *osseous grafting* is anticipated. Sulcular incisions allow the preservation of all of the keratinized tissue, therefore allowing complete closure of the wound and protection of the graft (Figs. 16-76a through 16-76h). There are minimal data on the quality of flap closure with the success of bone grafting results.[106] However, in the author's clinical experience, complete closure appears to enhance therapeutic results. Numerous studies report success in the placement of bone grafts.[107] However, long-term studies utilizing adequate controls, standardization of therapy, controls, histological evidence, and reproducibility have not been done. Osseous grafting is performed by most periodontists and clinically touted as a means of providing regeneration of the attachment apparatus. However, clinicians still await firm scientific evidence to support this commonly used therapy.

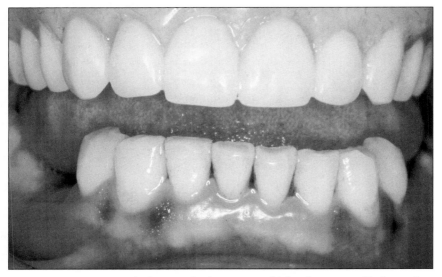

Fig. 16-76a Presurgical photograph of a 60-year-old female patient. She has only eight teeth remaining. She wears a complete maxillary denture. The goal of therapy is to maintain the mandibular teeth to support a removable partial denture

635

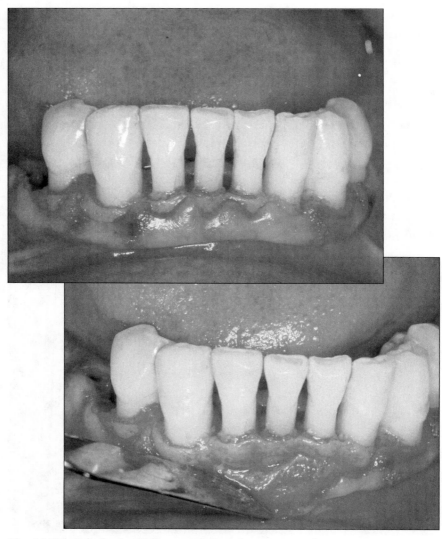

Fig. 16-76b Sulcular incisions are made in order to preserve the attached gingiva in anticipation of a bone-grafting procedure

Fig. 16-76c A full thickness flap is elevated, exposing the underlying alveolar bone. Interproximal defects are evident

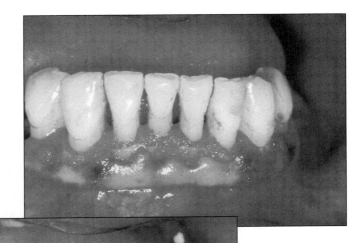

Fig. 16-76d
Autogenous bone
is harvested and
packed into the
interproximal
craters once they
have been
debrided and the
root meticulously
root planed

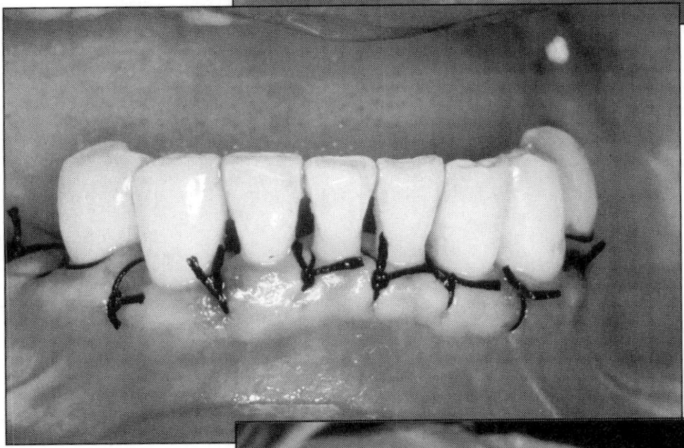

Fig. 16-76e The
facial and lingual
flaps are elevated
to achieve primary
closure with inter-
rupted sutures

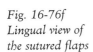

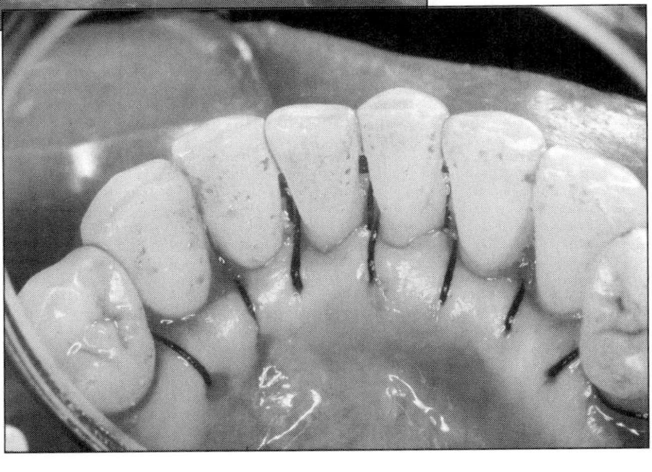

Fig. 16-76f
Lingual view of
the sutured flaps

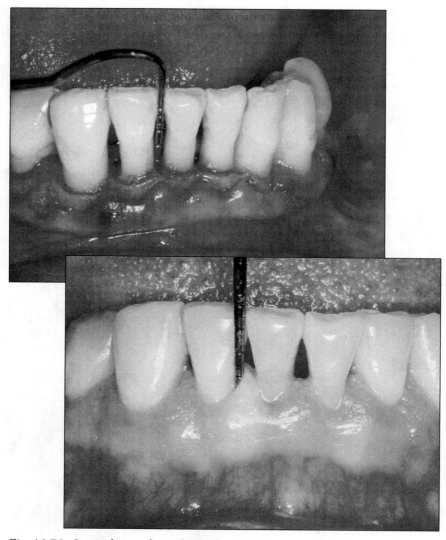

Fig. 16-76g *Surgical view of a probe in place measuring the attachment loss of approximately 3.5 mm*

Fig. 16-76h *Five-year postoperative result. About 3 mm of attachment has been regenerated, and the patient is stable. She is maintained on a three-month recall program*

Guided tissue regeneration (GTR) is a surgical procedure that attempts to regenerate lost periodontal structures through differential tissues responses, utilizing a barrier membrane. Gore-Tex, ePTFE, is perhaps the most scientifically researched of the barrier membranes. In 1976, Melcher[108] suggested that four components made up the connective tissue of the periodontium—gingiva, periodontal ligament, bone, and cementum. He hypothesized that progenitor cells for the formation of new connective tissue attachment reside in the periodontal ligament. This concept was proven by Gottlow,[109] who utilized barrier membranes in monkeys to regenerate new attachment. The following case demonstrates the clinical application of this procedure (Figs. 16-77a through 16-77i). Sulcular incisions are utilized and allow the membrane to remain beneath the gingiva, healing unmolested from the oral environment, and minimizing bacterial colonization of the membrane.[110] Studies have shown that GTR treatment is predictable and that the attachment gain can be maintained on a long-term basis.[111-112]

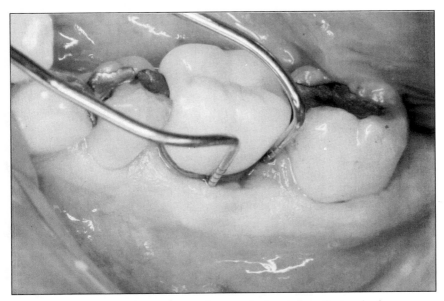

Fig. 16-77a Pretreatment photograph of periodontally-involved mandibular molar. Probing reveals a circumferential defect

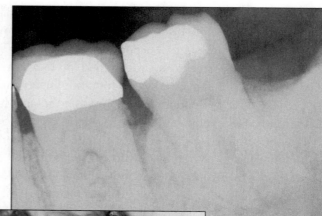

Fig. 16-77b Pretreatment radiograph demonstrates vertical bone loss and subgingival calculus

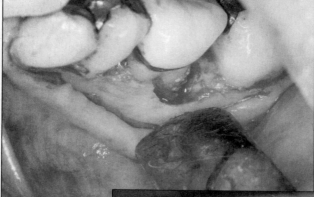

Fig. 16-77c Sulcular incisions with a full thickness flap expose the defect. Calculus is present on the distal of the mandibular first molar

Fig. 16-77d The root is meticulously debrided with high speed finishing burs to reveal a glossy white hard surface, free of endotoxins. It will now be treated with tetracycline paste for five minutes, prior to application of the bone grafting material

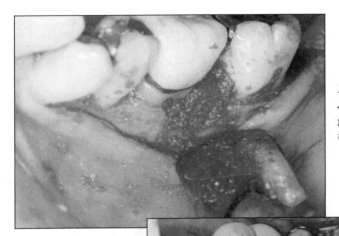

Fig. 16-77e Autogenous bone graft is placed into the defect

Fig. 16-77f A Gore-Tex (ePTFE) membrane is placed over the bone graft and sutured to place with two circumferential sutures

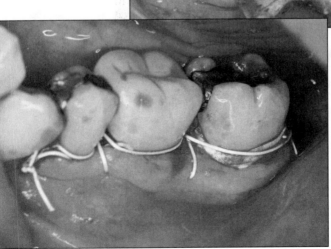

Fig. 16-77g The flap is coronally repositioned to obtain primary closure. Buccal periosteal releasing incisions are made to allow tension-free closure

641

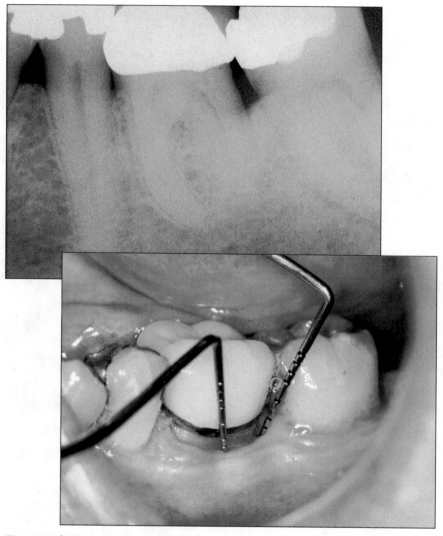

Fig. 16-77h Six year post-treatment radiograph
reveals bone fill and crestal cortication

Fig. 16-77i Post treatment, the mandibular molar
probes 1 to 2 mm, a 5 mm gain of probing attachment

Inverse bevel incisions

Indications for inverse bevel incisions include the following:

- Plenty of attached gingiva
- Pocket elimination
- Elimination of hyperplastic gingival, e.g., dilantin hyperplasia

An inverse bevel incision is one where the scalpel is angled to the tooth at a 45-degree apical to the free gingival margin. By definition, some keratinized tissue is removed (Fig. 16-78). This incision design assures that more tooth structure will be shown, for soft tissue is removed during the procedure. Contraindications for this incision include esthetics and minimal attached gingiva.

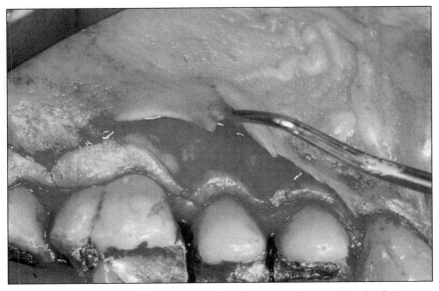

Fig. 16-78 An inverse bevel is used on the palate where pocket depth is present. Adequate keratinized tissue is always present on the palate; therefore, it is impossible to create a mucogingival defect. By design, gingival tissue is removed, and more of the root will be exposed

Where adequate keratinized gingiva exists (Fig. 16-78) and pocket elimination is the goal of therapy, an inverse bevel incision may be employed. The goal of treatment in cases of gingival hyperplasia is the removal of excess overgrown gingival tissues. The inverse bevel incision is the incision of choice when excess tissue is to be removed in conjunction with a gingival flap (Figs. 16-79a, 16-79b, and 16-79c).

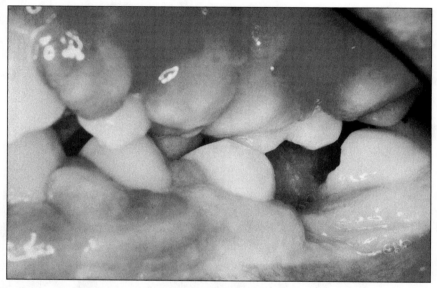

Fig. 16-79a Dilantin-induced gingival hyperplasia. Excess gingival tissue is present and is to be removed. An inverse bevel incision is the incision of choice

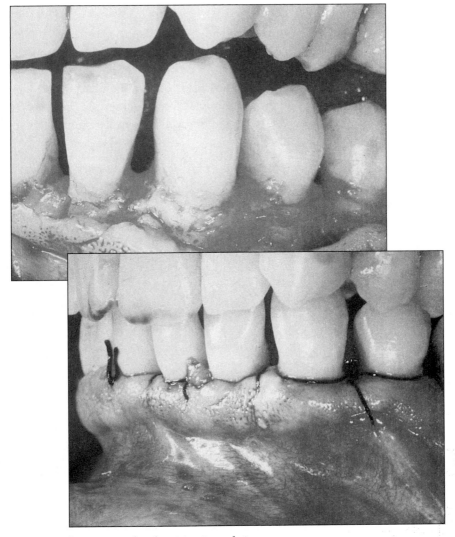

Fig. 16-79b *An inverse bevel incision is made in conjunction with a full thickness mucoperiosteal flap*

Fig. 16-79c *The flap is apically positioned with a continuous sling suture. Excess tissue has been removed, root debridement performed, and the pockets eliminated*

Full-thickness flap

A full-thickness flap is the most widely used flap to expose the underlying bone. The initial incision is made to the underlying bone and the flap is reflected along the crestal margin of bone, usually with the aid of a curette or a periosteal elevator. The periosteum is included in the flap, and the bone is left denuded. Full bony access is achieved (Fig. 16-80). Osseous resective surgery bone regeneration, or simple open debridement, is possible.

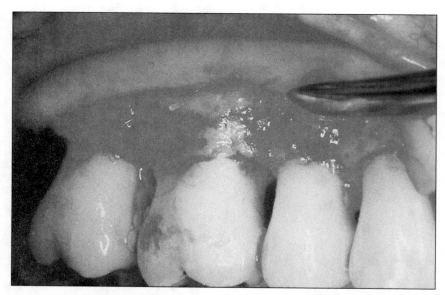

Fig. 16-80 Full thickness flap includes the periosteum and allows access to underlying alveolar bone. Bone grafting, osteoplasty, or simple debridement are possible

Osseous surgery is periodontal surgery involving modification of the bone. The principal goal of osseous surgery is the creation of a bony architecture, which is compatible with the maintenance of a physiologic gingival architecture.[113] An attempt is made to remove the most minimal amount of bone via osteoplasty (reshaping of the bone) rather than by osteotomy (removal of tooth supporting bone). It is better to err on the side of conservatism when performing osseous surgery (Figs. 16-81a through 16-81d). It is much more difficult to regenerate bone than to take it away. In the maxillary arch, a palatal approach[114] to osseous crater removal is employed. Advantages of this approach include:

- Better surgical access via the larger palatal embrasures

- Less post-surgical bone resorption on the palatal due to the presence of increased cancellous bone

- Avoidance of the buccal molar furcations, especially the maxillary first molar, which has a facial root trunk length that averages only 4 mm

A guiding surgical principle is to avoid the exposure of furcations. One does not want to make the patient more periodontally prone by performing surgery. *Above all do no harm!*

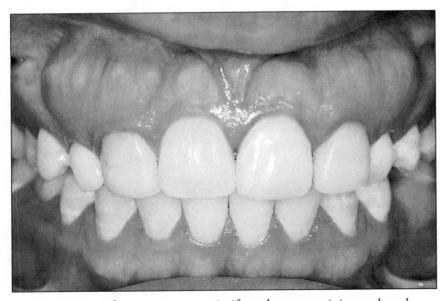

Fig. 16-81a Before osseous surgery, significant bony exostosis is seen throughout the buccal aspect of the maxilla. Patient has veneers on teeth #7, #8, #9, and #10. She is not satisfied with the cosmetics of the teeth. In addition, the alveolar bony overgrowth causes her to have a "cheeky" look. The patient feels that her face appears swollen due to the excess bone

Fig. 16-81b Full thickness flap reflection reveals the bony exostosis. The removal of the excess bone via osteoplasty was the goal of therapy

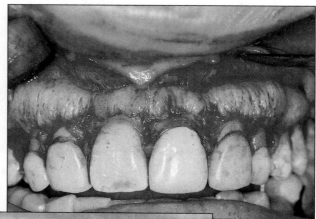

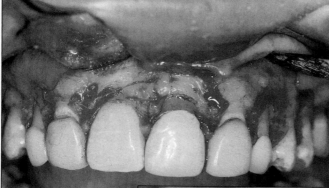

Fig. 16-81c Osteoplasty has been completed. In addition, crown lengthening was performed in order to allow the new veneers to be more harmonious

Fig. 16-81d Teeth #6 through #11 have new veneers. Cosmetically, they are more pleasing. Compare to Figure 16-81a. In addition, the excess bony overgrowth has been removed, and the patient is more pleased with her appearance (Restorative dentistry courtesy of Dr. Mark Samuels, Stratford, CT)

Partial-thickness flap

The partial-thickness flap is a split-thickness flap, in which the periosteum is left on the bone and the gingiva is split by sharp dissection apically (Fig. 16-82). Some therapists believe that crestal bone loss is diminished when partial-thickness flaps are employed and the exposure of alveolar bone is minimized. This is controversial, and the literature is unclear on this subject.[115] Partial-thickness flaps are used by some clinicians to protect the underlying bone from resorption, especially in areas of thin alveolar plates (Fig. 16-83).

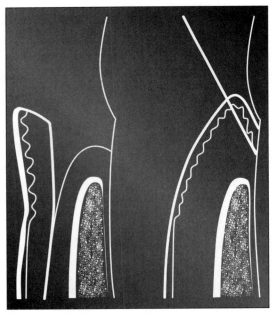

Fig. 16-82 Diagram of a split (partial) thickness flap. The flap is reflected by sharp dissection, and the periosteum is left attached to the bone

The partial-thickness flap is primarily utilized for pedicle tissue grafts, free gingival grafts, or for providing a base for precise suturing. Another indication is to increase the amount of keratinized tissue by apically moving the mucogingival junction without performing a mucogingival graft. [116] The split thickness flap is apically positioned and sutured to the (Figs. 16-84a, 16-84b, and 16-84c). This effectively increases the band of keratinized tissue.

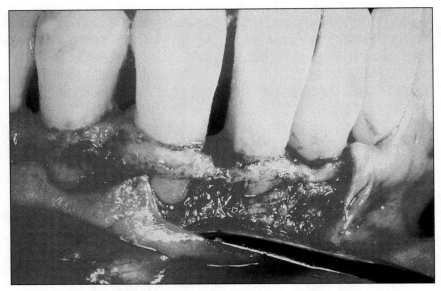

Fig. 16-83 Partial-thickness flap is used to protect the underlying bone from resorption. Note the tooth fenestration on the canine. Once this was observed, partial-thickness dissection was commenced in order to avoid further root exposure. An attempt was made to avoid buccal root recession

Apically-positioned versus repositioned flaps

Apically-positioned flaps are placed apical to the original free gingival margin. Indications include pocket elimination, crown lengthening procedures, increased zone of keratinized gingiva, and alteration of dental gingival margins for esthetics and dental harmony.

Repositioned flaps are replaced in their original position. Indications include guided bone regeneration, osseous grafting, subepithelial connective tissue grafts, ridge augmentation procedures, esthetics, and papilla preservation.

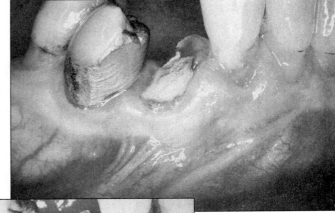

Fig. 16-84a Preoperative view of mandibular canine in need of crown lengthening. Minimal keratinized tissue is present

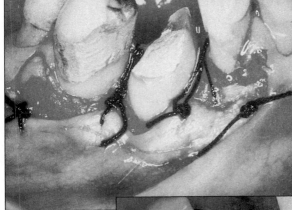

Fig. 16-84b A partial-thickness flap was elevated apical to the area of crown lengthening. The attached periosteum was used to apically tack the reflected flap. This technique is used in order to increase the band of keratinized gingiva. The use of a gingival graft is avoided

Fig. 16-84c One-week post crown lengthening surgery, the beginning of a new mucogingival junction is seen. The wound is still healing, but an increased band of keratinized tissue can clearly be seen

Today, an attempt is made to regenerate rather than resect bone in the treatment of periodontal disease. Esthetics is of paramount importance to patients. The emphasis on esthetics and regeneration has changed the philosophy of surgical therapy. Whenever possible, an attempt is made to reposition rather than apically position the flap.

Papillary retention procedure

Severe periodontal disease in the anterior maxilla can be very disfiguring. Bone loss and subsequent papillae loss lead to open gingival embrasures. Food impaction, problems with speech, and esthetic compromises are but a few of the negative sequella. In the past, periodontal surgery in this area exacerbated the cosmetic deformities (Fig. 16-1). In the 1980s, periodontists became more cosmetically oriented, and techniques were developed that minimized papillary loss post-surgically.[117] A modification of this procedure has been very effective in eliminating maxillary periodontal disease without causing additional esthetic disfigurement.[118]

Indications for the papillary retention procedure include:

- Severe maxillary anterior periodontal disease and attachment loss
- Prosthetic anterior maxillary treatment is not planned
- Root planing and scaling have been completed
- Oral hygiene is excellent
- Pocket depth is greater than 5 mm interproximally and palatally
- Labial pocket depth is minimal
- Patients are committed to a three-month maintenance program

The surgical approach is palatal. Minimal to no surgery is done on the labial surfaces of these teeth, for minimal pocket depth is present labially, due to the anatomy of the anterior maxilla. Bone loss on the labial aspect of maxillary anterior teeth usually results in gingival recession. An inverse bevel incision is made palatally, and the palatal granulation tissue is removed. Access is gained for root planing palatally and interprox-

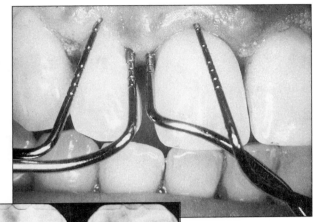

Fig. 16-85a Probing of a patient post initial therapy and pre-periodontal surgery. Patient has generalized severe periodontitis

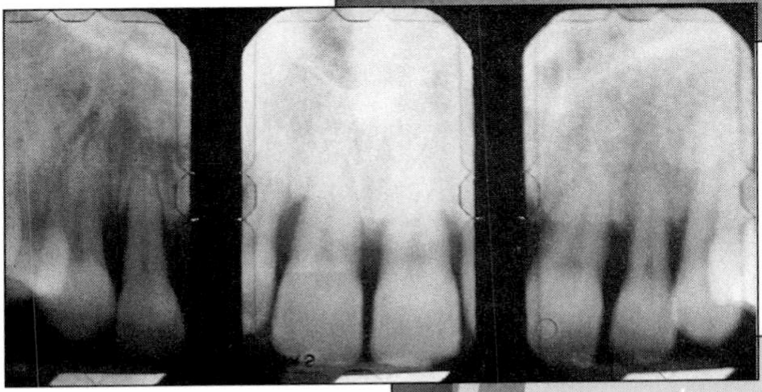

Fig. 16-85b Radiographs of the maxillary anterior teeth reveal 50 to 80% bone loss

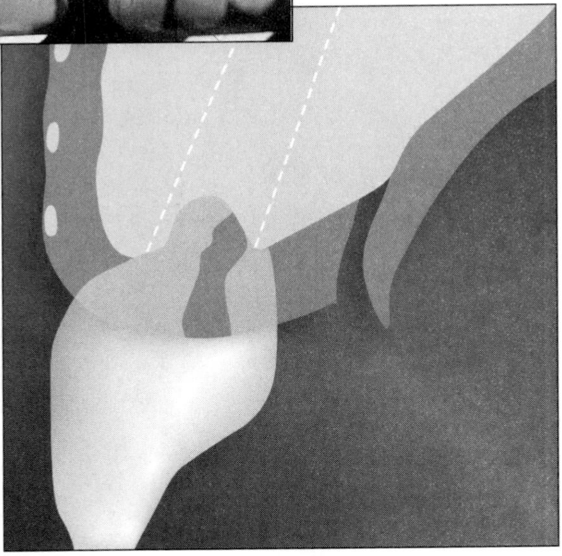

Fig. 16-85c Diagram of the initial incision, an inverse bevel palatal incision

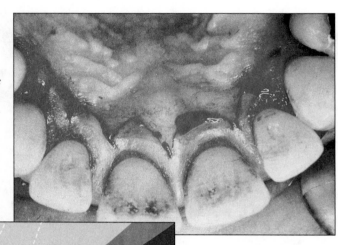

Fig. 16-85d
Clinical view of the
initial continuous
inverse bevel inci-
sion. Note the
papillae are
kept intact

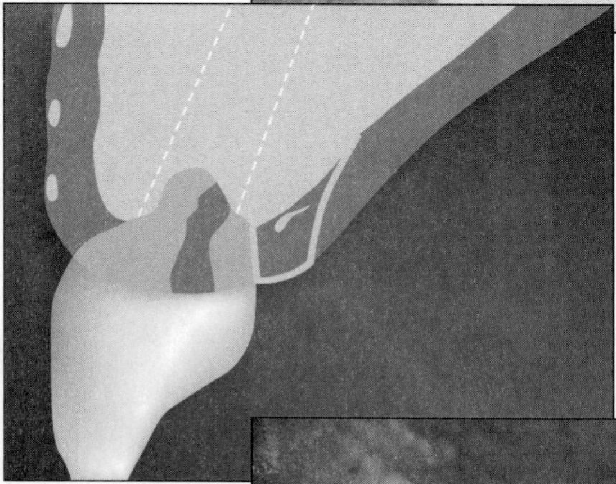

Fig. 16-85e Diagram of the
secondary incision, a continuous sulcular incision

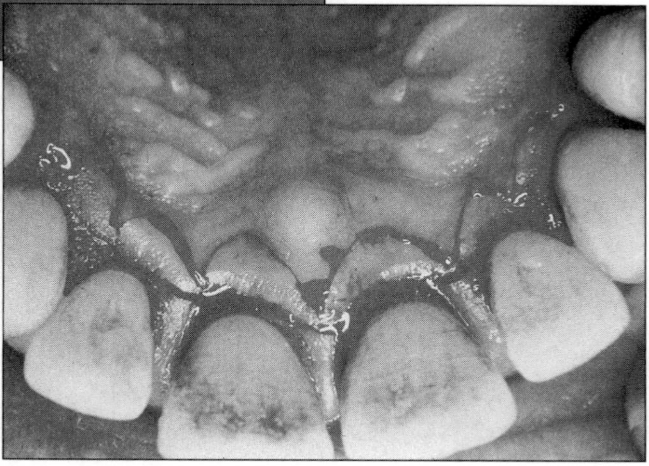

Fig. 16-85f
Clinical view of
the sulcular inci-
sion. The incision
begins in the sulcus
and connects to
adjacent teeth from
the palatal line
angles of the teeth,
so that the papil-
lae are not incised

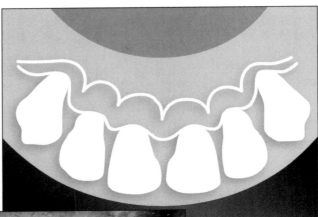

Fig. 16-85g Diagram of the two initial palatal incisions

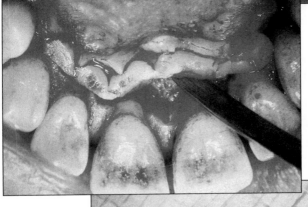

Fig. 16-85h The third incision connects the inverse bevel and sulcular incisions. An instrument is placed at the base of the sulcular incision and used to elevate the tissue defined by the two incisions off of the bone

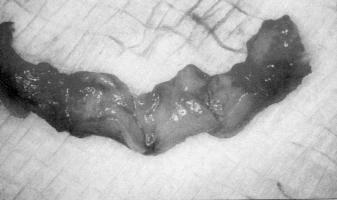

Fig. 16-85i The wedge of tissue is removed. It can be used for a connective tissue graft or discarded

655

Fig. 16-85j Access
is now possible to
root plane the
palatal and inter-
proximal surfaces.
The bone can be
treated with
osseous surgery,
bone grafting,
guided tissue
regeneration, or
simply debrided

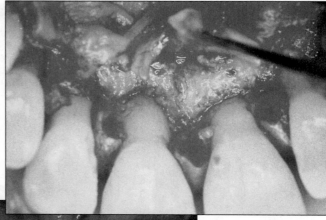

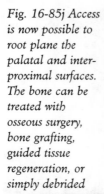

Fig. 16-85k Buccal
view of the suturing
technique. Since a
buccal flap was not
elevated, there is no
need to suture

Fig. 16-85l The
palatal tissues are
sutured with a con-
tinuous sling. In this
case, a horizontal
mattress suture is
also incorporated to
achieve good adap-
tation of the palatal
tissues to the under-
lying bone

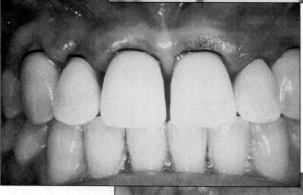

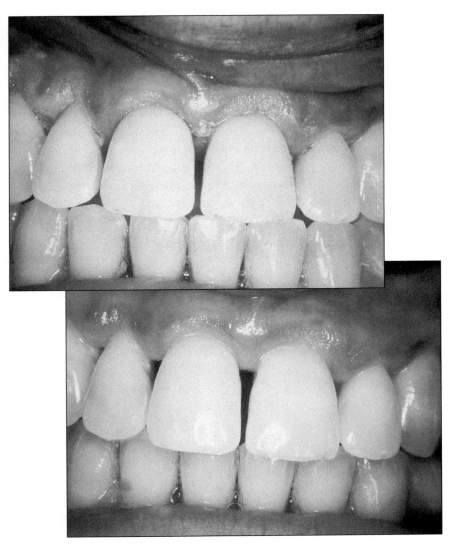

Fig. 16-85m Labial view of the patient prior to surgery

Fig. 16-85n Labial view of the patient three months following surgery. Pockets have been eliminated, and recession is minimal

imally (Figs. 16-85a through 16-85n). The bony defects can be treated with grafting, osteoplasty, or open debridement. The suturing technique can be a continuous sling or interrupted with a vertical mattress labially to maintain papilla position (Figs. 16-85k and 16-85l).

A study of 20 treated patients in the author's practice revealed that over five years, interproximal and palatal pockets could successfully be eliminated without causing labial gingival recession or any cosmetic compromise. Bony architecture remained stable or improved, although no bone grafting was performed (Figs. 16-86a through 16-86d). These patients are prone to periodontal disease, and placement on a maintenance program is essential for predictable success.

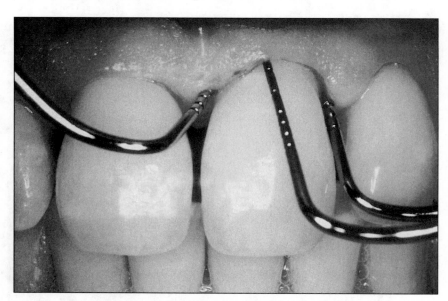

Fig. 16-86a Labial view of patient prior to periodontal surgery. Note that the labial pocket depth is minimal. Interproximally, the patient probes 7 to 8 mm

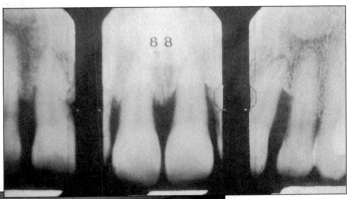

Fig. 16-86b Pretreatment radiograph reveals 60 to 80% bone loss

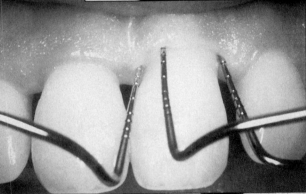

Fig. 16-86c Five years following peri- odontal papillary retention flap surgery, periodontal probing is 1 to 2 mm. Clinically, the patient is well main- tained. He is on a three-month recall program

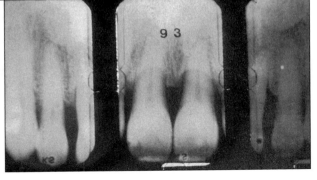

Fig. 16-86d Radiograph taken five years post periodontal surgery. Note that bone level has not appears to have regen- erated. Bone grafting was not performed. The author finds that some bone regenera- tion is possible when periodontally involved roots are debrided, excellent oral hygiene is maintained, and the patient is on a frequent recall program

Mucogingival Surgery

In 1950, Friedman first introduced the term "mucogingival surgery."[119] This was the early era of resective periodontal therapy. Oral health was the primary surgical objective. Most mucogingival procedures at that time were aimed at increasing the amount of keratinized tissue (Fig. 16-87). The question of what constituted an "adequate" band of attached gingival tissue was debated. Over the past two decades, the field of mucogingival surgery has undergone dramatic refinement. New techniques for achieving periodontal regeneration have also encompassed the field of mucogingival surgery. The multiplicity of mucogingival surgical procedures in the periodontist's armamentarium has led P. D. Miller to coin the term "periodontal plastic surgery."[120]

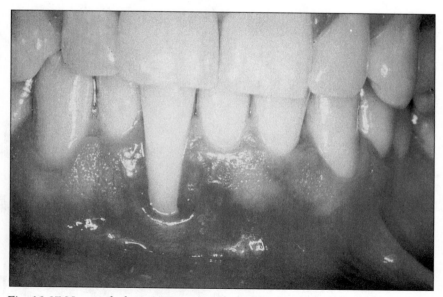

Fig. 16-87 No attached gingiva is present on the labial surface of the right mandibular central incisor. The tissue is inflamed, and oral hygiene is difficult to perform. There is no question that this tooth needs to be repaired. Recession has approached the apex of the incisor, and the tooth may soon be lost. The prognosis for this tooth is guarded

Health and esthetics are the two main indications for mucogingival surgery. Much is published on what categorizes an adequate band of attached tissue. However, no absolute truth exists. In general, one would like to see 2 mm of healthy, non-inflamed, attached, keratinized tissue about teeth, but this is also debatable.

The rationale for the treatment of mucogingival deformities comes down to clinical judgment. Some indications for mucogingival surgery include—increasing recession and/or inflammation despite good oral hygiene, a predisposition to recession, thin tissue in a patient about to undergo orthodontic treatment, a shallow vestibule preventing adequate oral hygiene, root sensitivity, aesthetics, and root caries. A number of mucogingival considerations are outlined in Table 16-13.

Three of the most common mucogingival procedures will be reviewed. These include the free gingival graft, the subepithelial connective tissue graft, and connective tissue ridge augmentation. Many others exist and they may be reviewed by the interested reader.[121-122]

Free gingival graft

The free gingival graft was introduced in 1963.[123] Sullivan and Atkins[124] first described its potential for achieved root coverage in area of gingival recession.

- No attached gingiva
- Thinness of the attached gingiva
- Increasing inflammation
- Increasing loss of attachment
- Prophylactic prevention of attachment loss
- Prosthetic concerns
- Orthodontic movement
- Shallow vestibule
- Elimination of frenum and muscle attachments
- Oral hygiene considerations
- Root coverage
- Improved esthetics
- Root sensitivity
- Root caries
- Ridge deficiency

Table 16-13 Mucogingival considerations

The free gingival graft placed on periosteum is a very predictable procedure and has a success rate close to 100%. In 1982, Miller reported excellent root coverage, utilizing what was at the time an innovative surgical technique.[125] Although technique sensitive, Miller's procedure is still a viable one today.

Indications for the free gingival graft include:[126]

- Progressive recession
- Root sensitivity
- Caries proclivity
- Oral hygiene facilitation
- Pre-orthodontic gingival stabilization
- Esthetic considerations
- Minimization of further recession in the presence of restorative dentistry
- Increase vestibular depth

Performance of the free gingival graft requires two surgeries—harvesting the graft from the palate and placing the graft upon its recipient site. The free gingival graft may be used to increase the zone of keratinized gingiva or for root coverage of a denuded root. Root coverage is the more technique sensitive. The first step in the procedure is to prepare the recipient site. The mucoperiosteal bed is prepared so that it extends approximately 5 mm past the apical margin of the denuded root. Vertical incisions are made a least one papilla mesial and distal to the recipient site (Figs. 16-88a through 16-88f). The exposed root is root planed with rotary finishing burs and treated with a tetracycline paste for five minutes.

The graft dimensions are determined, and the donor tissue is harvested from the palate, care being taken not to include rugae, for the esthetic result will be compromised. The epithelium and connective tissue are taken, the graft having a thickness of 1.0 to 1.5 mm. The graft should be in as much contact with the bleeding recipient periosteum as

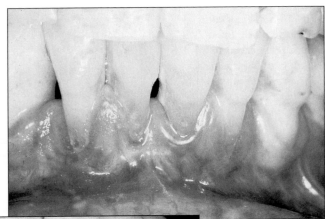

Fig. 16-88a A 50-year-old woman presents with recession of the mandibular anterior teeth

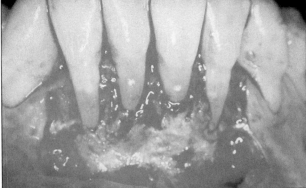

Fig. 16-88b The recipient site is prepared. The mucoperiosteal bed extends 5 mm past the denuded roots apically and one papilla past the roots to be covered. This ensures an adequate blood supply to the graft

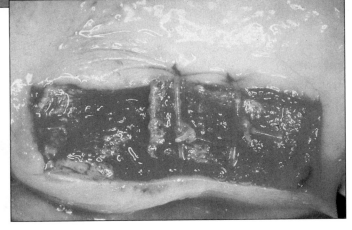

Fig. 16-88c The graft is harvested from the palate. Note the size of the wound. Healing must occur by secondary intention

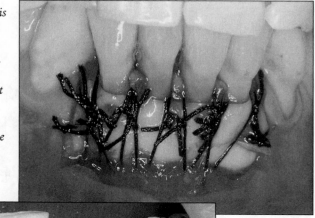

Fig. 16-88d The graft is sutured to place. Initial stabilization occurs by suturing to the papillae. Circumferential sutures sync the graft to the root surface and the periosteal bed, assuring good blood supply to the graft and eliminating a dead space between the graft and the root

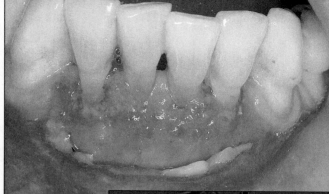

Fig. 16-88e One week post-operatively, the graft is edematous and red. This is a positive sign of graft vitality

Fig. 16-88f Five-year post operative result. The graft is healthy, does not probe, and 5 mm of root coverage has been achieved

possible. This ensures a better blood supply and improves the likelihood that the graft will "take." The donor site is dressed with sterile gauze soaked in cyanoacrylate and covered with a periodontal dressing (Figs. 16-89a, 16-89b, and 16-89c). The graft is then transferred to the previously prepared bed and sutured in place at the papillae. A continuous horizontal suture is positioned in a mesial to distal direction across the graft surface to stretch the graft and synch it to the underlying periosteum. Circumferential sutures are also placed to eliminate dead space between the graft and the perisoteal bed (Fig. 16-88d). Gauze pressure is applied for five minutes. Periodontal dressing is optional.

The patient is seen at one week for suture removal. The patient is placed on a liquid diet for two days and then a soft diet for three weeks, and instructed not to brush the graft for four weeks. Chlorhexidine, 0.12 % mouthwash is used until regular toothbrushing can be reestablished.

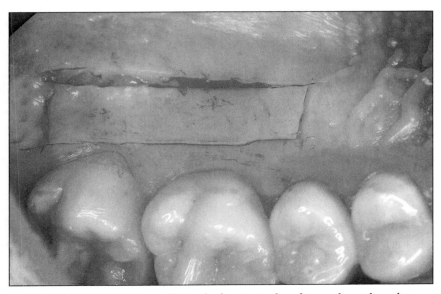

Fig. 16-89a An incision outlining the free gingival graft is made on the palate

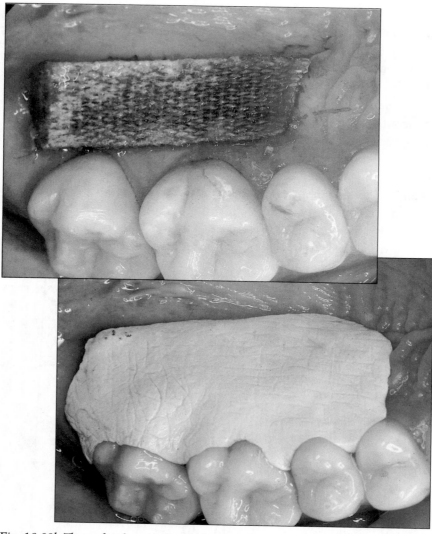

Fig. 16-89b *The graft is harvested, and the wound is dressed with a piece of iodoform gauze soaked in cyanoacrylate. This serves as an immediate "scab" and helps hemostasis*

Fig. 16-89c *A periodontal dressing is applied to the iodoform gauze. Once the gauze is soaked in the cyanoacrylate, it harden, thus allowing the periodontal dressing to adhere to it. The purpose of the dressing is patient comfort and hemostasis*

The free gingival graft placed without an attempt at root coverage does not require the surgical precision of the graft placed for root coverage. The success rate is also greater. The suturing technique does not require the circumferential and horizontal sutures (Figs. 16-90a through 16-90d).

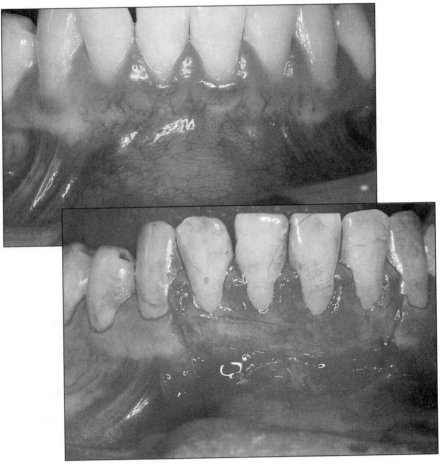

Fig. 16-90a Preoperative view of minimal keratinized gingiva

Fig. 16-90b Bed preparation via split thickness flap. Periosteum is left as a base for the free gingival graft

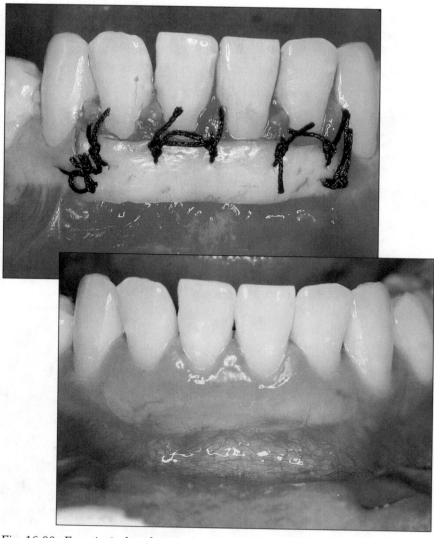

Fig. 16-90c Free gingival graft sutured to place with simple interrupted sutures at the papilla. Additional sutures are not necessary when root coverage is not attempted

Fig. 16-90d Six-month post-operative result. A healthy thickened band of keratinized tissue is evident. The graft blends with the papilla, for they were de-epithelialized as part of the procedure

Subepithelial connective tissue graft

Langer and Langer introduced the subepithelial connective tissue graft in 1985.[127] Indications for the subepithelial connective tissue graft are:[126]

- Root coverage when a gingival color match is aesthetically important
- Similar coverage for multiple root exposures
- Avoidance of "keloid" formation
- Recession adjacent to an edentulous area that also requires ridge augmentation
- Same indications as the free gingival graft, with the exception of increasing vestibular depth. This technique *will not increase* the vestibular depth

This technique revolutionized gingival grafting. In comparison to the free gingival graft, better color match can be achieved since the epithelium covering the graft is from adjacent tissue, not from the palate. Larger areas can be covered due to the surgical design. The free gingival graft obtains its blood supply from only the underlying periosteum. In contrast, the subepithelial connective tissue graft has a *dual* blood supply. In addition to the underlying periosteum, the coronally-repositioned pedicle flap nourishes the graft on the facial surface. A larger blood supply leads to a better, well-nourished graft, and the potential now exists for increased success and the ability to graft larger areas.

Similar to other gingival grafting, two surgeries are required. The area of recession is identified, and the graft bed is prepared (Figs. 16-91a through 16-91g). A partial thickness flap is elevated with two vertical incisions placed one papilla mesial and distal to the area of recession. The partial-thickness flap is dissected apically past the mucogingival junction, taking care not to perforate. root planing is performed with rotary finishing burs and then chemically conditioned with tetracycline for five minutes. The donor tissue is harvested from the anesthetized hard palate. An inverse bevel horizontal incision is made 3 mm from the teeth. A second

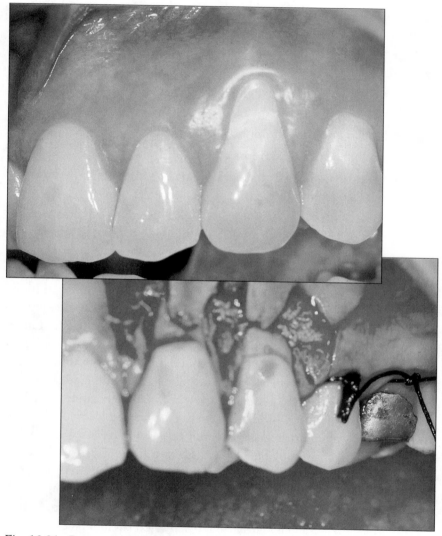

Fig. 16-91a Pre-operative view of recession of teeth #11 and #12.
Patient complains of sensitivity and is unhappy with the cosmetics

Fig. 16-91b Preparation of the recipient site. A partial-thickness flap is elevated
from the line angles of the teeth adjacent to the teeth that are to be grafted. Vertical
incisions are made at the ends of the flap to assure coverage of the graft

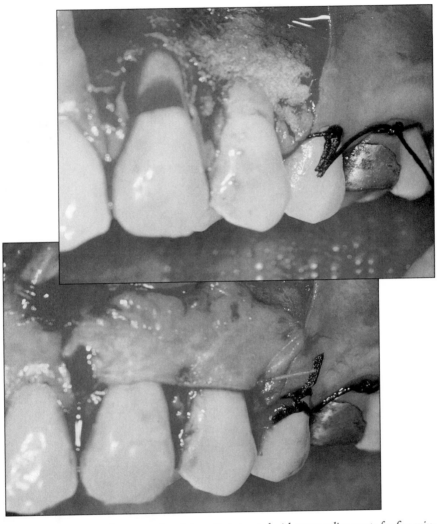

Fig. 16-91c The prepared recipient site is treated with tetracycline paste for five minutes. Note the yellowish color of the periosteum. Tetracycline treatment is performed in order to disinfect the wound, inhibit tissue collagenases, detoxify the root, and open up the dentinal tubules in preparation for the connective tissue graft

Fig. 16-91d The connective tissue graft is transferred to the recipient site and sutured with (5-0) gut to the papillae. Additional sutures may be placed laterally to stabilize and secure the graft

Fig. 16-91e The flap is coronally positioned in order to cover the connective tissue graft. This serves as an additional blood supply to nourish the graft. Vertical and periosteal releasing incisions assure that the flap will lie passively over the graft

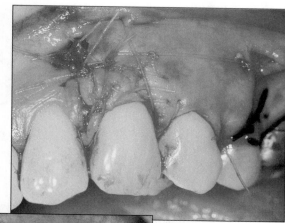

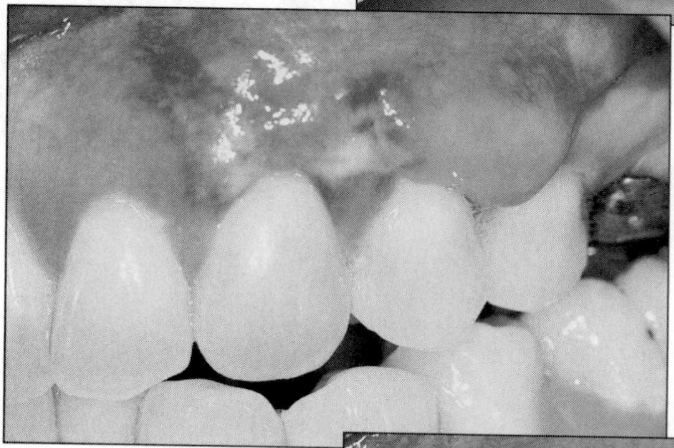

Fig. 16-91f At one week post surgery, excellent healing is evident. Hemorrhagic edematous tissues at one week are a sign of good healing

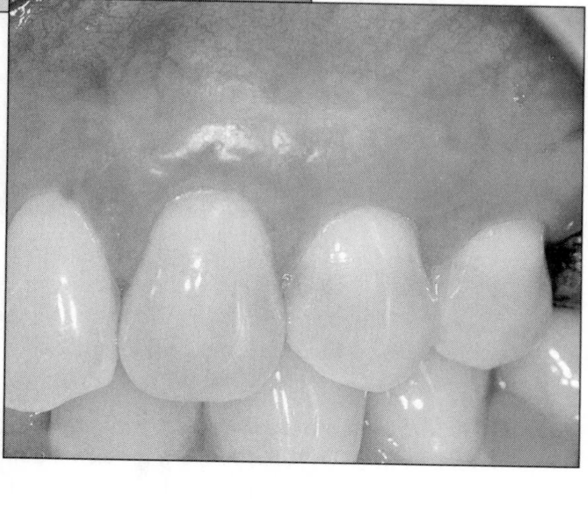

Fig. 16-91g At two years post surgery, complete root coverage is achieved. It is difficult to demarcate the graft from the surrounding tissues. A significant benefit of this procedure is the excellent color match of the graft

horizontal incision is made parallel to and 2 mm from the initial incision. The incisions are extended to the hard palate and connected. The connective tissue defined by the two incisions and the 2-mm band of palatal epithelium is now removed. The palatal wound can usually be sutured so that primary closure is obtained (Figs. 16-92a through 16-92f).

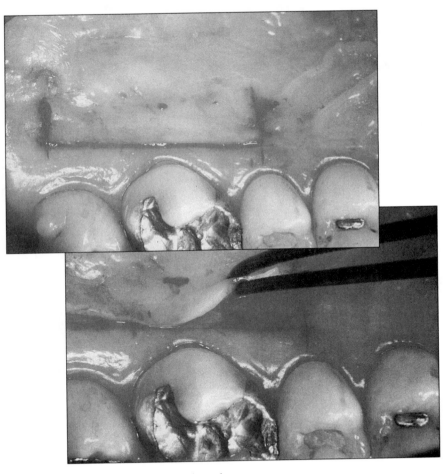

Fig. 16-92a Harvesting of the graft from the palate begins with an incision outline

Fig. 16-92b The epithelium is reflected in order to expose the underlying connective tissue that will be harvested

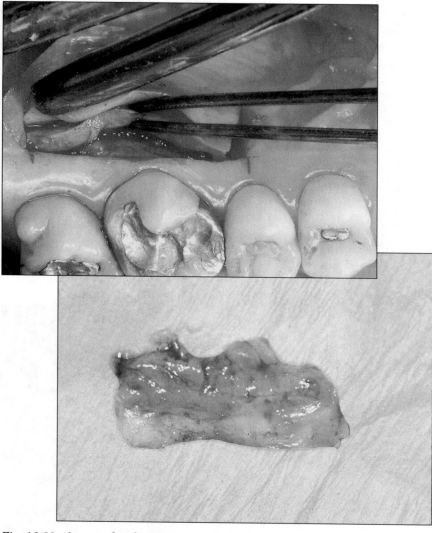

Fig. 16-92c A surgical pick up is used to delineate the
connective tissue graft from the surrounding palate

Fig. 16-92d Connective tissue graft placed on sterile drape

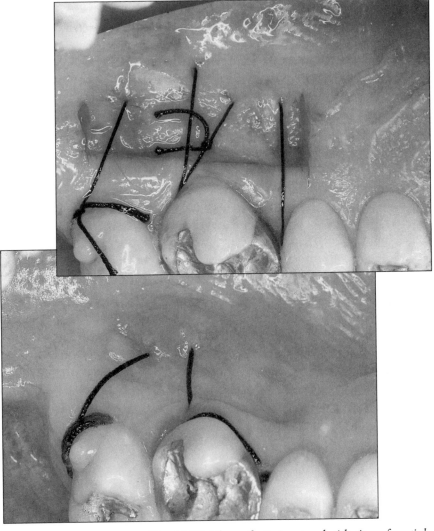

Fig. 16-92e The graft site is sutured with circumferential black silk sutures. Primary closure is almost achieved

Fig. 16-92f At one week, complete healing is almost achieved. This is an additional benefit of this procedure. A free gingival graft creates a much more significant wound (see Fig. 16-88c), and healing of the palate takes much longer

The graft is now transferred to the recipient site. The site is irrigated with saline, and the graft is stabilized with (5-0) gut sutures at the papillae. Additional sutures may be used to stabilize the graft and achieve more intimate adaptation to the periosteum. The partial-thickness flap is coronally elevated over the connective tissue graft and sutured with a sling or interrupted sutures. Five minutes of pressure with saline-soaked gauze is applied to achieve initial stabilization. The patient is placed on a liquid diet for two weeks. Sutures are removed at seven days. The patient is instructed to rinse with chlorhexidine and not brush the grafted area for four weeks.

Both the free gingival graft and the subepithelial graft work well. If successful, they do not probe. Few histological studies have been performed on these procedures. However, the three or four histologically documented cases performed on patients who submitted to extraction of these successfully grafted teeth reveal new attachment of the graft to the root.[128] It has been the author's experience that once the graft has been treated successfully, recession does not reoccur (Figs. 16-93a, 16-93b, and 16-93c).

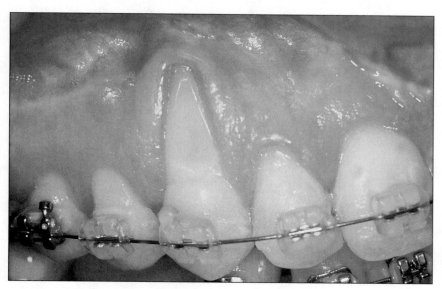

Fig. 16-93a Pre-operative view of recession on tooth #11. It was recommended that this tooth be extracted, for the patient was going through orthodontic treatment as well as orthognathic surgery. The patient opted to save the tooth, and a subepithelial connective tissue graft was performed

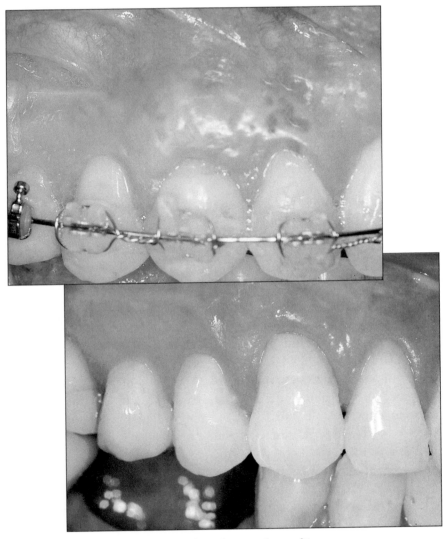

Fig. 16-93b One year post operatively and post orthognathic surgery, the graft is still stable, and good root coverage is maintained

Fig. 16-93c Two years later, orthodontics is completed, and the tooth is still stable

Connective Tissue Ridge Augmentation

The first documented case of connective tissue being used for ridge augmentation was published in a prosthetic journal by a prosthodontist, Calagna, and a periodontist, Langer.[129] Connective tissue harvested from the palate was used to augment a facial gingival concavity in an edentulous area where a future pontic was to be placed. This technique has a 100% success rate, providing the connective tissue is completely encased in a bleeding connective tissue bed.

Reconstruction of deformed edentulous ridges can be performed in three ways:

- Connective tissue augmentation
- Osseous grafting
- Guided bone regeneration

This discussion will be limited to reconstruction with connective tissue. Edentulous ridges may become deformed for many reasons. The loss of a tooth or teeth leads to bone resorption. A patient with aggressive periodontitis as a child who loses the tooth at a young age will have significant bone resorption as he/she ages. Traumatic injury, multiple surgical procedures resulting in the eventual loss of the tooth, and congenital abnormalities can all lead to an atrophic ridge. If the area is to be restored with a fixed prosthesis, asymmetry will result, unless the gingival pontic area is altered so that the prosthesis is in harmony with the adjacent teeth (Figs. 16-94a and 16-94b).

Seibert[130] described the principles, classifications, and surgical procedures involved in reconstructing deformed, partially edentulous ridges with connective tissue. This procedure is only useful when a pontic is the restoration replacing the tooth. If an implant is contemplated, the bone must be reconstructed as well as the soft tissue. Pontics frequently create esthetic problems for the restorative dentist. They may lack a root eminence and therefore create a dark shadow, lack marginal gingiva and interdental papillae, and give the impression that they rest on top of the

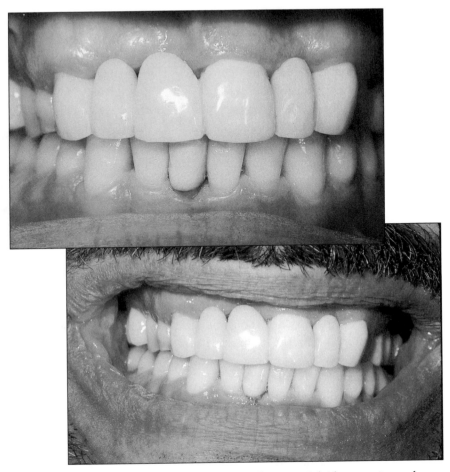

Fig. 16-94a Anterior view of a 40-year-old man with a six-unit bridge spanning teeth #6 through #11. Teeth #7, #8, and #10 were lost in his early 20s due to localized aggressive periodontitis (juvenile periodontitis). Significant bone loss had occurred, and the alveolar ridge resorbed. Subsequently, the pontics replacing these teeth were longer than normal. The result is an asymmetrical smile. The central incisors are of different lengths. The lateral incisors are also asymmetrical and not in proper proportion to the central incisors and canines. Labial concavities are noted over the pontics #7, #8, and #10. A shadow is seen that draws the eye to these areas

Fig. 16-94b Smile view reveals an asymmetrical smile. Esthetic harmony is not present. Even an untrained eye realizes that something is "just not right"

ridge instead of emerging from the gingiva like a natural tooth (Fig. 16-94a). Without a "normal" ridge, an ideal prosthesis may be impossible.

Prior to the reconstruction of the ridge, the size and shape of the ideal final restoration need to be determined. If the defect is large, reconstruction may need to be done in stages. The patient seen in Figure 16-94 is in his mid-40s and is unhappy with his smile. It was determined that connective tissue would be harvested from the palate at the same time posterior periodontal surgery was being performed. This saves the patient the discomfort of going through a second procedure. A pouch is made in the edentulous areas of the anterior maxilla, and two connective tissue grafts are harvested with a band of epithelium. The hemorrhagic connective tissue graft is placed within the bleeding connective tissue prepared donor site. The graft is sutured internally with (5-0) gut and externally with (4-0) silk (Figs. 16-94c through 16-94h). Currently, the author rarely uses silk suture material. Silk sutures have a tendency to wick, and the accumulated bacteria can cause an inflammatory response.

The final restoration reveals dental harmony and symmetry (Fig. 16-94j). The lateral incisors are the same size. The lateral incisors are no longer more apical than the central incisors, and the concepts of anterior esthetic harmony are present.[131-133]

Esthetic crown lengthening

Until recently, most of dentistry dealt with the management of disease, controlling periodontitis, filling cavities, performing endodontic treatment, and exodontia. Today, patients come to the dentist requesting cosmetic procedures. Dentists have become the "plastic surgeons of the oral cavity." Patients actively seek out dentists to "make over" their smile. Patients demand and expect more from their dentists. Dentists are in a unique position of being able to change people's appearances by changing their smiles. Success is associated with looking good—looking good is associated with feeling good. Better-looking people achieve more financial success and achieve greater awards in American society.[134-135]

Previously, crown lengthening was only performed for restorative and periodontal purposes. Crown margins should be at least 3 mm from the

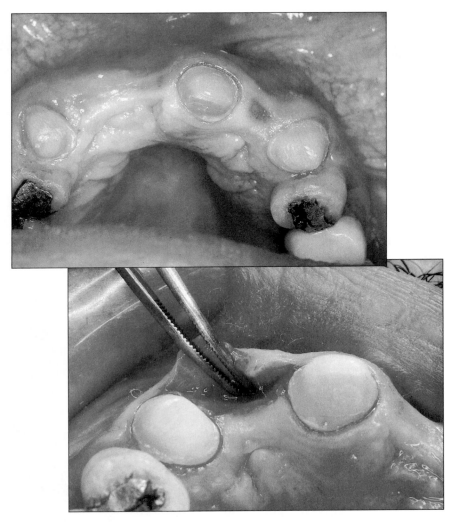

Fig. 16-94c Occlusal view with the provisional restoration removed. Concavities are seen in the areas of the missing teeth. Note the root prominence of the natural teeth

Fig. 16-94d A midcrestal incision is made in the pontic area of tooth #10, and an envelope pouch is made. This is to be the recipient site of the connective tissue graft

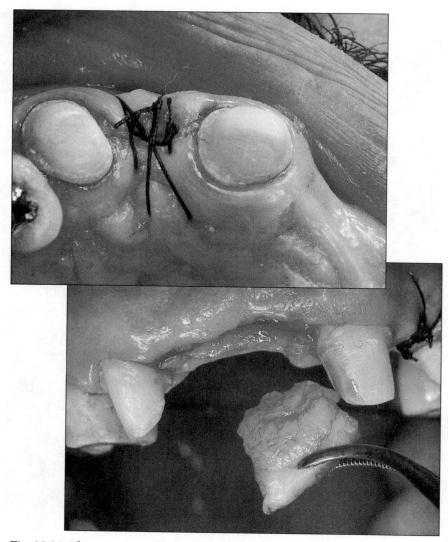

Fig. 16-94e *The connective tissue graft is placed into the recipient site. A small band of epithelium is kept on the graft, which is placed occlusally. The prepared pouch is filled with bleeding connective tissue. Externally, two sutures secure the graft*

Fig. 16-94f *The connective tissue graft with a small band of epithelium is being transferred to the prepared recipient site of the pontic area #7 and #8*

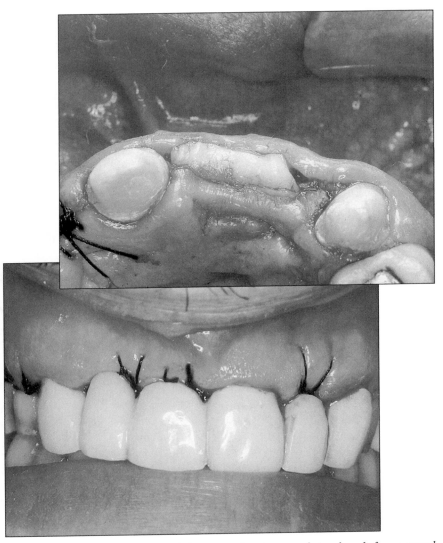

Fig. 16-94g *Occlusal view of the connective tissue graft in place before external suturing. A resorbable suture is used to tack the graft in place and prevent it from being dislodged. Note that the beginning of root prominences is already evident*

Fig. 16-94h *The provisional is replaced immediately after surgery. The provisional had to be altered to accommodate the connective tissue grafts. Compare to Figure 16-94a*

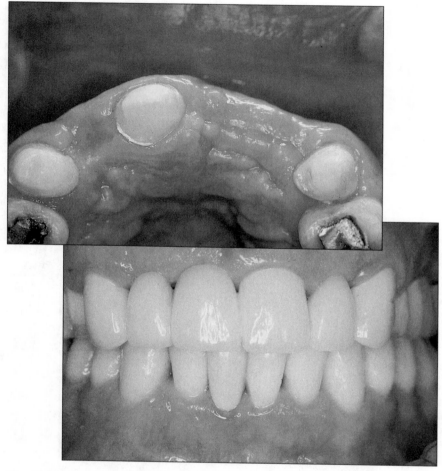

Fig. 16-94i *Two months following surgery, the connective tissue grafts have healed. Compare this occlusal view to the pre-operative view in Figure 16-94c. Significant ridge augmentation has been achieved*

Fig. 16-94j *Final restoration is in place; a 6-unit fixed bridge, spanning teeth #6 through #11. Harmony has been achieved. Central incisors are of equal length. Root prominences are seen in the pontic sites #7, #8, and #10. The gingival height of contour of the canines and central incisors are on the same plane. The gingival height of contour of the lateral incisors is approximately 1.5 mm incisal to the centrals and canines. Ten years post-operatively, the connective grafts remain stable (Restorative dentistry courtesy of Dr. Keith Rudolph, Westport, CT)*

gingival margin to avoid invading the body's biologic width.[136-137] Broken down teeth were in need of crown lengthening in order to create a retentive crown. Today, a crown-lengthening indication is to enhance the appearance of the anterior maxillary sextant. Patients want to eliminate their gummy smiles. Ideal relationships have been established that are associated with harmony and esthetics.[131,133,138-139]

When proper relationships are established between the lips and the teeth, the incisal plane and the occlusal plane, the occlusal plane and the interpupillary line, the gingiva and the teeth, the height of the gingival margins, the harmony of the teeth, the symmetry of the lips and face while smiling and in repose, etc., dramatic changes in a patient's overall appearance are possible (Figs. 16-95a through 16-95f).

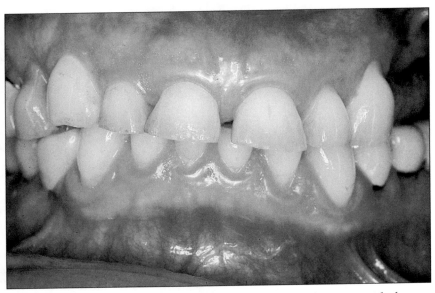

Fig. 16-95a Intraoral pre-operative view reveals many alterations in ideal dental and dental gingival relationships. Anterior flaring, diastemata, alterations in dental gingival heights, and teeth discolorations are evident

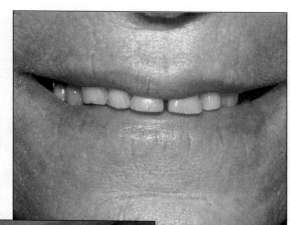

Fig. 16-95b Smile view shows minimal display of teeth due to tooth wear and decreased vertical dimension

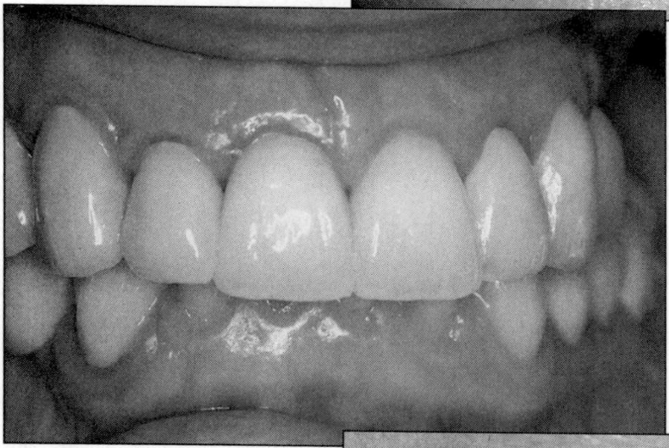

Fig. 16-95c Postoperative restoration displays re-establishment of proper dental and gingival relationships. Cosmetic and functional improvement has been achieved through periodontal crown lengthening and crowning of maxillary teeth

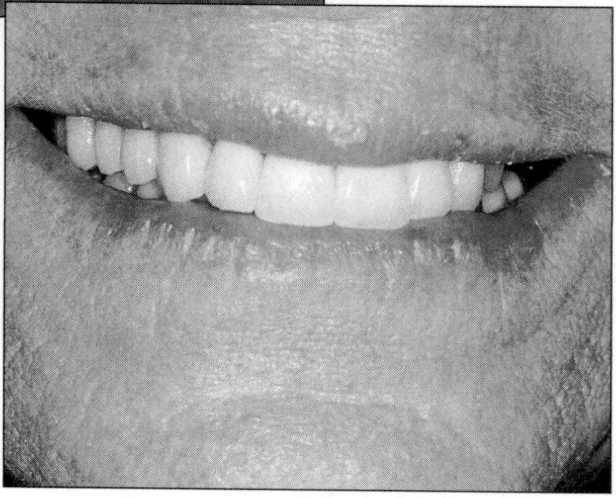

Fig. 16-95d Post-operative smile view reveals improved appearance. Teeth are in better balance, and more tooth structure is shown

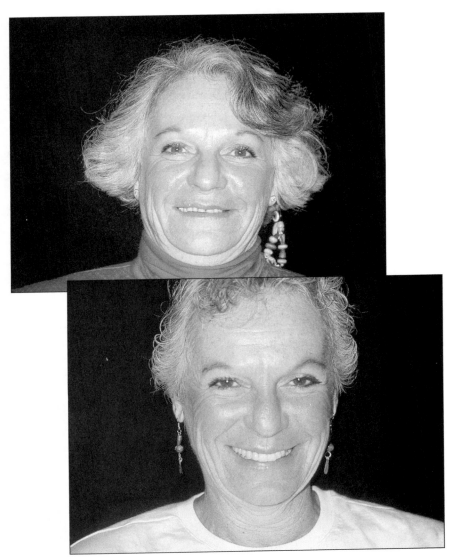

Fig. 16-95e Pre-operative facial appearance prior to beginning dental reconstruction

Fig. 16-95f Post-operative facial view. Esthetic appearance is greatly improved. Patient appears happier and more confident (Restorative dentistry courtesy of Dr. Stephen Rothenberg, Darien, CT)

687

The initial stage in smile makeovers, as it is with a routine periodontal treatment, is the examination and esthetic diagnosis. It begins with an analysis of the patient's smile. A treatment plan is then developed, and the goals of therapy are identified. When restorative treatment is to be performed, communication and excellent coordination between the periodontist and restorative dentist are essential, if a predictable final cosmetic result is to be achieved.

The patient in Figure 16-96 was unhappy with the amount of gingiva she showed when smiling. In conjunction with her restorative dentist, it was determined that the crowns on her six anterior teeth would be redone in conjunction with maxillary anterior crown lengthening. The sequence of therapy was as follows:

- Periodontal examination
- Restorative examination
- Joint consultation between periodontist, restorative dentist, and patient
- Development of a restorative and periodontal treatment plan
- Provisionalization of the maxillary anterior teeth
- Template and model fabrication
- Stage 1 periodontal crown lengthening—ostectomy and repositioned flap
- Healing for six weeks
- Stage 2 periodontal crown lengthening— aesthetic gingivectomy
- Healing for two weeks
- Final tooth preparation
- Final impressions
- Delivery of final prosthesis
- Maintenance

Photographic documentation of this patient's treatment plan allows for an understanding of the coordination of care that was necessary to achieve a predictable final result (Figs. 16-96a through 16-96s). The provisional restorations were not merely temporary crowns. They served a greater purpose. The provisional (temporary) crowns were a dress rehearsal for the final restoration. If the proper dental, gingival, and esthetic relationships are not achieved in the provisional restoration, they will never be achieved in the final restoration. The importance of an excellent set of provisional restorations cannot be over-emphasized. They are invaluable in determining where the gingival should be in relationship to the teeth.

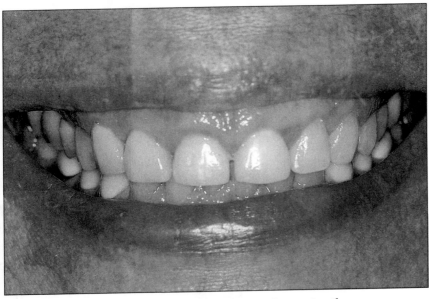

Fig. 16-96a Initial view of patient's "gummy" smile

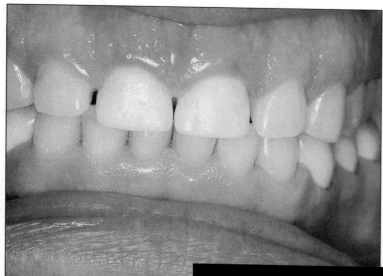

Fig. 16-96b Intraoral anterior view
reveals slightly altered dental gingival relationships. The central incisors are short in relationship to the
lateral incisors

Fig. 16-96c Extraoral facial
view of patient smiling. Excess
gingival tissue is evident

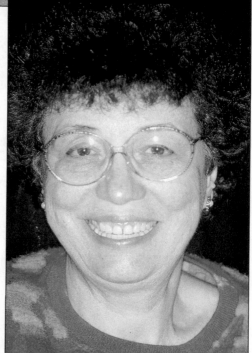

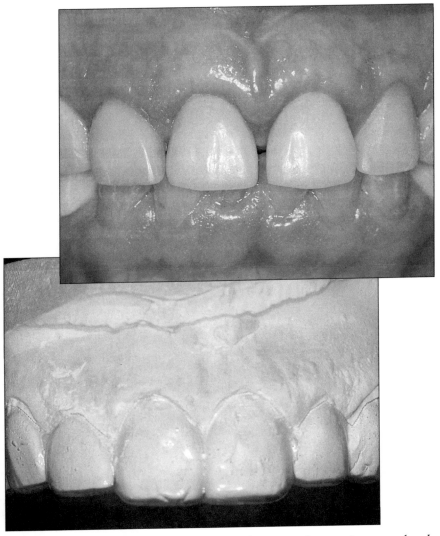

Fig. 16-96d Provisional restorations were placed
in anticipation of anterior crown lengthening

Fig. 16-96e A diagnostic model was made. Ideal dental
gingival relationships were determined and were used to
guide the surgeon during the crown-lengthening procedure

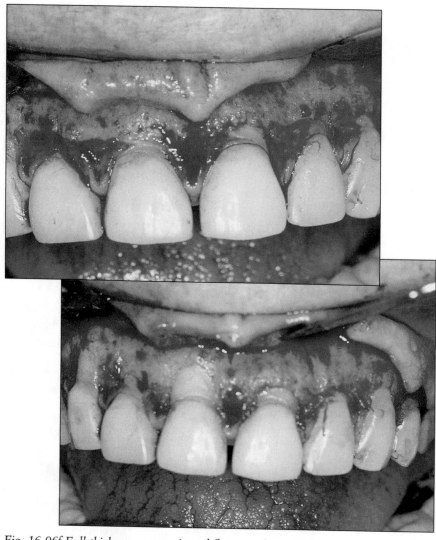

Fig. 16-96f Full thickness mucoperiosteal flap was elevated from bicuspid to bicuspid. Care was taken to preserve the papillae

Fig. 16-96g Ostectomy was begun on teeth #6, #7, and #8. Compare to the contralateral side

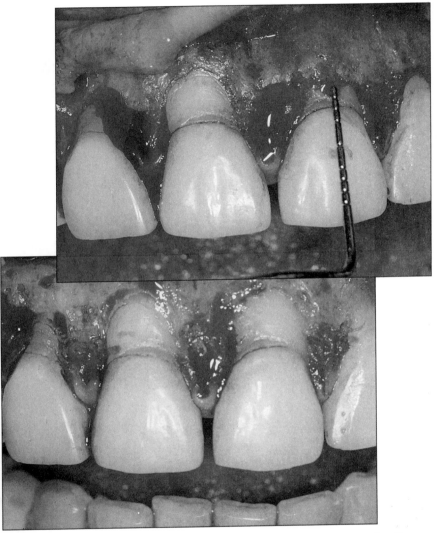

Fig. 16-96h A periodontal probe measures the distance from crown margin to bone. This crown had invaded the biologic width, for it is only 2 mm from the alveolar crest

Fig. 16-96i Ostectomy is complete. Bony profiles are symmetrical. Ideal bony relationships are established, for the soft tissue follows the bony architecture

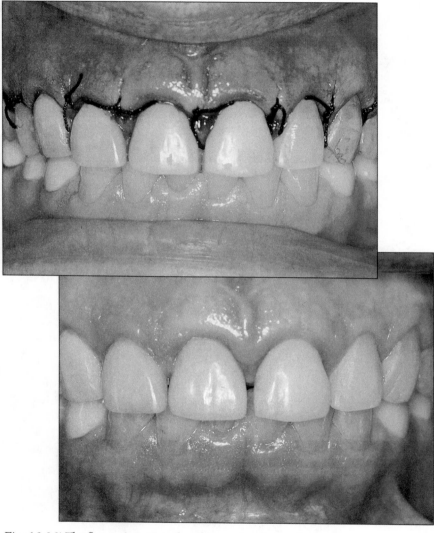

Fig. 16-96j *The flap is repositioned and sutured to the papilla. No attempt is made to reposition the gingiva at this time*

Fig. 16-96k *The tissue is allowed to heal unmolested for eight weeks*

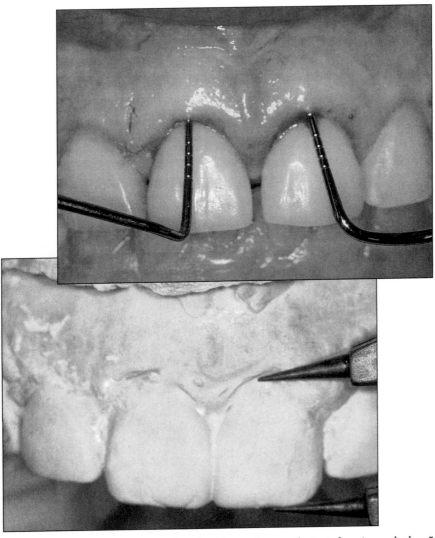

Fig. 16-96l Sounding (probing under anesthesia to bone) reveals that 5 mm exist from the free gingival margin to the alveolar crest. Two millimeters of gingiva can be removed without violating the biologic width

Fig. 16-96m A caliper is used to measure the length of the central incisor on the diagnostic model

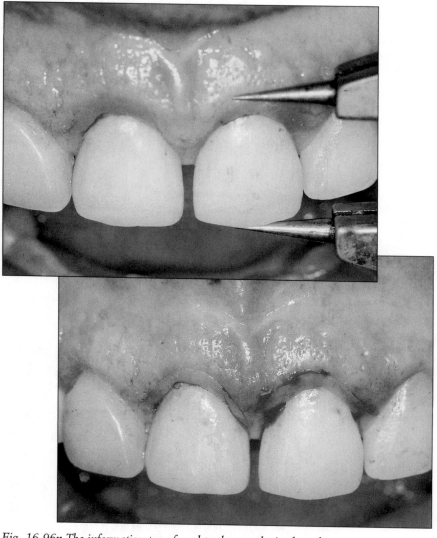

Fig. 16-96n The information transferred to the mouth via the caliper

Fig. 16-96o The gingiva is marked with the caliper, and an inverse bevel gingivectomy is performed

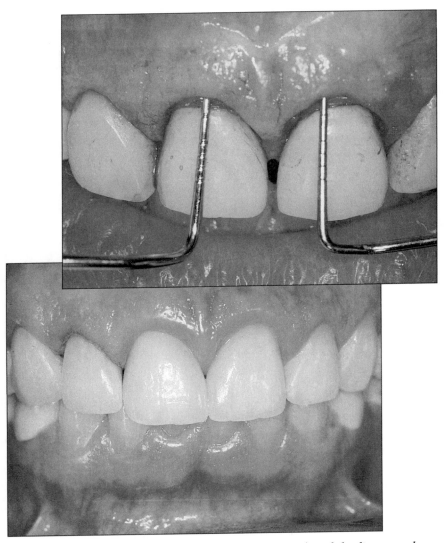

Fig. 16-96p *The collar of tissue is removed, and the distance to bone from free gingival margin evaluated. Three millimeters now exist*

Fig. 16-96q *The gingiva is allowed to heal for two weeks before final impressions are taken and the final crowns completed. Ideal harmony and esthetics are present in the final restoration*

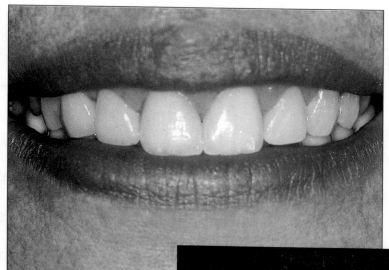

Fig. 16-96r Close up of smile shows ideal amount of teeth. Compare to Figure 16-96a. The gummy smile has been eliminated

Fig. 16-96s Full facial view. Patient is much happier with her new smile. A twinkle is present in her eyes. Compare to her initial photograph in Figure 16-96c. (Restoration courtesy of Dr. Fred Kriegle, Hartsdale, NY)

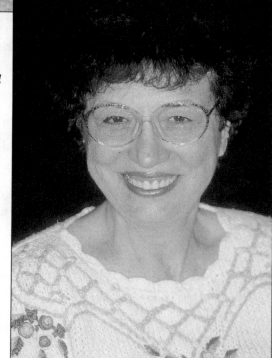

Notes

[1] Orban, B. Clinical and histologic study of the surface characteristics of the gingiva. *Oral surg*, 1:827, 1948

[2] Ainamo, J., and Loe, H. Anatomical characteristics of gingiva. A clinical and microscopic study of the free and attached gingiva. *J Periodontal*, 37:5, 1966

[3] Dumbest, C.O., and Barens, C. Oromucosal pigmentation: an updated literary review. *J Periodontal*, 42:726, 1971

[4] Morris, M.L. The position of the margin of the gingiva. *Oral Surg*, 11:969, 1958

[5] Kois, J. Altering gingival levels: The restorative connection part I: Biologic variables. *J Esthet Dent*, 6(1):3-9, 1994

[6] Socransky, S.S. Microbiology of periodontal disease. Present status and future considerations. *J. Periodontal*, 48:497, 1977

[7] Lindhe, J., Hamp, S. E., and Loe, H. Experimental periodontitis in the beagle dog. *J Periodont Res*, 8:1, 1973

[8] *Proceedings of the World Workshop in Clinical Periodontics*, American Academy of Periodontalogy, Chicago, 1989

[9] *Annals of Periodontalogy, 1996 World Workshop in Periodontics*, American Academy of Periodontalogy, Chicago, 1996

[10] Armitage, G.C. Development of a classification system for periodontal diseases and conditions. *An Periodontal*, 4:1-6, 1999

[11] Clerehugh, V. The changing face of periodontal epidemiology. *Community Dent Health*, 1993, 10 (suppl. 2): 19-28

[12] *Annals of Periodontalogy, 1999 International workshop for a classification of Periodontal Diseases and Conditions*, 4:1, December, 1999

[13] Loe, H., Theilade, E., and Jensen, S. B. Experimental gingivitis in man. *J Periodontal*, 36:177, 1965

[14] Page, R.C. Oral health status in the United States: Prevalence of inflammatory periodontal diseases. *J Dent Educ*, 49:354-367, 1985

[15] Loe, H. Periodontal changes in pregnancy. *J Periodontal*, 36: 209, 1965

[16] Kalkwarf, L. Effect of oral contraceptive therapy on gingival inflammation in humans. *J Periodontal*, 49:560, 1978

[17] Lindhe, J., and Attstrom, R. Gingival exudation during the menstrual cycle. *J Periodontal*, Res 2:194, 1967

[18] Sutcliffe, P. A longitudinal study of gingivitis and puberty. *J Periodontal Res* 7:52, 1972

[19] Kornman, K.S., and Loesche, W.J. The subgingival microbial flora during pregnancy. *J Periodontal Res* 15:111, 1980

[20] Cianciola, L.J., Parlk, B.H., Bruck, E., Mosovich, L., and Genco, R.J. Prevalence of periodontal disease in insulin-dependent diabetes mellitus (juvenile diabetes.) *JADA*, 104, 653-660, 1982

[21] Steinberg, S.C., and Steinberg, A.D. Phenytoin-induced gingival overgrowth in severely retarded children. *J Periodontal*, 53:429, 1982

[22] Rateitschak-Pluss, E.M., Hefti, A., Lortscher, R., and Thiel, G. Initial observation that cyclosporin-a induces gingival enlargement in man. *J Clin Periodontal*, 10: 237, 1983

[23] Lucas, R.M., Howell, L.P., and Wall, B.A. Nifedipine-induced gingival hyperplasia. A histochemical and ultrastructural study. *J Periodontal*, 56:211, 1985

[24] McCarthy, P.L., and Shklar, G. *Diseases of the Oral Mucosa*, 2nd ed. Philadelphia, PA: Lea and Ferbiger, 1980

[25] Rivera-Hidalago, F., and Stanford, T.W. Oral mucosal lesions caused by infective microorganisms. I. Viruses and bacteria. *J Periodontal*, 2000, 1999, 21:106-124

[26] Scully, C., Monteil, R., and Sposto, M.R. Infectious and tropical disease affected the human mouth. *J Periodontal*, 2000, 1998, 18:47-40

[27] Miller, C.S., and Redding, S.W. Diagnosis and management of orofacial herpes simplex virus infections. *Dent Clin North Am*, 1992, 36:879-895

[28] Grbic, J.T., Mitchell-Lewis, D.A., Fine, J.B., et al. The relationship of candadisis to linear gingival erythema in HIV-infected homosexual men and parental drug users. *J Periodontal*, 1995, 66:30-37

[29] Nisengard, R.J., and Neiders, M. Desquamative lesions of the gingiva. *J Periodontal*, 1981, 52:500-510

[30] Rosenberg, S., and Arm, R. *Clinician's guide to Treatment of Common Oral Conditions*. The American Academy of Oral Medicine, 4th ed., 1997, 19-20

[31] Loe, H., Anerud, A., Boysen, H., and Smith, M. The natural history of periodontal disease in man. The rate of periodontal destruction before 40 years of age. *J Periodontal*, 49:07, 1978

[32] Van Dyke, T.E., Levine, M.J., and Genco, R.J. Periodontal diseases and neutrophil abnormalities. In *Host-Parasite Interactions in Periodontal Diseases*, Washington, D.C.: American Society for Microbiology, 1982, 235-245 edited by Genco, R.J., and Mergenhagen, S.E.

[33] Haffajee, A.D., and Socransky, S.S. Microbial etiological agents of destructive periodontal diseases. In *Microbiology and Immunology of Periodontal Diseases*, edited by Socransky, S.S., and Haffajee, A.D. Periodontalogy, 2000, 5, 78-111

[34] Flemming, T.F. Periodontitis. *Annals of Periodontalogy*, 4:1, 32-38, 1999

[35] Consensus Report: Aggressive Periodontitis. *Annals of Periodontalogy*, 4:1, 53, 1999

[36] Saxen, L., and Nevanlinna, H.R. Autosomal recessive inheritance of juvenile periodontitis: test of a hypotheses. *Clin Genet*, 25:332, 1984

[37] Savitt, E.D., and Socransky, S.S. Distribution of certain subgingival microbial species in selected periodontal conditions. *J Periodontal Res* 19:111,1984

[38] Van Dyke, T.E., Levine, M.J., and Genco, R.J. neutrophil function and oral disease. *J Oral Pathol*, 14:95, 1985

39 Zambon, J.J., Grossi, S., Dunfor, R, Haraszthy, Vi, Presus, H., and Genco, R.J. Epidemiology of subgingival bacterial pathogens in periodontal disease. In *Molecular Pathogenesis of Periodontal disease*, edited by Genco, R., Hamada, S., Lehrner, T., McGhee, J., Mergenhagen S. Washington D.C.: American Society for Microbiology, 1994, 3-12

40 Kianane, D. Periodontitis modified by systemic factors. *Annals of Periodontalogy*, 4:1, 54-64, 1999

41 Johnson, B.D., and Engel, D. Acute necrotizing ulcerative gingivitis. A review of diagnosis, etiology, and treatment. *J Periodontal*, 1086, 57, 141-150

42 Prichard, J.F. Management of the periodontal abscess. *Oral Surg*, 6:474, 1953

43 Abiko, Y., Shimizu, N., Yamaguchi, M., Suzuki, H., and Takiguchi, H. Effect of aging on functional changes of periodontal tissue cells. *Annuals of Periodontalogy*, 3:1 350-369, 1998

44 1997 Guidelines for Antibiotic Prophylaxis for the Prevention of Bacterial Endocarditis for Dental and Oral Procedures. *JADA*, Vol. 277, No. 22, June, 1997

45 Tonnetti, M.S. Cigarette smoking and periodontal diseases: etiology and management of disease. *Annuals of Periodontalogy*, 3:1, 88-101, 1998

46 Bain, C. and Moy, P. The association between the failure of dental implants and cigarette smoking. *Int J Oral Maxillofac Implants*, 8:609-615, 1993

[47] Nyman, S., Lindhe, J., and Rosling, B. Periodontal surgery in plaque-infected dentitions. *J Clin Periodontal*, 4, 240-249, 1977

[48] Prichard, J. Interpretation of radiographs in periodontics. *Int J Periodontics Restorative Dent*, 1983, 3:8-39)

[49] Sonick, M. Abrahams, J., and Faiella, R. A Comparison of the accuracy of periapical, panoramic, and computerized tomographic radiographs in locating the mandibular canal. *Int J Oral Maxillofacial Impl*, 9:455-460, 1994

[50] Lang, N.P., Joss, A., Orsanic, T., Gusberti, F.A., and Siegrist, H.E. Bleeding on probing is a predictor for the progression of periodontal disease. *J Clin Periodontal*, 1986, 13:590-596

[51] Van der Velden, U. Influence of probing force on the reproducibility of bleeding tendency measurements. *J Clin Periodontal*, 1980, 7:421-427

[52] Schluger, S., Yudodelis, R., Page, R., and Johnson, R. *Periodontal Diseases*, Philadelphia: Lea & Febiger, 1990

[53] Kogon, S.L. The prevalence, location and conformation palato-radicular grooves in maxillary incisors. *J Periodontal*, 1986, 57:231-234

[54] Bower, R.C. Furcation morphology relative to periodontal treatment. Furcation entrance architecture. *J Periodontal*, 1979, 50:23-27

[55] Egelberg, J. *Periodontics, The Scientific Way*. OdontoScience, 1999, 346

56 Gantes, B.G., Synowski, B.N., Garrett, S., and Egelberg, J.H. Treatment of periodontal furcation defects. Mandiular class III defects. *J Periodontal*, 62:361-365, 1991

57 Langer, B., Stein, S., and Wagenberg, B. An evaluation of root resections. Ten-year study. *J Periodontal*, 52:719-722, 1981

58 Hamp, S.E., Nyman, S., and Lindhe, J. Periodontal treatment of multirooted teeth results after 5 years. *J Clin Periodontal*, 2:126-135,1975

59 Miller, S.C. *Textbook of Periodontia*, 3rd ed. Philadelphia: Blackston, 1950, 125

60 Lindhe, J., Karring, T., and Lang, N.P. *Clinical Periodontalogy and Implant dentistry*, 3rd ed., Munsgaard, 1998, 279-295

61 Dr. Harold Shavel, personal communication, 1996

62 Bergenholtz, A., Gustafsson, L.B., Segerlund, N., Hagberg, C. and Nygaard Ostby, P. Role of brushing technique and toothbrush design in plaque removal. Scandinavian Journal of Dental Research 92, 344-351, 1984.

63 Egelberg, Jan. *Oral Hygiene Methods, The Scientific Way*. OdontoScience, 1999, 13-19

64 Cyanic, S.G., Shibley, O., and Farber, G.A. Clinical evaluation of the effect of two types of dental floss on plaque and gingival health. *Clinical Preventative Dentistry*, 14(3), 14-18, 1992

65 Egelberg, Jan. *Oral Hygiene Methods, The Scientific Way*. OdontoScience, 1999, 45-66

[66] Egelberg, Jan. *Oral Hygiene Methods, The Scientific Way.* OdontoScience, 1999, 67-90

[67] Kiger, R.D., Nylund, K., and Feller, R.P. A comparison of proximal plaque removal using floss and interdental brushes. *J Clin Periodontal,* 18, 681-684, 1991

[68] Egelberg, Jan. *Oral Hygiene Methods, The Scientific Way.* OdontoScience, 1999, 197-223

[69] Axelsson, P., and Lindhe, J. Efficacy of mouthrinses in inhibiting dental plaque and gingivitis in man. *J Clin Periodontal,* 14:205-212, 1987

[70] Siegrist, B.E., Busberti, F.A., Brecx, M.C., Weber, H.P., and Lang, N.P. Efficacy of rinsing with chlorhexidine gluconate in comparison to phenolic and plant alkaloid compounds. *J Periodontal Res,* suppl., 60-73, 1986

[71] Caffesse, R., Sweeney, P.L., and Smith B.A. Scaling and root planning with and without periodontal flap surgery. *J Clin Periodontal,* 13:205, 1986

[72] Buchanan, S.A., and Robertson, P.A. Calculus removal by scaling/root planning with and without surgical access. *J Periodontal* 58:159-163, 1987

[73] Rabin, G.M., Ash, M.M., and Caffesse, R.G. The effectiveness of subgingival scaling and root planing in calculus removal. *J Periodontal,* 52:119, 1981

[74] Stambaugh, R., Dragoo, M., Smith, D., and Carasali, L. The limits of subgingival scaling. *Int J Periodontics Restorative Dent,* 1(5):30-41, 1981

[75] Torfason, T., Kiger, R., Selvig, K.A., and Egelberg, J. Clinical improvement of gingival conditions following ultrasonic versus hand instrumentation of periodontal pockets. *J Clin Periodontal*, 6, 165-176, 1979

[76] Badersten, A., Nilveus, R., and Egelberg, J. Effect of nonsurgical periodontal therapy. I. Moderately advanced periodontitis. *J Clin Periodontal*, 8, 57-72, 1981

[77] Oosterwaal, P.J.M., Matee, M.I., Mikx. F.H.M., Van't Hof, M.A., and Renggli, H.H. The effect of subgingival debridement with hand and ultrasonic instruments on the subgingival mircroflora. *J Clin Periodontal*, 14, 528-533, 1987

[78] Boretti, G., Zappa, U., Graf, H., and Case, D. Short-term effects of phase 1 therapy on crevicular cell populations. *J Periodontal*, 66, 235-240, 1995

[79] Loos, B., Kiger, R., and Egelberg, J. An evaluation of basic periodontal therapy using sonic and ultrasonic scalers. *J Clin Periodontal*, 14, 29-33, 1987

[80] Laurell, L., and Pettersson, B. Periodontal healing after treatment with either the Titan-S sonic scaler or hand instruments. *Swedish Dental Journal* 12, 187-192, 1988

[81] Bjorn, H., and Lindhe, J. The influence of periodontal instruments on the tooth surfaces. A methodological study. *Odontologisk Revy*, 13, 355-369, 1962

[82] Dr. Sal Sqautrito, Manchester, Connecticut, personal communication 1990

[83] Parashis, A.O., Anagnou-vareltzides, A., and Demetriou, N. Calculus removal from multirooted teeth with and without surgical access. I. Efficacy on external and furcation surfaces in relation to probing depth. *J Clin Periodontal*, 20, 63-68, 1993

[84] Egelberg, Jan. *Periodontics, The Scientific Way*. OdontoScience, 113-139, 1999

[85] Barrington, E. An overview of periodontal surgical procedures. *J Peridontol*, 52:518-528,1981

[86] Axelsson, P., and Lindhe, J. The significance of maintenance care in the treatment of periodontal disease. *J Clin Periodontal*, 8,281-294, 1981

[87] Rothwell, B.R., and Richard, E.L. Diabetes mellitus: Medical and dental considerations. *Spec Are Dent*, 4:58,1984

[88] Parnell, A.G. The medically compromised patient. *Int Dent J*, 36:77, 1986

[89] Machtei, E.E., Hausmann, E., Schmidt, M., Grossi, S.G., Dunford, R., Schifferle, R. Munoz, K., Davies, G., Chandler, J., and Genco, R.J. Radiographic and clinical responses to periodontal therapy. *J Periodontal*, 69, 590-595, 1998

[90] Mayfield, L., Soderhoml, G., Hallstrom, H., Kullendorff, B., Edwardsson, S., Bratthall, G., Bragger, U., and Attstrom, R. Guided tissue regeneration for the treatment of intraosseous defects using a bioabsorbable membrane, a controlled clinical study. *J Clin Periodontal*, 25, 585-595, 1998

91 Trombelli, L., and Scabbia, A. Healing response of gingival recession defects following guided tissue regeneration procedures in smokers and non-smokers. *J Clin Periodontal*, 24, 529-533, 1997

92 Scott, T.A., Towle, H.J., Assad, D.A., and Nicoll, B.K. Comparison of bioabsorbable laminar bone membrane and non-resorbable ePTFE membrane in mandibular furcations. *J Periodontal*, 68, 679-686, 1997

93 Wallace, R. The relationship between cigarette smoking and dental implant failure, *Euro. J Prosth & Rest Dent*, 8:103-108, 2001

94 O'Brien, T.P., Roszkowski, M.T., Wolff, L.F., Hinrichs, J.E., and Hargreaves, K. M. Effect of a non-steroidal anti-inflammatory drug on tissue levels of immunoreactive prostaglandin e2, immunoreactive leukotriene, and pain after periodontal surgery. *J Periodontal*, 67, 1307-1316, 1996

95 Vogel, R. I., and Desjardins, P.J., 7 Major, K.V.O. Comparison of pre-surgical and immediate post-surgical ibuprofen on postoperative periodontal pain. *J Periodontal*, 63, 914-918, 1992

96 Ariaudo, A.A. The efficacy of antibiotics in periodontal surgery. *J Periodontal* 40:150, 1969

97 Pack P., and Haber, J. The incidence of clinical infection after periodontal surgery. A retrospective study. *J Periodontal*, 54: 441-443, 1983

98 Gordon, J.M., Walker, C.B., Murphy, J.C., Goodson, J.M., and Socransky, S.S. Tetracycline: levels achievable in gingival crevice fluid and in vitro effect on subgingival organisms. Part I. *J Periodontal*, 52:609, 1981

[99] Dr. William MacDonnell, personal communication, 2001

[100] Bennett, C. R. *Monheim's local anesthesia and pain control in dental practice*, 7th ed., St. Louis: C.V. Mosby Co., 1983

[101] Malamed, S. *Handbook of Local Anesthesia*, 2nd ed., St. Louis: C.V. Mosby, 1986

[102] Malamed, S. *Handbook of Local Anesthesia*, 2nd ed, St. Louis: C.V. Mosby, 1986, p. 51-52

[103] Sonick, M. *Surgical Designs and Techniques*, Yankee Dental Congress, Boston, MA, 1994

[104] Ochsenbein, C. A primer for osseous surgery. *Int J Periodontics Restorative Dent*, 6(1): 9-47, 1986

[105] Tarnow, D., Magner, A., and Fletcher, P. The effect of the distance from the contact point to the crest of the bone on the presence or absence of the interproximal papilla. *J Periodontal*, 63:995-996, 1993

[106] Egelberg, Jan. *Periodontics, The Scientific Way, Synopses of Clinical Studies*. OdontoScience, 304-306, 1999

[107] Hallmon, W., Drisko, C., Rapley, J., and Robinson. *Periodontal Literature Reviews*, American Academy of Peridontology, Chicago, IL, Osseous Grafting, 167-171, 1996

[108] Melcher, A.H. On the repair potential of periodontal tissues. *J Peridontol*, 47:256-260, 1976

109 Gottlow, J., Nyman, S., Karring, T., and Lindhe, J. New attachment formation as the result of controlled tissue regeneration. *J Clin Periodontal*, 19, 315-317, 1984

110 Murphy, K. Post-operative healing complications associated with Gore-Tex periodontal material. Part 2. Effect of complications on regeneration. *Int J Periodontics Rest Dent*, 15, 549-561, 1995

111 Becker, W., and Becker, B. Treatment of mandibular 3-wall intrabony defects by flap debridement and expanded polytetrafluoroethylene barrier membranes. Long term evaluation of 2 treated patients. *J Periodontal*, 64:1138-1144, 1993

112 McClain, P., and Schallhorn, R. Long term assessment of combined osseous composite grafting, root conditioning and guided tissue regeneration. *Int J Periodontics Rest Dent*, 13, 9-27, 1993

113 Schluger, S. Osseous resection—a basic principle in periodontal surgery. *Oral Surg Oral Med Oral Pathol*, 2:316-325, 1949

114 Ochsenbein, C, and Bohannan H., The palatal approach to osseous surgery I. Rationale *J Periodontal* 34:60-68, 1963

115 Johnson, R.H. Basic flap management. *Dent. Clin. North Am.*, 20:3, 1976

116 Kramer, G.M., Nevins, M., and Kohn, J.D. The utilization of periosteal suturing in periodontal surgical procedures. *J Periodontal*, 41:457, 1970

117 Evian, C., Corn, H., and Rosenberg, E. Papillary retention procedure. *Compend Contin Educ Dent*, 6:38,1985

[118] Sonick, M. *Surgical management of patients with severe periodontal disease of the maxillary anterior teeth*. Annual Meeting of the American Academy of Periodontology, Chicago, IL, 1993

[119] Friedman, N. Mucogingival surgery. *Texas Dent*, 1957, 75:358

[120] Miller, P.D. Regenerative and reconstructive periodontal plastic surgery. *Dent Clin North Am*, 1988, 32(2):287

[121] Hallmon, W., Drisko, C., Rapley, J., and Robinson: *Mucogingival Surgery*, 151-158, 1996

[122] Lindhe, J. *Mucogingival Therapy and Esthetics in Periodontal Therapy in Clinical Periodontology and Implant Dentistry*, Munsgaard, Copenhagen, 1998

[123] Bjorn, H. Free transplantation of gingiva propria. *Odont Revy*, 1963, 14, 523

[124] Sullivan, H.C., and Atkins, J.H. Free autogenous gingival grafts. III. Utilization of grafts in the treatment of gingival recession. *Peridontics*, 1968, 6:152

[125] Miller, P.D. Root coverage using a free soft tissue autograph following citric acid application. I. Technique *Int J Periodontal Rest Dent*, 1982, 2:65

[126] Sonick, M. Root Coverage: A comparison of techniques: the free gingival graft versus the subepithelial connective tissue graft. *Prac Periodont & Aesth Dent*, 1992, 4:39-48

[127] Langer, B., and Langer, L. Subepithelial connective tissue graft techniques for root coverage. *J Periodontal*, 1985, 56:715

128 Pasquinelli, K.L. The histology of new attachment utilizing a thick autogenous soft tissue graft in an area of deep recession. A case report. *Int J Periodontics Rest Dent*, 15, 248-257, 1995

129 Langer, B., and Calagna, L. Subepithelial graft to correct ridge concavities. *J Prosthet Dent*, 1980, 44:363

130 Seibert, J., and Lindhe, J. Esthetics in Periodontal Therapy 645-681 in Lindhe, J. *Clinical Periodontology and Implant Dentistry*, Munsgaard, Copenhagen, 1997

131 Sonick, M. Esthetic Crown Lengthening of the Maxillary Anterior Teeth. *Compend Contin Educ Dent*, 18(8):807-820, 1997

132 Rufenacht, C.R. *Fundamentals of Esthetics*. Chicago: Quintessence Publishing Co. Inc., 1990

133 Garber, D.A., and Salama, M.A. The aesthetic smile: diagnosis and treatment. *Periodontology*, 2000, 11:18-28, 1996

134 Berscheid, E., Walsteer, E., and Bohrnsstedt, G. Body image: The happy American body: A survey report. *Psychol Today*, Nov: 119-131, 1973

135 Patzer, G.L. Understanding the casual relationship between physical attractiveness and self-esteem. *J Esthet Dent*, 3:144-146, 1996

136 Ingber, J.S., Rose, L.F., and Coslet, J.G. The "Biologic Width"-a concept in periodontics and restorative dentistry. *Alpha Omegan*, 70:62-65, 1977

137 Kois, J. The restorative-periodontal interface: biologic parameters. *Periodontology*, 2000, 11:29-38, 1996

[138] Sonick, M. Esthetic Rehabilitation of the maxillary Anterior Sextant. The Periodontal-Restorative Connection, *Contemporary Esthetics and Restorative Practice* 5, (3): 1-6, 1998

[139] Rufenacht, C.R. *Fundamentals of Esthetics*. Chicago: Quintessence Publishing Co. Inc., 1990

Index

A

Abscesses (periodontium), 548-549: treatment, 548-549

Access and rubber dam isolation (endodontics), 142-143

Accessibility (office), 92-95: wheelchair patient, 93

Acetone solvent, 115

Adhesives use (restorations), 110-116: vs. composites, 110-111; bonding strength, 112-115; etching, 114; solvents, 115-116; acetone, 115; ethanol, 116; water, 116

Adhesives vs. composites, 110-111

Advanced life support measures, 187

Aggressive periodontitis, 529, 540-545: localized, 541-543; generalized, 544-545

Algorithms (software), 380-381

Allergic reactions, 182-184, 536-538

Allergies, 5, 162, 182-184, 536-538: allergic reactions, 182-184, 536-538

Alveoplasty, 321

Amalgam position (restorations), 110-111: composites vs. adhesives, 110-111

American Society of Anesthesiologists (ASA), 9-11: classifications, 11

Analgesics (surgery), 623

Anatomy (periodontium), 519-525

Anesthesia (endodontics), 140-142: anesthetic test, 140

Anesthesia, 140-142, 161-188, 314-315: endodontics, 140-142; effects, 161-188; oral surgery, 314-315

Anesthetic test, 140

Angina pectoris, 180-181: signs/symptoms, 180

Ankylosed tooth (root), 326

Anterior crossbites, 399-403

Antianxiety agents, 288-289

Antibiotics, 622-624: prophylaxis (oral surgery), 622; coverage, 623-624

Antidepressants, 291

Antidotal drugs, 187

Apical infection (root), 325

Apically-positioned flap, 650, 652: vs. repositioned flap, 650, 652

Appointment card, 197-198

Appointments, 96, 197-198: children, 96; card, 197-198

Arthrogenous TMD, 266, 273-276: synovitis/capsulitis/retrodiscitis, 274; deviation in form, 275; TMJ dislocation, 276

ASA classifications, 9-11

Attachment level (periodontal), 576

Auxiliary personnel, 73-75

B

Behavior (children), 41-44, 48-49, 51-52, 65-71: dilemma, 43-44; parameters, 43-44; time out concept, 48-49; drug therapy, 51-52; parents in operatory, 65-71; patient management, 66-68; separation, 66-69; trust, 70; premedication, 71

Behavior parameters (children), 43-44

Behavioral/psychotherapy, 294

Between-meal snacks, 54-56, 58-59

Biomechanics, 257-258, 266, 268, 273, 275-279: TMD, 266, 268

Blood dyscrasias, 621-622

Blood flow (cerebral), 165

Blood pH, 167

Blood pressure, 165-167: cardiac output, 166; postural hypotension, 166; blood vessel patency, 166; glucose, 166-167; blood pH, 167; electrical equilibrium, 167

Blood problems, 5-6, 165-167, 621-622: cerebral blood flow, 165; blood pressure, 165-167; blood vessel patency, 166; blood pH, 167; dyscrasias, 621-622

Blood vessel patency, 166

Body response (syncope), 169

Bonding (restoration), 122, 365-366

Bonding strength (adhesive), 112-115: etching, 114

Bonding, 112-115, 122, 365-366: bond strength (adhesive), 112-115; restoration techniques, 122, 365-366

Border molding, 456-460

Bottle feeding, 54-56, 90-92: nursing caries, 54-56; between-meal snacks, 54-56; goals, 91-92

Breast feeding, 53-54: nursing caries, 54

Bridge and crown, 341-367: materials, 342-348; preparations, 347-351; impressions, 352; laboratory communication, 352-359; posts and cores, 358-361; temporaries, 361-364; bonding, 365-366; notes, 367

Brochures/printed materials, 195, 237-238

Bruxism, 345-346

Buccal mucosa, 565

Business cards, 197

C

CAD/CAM ceramics, 344

Candidosis (oral), 500-508: medications, 506, 508

Capacity to consent, 242

Capsulitis/retrodiscitis/synovitis, 274

Cardiovascular conditions, 5, 12, 166, 179-182: cardiac output, 166; angina pectoris, 180-181; myocardial infarction, 181-182

Caries/teeth examination, 54-56, 600: nursing, 54-56; periodontics, 600

Case law (dental malpractice actions), 232-241: no cause of action for failure to treat, 232-233; custom and practice, 233-234; consent (written vs. oral), 234-236; individual patient factors, 236; timing of execution of consent, 236-237; brochures/printed materials, 237-238; referrals (consent), 238-241

Case presentation (children), 95-97: parent communication, 95; prevention, 95-96; financial/payment arrangements, 96; appointments, 96

Cast ceramics, 344

Categorization (TMD), 266-268: biomechanics, 266, 268

Cause of action, 224-228: elements, 224-225; codification, 225-228; separate pleading, 228; failure to treat, 232-233

Ceramic restorative materials, 344-348: powder slurry, 344; pressable, 344; cast, 344; CAD/CAM, 344; infiltrated, 344; bruxism, 345-346; flexural strength, 345-348

CEREC 2 CAD-CAM system, 371

Chair position, 79, 318: children, 79; teeth extractions, 318

Charging interest, 219-220

Charting, 13

Child patients, 39-103: vision, 39-44; motivation, 40; heredity vs. environment, 41-43; behavior dilemma, 43-44; learning, 44-49; feelings and self-esteem, 50; drug therapy, 51-52; diet and nutrition, 52-62; before-visit preparation, 62-63; parental consent, 63-64; medical history, 64-65; parents in operatory, 65-71; sedation and general anesthesia, 72-73; restraint of patient, 73-75; dentist meets child, 76-80; shot/local anesthesia, 80-86; voice control, 87-88; prizes/rewards, 88-89;

reinforcement and review, 88, 90; oral habits, 90-92; special child, 92-95; case presentation, 95-97; relationship, 98-99; notes, 100-103

Chronic periodontitis, 529, 538, 540

Chronic TMD, 281-283: fractures, 282

Clasp design (prosthodontics), 443-450

Classification/diagnosis (periodontal diseases), 525-526, 528-529: gingivitis, 526, 528; periodontitis, 526, 529

Cleaning and shaping (root canal), 143

Clearview system, 381-382

Clinical assistant, 22, 34-38, 80: communication, 34-35; education/training, 35; teamwork, 35-36; staff empowerment, 35-38; attributes, 36-37; delegation (team), 37

Clinical conditions (emergency), 161, 168-188: syncope, 161, 168-171, 179; hyperventilation syndrome, 161, 172-173; diabetic reactions, 161, 173-176; seizures, 161, 177-179; differential diagnosis (syncope vs. epilepsy), 179-187

Clinical evaluation (TMD), 257-265: temporomandibular joint (TMJ) assessment, 257-258; predisposing/initiating/perpetuating factors, 258-261; psychological factors, 261-262; nutrition and exercise, 262; trauma, 263; occlusal factors, 263-264; postural considerations/imbalances, 264-265; sleep disturbances, 265

Clinical features (TMD), 252-253

Clinical procedures (Spring Aligner), 395-400

Codification (cause of action), 225-228

Communicating financially, 189-221: financial responsibilities (dentist), 190-191; financial needs (consumer), 191-192; new patient telephone calls, 192-194; welcome packets, 194-198; reception room signs, 198-201; consultation program effectiveness, 202-206; financial options/commitment, 206-212; telephone shoppers, 212-215; emergencies, 216-217; minors, 217; no show charge, 218-219; charging interest, 219-220; check list, 221

Communication (laboratory), 352-359

Communication skills, 16-18: relationship with patient, 16-17; expectations, 17

Communication, 16-18, 34-35, 94-95, 189-221, 352-359: skills, 16-18; special child, 94; parent, 95; financial information, 191-221; laboratory, 352-359

Comparing providers, 242-244

Complications (extractions), 325-327: fracture of root, 325-327

Composite restorations, 110-111: vs. adhesives, 110-111

Compromise/confrontation, 80

Computer imaging, 370-373: personal digital assistant (PDA), 372-373

Condylar fracture, 282

Confidence (staff), 19

Connective tissue ridge augmentation, 678-698: esthetic crown lengthening, 680, 685-698

Consent (informed), 223-250: historical background, 224-232; case law in dental malpractice actions, 232-241; written vs. oral, 234-236; timing, 236-237; emerging issues, 242-244; notes, 245-250

Consent (written vs. oral), 234-236

Consent execution (timing), 236-237

Consultant referrals (consent), 238-241

Consultation appointment, 200-203: scheduling, 203; location, 203

Consultation program effectiveness, 202-206: patient information, 202; scheduling, 203; location, 203; spouse invited, 204; staff member involved, 205-206;

Consumer financial needs, 191-192: inform before perform, 191

Contracture, 272

Contraindications (periodontal surgery), 621

Contributors/authors, viii-xi

Co-payment (insurance), 200

Cost information (providing), 191-221: first contact, 192-194; welcome packets, 194-198; reception room signs, 198-201; consultation program effectiveness, 202-206; financial options/commitment, 206-212; telephone shoppers, 212-215; emergencies, 216-217; minors, 217-218; no show charge, 218-219; charging interest, 219-220; check list, 221

Cost issues, 108, 189-221: restorations, 108; cost of treatment, 189-221; providing cost information, 191-221

Cost of treatment, 189-221: financial responsibilities (dentist), 190-191; financial needs (consumer), 191-192; cost information, 191-221; new patient telephone calls, 192-194; welcome packets, 194-198; cost estimate, 195-196; terminology, 195-196; reception room signs, 198-201; consultation program effectiveness, 202-206; financial options/commitment, 206-212; dental financing, 209-210; telephone shoppers, 212-215; emergencies, 216-217; minors, 217; no show charge, 218-219; charging interest, 219-220; check list, 221

Credit card payment, 208-209

Critical care (supplies/equipment/drugs), 185-187

Crossbites, 399-409: anterior, 399-403; function, 404-407; dental, 404-405; skeletal posterior, 407-409

Crown and bridge, 341-367: materials, 342-348; preparations, 347-351; impressions, 352; laboratory communication, 352-359; posts and cores, 358-361; temporaries, 361-364; bonding, 365-366; notes, 367

Crown down technique (root canal), 144-150

Crown lengthening, 631-638, 680, 685-698: esthetic, 680, 685-698

Crying/whining (children), 49, 77, 79

Curing light, 116-117

Custom and practice, 233-234

Custom plan (financial), 210

D

Decision (restorations), 125-126

Degenerative joint diseases, 280-281

Delegation (team), 20, 37

Dental assistant. SEE Clinical assistant.

Dental crossbites, 404-405

Dental financing, 209-210

Dental history, 130-131, 196-197, 553-557: form, 196-197; endodontics, 130-131; periodontics, 553-557

Dental hygiene program, 26-28

Dental malpractice actions (case law), 232-241: no cause of action for failure to treat, 232-233; custom and practice, 233-234; consent (written vs. oral), 234-236; individual patient factors, 236; timing of execution of consent, 236-237; brochures/printed materials, 237-238; referrals (consent), 238-241

Dental plaque-induced gingivitis, 527-528, 530-532

Dentin adhesives, 112-116

Dentinal tubule, 117

Dentist meets child, 76-80: first impressions, 76; show and tell and do, 76-78; elective dentistry, 77; temper control, 77; crying/whining, 77, 79; upright chair position, 79; eyes open, 80; talking, 80; dental assistant, 80; compromise/confrontation, 80

Denture design, 438-450

Denture stability, 432-437

Dentures, 431-481: patient evaluation, 432-437; stability, 432-437; design, 438-450; tooth preparation, 438-468; prosthesis trial, 468-471; prosthesis delivery, 471-475; post-delivery adjustment, 475-477; success factors, 478; notes, 479-481

Deviation in form (TMD), 275

Diabetes mellitus, 161, 173-176, 533, 621: diabetic reactions, 161, 173-176; gingivitis, 533

Diabetic reactions, 161, 173-176: signs/symptoms, 174-176; hyperglycemic reaction, 174-175; hypoglycemic reaction, 176

Diagnosis and classification (periodontal diseases), 525-526, 528-529: gingivitis, 526, 528; periodontitis, 526, 529

Diagnosis and classification, 129, 525-526, 528-529: endodontics, 129; periodontics, 525-526, 528-529

Dialog/inquiry history, 5-6: cardiovascular system, 5; respiratory system, 5; allergies, 5; gastrointestinal/G.U., 5; endocrine and blood systems, 5-6; medications, 6; other conditions, 6

Diet and nutrition (children), 52-62: breast feeding, 53-54; bottle feeding, 54-56; food choices, 57-59; oral hygiene, 60-62

Differential diagnosis (clinical emergencies), 179-187: syncope vs. epilepsy, 179-187; cardiovascular conditions, 179-180; angina pectoris, 180-181; myocardial infarction, 181-182; hypersensitivity reactions, 182-184; emergency supplies/equipment/drugs, 185-187

Digital detectors, 370-377: charge-coupled device (CCD), 372-377; complementary metal oxide semiconductor (CMOS), 372-375, 377; how they work, 374-377

Digital image processing, 370, 380-384

Digital imaging technology (DIT), 369-385: solid-state imaging detectors, 370-377; computer imaging, 370-373; digital detectors, 370, 372-377; digital/electronic image processing, 370, 380-384; photostimulable phosphor (PSP) imaging, 373-374, 378-380; notes, 385

Direct bonding (orthodontic attachment/placement, 421-422: steps, 422

Disc derangement disorders, 273, 277-281: disc displacement with reduction, 277; disc displacement without reduction, 277-279; osteoarthritis (primary), 280; osteoarthritis (secondary), 280-281; degenerative joint diseases, 280-281

Disc displacement, 277-279: with reduction, 277; without reduction, 277-279

Discipline (children), 47-48: methods, 47-48

Discount for prepaying, 199-200

Drug therapy (children), 51-52, 71

Dry socket, 330

Dyscrasias (blood), 621-622

E

Edentulous ridge augmentation/reconstruction, 678-698: esthetic crown lengthening, 680, 685-698

Education/training (staff), 19, 35

Elective dentistry (children), 77

Electric pulp tests, 139-140

Electrical equilibrium, 167

Electronic image processing (EIP), 370, 380-384

Emergencies (in clinic), 161-188: syncope, 161, 168-171; hyperventilation, 161, 172-173; diabetic reactions, 161, 173-176; seizures, 161, 177-179; cardiovascular system problems, 162, 179-182; hypersensitivity reactions, 162; general considerations, 162-164; physiology basics, 164; oxygen supply, 164-165; cerebral blood flow, 165; blood pressure, 165-167; clinical conditions, 168-188; supplies/equipment/drugs, 185-187; notes, 188

Emergency patient, 33-34, 216-217: fee payment, 216-217

Emergency supplies/equipment/drugs, 185-187

Emerging issues (informed consent), 242-244: capacity to consent, 242; comparing providers, 242-244

Empowerment (staff), 35-38

Endocrine and blood systems, 5-6

Endocrine-induced gingivitis, 532-533: treatment, 533

Endodontic examination and testing, 132-140: radiographs, 134-135; thermal tests, 136-139; electric pulp tests, 139-140; anesthetic test, 140

Endodontics, 129-160: diagnosis, 129; medical history, 130; dental history, 130-131; examination and testing, 132-140; radiographs, 134-135; thermal tests, 136-139; electric pulp tests, 139-140; anesthetic test, 140; anesthesia, 140-142; access and rubber dam isolation, 142-143; root canal cleaning and shaping, 143; root canal length determination, 143-144; crown down technique, 144-150; nickel-titanium fracture (causes), 151-152; fracture minimization, 152-154; one-appointment therapy, 154; root canal obturation, 154-159; references, 159-160

Epidemiology (TMD), 253

Epilepsy (seizures), 177-179: petit mal seizure, 177; grand mal seizure, 177-178; management, 178-179; characteristics, 179

Equipment (clinical), 27, 185-187: hygiene, 27; critical care/emergency, 185-187

ESSIX removable appliances, 408-411

Esthetic crown lengthening, 680, 685-698

Esthetic posterior restorations, 105-128: issues of involvement, 106-108; ethics, 106-108; patient approach, 108-109; amalgam position, 110-111; adhesives use, 110-116; postoperative sensitivity, 116-118; technique (tips), 118-125; polishing, 125-126; decision to begin, 125-126; notes, 127-128

Etching (adhesive application), 114

Ethanol solvent, 116

Ethical issues (restorations), 106-108

Etiology (inflammatory periodontal diseases), 519-525: healthy periodontium, 519; macroscopic anatomy, 519-521; microscopic anatomy, 522-525

Exceptions (telephone fee quotation), 214-215

Exercise (TMD), 262, 285, 292-293: and nutrition, 262

Expectations (patient), 17

Expert testimony requirement, 228-229

Extracapsular TMD, 266, 269-272: myositis, 269; protective muscle splinting, 269-270; myospasm, 270; myofascial pain, 271-272; contracture, 272

Extra-oral/intra-oral examination, 563-570: lymph nodes, 563-565; neck and thyroid gland, 565; lips, 565-566; buccal mucosa, 565; vestibule, 567-568; hard palate, 568-569; soft palate and pharynx, 569; tongue, 569-570; floor of mouth, 570

Eyes open (children), 79

F

Failure to treat (cause/no cause of action), 232-233

Fee/cost/price terminology, 195-196

Feelings (children), 50

Fiberfill obturator system, 358-361

Financial goals (practice), 30-31

Financial information/communication, 191-221: consumer needs, 191-192; new patient, 192-194; welcome packets, 194-198; financial investment, 195-196; reception room signs, 198-201; consultation program effectiveness, 202-206; financial options/commitment, 206-212; telephone shoppers, 212-215; emergencies, 216-217; minors, 217-218; no show charge, 218-219; charging interest, 219-220; check list, 221

Financial investment/options, 195-196

Financial needs (consumer), 191-192

Financial options/commitment, 206-212: prepay, 206, 208; retail credit card, 208-209; dental financing, 209-210; custom plan, 210; potential problems, 210-212; pay as you go, 210; half down and balance at

appointment, 211; half down and three payments, 211; statements, 212

Financial problems, 210-212: pay as you go, 210; half down and balance at appointment, 211; half down and three payments, 211; statements, 212

Financial program, 96, 189-221: financial responsibilities (dentist), 190-191; financial needs (consumer), 191-192; new patient telephone calls, 192-194; welcome packets, 194-198; reception room signs, 198-201; consultation program effectiveness, 202-206; financial options/commitment, 206-212; financing dental services, 209-210; telephone shoppers, 212-215; emergencies, 216-217; minors, 217; no show charge, 218-219; charging interest, 219-220; check list, 221

Financial/payment arrangements, 96, 189-221: financial responsibilities (dentist), 190-191; financial needs (consumer), 191-192; new patient telephone calls, 192-194; welcome packets, 194-198; reception room signs, 198-201; consultation program effectiveness, 202-206; financial options/commitment, 206-212; telephone shoppers, 212-215; emergencies, 216-217; minors, 217; no show charge, 218-219; charging interest, 219-220; check list, 221

First contact financial information, 192-221: first contact, 192-194; welcome packets, 194-198; reception room signs, 198-201; consultation program effectiveness, 202-206; financial options/commitment, 206-212; telephone shoppers, 212-215; emergencies, 216-217; minors, 217-218; no show charge, 218-219; charging interest, 219-220; check list, 221

First impressions (children), 76

Fissurotomy, 106-107

Fixed orthodontic appliances, 416-417

Fixed sectional pieces (orthodontic attachment), 425

Flap surgery, 628-629, 646-652: designs/techniques, 628-629; full thickness, 646-648; partial thickness, 649-652

Flexural strength (restorative materials), 345-348

Floor of mouth, 570

Flossing (children), 62

Food choices, 57-59: introducing foods, 57-58; between-meal snacks, 58-59

Forced eruption (orthodontic procedures), 426-427

Forms (welcome packet), 196-197

Fracture minimization (root canal), 152-154

Fracture of root, 325-327: apical infection, 325; loose fragment of tooth, 325-326; amount of root left, 326; ankylosed tooth, 326

Fracture of tuberosity, 334-335

Fractured molars, 327-329: maxillary, 327-328; mandibular, 328-329

Fractures (TMD), 282: condylar fracture, 282

Free gingival graft, 661-668

Full-thickness flap, 646-648: osseous surgery, 646-648

Functional crossbites, 404-407: dental crossbites, 404-405

Fungal origin gingival lesions, 536

Furcation involvement, 576-579

Furcation therapy, 580-593: Class I, 580; Class II, 581-584; Class III, 585-593

G

Gastrointestinal/G.U., 5

Gender factors (TMD), 258-259

General anesthesia/sedation (children), 72-73

Generalized aggressive periodontitis, 544-545

Gingival diseases (gingivitis), 526-545: gingivitis, 527-545; dental plaque-induced gingivitis, 527-528, 530-532; chronic periodontitis, 529, 538, 540; aggressive periodontitis, 529, 540-545; endocrine-induced gingivitis, 532-533; diabetes mellitus, 533; medication modified, 533-534; non-plaque-induced gingival lesions, 535-536; systemic disorders manifestations, 536-539

Glucose, 166-167

Grafting, 661-677: free gingival graft, 661-668; subepithelial connective tissue graft, 669-677

Grand mal seizure, 177-178

Guided bone regeneration, 678

Guidelines (team), 21

Gum cleaning, 60

H

Handicapped accessibility (clinic), 92-95

Hard palate, 568-569

Health history, 3-6, 64-65, 130-131, 196-197, 551-557: questionnaire, 4; children, 64-65; endodontics, 130

Health status/history (patient), 1-14, 64-65, 130-131, 196-197, 551-557: questionnaire, 4; health history, 3-4, 64-65; dialog/inquiry history, 5-6; vital signs, 6-8; physical examination, 8-9; physical status classification, 9-10; treatment modifications, 11-14; notes, 14; children, 64-65; dental history, 130-131, 196-197, 553-557

Heart problems, 5, 12, 166, 179-182

Hemorrhage (oral surgery), 336-337

Heredity vs. environment, 41-43: personality, 41-43; behavior, 41-43

Herpes simplex virus infection, 484-490: herpes simplex virus, 484-486; recurrent herpetic infections, 486-490

Herpetic infections medications, 487

Historical background (informed consent), 224-232: cause of action (elements), 224-225; cause of action codification, 225-228; cause of action (separate pleading), 228; expert testimony requirement, 228-229; jury instructions, 229-232

History (TMD pain/dysfunction), 254-256: visual analog scale, 254; self-reporting, 254; screening questionnaire, 255

Hormonal factors (TMD), 260

Hospital environment, 94-95

Hygiene program, 26-28: time scheduling, 26-27; equipment, 27; periodontal therapy, 27-28

Hyperglycemic reaction, 174-175

Hypersensitivity reactions, 5, 162, 182-184, 536-538

Hyperventilation syndrome, 161,172-173: signs/symptoms, 172-173; management, 173

Hypoglycemic reaction, 175-176: management, 176

Hypotension (posture), 166

I

Imaging technology, 369-385: solid-state imaging detectors, 370-377; computer imaging, 370-373; digital detectors, 370, 372-377; digital/electronic image processing, 370, 380-384; photostimulable phosphor (PSP) imaging, 373-374, 378-380; notes, 385

Impression techniques (prosthodontics), 450-468: irreversible hydrocolloid, 451-452; polysulfide rubber base, 452-454; polyether, 454; vinyl polysiloxane, 455-456; border molding, 456-460; wax records, 460-468

Indirect bonding (orthodontic attachment/placement), 422-424

Infection (oral surgery), 337-339

Infections (oral), 337-339, 484-510: oral surgery, 337-339; herpes simplex virus, 484-486; recurrent herpetic infections, 486-490; recurrent aphthous ulceration, 491-495; lichen planus, 496-500; oral candidosis, 500-507; management, 507-510; notes, 511-515

Infiltrated ceramics, 344

Inflammatory periodontal diseases, 519-526, 528-529: healthy periodontium, 519; macroscopic anatomy, 519-521; microscopic anatomy, 522-525; diagnosis and classification, 525-526, 528-529

Inform before perform (cost), 191

Informed consent, 223-250: historical background, 224-232; case law in dental malpractice actions, 232-241; emerging issues, 242-244; notes, 245-250

Initial visit (periodontics), 550-551

Initiating factors (TMD), 258-261

Insight system, 383-384

Instanding extractions, 323-324

Instruments, 29-30

Insurance patient co-payment, 200

Interest charge, 219-220

Interproximal contact, 122-124

Intracapsular TMD, 266, 273-276: synovitis/capsulitis/retrodiscitis, 274; deviation in form, 275; TMJ dislocation, 276

Introducing foods (children), 57-58

Inverse bevel incisions, 643-645

Invisalign, 412-416

Involvement in restorations, 106-108: technical issues, 106-108; ethical issues, 106-108; pain control, 106; cost issues, 108

Irreversible hydrocolloid, 451-452

Issues (children), 47

J

Jaw exercises, 292-293

Joint mobilization therapy, 292

Jury instructions, 229-232

L

Laboratory communication (restoration), 352-359

Leadership (team), 18

Learning (children), 44-49: social skills, 45-46; safety, 46; issues, 47; discipline, 47-48; time out concept, 48-49; crying, 49

Legal issues, 223-250: historical background, 224-232; case law in dental malpractice actions, 232-241; emerging issues, 242-244; notes, 245-250

Length determination (root canal), 143-144

Lichen planus, 496-500: medications, 498

Life support measures, 186-187: emergency equipment/drugs, 186-187

Lips, 565-566

Local anesthesia, 80-86, 106, 290, 625-626: children, 80-86

Local anesthesia/shot (children), 80-86: learning experience, 81-82; painless, 82-85; post-operative instructions, 86

Localized aggressive periodontitis, 541-543

Logistical signs (office), 198-199

Lymph nodes, 563-565

M

Malpractice, 223-250: historical background, 224-232; case law in dental malpractice actions, 232-241; emerging issues, 242-244; notes, 245-250

Management considerations, 283-284, 507-510: orofacial pain, 283-284; TMD, 283-284; oral mucosal disorders, 507-510

Mandibular extractions, 321-322

Margin placement, 350-351

Massage therapy, 292-293

Masticatory system conditions, 251

Material instructions, 116-117

Materials (restorative), 342-348: powder slurry ceramics, 344; pressable ceramics, 344; cast ceramics, 344; CAD/CAM ceramics, 344; infiltrated ceramics, 344; bruxism, 345-346; flexural strength, 345-348

Matrix band wedging, 120-121

Maxillary extractions, 318-320: chair position, 318; operator position, 318-320

Medical considerations (periodontal surgery), 621-622: contraindications, 621; diabetes mellitus, 621; blood dyscrasias, 621-622; pregnancy, 621-622; antibiotic prophylaxis, 622; smoking, 622

Medical emergencies, 161-188: syncope, 161, 168-171, 179; hyperventilation syndrome, 161, 172-173; diabetic reactions, 161, 173-176; seizures, 161, 177-179; cardiovascular system problems, 162, 179-182; hypersensitivity reactions, 162, 182-184; general considerations, 162-164; physiology basics, 164; oxygen supply, 164-165; cerebral blood flow, 165; blood pressure, 165-167; clinical conditions (emergency), 168-188; notes, 188

Medical history, 3-6, 64-65, 130, 196-197, 312-313, 551-553: questionnaire, 4; children, 64-65; endodontics, 130

Medication-modified gingivitis, 533-534

Medications (oral mucosal disorders), 487, 494, 498, 506, 508, 510: herpetic infections, 487; recurrent aphthous ulceration, 494; lichen planus, 498; candidosis, 506, 508

Medications (patient), 6, 51-52: children, 51-52

Metal restoration materials, 342-343

Micro-hybrid composites, 110

Milk (children), 53-56, 59: breast feeding, 53-54; bottle feeding, 54-56

Minors (payment), 217

Mission statement (practice), 198

Molar banding (orthodontic attachment/placement), 419-420

Motivation (treating child patient), 40

Motivation/reward (employees), 19-20

Mouth prop, 324

Mouth rinse/mouthwash, 62

Mucocutaneous disorders, 536-537

Mucogingival assessment, 594

Mucogingival surgery, 660-677: free gingival graft, 661-668; subepithelial connective tissue graft, 669-677

Mucosal disorders, 483-515: herpes simplex virus infection, 484-486; recurrent herpetic infections, 486-490; medications, 487, 494, 498, 506, 508, 510; recurrent aphthous ulceration, 491-495; lichen planus, 496-500; oral candidosis, 500-508; management, 507-510; notes, 511-515

Muscle relaxants, 288

Myocardial infarction, 181-182: signs/symptoms, 182

Myofascial pain, 271-272

Myogenous TMD, 266, 269-272: myositis, 269; protective muscle splinting, 269-270; myospasm, 270; myofascial pain, 271-272; contracture, 272

Myositis, 269

Myospasm, 270

Necrotizing ulcerative gingivitis (NUG), 546-548: treatment, 546-548

Necrotizing ulcerative periodontitis (NUP), 548

Nerve growth factor (TMD), 260-261

New patient financial information, 192-221: first contact, 192-194; welcome packets, 194-198; reception room signs, 198-201; consultation program effectiveness, 202-206; financial options/commitment, 206-212; telephone shoppers, 212-215; emergencies, 216-217; minors, 217-218; no show charge, 218-219; charging interest, 219-220; check list, 221

New patient process, 21-26: clinical assistant, 22; interview, 23; relationship, 23-25; clinical examination, 24; treatment planning, 24-25; treatment conference, 25; treatment acceptance, 25-26

Nickel-titanium fracture, 151-152

No show charge, 199, 218-219: policy, 199

Non-metal restoration materials, 342-348

Non-plaque-induced gingival lesions, 535-536: viral origin, 535-536; fungal origin, 536

Non-steroidal anti-inflammatory drugs (NSAID), 286-287

Nursing caries, 54-56

Nutrition and exercise (TMD), 262

Nutrition/diet (children), 52-62: breast feeding, 53-54; bottle feeding, 54-56; food choices, 57-59; milk, 59; oral hygiene, 60-62

N

Neck and thyroid gland, 565

Necrotizing ulcerative diseases, 546-549: necrotizing ulcerative gingivitis (NUG), 546-548; necrotizing ulcerative periodontitis (NUP), 548; abscesses of periodontium, 548-549

O

Obturation (root canal), 154-159

Occlusal appliance therapy, 294-297

Occlusal examination, 595-600

Occlusal factors (TMD), 263-264

Occlusal reduction, 350-351

One-appointment therapy (endodontics), 154

Operator position (teeth extractions), 318-320

Opiods, 289

Options (financial), 195-196, 213-214: telephone fee quotation, 213-214

Oral candidosis, 500-508: medications, 506, 508

Oral examination, 563-570: lymph nodes, 563-565; neck and thyroid gland, 565; lips, 565-566; buccal mucosa, 565; vestibule, 567-568; hard palate, 568-569; soft palate and pharynx, 569; tongue, 569-570; floor of mouth, 570

Oral habits, 90-92: bottles, pacifiers, and thumbs, 90-92; goals, 91-92

Oral hygiene (children), 60-62: parental counseling, 60; gum cleaning, 60; tooth brushing, 60-62; toothbrush, 60-61; toothpaste, 61; flossing, 62; mouth rinse/mouthwash, 62

Oral mucosal disorders, 483-515: herpes simplex virus infection, 484-486; medications, 487, 494, 498, 506, 508, 510; recurrent herpetic infections, 486-490; recurrent aphthous ulceration, 491-495; lichen planus, 496-500; oral candidosis, 500-508; management, 507-510; notes, 511-515

Oral surgery, 311-340: assessment, 312-314; anesthesia, 314-315; teeth extraction, 315-329; fractured maxillary molars, 327-328; fractured mandibular molars, 328-329; maxillary and mandibular roots, 329; dry socket, 330; torn tissues, 331; suturing, 331-332; tissue emphysema, 332; oro-antral perforation, 333-334; fracture of tuberosity, 334-335; syncope, 335-336; hemorrhage, 336-337; infection, 337-339; notes, 340

Oro-antral perforation, 333-334

Orofacial pain, 251-309: masticatory system conditions, 251; TMD definition, 252-253; clinical features, 252-253; associated features, 253; epidemiology, 253; patient evaluation, 254-265; categorization, 266-268; myogenous TMD, 266, 269-272; arthrogenous TMD, 266, 273-276; disc derangement disorders, 273, 277-281; chronic TMD, 281-283; management considerations, 283-284;

patient education/self-care, 284-286; pharmacotherapy, 286-297; notes, 298-309

Orthodontic attachments (placement), 417-427: separation, 417-420; molar banding, 419-420; direct bonding, 421-422; indirect bonding, 422-424; wire placement, 424-425; fixed sectional pieces, 425; tooth movement, 424, 426-427; forced eruption, 426-427; uprighting molars, 426-427

Orthodontics, 387-430: removable appliances, 388-400, 408-411; Spring Aligner, 390-400; clinical procedures, 395-400; anterior crossbites, 399-403; functional crossbites, 404-407; skeletal posterior crossbites, 407-409; ESSIX removable appliances, 408-411; Invisalign, 412-416; fixed appliances, 416-417; orthodontic attachments placement, 417-427; notes, 429-430.

Osseous grafting, 678

Osseous surgery, 646-648

Osteoarthritis, 280-281: primary, 280; secondary, 280-281

Oxygen supply, 164-165

P

Pacifiers/bottles/thumbs, 90-92: goals, 91-92

Pain control, 82-85, 106, 283-284: shot/local anesthesia, 82-85; TMD, 283-284

Papillary retention procedure, 652-659

Parental consent, 63-64

Parental counseling, 60

Parental discipline, 47-48: methods, 47-48

Parenting issues, 41-63, 90-92: heredity vs. environment, 41-43; behavior parameters, 43-44; learning and development, 44-49; discipline, 47-49; crying, 49; feelings/self-esteem, 50; drugs for children, 51-52; diet and nutrition, 52-59; oral hygiene, 60-62; preparation before first visit, 62-63; oral habits, 90-92

Parents in operatory, 65-71: management of patient, 66-68; separation, 66-69; trust, 70; premedication, 71

Partial payment options, 210-211

Partial-thickness flap, 649-652: apically-positioned vs. repositioned flaps, 650, 652

Patient approach (restorations), 108-109: patient education, 108-109

Patient billing/statements, 212

Patient education, 108-109, 202, 284-286, 293, 600: TMD self-care, 284-286; postural, 293

Patient evaluation (TMD), 254-265: history (pain/dysfunction), 254-256; clinical evaluation, 257-265

Patient examination/evaluation, 8-10, 24, 132-133, 162-164, 254-265, 312-314, 432-437, 550-551, 563-579: physical status classification, 9-10; endodontics, 132-133; TMD, 254-265; oral surgery, 312-314; prosthodontics, 432-437; periodontics, 550-551, 570-579; oral, 563-570

Patient factors (individual), 236

Patient health status, 1-14, 23, 64-65, 130-131, 196-197, 553-557: health history, 3-4, 64-65; dialog/inquiry history, 5-6; vital signs, 6-8; physical examination, 8-9; physical status classification, 9-10; treatment modifications, 11-14; notes, 14; children, 64-65; dental history, 130-131, 196-197, 553-557

Patient information (case and cost), 202

Patient management (children), 39-103: vision, 39-44; motivation, 40; heredity vs. environment, 41-43; behavior dilemma, 43-44; learning, 44-49; feelings and self-esteem, 50; drug therapy, 51-52; diet and nutrition, 52-62; before-visit preparation, 62-63; parental consent, 63-64; medical history, 64-65; parents in operatory, 65-71; sedation and general anesthesia, 72-73; restraint of patient, 73-75; dentist meets child, 76-80; shot/local anesthesia, 80-86; voice control, 87-88; prizes/rewards, 88-89; reinforcement and review, 88, 90; oral habits, 90-92; special child, 92-95; case presentation, 95-97; relationship, 98-99; notes, 100-103

Patient monitoring (oral surgery), 337-339: improvement, 338; worsening, 338-339; not improving, 339

Pay as you go option, 210

Payment options/commitment, 206-212

Perfect day scenario, 31-33

Periodontal disease treatment, 27-28, 550-557, 601-618: patient examination, 550-551; initial visit, 550-551; medical history, 551-553; dental history, 553-557; treatment planning, 601-618

Periodontal diseases, 27-28, 519-526, 528-529, 550-557, 601-618: treatment, 27-28, 550-557, 601-618; healthy periodontium, 519; macroscopic anatomy, 519-521; microscopic anatomy, 522-525; diagnosis and classification, 525-526, 528-529

Periodontal examination/evaluation, 550-551, 570-579: visual inflammation/bleeding (probing), 571-572; suppuration, 571-573; pocket depth and probing, 571, 573-575; attachment level, 576; furcation involvement, 576-579

Periodontal surgery, 618-659: indications, 619-620; principles, 621-659; medical considerations, 621-622; pre-surgical instructions, 622-626; surgical instruments and setup, 626-627; surgical procedures, 628; flap surgery (designs/techniques), 628-629; sulcular incisions, 629-642; inverse bevel incisions, 643-645; full-thickness flap, 646-648; partial-thickness flap, 649-652; papillary retention procedure, 652-659

Periodontics, 27-28, 517-714: therapy, 27-28; etiology of inflammatory periodontal diseases, 519-525; diagnosis and classification (periodontal diseases), 525-526, 528-529; gingival diseases, 527-545; periodontitis (systemic disease manifestation), 545-549; treatment of periodontal disease, 550-557; dental history, 553-557; full mouth radiographs, 557-562, 595; extra-oral/intra-oral examination, 563-570; periodontal examination, 570-579; furcation therapy, 580-593; mucogingival assessment, 594; tooth mobility, 594-600; treatment planning, 601-618; surgical therapy, 618-620; principles of periodontal surgery, 621-659; mucogingival surgery, 660-677; connective tissue ridge augmentation, 678-698; notes, 699-714

Periodontitis (systemic disease manifestation), 545-549: necrotizing ulcerative diseases, 546-549

Periodontitis, 140-141, 526, 529, 538, 540-549: chronic, 529, 538, 540; aggressive, 520. 540-545; systemic disease manifestation, 545-549; necrotizing ulcerative diseases, 546-549

Periodontium, 140-141, 519-526, 538, 540-549: macroscopic anatomy, 519-521; microscopic anatomy, 522-525; abscesses, 548-549

Perpetuating factors (TMD), 258-261

Personal digital assistant (PDA), 372-373

Personal history form, 196-197

Personality (children), 41-43

Personality attributes (clinical assistant), 36-37

Petit mal seizure, 177

Ph range (blood), 167

Pharmacotherapy (orofacial pain), 286-297: non-steroidal anti-inflammatory drugs (NSAID), 286-287; steroids, 286-287; muscle relaxants, 288; antianxiety agents, 288-289; opiods, 289; local anesthetics, 290; antidepressants, 291; physical therapy/physical medicine, 292-293; behavioral/psychotherapy, 294; occlusal appliance therapy, 294-297

Pharmacotherapy (TMD), 286-297: non-steroidal anti-inflammatory drugs (NSAID), 286-287; steroids, 286-287; muscle relaxants, 288; antianxiety agents, 288-289; opiods, 289; local anesthetics, 290; antidepressants, 291; physical therapy/physical medicine, 292-293; behavioral/psychotherapy, 294; occlusal appliance therapy, 294-297

Pharynx, 569

Phosphors/phosphor plates, 378-380

Photographs (periodontics), 600

Photostimulable phosphor (PSP) imaging, 373-374, 378-380: phosphors/phosphor plates, 378-380

Physical examination (oral), 563-570: lymph nodes, 563-565; neck and thyroid gland, 565; lips, 565-566; buccal mucosa, 565; vestibule, 567-568; hard palate, 568-569; soft palate and pharynx, 569; tongue, 569-570; floor of mouth, 570

Physical examination/evaluation, 8-10, 162-164, 254-265, 432-437, 550-551, 563-579: physical status classification, 9-10; TMD, 254-265; prosthodontics, 432-437; periodontics, 550-551, 570-579; oral, 563-570

Physical modalities, 293

Physical status classification, 9-10

Physical therapy/physical medicine, 292-293: massage, 292; joint mobilization, 292; jaw exercises, 292-293; physical modalities, 293; postural re-education, 293

Physiologic factors (TMD), 259-260

Physiology basics, 164

Pocket depth and probing, 571, 573-575

Polishing, 123-126

Polyether, 454

Polysulfide rubber base, 452-454

Post-delivery adjustment (prosthesis), 475-477

Posterior restorations, 105-128: issues of involvement, 106-108; patient approach, 108-109; amalgam position, 110-111; adhesives use, 110-116; postoperative sensitivity, 116-118; technique (tips), 118-125; polishing, 125-126; decision to begin, 125-126; notes, 127-128

Postoperative instructions, 86, 324-325: extractions, 324-325

Postoperative sensitivity, 116-118: curing light, 116-118; material instructions, 116-118; dentinal tubule, 117

Posts and cores, 358-361

Postural considerations, 166, 264-265, 293: hypotension, 166; imbalances (TMD), 264-265; re-education, 293

Powder slurry ceramics, 344

Practice brochure, 195, 237-238

Practice efficiency/profitability, 15-38: communication skills, 16-18; teamwork, 18-21; new patient process, 21-26; hygiene program, 26-28; scheduling system, 28-34; clinical assistant, 34-38

Predisposing factors (TMD), 258-261: gender, 258-259; physiologic factors, 259-260; hormonal factors, 260; nerve growth factor, 260-261; pressure differential, 261

Pregnancy, 621-622

Premedication, 71, 622-623: children, 71; oral surgery, 622-623

Preparations, 62-63, 118-125, 347-351: child patient, 62-63; restorations, 118-125, 347-351

Prepay option, 206, 208

Pressable ceramics, 344

Pressure differential (TMD), 261

Pre-surgical instructions (periodontics), 622-626: premedication, 622-623; analgesics, 623; antibiotic coverage, 623-624; sedation, 624-625; local anesthesia, 625-626

Prevention (children), 95-96

Price/fee/cost terminology, 195-196

Printed materials/brochures, 195, 237-238

Prizes/rewards (children), 88-89

Problematic patient identification, 1-14: health history, 3-4; dialog/inquiry history, 5-6; vital signs, 6-8; physical examination, 8-9; classification, 9-10; treatment modifications, 11-14; notes, 14

Productivity, 15-38: communication skills, 16-18; teamwork, 18-21; new patient process, 21-26; hygiene program, 26-28; scheduling system, 28-34; clinical assistant, 34-38

Prostheses, 432-450, 468-477: stability, 432-437; design, 438-450; trial, 468-471; delivery, 471-475; post-delivery adjustment, 475-477

Prosthodontics, 431-481: patient evaluation, 432-437; prothesis stability, 432-437; prosthesis design, 438-450; tooth preparation, 438-468; prosthesis trial, 468-471; prosthesis delivery, 471-475; post-delivery adjustment, 475-477; success factors, 478; notes, 479-481

Protective muscle splinting, 269-270

Provider comparison, 242-244

Psychological assessment (children), 64

Psychological factors (TMD), 261-262

Psychotherapy, 294

Pulp calcification, 139-140

Pulp tests, 139-140

Pulpal inflammation, 136-139

R

Radiographs, 134-135, 557-562, 595: full mouth, 557-562, 595

Reception room signs, 198-201: mission statement, 198; logistical, 198-199; financial, 199; no show charge policy, 199; offering percentage discount for prepaying, 199-200; returned check charge, 200; insurance patient co-payment, 200; scheduling consultation, 200-201

Reconstruction (edentulous ridge), 678-698: esthetic crown lengthening, 680, 685-698

Recurrent aphthous ulceration, 491-495: medications, 494

Recurrent herpetic infections, 486-490: recurrent herpes labialis (RHL), 486-489; recurrent intraoral herpes (RIH), 486-487, 489-490

Reevaluation (periodontics), 617-618

Referrals (consent), 238-241

Reinforcement/review (children), 88, 90

Relationship with patient, 16-17, 23-25, 98-99: children, 98-99

Removable orthodontic appliances, 388-400, 408-416: Spring Aligner, 390-400; ESSIX removable appliances, 408-411; Invisalign, 412-416

Removable prosthodontics, 431-481: patient evaluation, 432-437; tooth preparation, 438-468; prosthesis trial, 468-471; prosthesis delivery, 471-475; post-delivery adjustment, 475-477; success factors, 478; notes, 479-481

Repositioned flap, 650, 652: vs. apically-positioned flap, 650, 652

Respiratory system, 5

Restoration bonding, 365-366

Restorations (crown/bridge), 341-367: materials, 342-348; preparations, 347-351; impressions, 352; laboratory communication, 352-359; posts and cores, 358-361; temporaries, 361-364; bonding, 365-366; notes

Restorations (posterior), 105-128: issues of involvement, 106-108; patient approach, 108-109; amalgam position, 110-111; adhesives use, 110-116; postoperative sensitivity, 116-118; technique (tips), 118-125; polishing, 125-126; decision to begin, 125-126; notes, 127-128

Restorative materials, 342-348: powder slurry ceramics, 344; pressable ceramics, 344; cast ceramics, 344; CAD/CAM ceramics, 344; infiltrated ceramics, 344; bruxism, 345-346; flexural strength, 345-348

Restraint (children), 73-75: auxiliary personnel, 73-75

Retail credit card, 208-209

Retainers (orthodontic appliances), 388-400, 408-411, 416: removable, 388-400, 408-416; Spring Aligner, 390-400; ESSIX removable appliances, 408-411; Invisalign, 412-416; fixed, 416-417

Retrodiscitis/synovitis/capsulitis, 274

Returned check charge, 200

Reward/motivation (employees), 19-20

Ridge augmentation/reconstruction, 678-698: esthetic crown lengthening, 680, 685-698

Risk/risk analysis, 223-250

Root canal fracture, 151-154: nickel-titanium fracture, 151-152; fracture minimization, 152-154

Root canal length, 143-144

Root canal obturation, 154-159

Root canal preparation, 144-150

Root canals, 129-160: diagnosis, 129; medical history, 130; dental history, 130-131; examination and testing, 132-140; radiographs, 134-135; thermal tests, 136-139; electric pulp tests, 139-140; anesthetic test, 140; anesthesia, 140-142; access and rubber dam isolation, 142-143; cleaning and shaping, 143; length determination, 143-144; preparation, 144-150; crown down technique, 144-150; nickel-titanium fracture (causes), 151-152; fracture minimization, 152-154; one-appointment therapy, 154; obturation, 154-159; references, 159-160

Root planing/scaling, 609-616

Roots, 326, 329, 609-616: amount remaining, 326; maxillary/mandibular, 329; planing and scaling, 609-616

Rubber dam isolation (endodontics), 142-143

S

Safety (children), 46

Salary (employees), 20

Scheduling system, 28-34: time management, 28-34; instruments, 29-30; time analysis, 30; financial goals, 30-31; perfect day scenario, 31-33; emergency patient, 33-34

Scintillator/scintillation, 374-376

Screening questionnaire (TMD), 255

Second opinion, 215, 238-241: referrals, 238-241

Secondary/non-critical equipment/drugs, 187

Sedation, 72-73, 624-625: children, 72-73; oral surgery, 624-625

Seizure disorders, 177-178: petit mal seizure, 177; grand mal seizure, 177-178

Seizures, 161, 177-179: seizure disorders, 177-178; management, 178-179

Self-care (TMD), 284-286

Self-esteem (children), 50

Self-reporting (TMD), 254

Sensitivity (postoperative), 116-118: curing light, 116-117; material instructions, 116-118; dentinal tubule, 117

Separate pleading (cause of action), 228

Separation (orthodontic attachment/placement), 417-420

Separation (parent-child), 66-69

Shade taking (color), 353, 355-359

Shot/local anesthesia (children), 80-86: learning experience, 81-82; painless, 82-85; post-operative instructions, 86

Show and tell and do (children), 76-78

Signs/symptoms (patient condition), 161, 168-187, 335-336: syncope, 161, 168-171, 335-336; hyperventilation, 172-173; diabetic reactions, 174-176; seizure disorders, 177-179; cardiovascular conditions, 179-182; diagnosis, 179-187; angina pectoris, 180-181; myocardial infarction, 181-182; hypersensitivity reactions, 182-184; emergency supplies/equipment/drugs, 185-187

Skeletal posterior crossbites, 407-409

Sleep disturbances (TMD), 265

Smoking, 622

Social skills (children), 45-46

Soft palate and pharynx, 569

Software (image processing), 370, 380-384: algorithms, 380-381

Solid-state imaging detectors, 370-377

Solvents (adhesive), 115-116: acetone, 115; ethanol, 116; water, 116

Special child, 92-95: accessibility of office, 93; wheelchair, 93; communication, 94; hospital environment, 94-95

Spouse at consultation, 204

Spring Aligner, 390-400: clinical procedures, 395-400

Staff at consultation, 205-206

Staff education/training, 19, 35

Statement billing (patient), 212

Steroids, 286-287

Subepithelial connective tissue graft, 669-677

Success factors (prosthodontics), 478

Sulcular incisions, 629-642: crown lengthening, 631-638; guided tissue regeneration, 639-642

Supplies/equipment/drugs, 185-187: emergency, 185-187; secondary, 187

Suppuration, 571-573

Surgery assessment, 312-314

Surgical instruments and setup, 626-627

Surgical procedures (periodontics), 628

Surgical therapy (periodontics), 618-622: indications, 619-620; contraindications, 621; diabetes mellitus, 621; blood dyscrasias, 621-622; pregnancy, 621-622; antibiotic prophylaxis, 622

Suturing, 331-332

Symptoms/signs (patient condition), 161, 168-187, 335-336: syncope, 161, 168-171, 335-336; hyperventilation, 172-173; diabetic reactions, 174-176; seizure disorders, 177-179; cardiovascular conditions, 179-182; diagnosis, 179-187; angina pectoris, 180-181; myocardial infarction, 181-182; hypersensitivity reactions, 182-184; emergency supplies/equipment/drugs, 185-187

Syncope vs. epilepsy (diagnosis), 179-187: cardiovascular conditions, 179-182; angina pectoris, 180-181; myocardial infarction, 181-182; hypersensitivity reactions, 182-184; emergency supplies/equipment/drugs, 185-187

Syncope, 161, 168-171, 179-187, 335-336: body's response, 169; signs/indications, 169; symptoms/indications, 170; management, 170-171; characteristics, 179; diagnosis, 179-187; oral surgery, 335-336

Synovitis/capsulitis/retrodiscitis, 274

Systemic disease manifestation (periodontitis), 545-549: necrotizing ulcerative diseases, 546-549

Systemic disorders manifestations (gingivitis), 536-539: mucocutaneous disorders, 536-537; allergic reactions, 536-538; traumatic lesions, 538-539

Systemic manifestations (oral), 536-539, 545-549: gingivitis, 536-539; periodontitis, 545-549

T

Talking to children, 80, 82, 87-88, 94

Teamwork, 18-21, 35-36: leadership, 18; trust, 18-19; confidence, 19; education/training, 19; reward/motivation, 19-20; salary, 20; delegation, 20; guidelines, 21

Technical issues (restorations), 106-108

Technique (restorations), 118-125: tooth preparation, 118-120; wedging of matrix band, 120-121; bonding technique, 122; interproximal contact, 122-124; polishing, 123-125

Teeth extractions, 315-329: maxillary, 318-320; alveoplasty, 321; mandibular, 321-322; instanding, 323-324; mouth prop, 324; postoperative instructions, 324-325; complications, 325-327; fractured molars, 327-329; maxillary/mandibular roots, 329

Telephone shoppers, 212-215: fee quotation, 212-215; options, 213-214; exceptions, 214-215; second opinion, 215

Temper control (treating children), 77

Temporaries (restoration), 361-364

Temporomandibular disorders (TMD), 251-309: masticatory system conditions, 251; TMD definition, 252-253; clinical features, 252-253; associated features, 253; epidemiology, 253; patient evaluation, 254-265; TMJ assessment, 257-258; categorization, 266-268; myogenous TMD, 266, 269-272; arthrogenous TMD, 266, 273-276; disc derangement disorders, 273, 277-281; chronic TMD, 281-283; management considerations, 283-284; patient education/self-care, 284-286; pharmacotherapy, 286-297; notes, 298-309

Temporomandibular joint (TMJ) assessment, 257-258

Therapy reevaluation, 617-618

Thermal tests, 136-139

Thumb sucking, 90-92: goals, 91-92

Thyroid gland, 565

Time management, 28-34: instruments, 29-30; time analysis, 30; financial goals, 30-31; perfect day scenario, 31-33; emergency patient, 33-34

Time out concept, 48-49: behavior, 48-49

Time scheduling (hygiene), 26-27

Timing (execution of consent), 236-237

Tissue emphysema, 332

TMD definition, 252-253: clinical features, 252-253; associated features, 253; epidemiology, 253

TMD self-reporting, 254

TMJ dislocation, 276

Tongue, 569-570

Tooth brushing (children), 60-62: toothbrush, 60-61; toothpaste, 61; flossing, 62; mouth rinse/mouthwash, 62

Tooth fragment (root), 325-326

Tooth mobility, 594-600: occlusal examination, 595-600; caries/teeth examination, 600; photographs, 600; patient education, 600

Tooth movement (orthodontic procedures), 424, 426-427

Tooth preparation (prosthodontics), 438-468: clasp design, 443-450; impression techniques, 450-468

Tooth preparation, 118-120; 438-468: restorations, 118-120; prosthodontics, 438-468

Toothbrush choice, 60-61

Toothpaste choice, 61

Torn tissues, 331

Training/education (staff), 19, 35

Trauma (TMD), 263

Traumatic lesions, 538-539

Treatment (abscesses of periodontium), 548-549

Treatment (endocrine-induced gingivitis), 533

Treatment (necrotizing ulcerative gingivitis), 546-548

Treatment (periodontal disease), 550-557, 601-618: patient examination, 550-551; initial visit, 550-551; medical history, 551-553; dental history, 553-557; planning, 601-618

Treatment conference, 25-26: acceptance of treatment, 25-26

Treatment modifications, 11-14: ASA classifications, 11; heart problems, 12; charting, 13

Treatment planning (periodontics), 601-618: initial therapy, 602-609; root planing and scaling, 609-616; reevaluation, 617-618

Treatment planning, 24-25, 601-618: periodontics, 601-618

Trust issues, 18-19, 70: staff, 18-19; patient, 70

Tuberosity fracture, 334-335

U

Ulceration (aphthous), 491-495

Uprighting molars (orthodontic procedures), 426-427

V

Vestibule, 567-568

Vinyl polysiloxane, 455-456

Viral origin gingival lesions, 535-536

Visual analog scale (TMD), 254

Visual examination (inflammation/bleeding), 571-572

Vital signs, 6-8

Voice control (children), 87-88

W-X-Y-Z

Water solvent, 116

Wax records, 460-468

Wedging (matrix band), 120-121

Welcome packets, 194-198: welcome letter, 194-195; practice brochure, 195; fee/cost/price terminology, 195-196; forms (dental/medical/personal history,), 196-197; business cards, 197; appointment card, 197-198

Wheelchair patient, 93

Wire placement (orthodontic attachment), 424-425

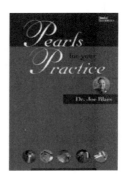
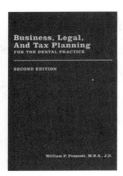
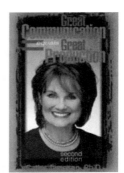